Advances in Veterinary Dermatology

Volume 5

Proceedings of the Fifth World Congress of Veterinary Dermatology, Hofburg Conference Centre, Vienna, Austria, 25–28 August 2004

Edited by

Andrew Hillier

College of Veterinary Medicine, The Ohio State University, Columbus, Ohio, USA

Aiden P. Foster

American College of Veterinary Dermatology, VLA Shrewsbury, Shropshire, UK

Kenneth W. Kwochka

American College of Veterinary Dermatology, DVM Pharmaceuticals, Inc., Miami, Florida, USA

Blackwell
Publishing

Editorial Offices:
Blackwell Publishing Ltd, 9600 Garsington Road, Oxford OX4 2DQ, UK
    Tel: +44 (0)1865 776868
Blackwell Publishing Professional, 2121 State Avenue, Ames, Iowa 50014-8300, USA
    Tel: +1 515 292 0140
Blackwell Publishing Asia, 550 Swanston Street, Carlton, Victoria 3053, Australia
    Tel: +61 (0)3 8359 1011

First published 2005 by Blackwell Publishing Ltd

ISBN-10: 1-4051-3196-9
ISBN-13: 978-1-4051-3196-4

Library of Congress Cataloging-in-Publication Data is available

A catalogue record for this title is available from the British Library

Set in 10/12 pt Minion by Sparks Computer Solutions, Oxford – www.sparks.co.uk
Printed and bound in Denmark by Narayana Press, Odder

While every care has been taken to ensure the accuracy of the information contained in this book, neither the authors or the publishers can accept liability for any inaccuracies in or omissions from the information provided or any loss or damage arising from or related to its use.

The publisher's policy is to use permanent paper from mills that operate a sustainable forestry policy, and which has been manufactured from pulp processed using acid-free and elementary chlorine-free practices. Furthermore, the publisher ensures that the text paper and cover board used have met acceptable environmental accreditation standards.

For further information on Blackwell Publishing, visit our website:
www.blackwellpublishing.com

Front cover images:
The images portrayed on the front cover reflect the broad range of clinical, diagnostic and basic science presentations at the Fifth World Congress of Veterinary Dermatology.

Background picture:
Primer sequences used for detection of *Anaplasma* spp. by PCR (Chapter 6.5).

Other pictures (clockwise from top left):
Collie dog with facial dermatitis due to self trauma associated with atopic dermatitis (Chapters 1.1 and 1.2).
Electron microscopic appearance of eosinophilic cytolysis in feline eosinophilic granuloma complex lesions (Chapter 6.5).
Macrophages with intracellular acid-fast *Mycobacteria* spp. (carbol fuchsin stain) from a cat with feline leprosy (Chapter 5.1).
Histopathological appearance of lesional skin from a dog with staphylococcal toxic shock-like syndrome (Chapter 5.7).

Contents

Sponsors of the Fifth World Congress of Veterinary Dermatology

Principal sponsors

Virbac Animal Health
Royal Canin
Bayer Animal Health
Novartis Animal Health

Major sponsors

Vetoquinol Veterinary Pharmaceuticals
Hill's Pet Nutrition
Schering-Plough Animal Health
Merial Animal Health
Intervet International
Janssen Animal Health
ICF Veterinary Products

Supporting sponsors

DVM Pharmaceuticals
Heska Corporation
Pfizer Animal Health
The Iams Company

Sponsors

Toray Industries
Phytopharm
Zenoaq
Interzoo Publishing

Officers and Organizing Committees of the Fifth World Congress of Veterinary Dermatology

Officers

President: Dr David Lloyd
Secretary: Dr Regina Wagner
Treasurer: Mr Craig Harrison

Executive Organizing Committee

The Officers and:

Dr Otto Fischer
Dr Andrew Hillier
Prof. Richard Halliwell
Prof. Toshiro Iwasaki
Dr Chiara Noli
Dr Kristian Pedersen
Dr Stephen White

Committees

Finance and Fundraising Committee

Dr David Lloyd (Chairperson)
Mr Craig Harrison (Co-chairperson)
Dr Wayne Rosenkrantz (Co-chairperson, USA)
Prof. Toshiro Iwasaki (Co-chairperson, Asia)
Dr Hans-Joachim Koch

Local Organizing Committee

Dr Otto Fischer (Chairperson)
Dr Maurizio Colcuc
Dr Trix Grund
Dr Klemens Alton
Dr Christa Horvath
Dr Janina Tran
Dr Robert Stiel
Dr Gabi Luckinger
Dr Nina Stallmeister
Dr Kurt Sick

Programme Committee

Dr Chiara Noli (Chairperson)
Dr Manon Paradis (Co-chairperson)
Dr Didier Carlotti
Dr Leena Saijonmaa-Koulumies
Dr Peter Ihrke
Dr Stephen White
Dr Jan Hall
Dr Zeineb Alhaidari
Dr Manfred Kietzmann

Publications Committee

Dr Andrew Hillier (Chairperson)
Dr Aiden Foster
Dr Kenneth Kwochka

Publicity Committee

Dr Kristian Pedersen (Chairperson)
Dr Craig Griffin (Co-chairperson, USA)
Dr Genevieve Marignac
Dr Guillermina Manigot
Dr Hans-Joachim Koch
Dr Maurizio Colcuc
Prof. Toshiro Iwasaki

Preface

The Fifth World Congress of Veterinary Dermatology was held in Vienna, Austria on 25–28 August 2004. The congress was organized under the auspices of the World Congress of Veterinary Dermatology Association and the Austrian Small Animal Veterinary Association, and included the annual congress of the Veterinary Wound Healing Association.

Veterinary dermatology has become truly global, with 56 countries from 6 continents being represented at the congress. Interest in veterinary dermatology continues to grow, and the congress attracted over 1000 delegates and a total of over 1500 participants. To accommodate the diverse backgrounds and interests of delegates, a significantly expanded programme was organized and offered at this congress. In addition to the traditional plenary sessions, free communications, poster abstracts, workshops and continuing education sessions, several new features were introduced. These included special sessions for nurses, technicians, equine veterinarians and dermatopathologists, as well as hands-on courses for otoscopy, parasitology, cytology and wound dressing.

Advances in Veterinary Dermatology Volume 5 is the peer-reviewed proceedings of the congress and includes the State of the Art, Supporting Review and Supporting Original Study presentations. Manuscripts were subject to rigorous and strict review in accordance with the conress's commitment to scientific integrity and excellence. As in previous volumes, transcripts of the workshops are also included, whereas the free communications and poster abstracts were published in a special supplement of the journal *Veterinary Dermatology* (Volume 15, Supplement 1, 2004).

The success of the Fifth World Congress of Veterinary Dermatology would not have been realized if not for the commitment, dedication and energy of the officers and members of all the organizing committees. Further, we would like to recognize the generous assistance and support of our sponsors and colleagues in the pharmaceutical, pet food and diagnostic industries.

Andrew Hillier
Columbus, USA

Aiden P. Foster
Shrewsbury, UK

Kenneth W. Kwochka
Miami, USA

Contributors

F. Abramo Dipartimento di Patologia Animale, Pisa, Italy

Z. Alhaidari Clinique Vétérinaire, Roquefort les Pins, France

J.P. Allam Department of Dermatology and Allergy, Faculty of Medicine, Friedrich-Wilhelms-University, Bonn, Germany

E. Anacleto School of Veterinary Medicine, Center for Vectorborne Diseases, University of California, Davis, California, USA

B. Baddaky-Taugbøl Dr. Baddakys Hudpraksis as, Skotterud, Norway

W. Bäumer Department of Pharmacology, Toxicology and Pharmacy, University of Veterinary Medicine Hannover Foundation, Hannover, Germany

A.C. Beynen Department of Nutrition, Faculty of Veterinary Medicine, Utrecht University, Utrecht, The Netherlands

T. Bieber Department of Dermatology and Allergy, Faculty of Medicine, Friedrich-Wilhelms-University, Bonn, Germany

M. Braun Department of Pharmacology, Toxicology and Pharmacy, University of Veterinary Medicine Hannover Foundation, Hannover, Germany

F.D. Brouta Faculty of Veterinary Medicine, Department of Infectious and Parasitic Diseases, Parasitology and Parasitic Diseases, University of Liège, Liège, Belgium

J. Brown Department of Veterinary Clinical Studies, University of Edinburgh, Scotland, UK

D.N. Carlotti Cabinet de Dermatologie Vétérinaire, Bordeaux-Mérignac, France

R. Cerundolo University of Pennsylvania, Philadelphia, Pennsylvania, USA

Z. Chen Beckman Laser Institute, School of Medicine, University of California, Irvine, California, USA

E. Clark Department of Veterinary Pathology, Western College of Veterinary Medicine, Saskatoon, Canada

L.K. Cole Department of Veterinary Clinical Sciences, College of Veterinary Medicine, The Ohio State University, Columbus, Ohio, USA

C.F. Curtis Dermatology Referral Service, Ware, Hertfordshire, UK

M.J. Day Division of Veterinary Pathology, Infection and Immunity, School of Clinical Veterinary Science, University of Bristol, Langford, North Somerset, UK

D.J. DeBoer Department of Medical Sciences, School of Veterinary Medicine, University of Wisconsin, Madison, Wisconsin, USA

F.F. Descamps Faculty of Veterinary Medicine, Department of Infectious and Parasitic Diseases, Parasitology and Parasitic Diseases, University of Liège, Liège, Belgium

E.J. Dick US Army Institute of Surgical Research, San Antonio, Texas, USA

N. Drazenovich School of Veterinary Medicine, Center for Vectorborne Diseases, University of California, Davis, California, USA

S.W. Eberhart Department of Large Animal Clinical Sciences, College of Veterinary Medicine, Michigan State University, East Lansing, Michigan, USA

M.A.C.M. Engelen Janssen Animal Health, Beerse, Belgium

G. Fall Unite d'Immunophysiologie et Parasitisme Intracellulaire, Institut Pasteur, Paris, France

M.W.J. Ferguson Faculty of Life Sciences, University of Manchester, Manchester, UK

K.V. Fieseler College of Veterinary Medicine and Biomedical Sciences, Colorado State University, Fort Collins, Colorado, USA

J.E. Foley School of Veterinary Medicine, Department of Medicine and Epidemiology, University of California, Davis, California, USA

P.J. Forsythe Veterinary Dermatology Referrals, Dunlop, Ayrshire, Scotland, UK

V.K. Ganjam Department of Veterinary Medicine and Surgery, College of Veterinary Medicine, University of Missouri, Columbia, Missouri, USA

L. Gardey Virbac SA, Carros, France

R.A. Garfield Animal Dermatology Referral Clinic, Dallas, Texas, USA

C.M. Gordon Royal (Dick) School of Veterinary Studies, University of Edinburgh, Roslin, Midlothian, Scotland, UK

C.A. Graham-Mize Allergy and Dermatology Veterinary Referral Center, Milwaukie, Oregon, USA

E.A. Graves Department of Large Animal Clinical Sciences, College of Veterinary Medicine, Michigan State University, East Lansing, Michigan, USA

C.E. Griffin Animal Dermatology Clinic, San Diego, California, USA

T.L. Gross IDEXX Veterinary Services and California Dermatopathology Service, West Sacramento, California, USA

J. Hall Ontario Veterinary College, University of Guelph, Guelph, Ontario, Canada

R.E.W. Halliwell Royal (Dick) School of Veterinary Studies, University of Edinburgh, Roslin, Midlothian, Scotland, UK

B. Hammerberg Department of Population Health and Pathobiology, College of Veterinary Medicine, North Carolina State University, Raleigh, North Carolina, USA

J. Hauptman Department of Small Animal Clinical Sciences, College of Veterinary Medicine, Michigan State University, East Lansing, Michigan, USA

M. Hecht Fraunhofer Institute of Toxicology and Experimental Medicine, Hannover, Germany

P.B. Hill Royal (Dick) School of Veterinary Studies, University of Edinburgh, Roslin, Midlothian, Scotland, UK

A. Hillier Department of Veterinary Clinical Sciences, College of Veterinary Medicine, The Ohio State University, Columbus, Ohio, USA

K. Horne Department of Small Animal Clinical Sciences, University of Minnesota, Saint Paul, Minnesota, USA

C. Horvath Veterinary University of Vienna, Vienna, Austria

C. Hou Royal (Dick) School of Veterinary Studies, University of Edinburgh, Roslin, Midlothian, Scotland, UK

R. Hovenier Department of Nutrition, Faculty of Veterinary Medicine, Utrecht University, Utrecht, The Netherlands

J.F. Huntley Division of Parasitology, Moredun Research Institute, Pentlands Science Park, Bush Loan, Penicuik, UK

T. Iwasaki Department of Veterinary Internal Medicine, Tokyo University of Agriculture and Technology, Tokyo, Japan

H.A. Jackson Department of Clinical Sciences, College of Veterinary Medicine, North Carolina State University, Raleigh, North Carolina, USA

P. Jasmin Virbac SA, Carros, France

S. Jessen Department of Small Animal Clinical Sciences, University of Minnesota, Saint Paul, Minnesota, USA

P.J. Johnson Department of Veterinary Medicine and Surgery, College of Veterinary Medicine, University of Missouri, Columbia, Missouri, USA

N. Kagawa Hokuai Animal Hospital, Sapporo, Japan

N. Kanazawa Department of Veterinary Internal Medicine, Tokyo University of Agriculture and Technology, Tokyo, Japan

N.T. Kelbick Center for Biostatistics, The Ohio State University, Columbus, Ohio, USA

M. Kietzmann Department of Pharmacology, Toxicology and Pharmacy, University of Veterinary Medicine, Hannover Foundation, Hannover, Germany

P.A. Knight Department of Veterinary Clinical Studies, Royal (Dick) School of Veterinary Studies, University of Edinburgh, Scotland, UK

D.C. Knottenbelt University of Liverpool, Liverpool, UK

J.J. Kowalski Department of Veterinary Clinical Sciences, College of Veterinary Medicine, The Ohio State University, Columbus, Ohio, USA

T. Kubo Hokuai Animal Hospital, Sapporo, Japan

K.W. Kwochka DVM Pharmaceuticals, Inc., Miami, Florida, USA

J.R. Lamb MRC Centre for Inflammation Research, University of Edinburgh, Scotland, UK

M. Lebastard Unite d'Immunophysiologie et Parasitisme Intracellulaire, Institut Pasteur, Paris, France

M.H.G. Leistra Dierenarts Specialisten Amsterdam, Amsterdam, The Netherlands

K. Lelieur Department of Pharmacology, Toxicology and Pharmacy, University of Veterinary Medicine Hannover Foundation, Hannover, Germany

B.J. Losson Faculty of Veterinary Medicine, Department of Infectious and Parasitic Diseases, Parasitology and Parasitic Diseases, University of Liège, Liège, Belgium

S.M. McAleese Royal (Dick) School of Veterinary Studies, Department of Veterinary Clinical Studies, University of Edinburgh, Roslin, Midlothian, Scotland, UK

H.C. McArdle University of Liverpool, Faculty of Veterinary Science, Liverpool, UK

A. Mackellar Division of Parasitology, Moredun Research Institute, Pentlands Science Park, Bush Loan, Penicuik, UK

S. Maeda Laboratory of Internal Medicine, Division of Veterinary Medicine, Faculty of Applied Biological Science, Gifu University, Japan

R. Malik Post Graduate Foundation in Veterinary Science, University of Sydney, New South Wales, Australia

G. Marignac École Nationale Vétérinaire d'Alfort, Paris, France

R. Marsella Department of Small Animal Clinical Sciences, College of Veterinary Medicine, University of Florida, Gainesville, Florida, USA

N.T. Messer Department of Veterinary Medicine and Surgery, College of Veterinary Medicine, University of Missouri, Columbia, Missouri, USA

B.R. Mignon Faculty of Veterinary Medicine, Department of Infectious and Parasitic Diseases, Parasitology and Parasitic Diseases, University of Liège, Liège, Belgium

H.R.P. Miller Royal (Dick) School of Veterinary Studies, University of Edinburgh, Roslin, Midlothian, Scotland, UK

G. Milon Unite d'Immunophysiologie et Parasitisme Intracellulaire, Institut Pasteur, Paris, France

Y. Momoi Department of Veterinary Internal Medicine, Tokyo University of Agriculture and Technology, Tokyo, Japan

T. Mori Hokuai Animal Hospital, Sapporo, Japan

K.A. Moriello Department of Medical Sciences, School of Veterinary Medicine, University of Wisconsin, Madison, Wisconsin, USA

R.S. Mueller College of Veterinary Medicine and Biomedical Sciences, Colorado State University, Fort Collins, Colorado, USA (Current address: Ludwig-Maximilians University, Munich, Germany)

R.J. Nachreiner Diagnostic Center for Population and Animal Health, College of Veterinary Medicine, Michigan State University, East Lansing, Michigan, USA

J.S. Nelson Beckman Laser Institute, School of Medicine, University of California, Irvine, California, USA

L. Nicolas Unite d'Immunophysiologie et Parasitisme Intracellulaire, Institut Pasteur, Paris, France

A.F. Nikkels Faculty of Medicine, Department of Dermatopathology, University of Liège, Liège, Belgium

S.A.F. Nogueira Department of Small Animal Clinical Sciences, University of Minnesota, Saint Paul, Minnesota, USA

L. Nordberg Trollesminde Dyreklinik, Hillerød, Denmark

N. Novak Department of Dermatology and Allergy, Faculty of Medicine, Friedrich-Wilhelms-University, Bonn, Germany

T.J. Nuttall University of Liverpool, Faculty of Veterinary Science, Liverpool, UK

T. Olivry Department of Clinical Sciences, College of Veterinary Medicine, North Carolina State University, Raleigh, North Carolina, USA

M. Paradis University of Montreal, Quebec, Canada

S.J. Park Department of Veterinary Internal Medicine, Tokyo University of Agriculture and Technology, Tokyo, Japan

F.J.H. Pastoor LEO Animal Health, Ballerup, Denmark

G.M. Peavy Beckman Laser Institute, School of Medicine, University of California, Irvine, California, USA

E. Prina Unite d'Immunophysiologie et Parasitisme Intracellulaire, Institut Pasteur, Paris, France

C.M. Pucheu-Haston Department of Population Health and Pathobiology, College of Veterinary Medicine, North Carolina State University, Raleigh, North Carolina, USA

F. Ramiro-Ibanez Pfizer Global Research and Development, La Jolla Laboratories, San Diego, California, USA

K.R. Refsal Diagnostic Center for Population and Animal Health, College of Veterinary Medicine, Michigan State University, East Lansing, Michigan, USA

C.A. Rème Medical Department, Virbac SA, Carros, France

J.R. Rest Swaffham Prior, Cambridge, UK

C. Rivierre Marseille, France

W.S. Rosenkrantz Animal Dermatology Clinic, Tustin and San Diego, California, USA

E.J. Rosser Jr Department of Small Animal Clinical Sciences, College of Veterinary Medicine, Michigan State University, East Lansing, Michigan, USA

R.A.W. Rosychuk College of Veterinary Medicine and Biomedical Sciences, Colorado State University, Fort Collins, Colorado, USA

L. Saijonmaa-Koulumies Veterinary Clinic Mevet, Helsinki, Finland

A. Sanquer Virbac SA, Carros, France

R. Schenker Novartis Animal Health, Basel, Switzerland

H.C. Schott Department of Large Animal Clinical Sciences, College of Veterinary Medicine, Michigan State University, East Lansing, Michigan, USA

M. Shipstone Dermatology for Animals, Brisbane, Australia

C. Simou Royal (Dick) School of Veterinary Studies, University of Edinburgh, Roslin, Midlothian, Scotland, UK (Current address: University of Athens, School of Biology, Panepistimioupoli, Athens, Greece)

J.D. Sinke Dierenarts Specialisten Amsterdam, Amsterdam, The Netherlands

S.H. Slight Department of Veterinary Biomedical Sciences, College of Veterinary Medicine, University of Missouri, Columbia, Missouri, USA

M.M. Sloet van Oldruitenborgh-Oosterbaan University of Utrecht, Utrecht, The Netherlands

D.D. Smeak Department of Veterinary Clinical Sciences, College of Veterinary Medicine, Ohio State University, Columbus, Ohio, USA

J. Steffan Novartis Animal Health, Basel, Switzerland

B. Sülzle Department of Pharmacology, Toxicology and Pharmacy, University of Veterinary Medicine Hannover Foundation, Hannover, Germany

H. Tanikawa Department of Veterinary Pathology, Rakuno Gakuen University, Ebetsu, Hokkaido, Japan

M.A. Taylor Central Science Laboratory, Sand Hutton, York, UK

K.L. Thoday Royal (Dick) School of Veterinary Studies, University of Edinburgh, Roslin, Midlothian, Scotland, UK

S.M.F. Torres Department of Small Animal Clinical Sciences, University of Minnesota, Saint Paul, Minnesota, USA

S.I.J. Vandenabeele University of Ghent, Merelbeke, Belgium

A.H.M. van den Broek Royal (Dick) School of Veterinary Studies, University of Edinburgh, Roslin, Midlothian, Scotland, UK

S.M. Vermout Faculty of Veterinary Medicine, Department of Infectious and Parasitic Diseases, Parasitology and Parasitic Diseases, University of Liège, Liège, Belgium

K.M.J.A. Vlaminck Janssen Animal Health, Beerse, Belgium

L.M. Volk Novartis Animal Health, Basel, Switzerland

M.W. Vroom Veterinaire Specialisten Oisterwijk, Oisterwijk, The Netherlands

R. Wagner Vetderm-Service, Vienna, Austria

S. Waisglass Doncaster Animal Clinic, Veterinary Dermatology Service, Thornhill, Ontario, Canada

E.J. Walder An Independent Biopsy Service, Venice, California, USA

R.S. Walton US Army Institute of Surgical Research, San Antonio, Texas, USA

H. Weigt LipoNova GmbH, Hannover, Germany

S.D. White School of Veterinary Medicine, University of California, Davis, California, USA

G. Woong Beckman Laser Institute, School of Medicine, University of California, Irvine, California, USA

A. Yu Department of Clinical Studies, Ontario Veterinary College, University of Guelph, Guelph, Ontario, Canada

S. Zabel College of Veterinary Medicine and Biomedical Sciences, Colorado State University, Fort Collins, Colorado, USA

J. Zhang Beckman Laser Institute, School of Medicine, University of California, Irvine, California, USA

Part 1

Immunology

Pathophysiology of atopic eczema in humans

J.-P. Allam MD, N. Novak MD, T. Bieber MD, PhD

Department of Dermatology and Allergy, Faculty of Medicine, Friedrich-Wilhelms-University, Bonn, Germany

Summary

Atopic eczema is a common inflammatory and pruritic disease affecting infants in particular, but may persist or start in adulthood. At least two types of the disease have been recognised. The extrinsic (or allergic) type is most common and is associated with IgE-mediated sensitisation, whereas the intrinsic (or non-allergic) type has no detectable sensitisation and low serum IgE levels. The major factors associated with the development of atopic eczema include genetic predisposition, immunologic abnormalities and environmental factors. Numerous candidate genes for atopic eczema have recently been identified. Studies of the systemic immune response, cytokine expression in skin lesions, antigen-presenting cells and the inflammatory infiltrate in the skin, have elucidated some of the immunologic abnormalities involved in the disease. Food allergens, aeroallergens, autoallergens and colonisation of affected skin with Staphylococcus aureus have been documented as triggers of the immunologic response. This chapter provides an update of the current understanding of the pathomechanisms involved in the development of atopic eczema in humans.

Introduction

Atopic eczema (AE) describes a highly pruritogenic inflammatory skin disease which typically affects individuals during early infancy, but may also continue into adulthood, or may occur for the first time during adulthood. Atopic eczema is reported to affect 10–20% of infants and around 1–3% of adults, with an increasing prevalence in recent years.[1] Higher prevalence has been recorded in urban regions of industrialised nations and has been associated with the so-called western lifestyle (i.e. small family size, increased income and education, migration from rural to urban areas, and increased use of antibiotics).

Allergic or non-allergic disease?

Atopic eczema, allergic bronchial asthma and allergic rhinoconjunctivitis represent a group of atopic diseases which are associated with elevated serum IgE levels, positive skin prick testing (SPT) for aeroallergens, and the presence of elevated levels of allergen-specific IgE in the serum as measured by radioallergosorbent tests (RAST).[2] In contrast, clinically similar forms of allergic diseases, especially AE, may exist without increased serum IgE levels and without IgE-sensitisation to common aeroallergens. These forms have formerly been classified as intrinsic, or non-allergic, variants of atopic disorders. Approximately 20–30% of patients with AE fall into this group, with almost all these patients being female.[3] Similarities and differences in clinical and immunologic parameters that define the two variants of AE are presented in Table 1.1.1 and Figure 1.1.1.

Clinical course

The major clinical features of AE are severe pruritus and eczematous skin lesions which show a typical distribution pattern affecting the flexural surfaces of the extremities preferably, but also affecting the face. The pruritus usually peaks in the evening and at night, but it may also occur throughout the day. Scratching episodes may be provoked by allergens, humidity, sweat and irritants.

Table 1.1.1 Similar and distinguishing features of non-allergic (intrinsic) and allergic (extrinsic) atopic eczema (dermatitis)

	Non-allergic atopic dermatitis	Allergic atopic dermatitis
Clinical parameters		
Skin manifestation	Similar	Similar
Onset of eczema	Early (in childhood)	Early (in childhood)
Sex	Female predominance	No female predominance
Frequency	16–45% of atopic dermatitis patients	55–84% of atopic dermatitis patients
Skin prick test	Negative	Positive
Parameters in the peripheral blood		
Total serum IgE	<150 kU/L	>150 kU/L
Specific IgE	Negative	Positive
Blood eosinophilia	↑	↑
Eosinophil survival	↑	↑
CD137 expression of eosinophils	↑	↑↑
Eosinophilic cationic protein in the blood	↑	↑
T cells in the peripheral blood	HLA-DR expression similar	HLA-DR expression similar
Cytokines in the peripheral blood	↑ IL-5	↑ IL-5
	↑ IL-4	↑ IL-4
	↑ IL-13	↑ IL-13
	↑ sIL-4R	↑ sIL-4R
B-cell activation	CD23+ B cells	CD23+ B cells ↑↑
Stimulated PBMCs	↑↑ IL-13 release	↑ IL-13 release
Phenotype of monocytes	↓ Fc RI, Fc RII	↑ Fc RI, Fc RII
	↓ IL-4R	↑ IL-4R
	↓ CD40	↑ CD40
Parameters in the skin		
Phenotype of epidermal dendritic cells	↑ Fc RI	↑↑ Fc RI
	Fc RI/Fc RII ratio <0.5	Fc RI/Fc RII ratio >1.5
Cytokines derived from lesional skin	↑ IL-5, IL-13	↑↑ IL-5, IL-13
Parameters at the genetic level		
IL-4R promoter polymorphism C-3223-T	↑↑ frequency	↓ frequency
IL-4 promoter polymorphism C-590-T	↓ frequency	↑ frequency

Acute and subacute lesions are characterised by erythematous papules with excoriations and serous exudates, while chronic lesions are characterised by lichenification, which may be severe. Importantly, during all stages of AE, patients usually suffer from dry skin.[1]

Acute episodes of AE frequently affect infants, with lesions usually located on the face, scalp and extensor surfaces of the extremities. Persistent AE often occurs during childhood, with lichenification of the flexural surfaces of the extremities. In adults, AE is usually chronic and is associated with dyshydrotic eczema of the hands.

Pathophysiology

Significant progress has been made in understanding the pathophysiological mechanisms underlying AE. Genetic predisposition, immunological abnormalities and the environment are the major factors contributing to the development of AE, and thus have a great

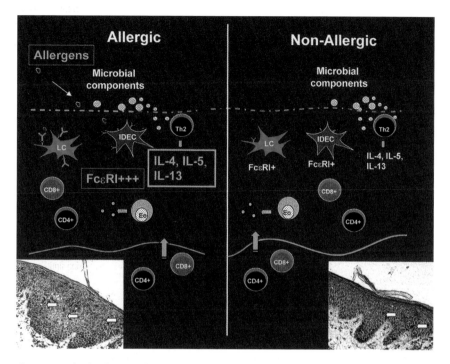

Fig. 1.1.1 Pathophysiologic mechanisms involved in the development of allergic (extrinsic) and non-allergic (intrinsic) atopic eczema. Differences between the two types of disease are indicated in yellow. Immunohistochemical staining of FcεRI on CD1a+ Langerhans cells and inflammatory dendritic epidermal cells is indicated by arrows inset at the bottom of each figure. FcεRI = high affinity receptor for IgE; Eo = eosinophils. Reprinted from *Journal of Allergy and Clinical Immunology*, **112**, Allergic and nonallergic forms of atopic diseases, pp. 252–262, ©2003, with permission from the American Academy of Allergy, Asthma and Immunology.

impact on the manifestation, severity, progression and duration of the clinical disease.

Genetics

AE is a genetically complex hereditary disease with a strong influence of maternal genes. Infants from families where both parents suffer from AE are at increased risk of developing the disease and this risk is greater than for infants whose parents suffer from other atopic diseases (such as allergic rhinoconjunctivitis or allergic asthma), but not AE. Thus, it stands to reason that specific genes contribute to the development of AE. In recent years, many reports have been published identifying so-called candidate genes for AE (Table 1.1.2). Loci in the region of the genes encoding for the Th2-cytokines interleukin (IL)-3, IL-4, IL-5, IL-13 and GM-CSF on chromosome 5q31 have been postulated to predispose individuals to atopic disease, and AE in particular.[4] Other studies have related AE to variants of the IL-13-coding region, functional muta-

tions of the promotor region of RANTES (chromosome 17q11) and gain-of-function polymorphisms in a subunit of IL-4 (chromosome 16q12).[5] Polymorphisms in a subunit of the IL-4 receptor have also been linked to the intrinisic form of AE.[6] Further, genes encoding for the β-chain of the high-affinity receptor for IgE (FcεRI) on chromosome 11q13 have also been associated with AE, although this is still controversial.[7] In a genome-wide linkage study, regions on chromosome 3q21 carrying genes encoding the co-stimulatory molecules CD80 and CD86 have been proposed to be linked to AE.[8] Another study associated psoriasis and AE to loci on chromosomes 1q21 and 17q25,[9] suggesting that common candidate genes are involved in both these skin inflammatory processes. Recently, a low-producer transforming growth factor β (TGF-β) cytokine phenotype has also been linked to the development of AE.[10] As TGF-β is critically involved in tolerogenic immune mechanisms, a decrease in production of this cytokine could result in an accelerated inflammatory response.

Table 1.1.2 Postulated and identified candidate genes for atopic diseases and atopic eczema (dermatitis).

Region	Candidate gene	Phenotype
1q21	?	Atopic eczema
2q21-23	Unknown	Specific IgE
3q21	CD 86?	Atopic eczema
5q31.1	IL-4 cluster	Total IgE
5q32-33	GC-R, β2-adren-R	Total IgE, asthma
6p21.3	MHC class II	Specific IgE
11q13	FcεRIβ	Total IgE, asthma
12q15-24.1	IGF1, SCF	Total IgE, atopy
14q11.2	Mast cell chymase	Atopic eczema
14q32	IgG heavy chain	Atopy
16p11.2-12.1	IL-4Rα	Total IgE
17q11.2-12	RANTES	Atopic eczema
17q25	?	Atopic eczema
20p	?	Atopic eczema

Immunological abnormalities

Systemic immune response

Patients with AE often display peripheral blood eosinophilia and increased serum IgE levels. Almost 80% of children with AE develop allergic rhinitis or allergic asthma, suggesting that sensitisation to allergens through the skin increases the risk of developing respiratory diseases such as allergic bronchial asthma and allergic rhinoconjunctivitis in AE patients.[1] Decreased serum levels of interferon-γ (IFN-γ) observed in AE patients may result from the deficiency of IL-18, a cytokine known to induce production of IFN-γ.[11] The increased frequency of allergen-specific T cells which produce IL-4, IL-5 and IL-13, but little IFN-γ, may also contribute to the predominance of Th2-type response seen in AE patients.[12] Accelerated apoptosis of circulating Th1 cells in AE patients could further enhance the Th2 predominance.[13] The Th2-cytokines IL-4 and IL-13 are of great importance as they induce isotype switching to IgE production. Further, IL-5, which is critically involved in the development and activation of eosinophils, also contributes to the survival of eosinophils which is reported to be prolonged in patients with atopic dermatitis.[14]

Cytokine expression in skin lesions

Many studies have investigated the expression of cytokine mRNA in affected and unaffected skin of AE patients. Increased mRNA for the Th2-cytokines IL-4 and IL-13 is seen in the unaffected skin of AE patients, compared with the skin of healthy non-atopic individuals.[15,16] Further, increased mRNA expression of IL-4, IL-5 and IL-13 in acute AE skin lesions, compared with unaffected skin of AE patients, has been demonstrated. However, mRNA for the Th1-related cytokines IFN-γ or IL-12 was not significantly increased in acute AE lesions, whereas mRNA for IFN-γ, IL-12, IL-5 and GM-CSF has been demonstrated in chronic AE lesions. Comparative immunohistochemical investigations revealed increased IL-17 in acute lesional skin, while more IL-11 was demonstrated in chronic lesions. These cytokines are known to play a role in tissue remodelling.[17]

Cytokine production in the initial development of AE skin lesions has been studied utilising the atopy patch test (APT), whereby allergens are applied to the skin to provoke an eczematoid reaction. After application of house dust mite allergens, an increased level of the Th2-cytokine IL-4 was detected in the initial phase, whereas a predominance of the Th1-cytokine IFN-γ was detected after 24–48 hours.[18] Investigations utilising the APT in cats have also been performed with similar results to those seen in humans, with an increase in IL-4-secreting T cells after APT.[19]

Antigen-presenting cells

Dendritic cells (DCs) are professional antigen-presenting cells that play a central role in the initiation of the primary and secondary immune responses. Two distinct populations of DCs have been described in the lesional skin of AE patients: classical resident Langerhans cells (LCs), and a second population of so-called inflammatory dendritic epidermal cells (IDECs). Significant numbers of IgE-bearing LCs and IDECs expressing the high-affinity receptor for IgE (FcεRI) were detectable in the lesional skin of AE patients.[20,21] These cells play a central role in the uptake and presentation of antigens to Th1 and Th2 cells.[22] Allergens can be internalised via FcεRI and processed for antigen presentation to T cells in atopic skin, or LCs may migrate to regional lymph nodes and present antigen to naive T cells. Thus, LCs may contribute to the expansion of the Th2-cell repertoire by activation of naive T cells. Recently, FcεRI-activated LCs have been demonstrated to release chemotactic signals that increase the migratory capacity of IDEC precursor cells and naive T cells *in vitro*. Further, *in vitro* studies demonstrate that activation of FcεRI on IDEC appears to prime naive T cells into production of IFN-γ and release of IL-12 and IL-18, which may facilitate the observed switch *in vivo* of a Th2-type immune response into a Th1-type response.[22] FcεRI expression on LCs and IDECs may result from high serum IgE levels or a low TGF-β-producing phenotype, as both conditions have been demonstrated to stabilise FcεRI on LCs and IDECs *in vitro*.[23,24] The clinical relevance of FcεRI-positive LCs is reflected by the observation that they are essential components provoking the eczematous reaction observed with the APT.[25] Interestingly, FcεRI-bearing LCs have also been detected in unaffected skin of patients suffering from allergic rhinitis, allergic asthma and atopic dermatitis during the active phase of disease.[26]

Infiltration of inflammatory cells

Soluble factors play a central role in determining the cellular infiltrate in AE lesional sites. Elevated expression of IL-16, which attracts CD4+ T cells, has been demonstrated in acute AE lesions.[27] Further, the CC chemokines RANTES, monocyte chemoattractant protein 4 (MCP4), and eotaxin were detected in significant quantities in the lesional skin of AE patients, and likely contribute to the chemotaxis of CCR3+ eosinophils and Th2 cells into the lesions.[28,29] Keratinocytes of AE patients produce increased levels of the chemokines thymic stromal lymphopoeitin (TSLP) and macrophage-derived chemokine (MDC), which activate CD11c+ DC. These DCs, in turn, produce significant quantities of MDC and thymus and activation-regulated chemokine (TARC).[30,31] Selective recruitment of CCR4+ Th2 cells into the skin may result from the presence of MDC and TARC.[30,31] In chronic lesions with signs of persistent inflammation, increased IL-5 and GM-CSF have been detected.[32] These cytokines are known to promote survival of eosinophils, macrophages, monocytes and LCs. Mechanical skin trauma (e.g. scratching) can result in release of tumour necrosis factor (TNF)-α which may stimulate keratinocytes to produce increased quantities of RANTES in patients with AE.[33]

Environmental factors

Environmental factors such as foods, allergens and *Staphylococcus aureus* are well-known immunological triggers which can lead to the exacerbation of disease in patients with AE.

Foods

Approximately 40% of skin rashes seen in children with moderate to severe AE are caused by food allergens. Infants and young children with food allergies have positive prick tests and/or detectable specific IgE to causative food allergens. The most frequently identified food allergens include peanuts, eggs, milk, wheat and soy.

Furthermore, specific T-cell clones against food allergens have been isolated from the skin lesions of AE patients, suggesting a direct association between the food allergens and skin inflammation. In an AE mouse model, oral sensitisation of mice with food allergens results in the development of eczematous skin lesions after oral re-exposure to the sensitised food allergen.[1]

Aeroallergens

It has been shown that either bronchial or intranasal challenge with aeroallergens can provoke pruritus and eczematous skin lesions in AE patients with allergen-specific IgE to these aeroallergens. Further, epicutaneous application of aeroallergens (e.g. house dust mites, weeds, animal danders and moulds) by APT on non-lesional skin of AE patients provokes an eczematoid reaction in 30–50% of patients. However, APT does not provoke this reaction in healthy volunteers or patients with allergic respiratory diseases.

A significant improvement of AE lesions and pruritus may be observed by reduction of contact with house dust mites. A direct association between the degree of IgE-sensitisation to aeroallergens and the severity of AE has also been demonstrated. Further, house dust mite allergen-specific T-cell clones have been isolated from lesional skin and from sites of APT on AE patients, providing further evidence of the importance and relevance of aeroallergens in AE.[1,3]

Autoallergens

Specific IgE against human proteins (i.e. autoallergens) have been detected in the serum of most patients with AE.[34] The autoallergens characterised to date are intracellular proteins, which have also been detected in IgE-immune complexes in serum.[34] Observations suggest that the autoallergens are released following mechanical trauma (such as scratching), resulting in IgE sensitisation and the subsequent generation of T-cell and IgE-mediated immune response. The probable pathogenic role of autoallergens is further supported by the decrease in specific IgE against autoallergens following successful therapy of AE with cyclosporin.[3,34]

Staphylococcus aureus

Staphylococcus aureus is present on the skin in over 90% of AE patients. A possible explanation for colonisation of the skin with *S. aureus* is the reduced production of defensins in the skin of patients with AE. Defensins are produced by keratinocytes and have potent antimicrobial activity.[28] The importance of *S. aureus* is confirmed by the observation that AE patients with secondary *S. aureus* infections have a superior clinical response to antibiotic and topical corticosteroid combination therapy, compared to patients treated with topical corticosteroids alone.[1]

Some strains of *S. aureus* are known to produce enterotoxins (e.g. *S. aureus* enterotoxin A, B, C, D, E, G, and toxic shock syndrome toxin-1 [TSST-1]) which serve as superantigens. Typically, superantigens stimulate significant T-cell proliferation in an antigen-non-specific manner, leading to amplification of the inflammatory response.[35] In addition, the recent observation of specific IgE against these superantigens suggests that an antigen-specific reaction may also be involved in the inflammatory response seen in the skin of AE patients. To this end, specific IgE on mast cells against superantigens can lead to the release of histamine into the skin.[36] Interestingly, significant amounts of specific IgE against *S. aureus* enterotoxin A, B, C, D, E, G and TSST-1 have been detected in patients with clinical features of AE but who have normal allergen-specific serum IgE levels and thus are not sensitised to common aeroallergens.[37]

Conclusion

Despite recent progress in the understanding of the pathomechanisms involved in AE, its pathology remains very enigmatic. Atopic eczema is certainly a complex disease, resulting from interactions between genes, the immune system and environmental factors. Modern technical methods in the field of genetics combined with a better definition of clinical phenotypes of AE should facilitate the identification of genes involved with the development of AE in the near future. This new knowledge will have important consequences in our comprehension of the immunological mechanisms involved in AE, and finally for new and more specific therapeutic strategies.

References

1 Leung, D.Y., Bieber, T. Atopic dermatitis. *Lancet*, 2003; **361**: 151–160.

2 Johansson, S.G., Bieber, T., Dahl, R., *et al.* Revised nomenclature for allergy for global use: Report of the Nomenclature Review Committee of the World Allergy Organization, October 2003. *Journal of Allergy and Clinical Immunology*, 2004; **113**: 832–836.

3 Novak, N., Bieber, T. Allergic and nonallergic forms of atopic diseases. *Journal of Allergy and Clinical Immunology*, 2003; **112**: 252–262.

4 Forrest, S., Dunn, K., Elliott, K., *et al.* Identifying genes predisposing to atopic eczema. *Journal of Allergy and Clinical Immunology*, 1999;**104**:1066–1070.

5 Kawashima, T., Noguchi, E., Arinami, T., *et al.* Linkage and association of an interleukin 4 gene polymorphism with atopic dermatitis in Japanese families. *Journal of Medical Genetics*, 1998; **35**: 502–504.

6 Novak, N., Kruse, S., Kraft, S., *et al.* Dichotomic nature of atopic dermatitis reflected by combined analysis of monocyte immunophenotyping and single nucleotide polymorphisms of the interleukin-4/interleukin-13 receptor gene: the dichotomy of extrinsic and intrinsic atopic dermatitis. *Journal of Investigative Dermatology*, 2002; **119**: 870–875.

7 Cox, H.E., Moffatt, M.F., Faux, J.A., *et al.* Association of atopic dermatitis to the beta subunit of the high affinity immunoglobulin E receptor. *British Journal of Dermatology*, 1998; **138**: 182–187.

8 Lee, Y.A., Wahn, U., Kehrt, R., *et al.* A major susceptibility locus for atopic dermatitis maps to chromosome 3q21. *Nature Genetics*, 2000; **26**: 470–473.

9 Cookson, W.O., Ubhi, B., Lawrence, R., *et al.* Genetic linkage of childhood atopic dermatitis to psoriasis susceptibility loci. *Nature Genetics*, 2001; **27**: 372–373.

10 Arkwright, P.D., Chase, J.M., Babbage, S., Pravica, V., David T.J., Hutchinson, I.V. Atopic dermatitis is associated with a low-producer transforming growth factor beta(1) cytokine genotype. *Journal of Allergy and Clinical Immunology*, 2001; **108**: 281–284.

11 Higashi, N., Gesser, B., Kawana. S., Thestrup-Pedersen K. Expression of IL-18 mRNA and secretion of IL-18 are reduced in monocytes from patients with atopic dermatitis. *Journal of Allergy and Clinical Immunology*, 2001; **108**: 607–614.

12 van Reijsen, F.C., Bruijnzeel-Koomen, C.A., Kalthoff, F.S., *et al.* Skin-derived aeroallergen-specific T-cell clones of Th2 phenotype in patients with atopic dermatitis. *Journal of Allergy and Clinical Immunology*, 1992; **90**: 184–193.

13 Akdis, M., Trautmann, A., Klunker, S., *et al.* T helper (Th) 2 predominance in atopic diseases is due to preferential apoptosis of circulating memory/effector Th1 cells. *Federation of American Societies for Experimental Biology Journal*, 2003; **17**: 1026–1035.

14 Leung, D.Y., Boguniewicz, M., Howell, M.D., Nomura, I., Hamid, Q.A. New insights into atopic dermatitis. *Journal of Clinical Investigation*, 2004; **113**: 651–657.

15 Hamid, Q., Naseer, T., Minshall, E.M., Song, Y.L., Boguniewicz, M., Leung, D.Y. In vivo expression of IL-12 and IL-13 in atopic dermatitis. *Journal of Allergy and Clinical Immunology*, 1996; **98**: 225–231.

16 Hamid, Q., Boguniewicz, M., Leung, D.Y. Differential in situ cytokine gene expression in acute versus chronic atopic dermatitis. *Journal of Clinical Investigation*, 1994; **94**: 870–876.

17 Toda, M., Leung, D.Y., Molet, S., *et al.* Polarized in vivo expression of IL-11 and IL-17 between acute and chronic skin lesions. *Journal of Allergy and Clinical Immunology*, 2003; **111**: 875–881.

18 Kerschenlohr, K., Decard, S., Przybilla, B., Wollenberg, A. Atopy patch test reactions show a rapid influx of inflammatory den-

dritic epidermal cells in patients with extrinsic atopic dermatitis and patients with intrinsic atopic dermatitis. *Journal of Allergy and Clinical Immunology,* 2003; **111**: 869–874.

19 Roosje, P.J., Thepen, T., Rutten, V.P., Van Den Brom, W.E., Bruijnzeel-Koomen, C.A., Willemse, T. Immunophenotyping of the cutaneous cellular infiltrate after atopy patch testing in cats with atopic dermatitis. *Veterinary Immunology and Immunopathology,* 2004; **101**: 143–151.

20 Bieber, T., de la Salle.H., Wollenberg, A., *et al.* Human epidermal Langerhans cells express the high affinity receptor for immunoglobulin E (Fc epsilon RI). *Journal of Experimental Medicine,* 1992; **175**: 1285–1290.

21 Wollenberg, A., Kraft, S., Hanau, D., Bieber, T. Immunomorphological and ultrastructural characterization of Langerhans cells and a novel, inflammatory dendritic epidermal cell (IDEC) population in lesional skin of atopic eczema. *Journal of Investigative Dermatology,* 1996; **106**: 446–453.

22 Novak, N., Valenta, R., Bohle, B., *et al.* FcεRI engagement of Langerhans cell-like dendritic cells and inflammatory dendritic epidermal cell-like dendritic cells induces chemotactic signals and different T-cell phenotypes in vitro. *Journal of Allergy and Clinical Immunology,* 2004; **113**: 949–957.

23 Novak, N., Kraft, S., Haberstok, J., Geiger, E., Allam, P., Bieber, T. A reducing microenvironment leads to the generation of FcεRI-high inflammatory dendritic epidermal cells (IDEC). *Journal of Investigative Dermatology,* 2002; **119**: 842–849.

24 Allam, J.P., Klein, E., Bieber, T., Novak, N. Transforming growth factor-beta1 regulates the expression of the high-affinity receptor for IgE on CD34 stem cell-derived CD1a dendritic cells in vitro. *Journal of Investigative Dermatology,* 2004; **123**: 676–682.

25 Langeveld-Wildschut, E.G., Bruijnzeel, P.L., Mudde, G.C., *et al.* Clinical and immunologic variables in skin of patients with atopic eczema and either positive or negative atopy patch test reactions. *Journal of Allergy and Clinical Immunology,* 2000; **105**: 1008–1016.

26 Semper, A.E., Heron, K., Woollard, A.C., *et al.* Surface expression of Fc epsilon RI on Langerhans' cells of clinically uninvolved skin is associated with disease activity in atopic dermatitis, allergic asthma, and rhinitis. *Journal of Allergy and Clinical Immunology,* 2003; **112**: 411–419.

27 Reich, K., Hugo, S., Middel, P., *et al.* Evidence for a role of Langerhans cell-derived IL-16 in atopic dermatitis. *Journal of Allergy and Clinical Immunology,* 2002; **109**: 681–687.

28 Yawalkar, N., Uguccioni, M., Scharer, J., *et al.* Enhanced expression of eotaxin and CCR3 in atopic dermatitis. *Journal of Investigative Dermatology,* 1999; **113**: 43–48.

29 Morales, J., Homey, B., Vicari, A.P., *et al.* CTACK, a skin-associated chemokine that preferentially attracts skin-homing memory T cells. *Proceedings of the National Academy of Sciences of the United States of America,* 1999; **96**: 14470–14475.

30 Galli, G., Chantry, D., Annunziato, F., *et al.* Macrophage-derived chemokine production by activated human T cells in vitro and in vivo: preferential association with the production of type 2 cytokines. *European Journal of Immunology,* 2000; **30**: 204–210.

31 Kakinuma, T., Nakamura, K., Wakugawa, M., *et al.* Thymus and activation-regulated chemokine in atopic dermatitis: serum thymus and activation-regulated chemokine level is closely related with disease activity. *Journal of Allergy and Clinical Immunology,* 2001; **107**: 535–541.

32 Taha, R.A., Leung, D.Y., Ghaffar, O., Boguniewicz, M., Hamid, Q. In vivo expression of cytokine receptor mRNA in atopic dermatitis. *Journal of Allergy and Clinical Immunology,* 1998; **102**: 245–250.

33 Yamada, H., Matsukura, M., Yudate, T., Chihara, J., Stingl, G., Tezuka, T. Enhanced production of RANTES, an eosinophil chemoattractant factor, by cytokine-stimulated epidermal keratinocytes. *International Archives of Allergy and Immunology,* 1997; **114** (Suppl. 1): 28–32.

34 Valenta, R., Natter, S., Seiberler, S., *et al.* Molecular characterization of an autoallergen, Hom s 1, identified by serum IgE from atopic dermatitis patients. *Journal of Investigative Dermatology,* 1998; **111**: 1178–1183.

35 Beuer, K., Wittmann, M., Bosche, B., Kapp, A., Werfel, T. Severe atopic dermatitis is associated with sensitization to staphylococcal enterotoxin B (SEB). *Allergy,* 2000; **55**: 551–555.

36 Leung, D.Y., Harbeck, R., Bina, P., *et al.* Presence of IgE antibodies to staphylococcal exotoxins on the skin of patients with atopic dermatitis: evidence for a new group of allergens. *Journal of Clinical Investigation,* 1993; **92**: 1374–1380.

37 Novak, N., Allam, J.P., Bieber, T. Allergic hyperreactivity to microbial components: a trigger factor of "intrinsic" atopic dermatitis? *Journal of Allergy and Clinical Immunology,* 2003; **112**: 215–216.

Mechanism of lesion formation in canine atopic dermatitis: 2004 hypothesis

T. Olivry DrVet, PhD[1], R. Marsella DVM[2], S. Maeda BVSc, MS, PhD[3], C.M. Pucheu-Haston DVM[4], B. Hammerberg DVM, PhD[4]

[1] Department of Clinical Sciences, College of Veterinary Medicine, North Carolina State University, Raleigh, North Carolina, USA
[2] Department of Small Animal Clinical Sciences, College of Veterinary Medicine, University of Florida, Gainesville, Florida, USA
[3] Laboratory of Internal Medicine, Division of Veterinary Medicine, Faculty of Applied Biological Science, Gifu University, Japan
[4] Department of Population Health and Pathobiology, College of Veterinary Medicine, North Carolina State University, Raleigh, North Carolina, USA

Summary

The exact pathogenesis of canine atopic dermatitis (AD) remains elusive at this time. However, information can be derived from results of static (or fixed-point) and dynamic studies. Static studies yield data from samples collected at single time points and are therefore complicated by uncertainty regarding the immunological stage of the lesions sampled. In contrast, dynamic investigations provide information from sequential specimens collected after challenge by allergens or other stimuli.

The information obtained from both types of studies enables the generation of hypotheses for the pathogenesis of AD skin lesions. In the acute phase of AD, an epidermal barrier defect may facilitate contact of environmental (and microbial) allergens with epidermal immune cells at sites of friction and trauma. Epidermal Langerhans cells capture allergens with allergen-specific IgE, and then migrate to the dermis and regional lymph nodes. Keratinocytes are activated by microbial products and immune cell-derived inflammatory mediators, and in turn release more chemokines and cytokines. IgE-coated dermal mast cells release histamine, proteases, chemokines and cytokines. There is an early influx of granulocytes (neutrophils and eosinophils), allergen-specific Th2 lymphocytes and dermal dendritic cells. Eosinophils degranulate and release proteins inducing dermal and epidermal damage. Type-2 helper T lymphocytes release cytokines promoting IgE synthesis and eosinophil survival.

Microbes, self-trauma, and neuromediators might contribute to persistent inflammation in chronic canine AD lesions. There is a continuous cycle of chemokine release, leading to influx and activation of leukocytes, which further release chemokines and other mediators. Infiltrating T lymphocytes secrete type-2 and type-1 cytokines. The failure to down-regulate proinflammatory mechanisms leads to self-perpetuating cutaneous inflammation.

Introduction

Atopic dermatitis (AD) is one of the most common allergic skin diseases of dogs. This entity has recently been redefined as a 'genetically predisposed inflammatory and pruritic allergic skin disease with characteristic clinical features. It is associated most commonly with IgE antibodies to environmental allergens'.[1] The exact prevalence of canine AD is not known, but in a recent study of 31 484 dogs examined by veterinarians in 52 private veterinary practices in the USA, 8.7% of the dogs were diagnosed with atopic/allergic dermatitis, allergy or atopy.[2]

The specific pathogenesis of canine AD remains unknown at this time, but the remarkable similarity between the human and canine diseases at both epidemiological and clinical levels[3,4] suggests that immunological mechanisms leading to lesion generation are likely to be comparable.

The objective of this chapter is to analyse the results of static and dynamic studies, and propose a working hypothesis for the pathogenesis of canine AD skin lesions. A static investigation generates results from samples collected at single time points. However, interpretation of such studies is complicated by uncertainty regarding the immunological stage of the lesions sampled. These investigations have distinct limitations as cutaneous immunological abnormalities vary depending upon the age of the lesions.

In contrast, dynamic studies provide information from sequential samples collected after well-defined allergen challenges or immune stimuli. These experiments are likely to yield relevant information on the progression of the immunological response over time, as they should approximate more closely the natural course of spontaneous canine AD skin lesions. Evaluation of results from both static and dynamic investigations has allowed the identification of some aspects of the complex interplay of cells and mediators involved in the generation of acute and chronic lesions of canine AD. This review will focus on studies evaluating skin samples.

Observations from static studies

Epidermal changes

Skin lipids

A preliminary study using ruthenium tetroxide fixation documented that stratum corneum lipid lamellae appeared abnormal, at the ultrastructural level, in lesional skin of several dogs with AD compared with those of normal dogs.[5] Both continuity and thickness of lipid lamellae were significantly decreased compared with those of normal dogs. However, an abnormal extrusion of lamellar bodies was not found.

At the biochemical level, most studies have not reported differences between normal and atopic dogs in fatty acid composition of skin abrasion fluids,[6] subcutaneous fat,[7] plasma[7] or serum.[6,8] In contrast, a recent report suggested that non-lesional canine atopic thoracic skin contained higher linoleic acid levels than did similar samples of normal dog skin.[9] Finally, a recent abstract reported that the total amounts of ceramides were not significantly different between normal and atopic canine skin.[10]

Collectively, these studies have yielded conflicting information on whether biochemical lipid anomalies are associated with a defective epidermal barrier in the skin of dogs with AD, or not. Additional investigations are critically needed to resolve these contradictions.

Keratinocytes and leukocytes

Keratinocytes in lesional skin of dogs with AD express the adhesion molecule ICAM-1, which allows CD11a-expressing leukocytes to bind to these epidermal cells.[11] In the same areas, keratinocytes can express class II major histocompatibility (MHC II) molecules, a marker of activation.[11] Immunohistochemical studies of keratinocytes in lesional atopic skin have also demonstrated intracellular staining for inflammatory cytokines (e.g. tumour necrosis factor-alpha – [TNF-α])[12] and chemokines (e.g. thymus and activation-regulated chemokine [TARC], CCL-17).[13]

Epidermal Langerhans cells (LCs) in lesional skin of dogs with AD are hyperplastic, and are commonly seen in clusters.[14,15] These LCs frequently exhibit surface-bound IgE, especially when they are aggregated.[15] Epitheliotropic lymphocytes in lesional atopic skin possess either alpha-beta ($\alpha\beta$) or gamma-delta ($\gamma\delta$) T-cell receptors, and they express CD8 more often than CD4.[11]

Low numbers of epidermal neutrophils are seen in approximately half of skin sections of canine lesional AD skin.[11] Intact and degranulated eosinophils are occasionally detected singly or aggregated in subcorneal microabscesses.[11]

Microbial flora

Staphylococci are commonly found on the epidermal surface during microscopic evaluation of skin biopsy samples from dogs with 'allergy'.[16] There is a greater adherence by *Staphylococcus intermedius* to keratinocytes of dogs with AD compared with those of normal dogs.[17] Increased adherence occurs with epidermal cells collected from both inflamed and non-inflamed skin.[18] However, when AD skin lesions are in remission after low-dose oral glucocorticoid administration, the cutaneous carriage of *S. intermedius* is not significantly different from that of normal dogs.[19] Penetration of staphylococcal proteins through the stratum corneum has been demonstrated at the site of mast cell degranulation induced by compound 48/80.[20] Remarkably, anti-staphylococcal IgE is detected in the serum of dogs with recurrent pyoderma secondary to AD.[21] Finally, approximately one-quarter of canine *S. intermedius* isolates secrete superantigen exotoxins such as staphylococcal enterotoxins A (SEA), SEB, SEC, SED and toxic shock syndrome toxin-1 (TSST-1); both SEA and SEB can stimulate blastogenesis in canine lymphocytes.[22] Whether staphylococci isolated from canine atopic skin differ from those isolated from normal canine skin with regard to the amount and type of superantigens produced has not been reported at this time.

The commensal yeast *Malassezia pachydermatis* is found more commonly on the skin of atopic dogs than on that of normal dogs.[23] Yeast numbers are higher in superficial skin scrapings and skin cultures from dogs with AD than those of normal dogs, especially when the underlying skin is erythematous.[24] Humoral and cellular hypersensitivity toward *M. pachydermatis* has been shown in dogs with AD and cutaneous *Malas-*

sezia overgrowth. Indeed, various studies have revealed the existence of *Malassezia*-specific serum IgE,[25] skin wheal-and-flare reactions after intradermal injections of *Malassezia* extracts,[26,27] lymphocyte blastogenic responses to crude *Malassezia* extracts[28] and successful passive transfer of cutaneous hypersensitivity (positive Prausnitz-Küstner tests).[29]

In summary, there is evidence suggesting that stratum corneum carriage of both staphylococci and *Malassezia* is greater in lesional atopic canine skin than that of normal dogs. These microbes and/or their toxins have the potential to induce cutaneous inflammation not only by colonization and infection of the skin, but also by triggering microbe-specific hypersensitivity responses, or by non-specific polyclonal T-cell activation by superantigens. However, neither organism has been shown to directly induce the development of AD skin lesions in dogs, at this time.

Dermal changes

Leukocytes

Distinct differences are seen in the composition of the dermal cellular infiltrate in atopic skin compared with normal skin. Variations in granulocytes, mast cells and mononuclear cells have been reported.

Eosinophils are found more often in lesional than non-lesional canine atopic skin.[11,30] Dermal eosinophils commonly exhibit features of activation, such as aggregation of granules and paracellular granule release, in AD skin lesions.[11] Neutrophils usually represent less than 5% of the dermal infiltrate seen in lesional AD skin.[11]

Mast cell percentages, expressed per number of total nucleated dermal cells, are not significantly different between lesional AD and normal canine skin, or between non-lesional AD and normal canine skin.[11] However, as dermal cellularity is higher in lesional AD skin than normal canine skin, dermal mast cell numbers are higher in lesional canine AD skin.[11] Dermal mast cells express membrane-bound IgE,[15,31] and degranulation can be triggered by both IgE-dependent and IgE-independent mechanisms.[32,33] In one study, there were differences in the number of dermal cells that stained positive for tryptase and/or chymase in atopic skin compared with normal canine skin, and this observation was interpreted as selective protease degranulation in canine AD skin.[34]

The importance of mast cell-derived histamine as a major mediator of canine AD is controversial. Skin histamine levels are higher in dogs with AD compared with normal dogs, but they do not correlate with plasma histamine concentrations.[35] There is no significant difference in the percentage of total cell histamine released spontaneously from mast cells isolated from the skin of dogs with AD, ascaris-sensitive and normal dogs.[36] However, the total histamine content per isolated skin mast cell is higher in dogs with AD than in control subjects.[33] Mast cells isolated from canine AD skin release more histamine than those of normal skin when stimulated with either concanavalin-A or a calcium ionophore.[33]

Regarding mononuclear leukocytes, there are more numerous CD1-positive dendritic cells (DCs) in the dermis of lesional and non-lesional atopic skin than normal canine skin. Approximately 10% of lesional atopic dermal DCs express membrane IgE, while those of normal canine skin do not express surface IgE.[15] B lymphocytes and mature plasma cells compose less than 1% of dermal cells.[11] Lesional dermal CD3-positive T lymphocytes express the $\alpha\beta$ T-cell receptor ten times more often than the $\gamma\delta$ T-cell receptor,[11] and they stain for CD4 more commonly than CD8.[11,37]

Cytokine profile

Messenger RNA (mRNA) coding for the proinflammatory cytokine TNF-α is found at high levels in canine lesional AD skin specimens.[38–40] The translation of TNF-α protein has been shown in both epidermal and dermal cells.[12] Messenger RNA specific for interleukin-1-beta (IL-1β) is detected at high levels in chronically inflamed canine AD skin.[40]

Messenger RNA coding for the type-2 cytokines IL-4 and IL-5 is detected more commonly,[38] and at higher levels of expression,[39] in lesional AD than in normal canine skin biopsy specimens. However, this finding does not appear to be universal, as one study failed to detect mRNA for IL-4 in chronically inflamed canine AD skin samples.[40]

Messenger RNA specific for the type-1 cytokines IL-2 and IL-12 is less commonly detected in lesional AD than in normal canine skin.[38] However, when it is detected, IL-2 mRNA is present at higher levels in lesional AD skin than in normal skin.[39] Messenger RNA encoding IFN-γ is detected variably in canine lesional AD skin, but it is found more frequently in biopsies from chronic lesions.[38,39] Levels of transcription of IFN-γ can be three to six times higher in AD skin lesions compared with those of normal skin.[39,40]

The level of expression of mRNA encoding transforming growth factor-beta (TGF-β), a regulatory/suppressive cytokine, is higher in normal than in lesional canine AD skin.[39] There are conflicting data regarding the frequency of transcription of IL-10 mRNA in canine AD skin.[38,39]

Stem cell factor (SCF), a mast cell growth factor, is secreted in the dermis of lesional and non-lesional canine AD skin.[41] Messenger RNA encoding CC-chemokine ligand 17 (CCL-17/TARC), a chemokine involved in Th2 lymphocyte chemotaxis, is detected in lesional canine AD skin, but is absent from non-lesional AD skin,[40] and expression of CCL-17 protein can be detected in keratinocytes from lesional areas.[13] Messenger RNA coding for the CCL-17 receptor CCR4, which is specifically expressed on Th2 lymphocytes, also can be detected in canine AD lesional skin.[42] Although both CCL-17 mRNA and protein can readily be detected in lesional atopic dog skin, the transcription of macrophage-derived chemokine (MDC/CCL-22), another CCR4-ligand, is only rarely observed.[43]

Observations from 'dynamic' studies

Intradermal challenge with allergens and anti-IgE antibodies in normal or allergic dogs

Late-phase reactions (LPRs) develop in the skin of atopic dogs after intradermal challenge with allergens to which they are hypersensitive.[44,45] Similar reactions can be induced in normal and atopic dogs by intradermal injections of anti-canine IgE antibodies.[44,46]

Allergen- and anti-IgE-induced LPRs are macroscopically characterized by erythema, oedema and induration.[44] Microscopically, LPRs are associated with the sequential migration of neutrophil and eosinophil granulocytes, followed by an infiltration of T lymphocytes and dermal DCs.[44]

In normal dogs challenged intradermally with anti-canine IgE antibodies, there is an increase in mRNA expression encoding for IL-13, IL-5, monocyte chemoattractant protein-1 (MCP1/CCL-2), regulated upon activation, normal T cell expressed and secreted (RANTES/CCL-5) and TARC/CCL-17.[47] Levels of mRNA coding for IL-2, IL-4, IL-6 and IFN-γ remain negligible.[47]

In summary, allergen- and anti-IgE-induced dermal LPRs approximate skin lesions of canine AD both macroscopically and microscopically, and they are associated with a cytokine profile similar to that seen in spontaneous disease. However, neither stimulus produces the epidermal changes seen in naturally occurring AD, which limits their utility in studying the role of epidermal cells in the development of AD lesions.

Epicutaneous challenge of sensitized IgE-hyperresponsive beagle dogs

Genetically predisposed beagles can be sensitized to various allergens, such as *Dermatophagoides farinae* house dust mite, after repeated weekly epicutaneous applications of allergen extracts. In this line of dogs, allergen-specific serum IgE levels increase during sensitization, and inflammation develops at the site of epidermal mite application.[48]

The epicutaneous application (patch test) of allergen extracts on these dogs results in visible inflammation if elevated serum levels of IgE specific for the challenging allergens are present. Inflammation occurs as early as 2 hours after provocation, and increases in severity with time. Microscopic examination of positive tests reveals epidermal microabscesses containing eosinophils, and eosinophil-rich superficial dermal inflammation.[49] Immunohistochemical studies reveal the presence of epidermal LC aggregates as well as co-clustering of dermal DCs and T lymphocytes in the superficial dermis.[49] At 48 and 96 hours after allergen challenge, the magnitude of the dermal infiltrate correlates with allergen-specific IgE serum levels. IgE-expressing epidermal and dermal DCs are seen in positive patch test reactions.[50]

A recent unpublished study evaluated the kinetics of cytokine gene transcription during patch test reactions performed in IgE-hyperresponsive beagle dogs sensitized to *D. farinae*. Messenger RNAs encoding CCL-5 and IL-5 were highest in the samples collected after 6 hours, while those coding for IL-6 and IL-13 were highest in the 24-hour specimens. Interleukin-8 (IL-8/CXCL-8) and CCL-17-specific mRNA values peaked after 48 hours. IL-2 and IFN-γ transcription was high after 6 hours, with a further increase at 96 hours. Transcription of mRNA for IL-12 was demonstrated in specimens collected at 24–48 hours. Of the cytokine transcripts evaluated, CCL-17 was expressed at the highest levels, while IL-4, IL-10 and TNF-α expression levels were somewhat lower.

In all, results from these studies suggest that epicutaneous application of relevant allergens to IgE-hyperresponsive beagle dogs produces many of the macroscopic, microscopic and cytokine/chemokine changes seen in spontaneous canine AD skin lesions.

Environmental allergen challenges of sensitized IgE-hyperresponsive beagle dogs

Dermatophagoides-sensitized beagle dogs, experimentally exposed to elevated levels of this allergen in their housing environment, develop an erythematous maculo-papular dermatitis suggestive of AD as early as the second day after exposure to mite allergens.[51] Microscopic examination of lesional skin biopsy specimens reveals early oedema and congestion followed by a superficial perivascular to diffuse dermatitis rich in mononuclear cells. Luna stain reveals the presence of degranulating eosinophils. Epidermal eosinophil exocytosis and abscess formation is seen in late lesions. Immunohistochemical studies further characterize the skin infiltration as including CD4- and CD8-positive αβ and γδ T lymphocytes as well as DCs. T lymphocytes and DCs are often seen co-localized in dermal and epidermal clusters. Mast cells and DCs express surface IgE.[51]

Results from these challenges suggest that this experimental model reproduces most, if not all, macroscopic and microscopic changes seen in spontaneously occurring canine AD skin lesions.

Hypotheses for the generation of canine atopic skin lesions

Acute phase

The following steps may occur sequentially, but they could overlap or occur concurrently:

- An epidermal barrier defect could facilitate the contact of environmental, and possibly microbial, allergens with epidermal immune cells at skin sites that have been subjected to friction and trauma.
- Epidermal LCs capture allergens with antigen-specific IgE and migrate to the dermis and regional lymph nodes.
- Keratinocytes are activated and release chemokines and cytokines, presumably in response to signals from LCs and/or microbes.
- Allergen-specific IgE-coated dermal mast cells release histamine, proteases, chemokines, cytokines and other mediators.

- There is a rapid influx of granulocytes (neutrophils and eosinophils), allergen-specific Th2 lymphocytes and dermal DCs.
- Eosinophils are activated and degranulate upon exposure to inflammatory mediators and allergens.
- Th2 lymphocytes and mast cells release type-2 cytokines promoting IgE synthesis and eosinophil survival.

Chronic phase

- Microbial overgrowth may contribute to chronic inflammation by producing polyclonal T-lymphocyte-activating superantigens, by activating keratinocytes and LCs through pathogen-associated molecular patterns and Toll-like receptors, and/or by acting as allergens.
- Self-trauma and neuromediators contribute to chronic inflammation. Pruritus resulting from the acute phase inflammation leads to self-trauma and the release of neuromediators, both of which may cause further tissue damage and exacerbate inflammation.
- There is a cycle of chemokine release (both allergen-dependent and allergen-independent) with subsequent further influx and activation of leukocytes, which in turn results in the release of additional chemokines and other mediators.
- There is an infiltration of T lymphocytes secreting type-2 and type-1 cytokines. Many of these lymphocytes are specific to the initial offending allergen(s), but other T cells may also be recruited and stimulated non-specifically.
- Normal regulatory mechanisms, which could include regulatory T lymphocytes, fail to inhibit cutaneous inflammation. Such an anomaly probably results in the persistence of chronic AD skin lesions.

References

1   Olivry, T., DeBoer, D.J., Griffin, C.E., *et al.* The ACVD task force on canine atopic dermatitis: forewords and lexicon. *Veterinary Immunology and Immunopathology*, 2001; **81**: 143–146.
2   Lund, E.M., Armstrong, P.J., Kirk, C.A., Kolar, L.M., Klausner, J.S. Health status and population characteristics of dogs and cats examined at private veterinary practices in the United States. *Journal of the American Veterinary Medical Association*, 1999; **214**: 1336–1341.
3   Thestrup-Pedersen, K. Clinical aspects of atopic dermatitis. *Clinical and Experimental Dermatology*, 2000; **25**: 535–543.
4   Hillier, A., Olivry, T. Spontaneous canine model of atopic der-

matitis. In: Chan, L.S., ed. *Animal models of human inflammatory skin diseases*, CRC Press, Boca Raton, FL, 2004: 353–369.

5 Inman, A.O., Olivry, T., Dunston, S.M., Monteiro-Riviere, N.A., Gatto, H. Electron microscopic observations of the stratum corneum intercellular lipids in normal and atopic dogs. *Veterinary Pathology*, 2001; **38**: 720–723.

6 White, P.D. Evaluation of serum and cutaneous essential fatty acid profiles in normal, atopic and seborrheic dogs (abstract). *Proceedings of the Annual Meeting of the American Academy of Veterinary Dermatology/American College of Veterinary Dermatology*, San Francisco, 1990: 37.

7 Taugbol, O., Baddaky-Taugbol, B., Saarem, K. The fatty acid profile of subcutaneous fat and blood plasma in pruritic dogs and dogs without skin problems. *Canadian Journal of Veterinary Research – Revue Canadienne de Recherche Veterinaire*, 1998; **62**: 275–278.

8 Saevik, B.K., Thoresen, S.I., Taugbol, O. Fatty acid composition of serum lipids in atopic and healthy dogs. *Research in Veterinary Science*, 2002; **73**: 153–158.

9 Mueller, R.S., Richardson, K., Miller, A., Magowitz, J., Ogilvie, G.K. Cutaneous fatty acid concentrations in normal and atopic dogs (abstract). *Proceedings of the 19th Annual Congress of the European Society of Veterinary Dermatology/European College of Veterinary Dermatology*, Tenerife, Spain, 2003: 167.

10 Segiguchi, M., Ikeno, K., Iwasaki, T. Ceramides in keratin layer of normal and atopic dogs (abstract). *Proceedings of the American Academy of Veterinary Dermatology/American College of Veterinary Dermatology Annual Meeting*, Monterey, CA, 2003: 235.

11 Olivry, T., Naydan, D.K., Moore, P.F. Characterization of the cutaneous inflammatory infiltrate in canine atopic dermatitis. *American Journal of Dermatopathology*, 1997; **19**: 477–486.

12 Olivry, T., Dunston, S.M., Rivierre, C., *et al.* A randomized controlled trial of misoprostol monotherapy for canine atopic dermatitis: effects on dermal cellularity and cutaneous tumor necrosis factor-alpha. *Veterinary Dermatology*, 2003; **14**: 37–46.

13 Maeda, S., Tsukui, T., Saze, K., *et al.* Production of a monoclonal antibody to canine thymus and activation-regulated chemokine (TARC) and detection of TARC in lesional skin of dogs with atopic dermatitis. *Veterinary Immunology and Immunopathology*, 2005; **103**: 83–92.

14 Day, M.J. Expression of major histocompatibility complex class II molecules by dermal inflammatory cells, epidermal Langerhans cells and keratinocytes in canine dermatological disease. *Journal of Comparative Pathology*, 1996; **115**: 317–326.

15 Olivry, T., Moore, P.F., Affolter, V.K., Naydan, D.K. Langerhans cell hyperplasia and IgE expression in canine atopic dermatitis. *Archives of Dermatological Research*, 1996; **288**: 579–585.

16 Scott, D.W. Bacteria and yeast on the surface and within non-inflamed hair follicles of skin biopsies from dogs with non-neoplastic dermatoses. *Cornell Veterinarian*, 1992; **82**: 379–386.

17 McEwan, N.A. Adherence by *Staphylococcus intermedius* to canine keratinocytes in atopic dermatitis. *Research in Veterinary Science*, 2000; **68**: 279–283.

18 McEwan, N.A. *Staphylococcus intermedius* adherence to canine corneocytes: a comparison of inflamed and non-inflamed skin (abstract). *Proceedings of the 19th Annual Congress of the European Society of Veterinary Dermatology/European College of Veterinary Dermatology*, Tenerife, Spain, 2003: 142.

19 Harvey, R.G., Noble, W.C. A temporal study comparing the carriage of *Staphylococcus intermedius* on normal dogs with atopic dogs in clinical remission. *Veterinary Dermatology*, 1994; **5**: 21–25.

20 Mason, I.S., Lloyd, D.H. The role of allergy in the development of canine pyoderma. *Journal of Small Animal Practice*, 1989; **30**: 216–218.

21 Morales, C.A., Schultz, K.T., DeBoer, D.J. Antistaphylococcal antibodies in dogs with recurrent staphylococcal pyoderma. *Veterinary Immunology and Immunopathology*, 1994; **42**: 137–147.

22 Hendricks, A., Schuberth, H.J., Schueler, K., Lloyd, D.H. Frequency of superantigen-producing *Staphylococcus intermedius* isolates from canine pyoderma and proliferation-inducing potential of superantigens in dogs. *Research in Veterinary Science*, 2002; **73**: 273–277.

23 Vitale, C., Ihrke, P.J., Kass, P., Yang, S. Quantification of *Malassezia pachydermatis* obtained from the skin of normal and atopic dogs (abstract). *Proceedings of the Annual Meeting of the American Academy of Veterinary Dermatology/American College of Veterinary Dermatology*, Santa Fe, 1995: 14.

24 White, S.D., Bourdeau, P., Blumstein, P., *et al.* Comparison via cytology and culture of carriage of *Malassezia pachydermatis* in atopic and healthy dogs. In: Kwochka, K.W., Willemse, T., VonTscharner, C., eds. *Advances in Veterinary Dermatology*, vol 3. Butterworth-Heinemann, Oxford, 1998: 292–298.

25 Chen, T.A., Halliwell, R.E.W., Pemberton, A.D., Hill, P.B. Identification of major allergens of *Malassezia pachydermatis* in dogs with atopic dermatitis and *Malassezia* overgrowth. *Veterinary Dermatology*, 2002; **13**: 141–150.

26 Morris, D.O., Olivier, N.B., Rosser, E.J. Type-1 hypersensitivity reactions to *Malassezia pachydermatis* extracts in atopic dogs. *American Journal of Veterinary Research*, 1998; **59**: 836–841.

27 Bond, R., Curtis, C.F., Hendricks, A., Ferguson, E.A., Lloyd, D.H. Intradermal test reactivity to *Malassezia pachydermatis* in atopic dogs. *Veterinary Record*, 2002; **150**: 448–449.

28 Morris, D.O., Clayton, D.J., Drobatz, K.J., Felsburg, P.J. Response to *Malassezia pachydermatis* by peripheral blood mononuclear cells from clinically normal and atopic dogs. *American Journal of Veterinary Research*, 2002; **63**: 358–362.

29 Morris, D.O., DeBoer, D.J. Evaluation of serum obtained from atopic dogs with dermatitis attributable to *Malassezia pachydermatis* for passive transfer of immediate hypersensitivity to that organism. *American Journal of Veterinary Research*, 2003; **64**: 262–266.

30 Nimmo Wilkie, J.S., Yager, J.A., Eyre, P., Parker, W.M. Morphometric analyses of the skin of dogs with atopic dermatitis and correlations with cutaneous and plasma histamine and total serum IgE. *Veterinary Pathology*, 1990; **27**: 179–186.

31 Halliwell, R.E.W. The localization of IgE in canine skin: an immunofluorescent study. *Journal of Immunology*, 1973; **110**: 422–430.

32 Garcia, G., Ferrer, L., De Mora, F., Puigdemont, A. Inhibition of histamine release from dispersed canine skin mast cells by cyclosporin-A, rolipram and salbutamol, but not by dexamethasone or sodium cromoglycate. *Veterinary Dermatology*, 1998; **9**: 81–86.

33 DeMora, F., Garcia, G., Puigdemont, A., Arboix, M., Ferrer, L. Skin mast cell releasability in dogs with atopic dermatitis. *Inflammation Research*, 1996; **45**: 424–427.

34 Welle, M.M., Olivry, T., Grimm, S., Suter, M. Mast cell density and subtypes in the skin of dogs with atopic dermatitis. *Journal of Comparative Pathology*, 1999; **120**: 187–197.

35 Helton-Rhodes, K., Kerdel, F., Soter, N.A., Chinnici, R. Investigation into the immunopathogenesis of canine atopy. *Seminars in Veterinary Medicine and Surgery – Small Animal*, 1987; **2**: 199–201.

36 Brazis, P., Queralt, M., deMora, F., Ferrer, L., Puigdemont, A. Comparative study of histamine release from skin mast cells dispersed from atopic, ascaris-sensitive and healthy dogs. *Veterinary Immunology and Immunopathology*, 1998; **66**: 43–51.

37 Sinke, J.D., Thepen, T., Bihari, I.C., Rutten, V.P.M.G., Willemse, T. Immunophenotyping of skin-infiltrating T-cell subsets in dogs

with atopic dermatitis. *Veterinary Immunology and Immuno-pathology,* 1997; **57**: 13–23.

38 Olivry, T., Dean, G.A., Tompkins, M.B., Dow, J.L., Moore, P.F. Toward a canine model of atopic dermatitis: amplification of cytokine-gene transcripts in the skin of atopic dogs. *Experimental Dermatology,* 1999; **8**: 204–211.

39 Nuttall, T., Knight, P.A., McAleese, S.M., Lamb, J.R., Hill, P.B. Expression of Th1, Th2 and immunosuppressive cytokine gene transcripts in canine atopic dermatitis. *Clinical and Experimental Allergy,* 2002; **32**: 789–795.

40 Maeda, S., Fujiwara, S., Omori, K., *et al.* Lesional expression of thymus and activation-regulated chemokine in canine atopic dermatitis. *Veterinary Immunology and Immunopathology,* 2002; **88**: 79–87.

41 Hammerberg, B., Olivry, T., Orton, S.M. Skin mast cell histamine release following stem cell factor and high-affinity immunoglobulin E receptor cross-linking in dogs with atopic dermatitis. *Veterinary Dermatology,* 2001; **12**: 339–346.

42 Maeda, S., Okayama, T., Omori, K., *et al.* Expression of CC chemokine receptor 4 (CCR4) mRNA in canine atopic skin lesion. *Veterinary Immunology and Immunopathology,* 2002; **90**: 145–154.

43 Tsukui, T., Maeda, S., Ohmori, K., *et al.* Expression analysis of macrophage-derived chemokine (MDC/CCL22) gene in canine atopic dermatitis (abstract). *Journal of Allergy and Clinical Immunology,* 2004; **113**: S55.

44 Olivry, T., Murphy, K.M., Dunston, S.M., Moore, P.F. Characterization of the inflammatory infiltrate during IgE-mediated late-phase reactions in the skin of normal and atopic dogs. *Veterinary Dermatology,* 2001; **12**: 49–58.

45 Hillier, A., Cole, L.K., Kwochka, K.W., McCall, C. Late-phase reactions to intradermal testing with *Dermatophagoides farinae* in healthy dogs and dogs with house dust mite-induced atopic dermatitis. *American Journal of Veterinary Research,* 2002; **63**: 69–73.

46 DeBoer, D.J., Cooley, A.J. Use of induced cutaneous immediate-type hypersensitivity reactions to evaluate anti-inflammatory effects of triamcinolone topical solution in three dogs. *Veterinary Dermatology,* 2000; **11**: 25–33.

47 Pucheu-Haston, C.M., Shuster, D., Olivry, T., *et al.* Evaluation of IgE-mediated late phase reactions in the skin of normal placebo and prednisolone treated dogs: cellular, cytokine and chemokine responses (abstract). *Veterinary Dermatology,* 2004; **15** (S1): 38.

48 McCall, C., Geoly, F., Clarke, K. Transdermal allergen exposure of genetically high IgE beagle puppies elicits allergen-specific IgE and dermatitis at the site of exposure (abstract). *Veterinary Dermatology,* 2001; **12**: 234.

49 Olivry, T., Geoly, F., Dunston, S.M., Clarke, K.B., McCall, C.A. Histological and immunohistochemical characterization of "atopy patch tests" in IgE hyperresponsive beagle dogs: a pilot study (abstract). *Veterinary Dermatology,* 2001; **12**: 235.

50 Olivry, T., Buckler, K.E., Dunston, S.M., Clarke, K.B., McCall, C. Positive "atopy patch tests" reactions in IgE-hyperresponsive beagle dogs are dependent upon elevated allergen-specific IgE serum levels and are associated with IgE-expressing dendritic cells (abstract). *Veterinary Dermatology,* 2002; **13**: 219.

51 Marsella, R., Olivry, T., Nicklin, C.F., Saglio, S., Lopez, J., Dunston, S.M. A model for canine atopic dermatitis: induction of dermatitis in IgE hyperresponsive beagle dogs after house dust mite challenge (abstract). *Veterinary Dermatology,* 2003; **14**: 219.

Expression of Th1-cytokine mRNA in canine atopic dermatitis correlates with severity of clinical lesions

T.J. Nuttall BSc, BVSc, PhD, CertVD, CBiol MIBiol MRCVS[1], P.A. Knight BSc, PhD[2], S.M. McAleese BSc, PhD[2], J. Brown BSc, PhD[2], J.R. Lamb BSc, PhD[3], P.B. Hill BVSc, PhD, DVD, MRCVS[2]

[1] Department of Veterinary Clinical Science, University of Liverpool, UK
[2] Department of Veterinary Clinical Studies, University of Edinburgh, UK
[3] MRC Centre for Inflammation Research, University of Edinburgh, UK

Summary

Previous studies indicate that lesional atopic skin is associated with mRNA expression for the T-helper 1 (Th1) cytokines interferon gamma (IFN-γ) and interleukin (IL)-2, and the proinflammatory cytokine tumour necrosis factor alpha (TNF-α). The aim of this study was to determine whether the level of gene transcription for these cytokines correlates with the clinical lesion severity of canine atopic dermatitis (AD).

Six-millimetre punch biopsies of non-lesional and lesional skin were collected from dogs with AD ($n = 23$) and healthy dogs ($n = 12$), where AD was diagnosed on clinical criteria. Clinical severity was assessed using a modified canine atopic dermatitis extent and severity index (CADESI)-type clinical scoring scheme. Semi-quantitative reverse transcriptase-polymerase chain reactions (RT-PCR) were used to determine the mRNA levels of IFN-γ, TNF-α, IL-2 and the Th2-cytokine IL-4. Duplicate biopsies were submitted for histopathology. Five images ($\times 400$ magnification) of the superficial interfollicular dermis were captured for quantitative analysis of cell infiltration by calculating the proportion of the image that consisted of cell nuclei.

There was a significant correlation between cellular infiltration and mRNA levels for IFN-γ ($p < 0.0001$, $n = 13$), TNF-α ($p = 0.046$, $n = 8$) and IL-2 ($p = 0.023$, $n = 12$) in lesional but not in non-lesional ($n = 23$) or healthy skin ($n = 12$). There was also a significant correlation between the clinical score and mRNA levels for IFN-γ ($p = 0.02$, $n = 13$), TNF-α ($p = 0.04$, $n = 8$) and IL-2 ($p = 0.008$, $n = 12$) in lesional skin, but not non-lesional skin ($n = 23$). There was no correlation between cellular infiltration or clinical score and IL-4 mRNA levels.

It appears that Th1 and proinflammatory cytokines are pivotal in the pathogenesis of chronic lesional AD. In contrast, IL-4 does not appear to be linked to the development of chronic lesions.

Introduction

Atopic dermatitis (AD) is a universally recognised inflammatory skin disease of dogs and humans. Recent interest has focused on the role of CD4[+] T-helper (Th) cells in the pathogenesis of the disease. Th1 cells were first differentiated from Th2 cells in rats and mice.[1,2] Unlike rodent Th cells, human Th cells secrete a complex variety of cytokines,[3] although Th1- and Th2-type populations can be distinguished.[4] Th1-cytokines such as interferon-gamma (IFN-γ), interleukin (IL)-2, IL-12, and the proinflammatory-cytokine tumour necrosis factor-alpha (TNF-α) promote cell-mediated immunity, whereas Th2 cytokines such as IL-4, IL-5, IL-6 and IL-13 promote humoral immunity and IgE production.[3,5]

Th2 polarisation and expression of IL-4 appears to be a hallmark of AD.[6–8] Several studies have detected Th2 polarisation in peripheral blood mononuclear cells and skin of atopic humans,[9–13] atopic dogs[6,8,14,15] and mouse models of AD.[16,17] Th2 and Th1 responses have been regarded as mutually exclusive[18] but the Th1-cytokines IL-2 and IFN-γ, as well as the proinflammatory-cytokine TNF-α, have been found in lesional canine AD.[8] In contrast, only low levels of these cytokines were detected in healthy and non-lesional skin. Another recent study also found that IFN-γ and TNF-α, as well as IL-1β and thymus and activation regulated chemokine (TARC), were up-regulated in lesional skin, compared with non-lesional and healthy canine skin.[19] Th1-cytokines are also found in chronic lesions of human AD,[20] and they dominate atopy patch test sites after 48 hours in both humans[21] and dogs.[14]

These findings suggest that Th1-cytokines participate in the pathogenesis of chronic lesional AD. Therefore, the aim of this study was to determine whether the level of gene transcription for IL-2, IFN-γ, TNF-α and IL-4 could be correlated with the clinical severity of lesional canine AD.

Materials and methods

Sample collection

Dogs with AD ($n = 23$) were recruited from the dermatology clinic at the University of Edinburgh Hospital for Small Animals. The diagnosis of AD was based on compatible history and clinical signs, and exclusion of other pruritic dermatoses.[22] Coat brushings, skin scrapes, trial therapy and a 6-week diet trial were used to eliminate ectoparasites and cutaneous adverse food reactions (food allergy/intolerance). Staphylococcal and *Malassezia* infections were managed appropriately. No anti-inflammatory medication was administered for at least 3 weeks prior to entry into the study. All dogs with a clinical diagnosis of AD underwent intradermal testing (IDT) with 54 allergens, including *Dermatophagoides farinae* and *D. pteronyssinus* (Greer Laboratories, Lenoir, NC, USA), according to a standard protocol.[8] The extent and severity of clinical lesions was scored using a modification of the original canine atopic dermatitis extent and severity index (CADESI) developed by Olivry and others.[23] Briefly, erythema, papules, scaling, seborrhoea (used to denote excessive greasiness), hyperpigmentation and lichenification at 36 body sites were subjectively scored from 0 to 5 by a single investigator. The clinical scores did not refer to the individual biopsy sites, but rather to the entire patient.

Control samples were taken from healthy dogs ($n = 12$) presented for euthanasia that had no history or clinical signs of pruritus, or any other condition likely to alter immune function. By definition, their clinical score was 0.

In dogs with AD, non-lesional skin samples ($n = 23$) were taken from the flank. Lesional skin samples ($n = 13$) were taken from areas of erythematous and macular-papular dermatitis. Six-millimetre diameter skin biopsies were placed immediately into RNA-later® (Ambion Inc., Austin, TX, USA). Skin ($n = 12$) and

positive control samples (popliteal lymph node and tonsil) from healthy dogs were collected into RNA-later® immediately after euthanasia. Samples in RNA-later® were kept at 4°C for 24 hours, before storage at −20°C. Duplicate skin biopsies were collected into 10% neutral buffered formalin for histopathology.

Primer design

Primers (Table 1.3.1) were designed from published canine sequences (Genbank®; National Center for Biotechnology Information, www.ncbi.nlm.nih.gov/Genbank/) using Oligo6® software (Molecular Biology Insights, Cascade, CO, USA). Cross-reactive oligonucleotides were eliminated by screening against known sequences (BLAST®; National Centre for Biotechnology Information; www.ncbi.nlm.nih. gov/BLAST/).

RNA extraction

Total RNA was extracted from the skin biopsies and control samples by homogenisation (Ultra-turrax 125; Janke and Kunkel IKA, Staufen, Germany) in TRI-reagent® (Sigma, Poole, UK).[24,25] DNA was removed by incubating with 4 IU DNAse I per 50 µl RNA solution according to the manufacturer's instructions (DNA-free®; Ambion Inc.). The RNA concentration was quantified by ultraviolet absorbance at 260 nm with a 260 nm:280 nm ratio >1.5 (DU650 spectrophotometer; Beckman-Coulter, Fullerton, CA, USA). Heparin was removed by incubating 4 µg RNA with 4 IU heparinase I (Sigma).[26] Heparinased RNA was stored at −70°C.

Reverse transcriptase-polymerase chain reaction (RT-PCR)

The cDNA generated from 1 µg heparinased RNA (Reverse Transcriptase System; Promega Corp., Madison, WI, USA) was diluted to 200 µl in RNAse-free water. One microgram of heparinased RNA was diluted to 200 µl without reverse transcription as a negative control. The cDNA and negative control preparations were stored at 20°C. PCRs were carried out in 50-µl volumes containing 10 mM Tris-HCl, 2.5 IU *Taq* deoxyribonucleic acid polymerase (Roche Molecular Biochemicals, Lewes, UK), 200 µM deoxynucleotide triphosphates, 200 nM of each primer pair and 50 ng cDNA. Reaction conditions consisted of initial denaturing at 94°C for 2 minutes, then 35 cycles of denaturing at 94°C for 30 seconds, annealing for 30 seconds and elongation at 72°C for 1 minute, before a final elongation at 72°C for

Table 1.3.1 Cytokine primers and optimum conditions for polymerase chain reactions

Cytokine	Primer sequence	Annealing temperature (°C)	MgCl$_2$ (mM)	pH	PCR cycles	Product size (bp)
GAPDH	Forward - CCTTCATTGACCTCAACTACAT Reverse - CCAAAGTTGTCATGGATGACC Internal - CCCTCAAGATTGTCAGCAATGCC	55	2.0	8.6	35	400
IL-4	Forward - TAAAGGGTCTCACCTCCCAACTG Reverse - TAGAACAGGTCTTGTTTGCCATGC Internal - CACCAGCACCTTTGTCCACGGA	55	1.5	9.2	36	317
IFN-γ	Forward - TCGGACGGTGGGTCTCTTTCG Reverse - CACTTTGATGAGTTCATTTATCGCC Internal - CAGCACCAGTAAGAGGGAGGAC	60	2.5	8.9	35	281
IL-2	Forward - CTCACAGTAACCTCAACTCCTGC Reverse - TTCTGTAATGGTTGCTGTCTCGTC Internal - ACACGCCCAAGAAGGCCACAGA	55	2.5	8.6	35	461
TNF-α	Forward - ACTCTTCTGCCTGCTGCACTTTGG Reverse - GTTGACCTTTGTCTGGTAGGAGACGG Internal - CACCCACACCATCAGCCGCTTCGCCG	55	2.5	8.9	35	366

GAPDH, glutaraldehyde-3-phosphate dehydrogenase; IL, interleukin; IFN-γ, interferon gamma; TNF-α, tumour necrosis factor alpha; PCR, polymerase chain reaction; bp, base pairs.

7 minutes (GeneAmp PCR System 2400; Perkin-Elmer, Cambridge, UK). Optimum MgCl$_2$ concentration and annealing temperatures for each primer pair were established prior to the study (Table 1.3.1).[8,15] The PCR products were run on 1.2% agarose gels containing 0.5 µg/ml ethidium bromide and imaged under 590 nm ultraviolet light (Image Station 400CF; Kodak, Rochester, NY, USA). The PCRs using glyceraldehyde-3-phosphate dehydrogenase (GAPDH)-specific primers were performed for each cDNA and negative-control preparation. Samples with no GAPDH signal, or a positive signal from a negative control, or insufficient mRNA for analysis, were discarded.

Southern blotting and hybridisation
The PCRs for each primer pair using positive-control cDNA (derived from popliteal lymph node and tonsil) were performed as described previously. Southern blotting and hybridisation was performed using specific digoxigenin-labelled internal oligonucleotides.[24]

Semi-quantitative PCR
To determine the optimum number of cycles for semi-quantitative PCR, 26–44 PCR cycles for each primer pair were performed using positive-control cDNA and the gels were imaged as described. Standard curves were generated by plotting the number of cycles against the log2 net band intensity. The optimum number of

cycles (Table 1.3.1) for each cytokine primer pair was selected from the straight-line portion of the plot.[15]

The PCRs for each cytokine primer pair were performed with cDNA from each skin sample, positive control cDNA and negative controls (water and heparinased RNA) for the appropriate number of cycles. The PCR products were run on gels and imaged as before. Gels with no positive-control signal or a negative-control signal were discarded. The relative abundance of cytokine mRNA was determined by dividing the cytokine PCR product signal intensity by that of GAPDH for each sample.

Histopathology and morphometric analysis of the skin biopsy specimens

Skin biopsy samples from non-lesional AD skin, lesional AD skin, and from healthy dog skin were fixed in 10% neutral buffered formalin and embedded in paraffin wax. Sagittal sections (4 µm thick) were cut parallel to the hair follicles and stained with haematoxylin and eosin.

A single investigator assessed all the histopathology sections. Five images (×400 magnification) of the superficial interfollicular dermis were captured using a Sony DXC-390P 3CCD colour video camera (Scion Corporation, Frederick, VI, USA) mounted on an Axiovert 100 inverted microscope and digitised using

Scion Image (www.scioncorp.com). Prior evaluation showed that five images could be obtained from most sections by starting at the left edge (epidermis uppermost) and moving across by half a graticule division per image. Fields that included adnexal structures were discarded. Images were prepared for quantitative analysis using Object-Image (Norbert Vischer, University of Amsterdam, The Netherlands; www.simon.bio.uva.nl/object-image.html). The image software was used to compute the proportion of each image area that consisted of cell nuclei compared to cytoplasm and extracellular matrix. This yields a reliable estimate of cell numbers.[15] Sections with insufficient non-adnexal dermis for analysis were discarded.

Data analysis

Data were tested for normality (Kolmogorov-Smirnov test with the Dallal and Wilkinson approximation of the p value). One-way ANOVA with Dunn's post-tests was used to compare the proportion of each histopathological image that consisted of cell nuclei. Spearman's rank test was used to correlate cytokine-mRNA levels with the clinical score and cellular infiltration (Instat®; Graphpad Inc., San Diego, CA, USA). Significance was set at $p < 0.05$.

Results

Intradermal tests and histopathology

All the dogs with AD had positive reactions on IDT to *D. farinae* and *D. pteronyssinus*. There were also individual reactions to other dust and forage (storage) mites, epithelia, pollens and moulds.

Healthy skin was characterised by a thin epidermis and basket-weave stratum corneum of normal appearance. Hair follicles, sebaceous glands, arrector pili muscles, sweat glands and blood vessels appeared normal. There was a loose array of collagen fibres with a sparse infiltrate of fibrocytes, mast cells and mononuclear cells in the dermis. There were few differences between non-lesional atopic and healthy skin. These included occasional mild hyperkeratosis, mild acanthosis, sparse lymphocyte exocytosis and a mild superficial perivascular mononuclear cell infiltrate. Lesional atopic skin was characterised by moderate to severe basket-weave to lamellar hyperkeratosis, moderate to severe acanthosis and spongiosis, frequent lym-

phocyte exocytosis, and a moderate to marked superficial perivascular to interstitial infiltrate. The infiltrate was largely composed of mononuclear and mast cells, with variable numbers of eosinophils and neutrophils. There were significantly greater numbers of inflammatory cells present in the dermis of lesional atopic skin than in either non-lesional or healthy skin ($p < 0.0001$; Fig. 1.3.1).

Correlation of cytokine gene transcripts with cell infiltration

Single bands of the expected size for each cytokine were seen on the PCR gel and hybridisation blots using positive-control material. This verified expression of mRNA for each cytokine in the positive-control samples and confirmed primer specificity (Fig. 1.3.2).

The mean, maximal and minimum mRNA levels and clinical scores for IFN-γ, IL-2, TNF-α and IL-4 in samples from healthy skin, and non-lesional and lesional skin from atopic dogs, are presented in Table 1.3.2. There was a significant correlation of mRNA levels for the Th1-cytokines IFN-γ, IL-2 and the proinflammatory-cytokine TNF-α with the degree of cellular infiltration in each biopsy sample when all skin samples were considered together, and for lesional skin samples (Fig. 1.3.3 and Table 1.3.3). There was no significant correlation between mRNA expression for any of the cytokines and cell infiltration in non-lesional and healthy skin samples, except for IL-2 mRNA expression which was significantly correlated with the degree of cellular infiltration in non-lesional skin biopsies (Fig. 1.3.3 and Table 1.3.3). There was a significant cor-

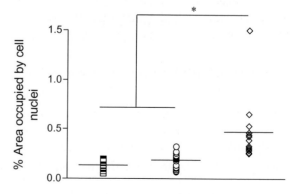

Fig. 1.3.1 The degree of cellular infiltration into lesional, non-lesional and healthy canine skin. ◇ Lesional atopic skin; ○ non-lesional atopic skin; □ healthy skin; bar = mean. *$p < 0.0001$.

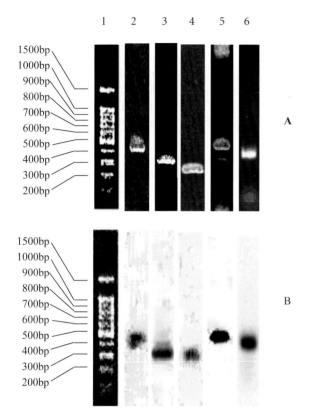

Fig. 1.3.2 Detection of cytokine gene transcription using positive-control cDNA (Image Station 440CF; Kodak). (A) 1.2% agarose gel with 0.5 µg/ml ethidium bromide. (B) Southern blotting and hybridization to digoxigenin-labelled internal probes. Lane 1, 100-bp DNA markers (Promega Corp.); lane 2, glutaraldehyde-3-phosphate dehydrogenase (GAPDH); lane 3, IL-4; lane 4, IFN-γ; lane 5, IL-2; lane 6, TNF-α.

Table 1.3.2 mRNA levels and clinical scores for IFN-γ, IL-2, TNF-α and IL-4 in samples from healthy skin, non-lesional and lesional skin from atopic dogs

	mRNA levels relative to GAPDH	Global clinical score
IFN-γ		
Healthy	0.07 (0.0005, 0.18 [12])	
Non-lesional	0.06 (0.0005; 0.16 [23])	76.2 (14, 213 [23])
Lesional	0.28 (0.03, 0.88 [13])	97.0 (34, 213 [13])
IL-2		
Healthy	0.07 (0.01, 0.2 [10])	
Non-lesional	0.05 (0.00006, 0.44 [19])	80.7 (14, 213 [19])
Lesional	0.29 (0.001, 0.49 [12])	100.0 (34, 213 [19])
TNF-α		
Healthy	0.6 (0.03, 1.87 [10])	
Non-lesional	0.82 (0.005; 2.0 [26])	82.0 (14, 213 [26])
Lesional	2.15 (0.95, 5.0 [8])	100.1 (34, 213 [8])
IL-4		
Healthy	0.03 (0.00006, 0.12 [10])	
Non-lesional	0.6 (0.002, 3.9 [23])	84.0 (14, 213 [23])
Lesional	1.0 (0.02, 3.1 [8])	100.1 (34, 213 [8])

Values are presented as mean (minimum, maximum [number evaluated]).

relation of mRNA levels of IL-4 and cellular infiltrate when all samples were considered together, but not for lesional, non-lesional and healthy skin when considered separately (Fig. 1.3.3 and Table 1.3.3).

Correlation of cytokine gene transcripts with clinical score

There was a significant correlation of mRNA levels for the Th1-cytokines IFN-γ, IL-2 and the proinflammatory-cytokine TNF-α with the clinical score in lesional skin samples, but not in non-lesional skin samples (Fig. 1.3.4 and Table 1.3.4). There was no significant correlation of IL-4 mRNA levels and clinical score in either lesional or non-lesional skin (Fig.1.3.4 and Table 1.3.4).

Discussion

This study demonstrates that Th1- and proinflammatory-cytokine mRNA expression is directly correlated with the inflammatory cell infiltrate in lesional skin samples. The Th1-cytokine mRNA levels in lesional, but not non-lesional skin, were also proportional to the clinical score. This is not a direct correlation as the clinical scores referred to global clinical score rather than a clinical score for each individual biopsy. CADESI-type clinical scores are, however, a reliable way to assess the severity of lesional AD,[15,23] and the skin biopsies were taken from representative areas of skin. Earlier studies have found Th1-cytokines in lesional atopic skin,[6,8,14,19]

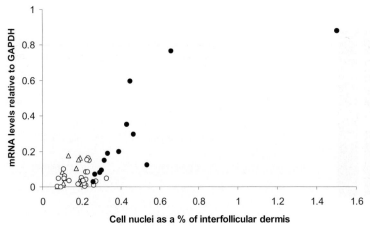

(a) IFN-γ

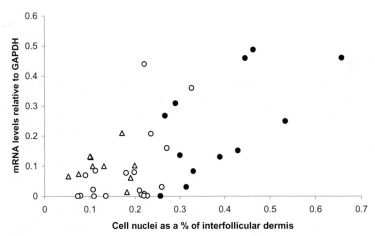

(b) IL-2

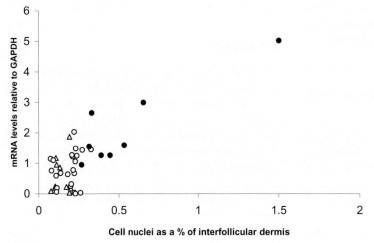

(c) TNF-α

Fig. 1.3.3 Correlation between cytokine gene transcription and degree of cellular infiltration. IFN-γ interferon gamma; TNF-α tumour necrosis factor alpha; IL, interleukin; ● lesional skin; ○ non-lesional skin; △ healthy skin.

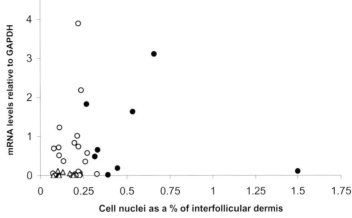

Fig. 1.3.3 (*Continued.*)   (d) IL-4

but our results provide evidence of an association with the degree of cellular infiltration and severity.

The findings imply that Th1 and proinflammatory cytokines likely play a key role in initiating and maintaining chronic cell-mediated inflammatory lesions in canine AD. The cytokines IL-2, IFN-γ and TNF-α recruit and activate lymphocytes and other mononuclear cells by inducing expression of intracellular adhesion molecule (ICAM)-1, vascular cell adhesion molecule (VACM)-1, class II major histocompatibility complex (MHC II) molecules, and other proinflammatory cytokines and chemokines.[4,18,27–29] Furthermore, activated lymphocytes and mononuclear cells are potent sources of Th1 cytokines and other proinflammatory mediators:[18] for example, autocrine secretion of IL-2 is a crucial factor in the activation and expansion of T cells.[27]

Our findings suggest an important role for TNF-α, a strongly proinflammatory cytokine, in the genera-

tion of inflammatory lesions of canine AD. In contrast, one small study in atopic dogs found no link between TNF-α expression and cellular infiltration, pruritus or lesional scores.[23] This study, however, was primarily concerned with therapeutic intervention and did not evaluate healthy dogs. In humans, TNF-α levels were found to correlate with the severity of allergic respiratory disease.[30]

A function of IFN-γ is the up-regulated expression of various proinflammatory mediators by inflammatory cells, keratinocytes and dermal cells.[4,31] Lesional skin in human AD is characterised by Fas-dependent keratinocyte apoptosis and disruption of the epidermal barrier, increasing exposure to allergens, irritants and microbes. In particular, IFN-γ induces expression of Fas on keratinocytes, which interacts with Fas-ligand present on infiltrating T cells.[32] In one study, keratinocytes from humans with AD were

Table 1.3.3 Correlation between cytokine gene transcription and degree of cellular infiltration

	IFN-γ	IL-2	TNF-α	IL-4
All skin samples	0.59 (*$p < 0.0001$; $n = 48$)	0.52 (*$p = 0.0005$; $n = 41$)	0.51 (*$p = 0.0006$; $n = 41$)	0.37 (*$p = 0.02$; $n = 41$)
Lesional skin	0.87 (*$p < 0.0001$; $n = 13$)	0.62 (*$p = 0.023$; $n = 12$)	0.73 (*$p = 0.046$; $n = 8$)	0.12 ($p = 0.79$; $n = 8$)
Non-lesional skin	0.25 ($p = 0.26$; $n = 23$)	0.5 (*$p = 0.028$; $n = 19$)	0.23 ($p = 0.29$; $n = 23$)	0.12 ($p = 0.96$; $n = 23$)
Healthy skin	0.53 ($p = 0.075$; $n = 12$)	0.067 ($p = 0.87$; $n = 10$)	0.08 ($p = 0.84$; $n = 10$)	0.08 ($p = 0.84$; $n = 10$)

IL, interleukin; IFN-γ, interferon gamma; TNF-α, tumour necrosis factor alpha. *$p < 0.05$.

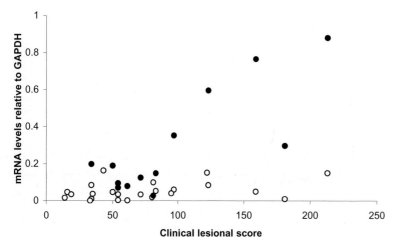

(a) IFN-γ

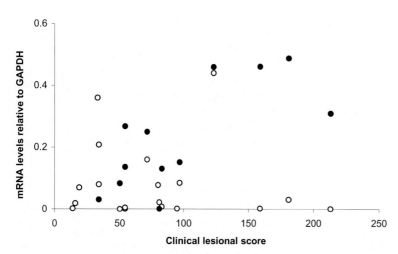

(b) IL-2

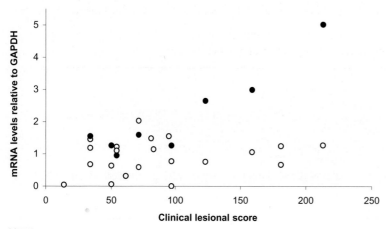

(c) TNF-α

Fig. 1.3.4 Correlation between cytokine gene transcription and CADESI score. IFN-γ, interferon gamma; TNF-α, tumour necrosis factor alpha; IL, interleukin; ● lesional skin; ○ non-lesional skin.

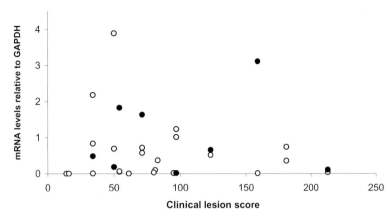

Fig. 1.3.4 (*Continued.*)   (d) IL-4

more sensitive to IFN-γ than those from healthy individuals.[31]

The findings from these studies suggest that Th1-cytokines and TNF-α are crucial in the pathogenesis of chronic lesional AD. Several papers, however, also state that expression of the archetypal Th2-cytokine IL-4 is a hallmark of canine AD,[6,8,14] although one study failed to demonstrate IL-4 mRNA in atopic canine skin.[19] In our study, IL-4 mRNA was detected in both lesional and non-lesional AD skin, but there was no significant correlation with the cellular infiltrate or clinical scores. These findings suggest that IL-4 is not directly involved in the recruitment of cells and the development of chronic lesions. However, it is likely that IL-4 expression underlies allergen sensitisation and IgE production. Subsequent IgE-mediated immediate-phase inflammatory reactions could then initiate a cascade of cellular activation and cytokine production, resulting in lesional AD. Canine AD, therefore, seems to involve the coordinated and sequential expression of Th2 and Th1-cytokines. The Th2 polarisation and allergic sensitisation are, furthermore, unlikely to be associated with a failure of Th1 differentiation. The activation of proinflammatory cytokines in AD may instead involve a loss of peripheral tolerance.[8]

The exact trigger for Th1-cytokine expression is not fully understood. Most authors conclude that chronic skin lesions result from self-trauma and microbial colonisation.[22,33] Self-trauma induces expression of inflammatory cytokines, including IL-1, TNF-α and GM-CSF, by keratinocytes.[29] Furthermore, histamine promotes Th1-cell proliferation *in vitro*.[34] Eosinophil- and mast cell-derived IL-12 may also drive Th1-cell differentiation.[14] The severity of human AD is also associated with staphylococcal colonisation.[35] Staphylococcal superantigens in humans may function to: induce cutaneous lymphocyte antigen expression on T cells; induce MHC II, IL-1, TNF-α, and IL-12 expression by mononuclear cells; and up-regulate endothelial ICAM-1 and VCAM-1.[7,35,36] *Staphylococcus aureus* preferentially binds to sites of IL-4-mediated inflammation in mice,[37] suggesting that they are important in

Table 1.3.4 Correlation between cytokine gene transcription and CADESI score

	IFN-γ	IL-2	TNF-α	IL-4
Lesional skin	0.63 (*$p = 0.02$; $n = 13$)	0.73 (*$p = 0.008$; $n = 12$)	0.75 (*$p = 0.04$; $n = 8$)	0 ($p = 1.0$; $n = 8$)
Non-lesional skin	0.34 ($p = 0.11$; $n = 23$)	−0.11 ($p = 0.66$; $n = 19$)	0.25 ($p = 0.22$; $n = 26$)	0.12 ($p = 0.58$; $n = 23$)

IL, interleukin; IFN-γ, interferon gamma; TNF-α, tumour necrosis factor alpha. *$p < 0.05$.

the switch from Th2- to Th1-inflammatory reactions. *Malassezia* organisms induce IgG, IgE, immediate- and late-phase skin reactivity, and PBMC proliferation in human[38–42] and canine[43–45] AD. *Malassezia* also induce IL-1β, IL-6, IL-8 and TNF-α production by human keratinocytes.[46] These findings suggest an important role for micro-organisms in enhancing leucocyte adhesion and migration, proinflammatory-cytokine release and the development of chronic skin lesions.

In summary, we hypothesise the following pathogenic sequence in canine AD. Early AD appears to be associated with increased expression of IL-4, sensitisation to environmental allergens and IgE-mediated acute inflammatory reactions.[6,8,14,47] Lesional skin, in contrast, exhibits a Th1- and proinflammatory-cytokine pattern that may be, in part, due to self-trauma and secondary infection. Gene transcription, however, does not necessarily equate with functional protein expression and further studies are needed to confirm these results. Further investigation could also identify targets for therapeutic intervention to block Th1-cytokine expression and the onset of chronic inflammatory lesions in AD.

Acknowledgements

The authors are grateful to Mrs Elisabeth Thornton and Mr Steven Wright (Department of Veterinary Clinical Studies, University of Edinburgh), Drs Sarah Howie, Karen Tan and Gillian Hall (MRC Centre for Inflammation Research), Prof. Michael Day (Department of Veterinary Pathology, University of Bristol), Dr John Huntley (Moredun Research Institute, Edinburgh) and Dr Sue Bell, Mrs Diane Isherwood and Prof. Stuart Carter (Department of Veterinary Clinical Science, University of Liverpool) for their help and support.

Funding

This study was funded, in part, by the Wellcome Trust.

References

1 Arthur, R.P., Mason, D. T-cells that help B-cell responses to soluble antigen are distinguishable from those producing interleukin 2 on mitogenic or allogeneic stimulation. *Journal of Experimental Medicine*, 1986; **163**: 774–786.

2 Mosmann, T.R., Coffman, R.L. Two types of mouse helper T-cell clone: implications for immune regulation. *Immunology Today*, 1987; **8**: 223–227.

3 Abbas, A.K., Murphy, K.M., Sher, A. Functional diversity of help-

4 Maggi, E. The TH1/TH2 paradigm in allergy. *Immunotechnology*, 1998; **3**: 233–244.

5 Romagnani, S., Parronchi, P., D'Elios, M.M., *et al.* An update on human Th1 and Th2 cells. *International Archives of Allergy and Immunology*, 1997; **113**: 153–156.

6 Olivry, T., Dean, G.A., Tompkins, M.B., Dow, J.L., Moore, P.F. Toward a canine model of atopic dermatitis: amplification of cytokine-gene transcripts in the skin of atopic dogs. *Experimental Dermatology*, 1999; **8**: 204–211.

7 Leung, D.Y.M. Atopic dermatitis: new insights and opportunities for therapeutic intervention. *Journal of Allergy and Clinical Immunology*, 2000; **105**: 860–876.

8 Nuttall, T.J., Knight, P.A., McAleese, S.M., Lamb, J.R., Hill, P.B. Expression of T-helper 1, T-helper 2 and immunosuppressive cytokines in canine atopic dermatitis. *Clinical and Experimental Allergy*, 2002; **32**: 789–795.

9 van der Heijden, F.L., Wierenga, E.A., Bos, J.D., Kapsenberg, M.L. High frequency of IL-4 producing CD4+ allergen-specific T lymphocytes in atopic dermatitis lesional skin. *Journal of Investigative Dermatology*, 1991; **97**: 389–394.

10 van Reijsen, F.C., Bruijnzeel-Koomen, C.A.F.M., Kalthoff, F.S., *et al.* Skin derived aeroallergen-specific T-cell clones of Th2 phenotype in patients with atopic dermatitis. *Journal of Allergy and Clinical Immunology*, 1992; **90**: 184–193.

11 Neumann, C., Gutgesell, C., Fliegert, F., Bonifer, R., Herrmann, F. Comparative analysis of the frequency of house dust mite specific and non-specific Th1 and Th2 cells in skin lesions and peripheral blood of patients with atopic dermatitis. *Journal of Molecular Medicine*, 1996; **74**: 401–406.

12 Koning, H., Neijens, H.J., Baert, M.R.M., Oranje, A.P., Savelkoul, H.F.J. T-cell subsets and cytokines in allergic and non-allergic children. II. Analysis of IL-5 and IL-10 mRNA expression and protein production. *Cytokine*, 1997; **9**: 427–436.

13 Koning, H., Neijens, H.J., Baert, M.R.M., Oranje, A.P., Savelkoul, H.F.J. T-cell subsets and cytokines in allergic and non-allergic children. I. Analysis of IL-4, IFNγ and IL-13 mRNA expression and protein production. *Cytokine*, 1997; **9**: 416–426.

14 Sinke, J.D., Rutten, V.P.M.G., Willemse, T. Immune dysregulation in atopic dermatitis. *Veterinary Immunology and Immunopathology*, 2002; **87**: 351–356.

15 Nuttall, T.J. *The immunopathogenesis of canine atopic dermatitis*. PhD thesis, University of Edinburgh, 2003: 229–262.

16 Spergel, J.M., Mizoguchi, E., Oettgen, H., Bhan, A.K., Geha, R.S. Roles of Th1 and Th2 cytokines in a murine model of allergic dermatitis. *Journal of Clinical Investigation*, 1999; **103**: 1103–1111.

17 Vestergaard, C., Yoneyama, H., Murai, M., *et al.* Overproduction of Th2-specific chemokines in NC/Nga mice exhibiting atopic dermatitis-like lesions. *Journal of Clinical Investigation*, 1999; **104**: 1097–1105.

18 Fiorentino, D.F., Bond, M.W., Mosmann, T.R. Two types of mouse T helper cell IV. Th2 clones secrete a factor that inhibits cytokine production by Th1 clones. *Journal of Experimental Medicine*, 1989; **170**: 2081–2095.

19 Maeda, S., Fujiwara, S., Omori, K., *et al.* Lesional expression of thymus and activation-regulated chemokine in canine atopic dermatitis. *Veterinary Immunology and Immunopathology*, 2002; **88**: 79–87.

20 Werfel, T., Morita, A., Grewe, M., *et al.* Allergen specificity of skin-infiltrating T-cells is not restricted to a type-2 cytokine pattern in chronic skin lesions of atopic dermatitis. *Journal of Investigative Dermatology*, 1996; **107**: 871–876.

21 Thepen, T., Langeweld-Wildschut, E.A.G., Bihari, I.C., *et al.* Biphasic response against aeroallergen in atopic dermatitis show-

er T lymphocytes. *Nature*, 1996; **383**: 787–793.

ing a switch from an initial TH2 response to a TH1 response *in situ*: an immunocytochemical study. *Journal of Allergy and Clinical Immunology*, 1996; **97**: 828–837.

22 Griffin, C.E., DeBoer, D.J. The ACVD task force on canine atopic dermatitis (XIV): clinical manifestations of canine atopic dermatitis. *Veterinary Immunology and Immunopathology*, 2001; **81**: 255–269.

23 Olivry, T., Dunston, S.M., Rivierre, C., *et al*. A randomized controlled trial of misoprostol monotherapy for canine atopic dermatitis: effects on dermal cellularity and cutaneous tumour necrosis factor-alpha. *Veterinary Dermatology*, 2003; **14**: 37–46.

24 McAleese, S.M., Pemberton, A.D., McGrath, M.E., Huntley, J.F., Miller, H.R.P. Sheep mast cell proteinases-1 and -3: cDNA cloning, primary structure and molecular modeling of the enzymes and further studies on substrate specificity. *Biochemical Journal*, 1998; **333**: 801–809.

25 Knight, P.A., Wright, S.H., Lawrence, C.E., Paterson, Y.Y.W., Miller, H.R.P. Delayed expulsion of the nematode *Trichinella spiralis* in mice lacking the mucosal mast cell-specific granule chymase, mouse mast cell protease-1. *Journal of Experimental Medicine*, 2000; **192**: 1849–1856.

26 Izraeli, S., Pfleiderer, C., Lion, T. Detection of gene expression by PCR amplification of RNA derived from frozen heparinized whole blood. *Nucleic Acids Research*, 1991; **19**: 6051.

27 Huston, D. The biology of the immune system. *Journal of the American Medical Association*, 1997; **278**: 1804–1814.

28 Kimber, I., Dearman, R.J., Cumberbatch, M., Huby, R.J.D. Langerhans cells and chemical allergy. *Current Opinion in Immunology*, 1998; **10**: 614–619.

29 Robert, C., Kupper, T.S. Inflammatory skin diseases, T cells, and immune surveillance. *New England Journal of Medicine*, 1999; **341**: 1817–1828.

30 Kobayashi, H., Ishizuka, T., Okayama, Y. Human mast cells and basophils as sources of cytokines. *Clinical and Experimental Allergy*, 2000; **30**: 1205–1212.

31 Pastore, S., Corinti, S., La Placa, M., Didona, B., Girolomoni, G. Interferon-γ promotes exaggerated cytokine production in keratinocytes cultured from patients with atopic dermatitis. *Journal of Allergy and Clinical Immunology*, 1998; **101**: 538–544.

32 Trautmann, A., Akdis, M., Kleemann, D., *et al*. T cell-mediated Fas-induced keratinocyte apoptosis plays a key pathogenetic role in eczematous dermatitis. *Journal of Clinical Investigation*, 2000; **106**: 25–35.

33 Rothe, M.J., Grant-Kels, J.M. Atopic dermatitis: an update. *Journal of the American Academy of Dermatology*, 1996; **35**: 1–13.

34 Jutel, M., Klunker, S., Akdis, M., *et al*. Histamine upregulates Th1 and downregulates Th2 responses due to different patterns of surface histamine 1 and 2 receptor expression. *International Ar-* *chives of Allergy and Immunology*, 2001; **124**: 190–192.

35 Herz, U., Bunikowski, R., Renz, H. Role of T cells in atopic dermatitis. New aspects on the dynamics of cytokine production and the contribution of bacterial superantigens. *International Archives of Allergy and Immunology*, 1998; **115**: 179–190.

36 Skov, L., Olsen, J.V., Giorno, R., Schlievert, P.M., Baadsgaard, O., Leung, D.Y.M. Application of staphylococcal enterotoxin B on normal and atopic skin induces up-regulation of T cells by a superantigen-mediated mechanism. *Journal of Allergy and Clinical Immunology*, 2000; **105**: 820–826.

37 Cho, S.H., Strickland, I., Tomkinson, A., Fehringer, A.P., Gelfand, E.W., Leung, D.Y.M. Preferential binding of *Staphylococcus aureus* to skin sites of Th2-mediated inflammation in a murine model. *Journal of Investigative Dermatology*, 2001; **116**: 658–663.

38 Kieffer, M., Bergbrant, I.-M., Faergemann, J., *et al*. Immune reactions to *Pityrosporum ovale* in patients with atopic and seborrhoeic dermatitis. *Journal of the American Academy of Dermatology*, 1990; **22**: 739–742.

39 Nordvall, S.L., Johansson, S. IgE antibodies to *Pityrosporum ovale* in children with atopic diseases. *Acta Paediatrica Scandinavica*, 1990; **79**: 343–348.

40 Rokugo, M., Tagami, H., Usaba, Y., Tomita, Y. Contact sensitivity to *Pityrosporum ovale* in patients with atopic dermatitis. *Archives of Dermatology*, 1990; **126**: 627–632.

41 Wessels, M.W., Doekes, G., van Ieperen-van Dijk, A.G., Koers, W.J., Young, E. IgE antibodies to *Pityrosporum ovale* in atopic dermatitis. *British Journal of Dermatology*, 1991; **125**: 227–232.

42 Tengvall Linder, M., Johansson, C., Bengtsson, A., Holm, L., Härfast, B., Scheynius, A. *Pityrosporum orbiculare* reactive T-cell lines in atopic dermatitis patients and healthy individuals. *Scandinavian Journal of Immunology*, 1998; **47**: 152–157.

43 Morris, D.O., Olivier, N.B., Rosser, E.J. Type-1 hypersensitivity reactions to *Malassezia pachydermatis* extracts in atopic dogs. *American Journal of Veterinary Research*, 1998; **59**: 836–841.

44 Chen, T.A., Halliwell, R.E.W., Hill, P.B. IgG responses to *Malassezia pachydermatis* antigens in atopic and healthy dogs. *Veterinary Dermatology*, 2000; **11** (Suppl. 1): 13.

45 Nuttall, T.J., Halliwell, R.E.W. Serum antibodies to *Malassezia* yeasts in canine atopic dermatitis. *Veterinary Dermatology*, 2001; **12**: 327–332.

46 Watanabe, S., Kano, R., Sato, H., Nakamura, Y., Hasegawa, A. The effects of *Malassezia* yeasts on cytokine production by human keratinocytes. *Journal of Investigative Dermatology*, 2001; **116**: 769–773.

47 Nuttall, T.J., Lamb, J.R., Hill, P.B. Characterisation of major and minor *Dermatophagoides* allergens in canine atopic dermatitis. *Research in Veterinary Science*, 2001; **71**: 51–57.

IgE and IgG antibodies to food antigens in sera from normal dogs, dogs with atopic dermatitis and dogs with adverse food reactions

R.E.W. Halliwell MA, VetMB, PhD[1], C.M. Gordon BSc[1], C. Horvath Dr med vet[2], R. Wagner Dr med vet[2,3]

[1] Royal (Dick) School of Veterinary Studies, University of Edinburgh, Roslin, Midlothian, UK
[2] Veterinary University of Vienna, Vienna, Austria
[3] Vetderm-Service, Döblinger Haupstr. 81, A-1190, Vienna, Austria

Summary

Food antigen-specific IgE and IgG were determined in sera from three well-defined canine populations: normal dogs (group 1), dogs with atopic dermatitis that failed to respond to a home-prepared limited-antigen diet trial (group 2), and dogs with confirmed adverse food reactions (group 3).

Positive IgE results were most frequently seen in group 3, followed by group 2, and then group 1. Multisensitivity was most often shown by dogs in group 3. IgE levels in group 3 were significantly higher than those in group 1 for 12/19 antigens, and than group 2 for 9/19 antigens, whereas IgE levels in group 3 were significantly lower than those in group 1 for 2/19 antigens, and than group 2 for 4/19 antigens. Results for IgG were arguably more discriminatory, with results in group 3 being significantly higher than in group 1 for 12/18 antigens, and than group 2 for 4/18 antigens.

The aetiological relevance of these results was not confirmed by antigen challenge studies, and indeed there are significant difficulties in such studies in the case of multisensitive dogs. Nonetheless, the results suggest that serology may be helpful in the management of dogs with suspected adverse food reactions by identifying suitable candidates for limited-antigen dietary trials, and in the selection of the most appropriate diet.

Introduction

Adverse reactions to dietary components in dogs are believed to result from both immunological and non-immunological mechanisms, although the relative incidence of both is unknown. Dogs suffering from adverse food reactions generally present with dermatological or gastrointestinal signs, or a combination of both. The true incidence of such reactions is speculative, but they have been reported as comprising 6% of canine and feline dermatoses, and 15% of all allergic dermatoses in a referral practice,[1] and as 19.6% and 30.6% of all dogs with non-seasonal pruritus.[2,3] Concomitant atopic dermatitis is frequently seen.[2,4] Although it is recognised that dermatological and gastrointestinal signs can be seen concomitantly, the proportion of cases in which this is documented may vary depending on the rigour with which these signs are observed and investigated. Thus, in one study involving 20 dogs with non-seasonal pruritus that were responsive to dietary change, only 4 of the owners had previously sought veterinary advice for gastrointestinal disease.[4] However, on careful questioning, a further 11 were judged to have abnormal gastrointestinal function, as evidenced by increased frequency of defecation (more than three times per day), presence of faecal mucus or blood, or tenesmus. Dermatological signs are varied, and often indistinguishable from those associated with atopic dermatitis,[4,5] although the presence of an unusual distribution or concomitant gastrointestinal signs may raise the index of suspicion for an adverse food reaction.

The definitive diagnosis of an adverse food reaction is dependent upon demonstrating resolution of the clinical signs following institution of dietary change, and relapse upon reinstitution of the original diet. However, as animals may be multisensitive,[4–6] it may be necessary to attempt dietary restriction more than once. Although the commercial hydrolysed protein diets should, in theory, provide the ultimate hypoallergenic diet for diagnostic purposes, only 3/14 dogs from a colony of known food-allergic dogs were symptomatic when fed a hydrolysed soy protein diet.[7] Use of a home-prepared limited-antigen diet is thus still favoured by many dermatologists for diagnostic purposes.[5]

In man, the double-blind placebo-controlled food challenge is generally regarded as the gold standard for diagnosis. Nonetheless, recent studies comparing results of such food challenges with food-specific IgE levels have shown that high antibody levels have a > 95% concordance with responses to food trials, thus obviating the need for food trials in some instances.[8] Serological tests for food allergen-specific IgE have been evaluated as diagnostic aids for canine food hypersensitivity in a number of studies and reported to be unreliable.[9,10] However, in earlier studies, the diagnosis was made by response to a 3-week limited-antigen diet trial, rather than the 6–8 week minimum that is now regarded as necessary in some cases.[11] No studies, however, have addressed the possible value of assaying for IgG antibodies.

The aim of this study was to assay sera for both IgE and IgG antibodies to food allergens under carefully controlled laboratory conditions, from three well-defined populations: normal dogs, dogs with atopic dermatitis who failed to respond to a limited-antigen diet trial, and dogs with confirmed adverse food reactions.

Materials and methods

Animals

Sera were obtained from the following animals:

- *Normal dogs (group 1):* group 1 comprised normal dogs owned by students and clients of the Hospital for Small Animals, University of Edinburgh, and sampled during the course of a study for which Home Office Approval was obtained.
- *Atopic dogs (group 2):* group 2 comprised dogs with atopic dermatitis that were patients of the University of Edinburgh Hospital for Small Animals. All had clinical signs compatible with atopic dermati-

tis, showed positive intradermal tests to one or more antigens (Greer Laboratories, Lenoir NC, USA), and failed to respond to a 6-week home-prepared limited-antigen diet trial.
- *Vienna dogs (group 3):* group 3 comprised dogs with confirmed adverse food reactions that were patients of the Veterinary University of Vienna. All had dermatological signs that responded to an 8-week limited-antigen diet trial with capelin and tapioca (Waltham Centre for Pet Nutrition, Melton Mowbray, Leicestershire, UK), and relapsed upon reinstitution of the original diet. Seven had concomitant gastrointestinal signs that were likewise diet-responsive.

Antisera

Monoclonal anti-canine IgE (E6-71; Custom Monoclonals, Sacramento CA, USA), alkaline phosphatase-conjugated polyclonal sheep anti-mouse IgG (Fc-specific, and non-reactive with canine IgG; Chemicon International, Temecula CA, USA), and alkaline phosphatase-conjugated polyclonal anti-canine IgG (Fc-specific; Bethyl Laboratories, Montgomery TX, USA) were purchased for use in the assays.

Food antigens

Extracts of beef, lamb, chicken, turkey, pork, codfish, soybean, potato, corn, wheat, rice, catfish, milk, egg white, egg yolk and milk (Greer Laboratories) were purchased as standardised antigens (protein nitrogen units, PNU). Additionally, purified milk proteins (lactoferrin, β-lactoglobulin A, casein) and bovine serum albumin (Sigma, Poole, Dorset, UK) were purchased as standardised antigens (µg/ml).

Performance of the ELISAs

IgE and IgG ELISAs were performed as described previously for our laboratory.[12] Briefly, microtitre trays (Thermo Lab Sciences, Basingstoke, Hampshire, UK) were coated with antigen at 200 PNU/ml, or 16 µg/ml in the case of the purified antigens. Plates were freshly coated for each assay, incubated with dilutions of sera for 2 hours at 37°C, and with each antiserum overnight at 4°C. Following addition of the conjugate, plates were incubated with substrate for periods ranging from 30 minutes to 2 hours, and read when optimal colour development was reached.

For each antigen, a serum was identified with a high level of IgE or IgG antibody, and dilutions were included on each plate to generate a standard curve. This was arbitrarily assigned a relative antibody unit (RAU) value of 1000. Sera were assayed at 1/10 dilution. In the event that the optical density (OD) fell above the midpoint of the standard curve, the assay was repeated at a higher dilution. In the case of the IgE assay, a positive was defined as >1.5 times the OD of the end-point of the standard curve.

Statistical methods

Results are depicted as mean ranks; the data from all groups were listed in ascending order and then each data point was allocated its rank in that ordering. The mean rank for each group was then the arithmetic mean of the ranks for that group.

Overall differences for each antigen were assessed by Kruskal–Wallis test, and pairwise differences by Mann–Whitney test. Correlations between IgE and IgG antibody levels and between results for BSA and beef were assessed by Spearman's rank correlation.

Results

Dogs

There were 24 dogs in group 1 with a mean age of 5 years (range, 9 months to 13 years), 32 dogs in group 2 with a mean age of 3.3 years (range, 9 months to 8 years), and 22 dogs in group 3 with a mean age of 5 years (range, 1 to 12 years).

IgE

Incidence of positive reactions

The IgE assay employed all 19 antigens. Overall, IgE results were positive to 3.51% of antigens in group 1, 7.07% in group 2 and 15.8% in group 3. Of the group 1 sera ($n = 24$), positive results to one or more antigen were seen in 11 sera (45.8%). The incidence was greater in group 2 with 19/32 (59%) sera positive to one or more antigens, and greater still in group 3 where 19/22 sera (86%) gave at least one positive reaction. When considering sera with three or more positive reactions, the distinction between the groups was greater, where 1/24 (4.2%) of group 1 sera, 5/32 (15.6%) of group 2 sera and 8/22 (36.4%) of group 3 sera were positive to three or more antigens (Fig. 1.4.1).

Comparison of sera from groups 1, 2 and 3

In comparing the IgE levels, the calculated RAU value was used. In many cases this approximated to the RAU value of the end-point of the standard curve. In the case of eight antigens, the levels were significantly greater in sera from group 2 than in those from group 1, and for eight antigens the reverse was the case. For three antigens, there were no significant differences (Fig. 1.4.2a and b, Table 1.4.1). In the case of nine antigens, levels were significantly greater in group 3 than in group 2, with the reverse situation in the case of four antigens. Levels in group 3 were significantly greater that those in group 1 for 12 antigens, with the reverse situation for two antigens.

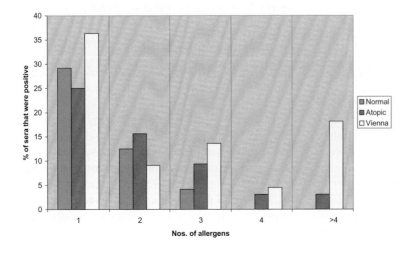

Fig. 1.4.1 Frequency of positive IgE results to 1, 2, 3, 4 and > 4 of 19 food allergens in normal dogs (group 1), atopic dogs (group 2) and Vienna dogs with confirmed adverse food reactions (group 3). Positive reaction is defined as a relative antibody unit level of at least 1.5 times the end-point of the standard curve.

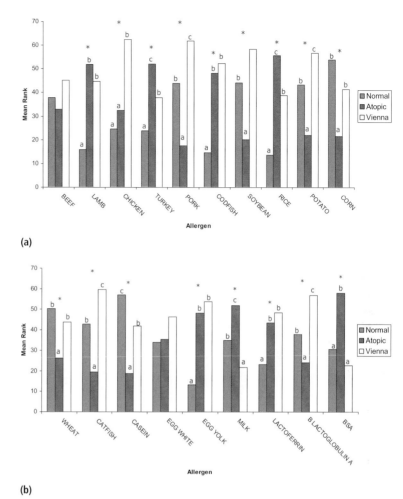

(a)

Fig. 1.4.2 (a, b) Mean rank of allergen-specific IgE antibody levels for normal dogs (group 1), atopic dogs (group 2) and Vienna dogs with confirmed adverse food reactions (group 3). Asterisks indicate allergens for which significant differences between groups were detected. Significant differences between groups ($p <$ 0.05) for each allergen are indicated by different letters; groups with the same letter were not significantly different.

(b)

IgG

Incidence of positive reactions

The IgG assay employed 18 antigens, with rice being omitted. Further, results were obtained in respect of 16 sera from group 1, 16 from group 2 and 13 from group 3, as some sera had become depleted. The incidence of positive reactions in the IgG assay was far greater, with positive values resulting from most sera to most antigens. However, levels were often low or undetectable in the case of potato, egg white and lactoferrin.

Comparison of sera from groups 1, 2 and 3

The IgG results showed a similar trend to those in the IgE assay, but with greater distinction between groups (Fig 1.4.3a and b, Table 1.4.2). The levels of IgG for

group 3 were significantly higher than group 2 in respect of four antigens, and than group 1 for 12 antigens. group 2 results were significantly greater group 1 in the case of five antigens. For all other antigens there was no significant difference. In contrast with the results for IgE, for no antigens were the results for groups 1 or 2 significantly greater than those for group 3.

Correlation between the levels of IgE and IgG

Overall, the levels of IgE and IgG were significantly correlated ($p = 0.001$). When the results for each antigen were examined, significant correlations were seen in respect of lamb (r = 0.39; $p = 0.008$), chicken (r = 0.44; $p = 0.002$), soybean (r = 0.34; $p = 0.024$), catfish

Table 1.4.1 Levels of significance of allergen-specific IgE between groups (group with the higher level in parentheses)

Antigen	Group 1 vs group 2	Group 2 vs group 3	Group 1 vs group 3
Beef	NS	NS	NS
Lamb	0.001 (2)	NS	0.001 (3)
Chicken	NS	0.001 (3)	0.001 (3)
Turkey	0.001 (2)	0.020 (2)	0.031 (3)
Pork	0.001 (1)	0.001 (3)	0.006 (6)
Codfish	0.001 (2)	NS	0.001 (3)
Soybean	0.001 (1)	0.001 (3)	0.029 (3)
Rice	0.001 (2)	0.006 (2)	0.001 (3)
Potato	0.001 (1)	0.001 (3)	0.040 (3)
Corn	0.001 (1)	0.001 (3)	NS
Wheat	0.001 (1)	0.004 (3)	NS
Catfish	0.001 (1)	0.001 (3)	0.009 (3)
Casein	0.001 (1)	0.001 (3)	0.019 (1)
Egg white	NS	NS	NS
Egg yolk	0.001 (2)	NS	0.001 (3)
Milk	0.005 (2)	0.001 (2)	0.042 (1)
Lactoferrin	0.001 (2)	NS	0.001 (3)
β-Lactoglobulin A	0.019 (1)	0.001 (3)	0.004 (3)
Bovine serum albumin	0.001 (2)	0.001 (2)	NS

NS, no significant difference; group 1, normal dogs; group 2, atopic dogs; group 3, Vienna dogs with confirmed adverse food reactions.

($r = 0.48$; $p = 0.001$), egg yolk ($r = 0.50$; $p = 0.001$), lactoferrin ($r = 0.44$; $p = 0.003$) and β-lactoglobulin A ($r = 0.36$; $p = 0.018$).

Correlation between the levels of anti-BSA and anti-beef antibody

In the case of IgG, BSA and beef antibody levels were highly correlated ($r = 0.5164$; $p = 0.001$), whereas there was no significant correlation for IgE ($r = 0.0854$; $p = 0.469$) against these two antigens.

Discussion

The results for each antigen are reported by mean ranks, which enables adjustment to be made for the varying RAU levels for each antigen. Assessment by median RAU levels gave very similar results, with the significant differences identical in each case (data not shown). In the case of IgE antibody, the mean ranks in group 3 were higher than those in group 1 for 14/19 allergens, and significantly so in the case of 12/19. The levels for the group 2 dogs fell generally in between the

other two groups. IgG antibody levels appeared to be even more discriminatory. The mean ranks for group 3 were higher that those for group 1 in all cases, and significantly so in the case of 12/18. Again, the levels in sera from group 2 fell in between the two. Similarly, when a positive reaction was defined as an OD >1.5 times the end-point of the standard curve, the incidence of positive reactions was greatest for group 3, with group 2 being intermediate. Although positive results were indeed seen in some normal dogs, multisensitivity was more frequently encountered in group 3.

In the case of the dogs with atopic dermatitis (group 2), a contribution from adverse food reactions had been excluded by failure to respond to a single home-prepared limited-antigen diet trial. Obviously, although chosen by reference to the current diet, it is possible that there were indeed dietary components to their disease, and that the use of two, or even three, different single source protein diets might have identified them. It is also possible that they may have been multisensitive in respect of their adverse food reactions, and react to both protein antigens and also to antigens that are predominantly carbohydrate (e.g. rice, potato). Thus the removal of one offending allergen might not have induced clinically evident improvement. The use of dietary trials can also be confused by cross-reacting antigens. It is, of course, possible that the presence of the generally higher levels of IgE and IgG antibody of different specificities in this group may merely be a reflection of generalised hyper-reactivity of the immune response in the dogs with atopic dermatitis.

The recent development of a colony of beagle/Maltese-cross dogs with food hypersensitivity has provided interesting data on this condition. In two reports, levels of serum allergen-specific IgE have been reported, as well as dynamic changes following challenge studies. These animals show sensitivity to a number of dietary components, including soybean and corn, manifested by both dermatological and gastrointestinal signs. In the first report,[13] institution of a hydrolysed protein diet led to a significant fall in the level of corn-specific IgE, which reversed upon reinstitution of the original corn-containing diet. There was no change in the level of wheat-specific IgE, an antigen absent from both diets. Institution of the hydrolysed protein diet was also accompanied by a fall in milk-specific IgE. These animals had never knowingly been exposed to oral cows' milk proteins. Challenge of the test dogs with milk

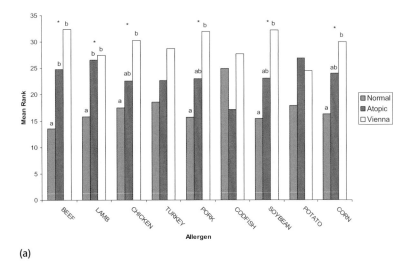

(a)

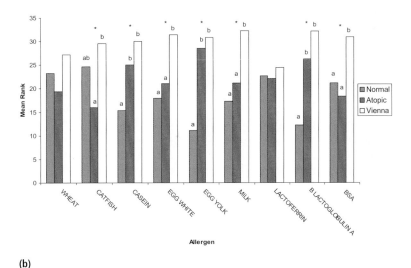

Fig. 1.4.3 (a, b) Mean rank of allergen-specific IgG antibody levels for normal dogs (group 1), atopic dogs (group 2) and Vienna dogs with confirmed adverse food reactions (group 3). Asterisks indicate allergens for which significant differences between groups were detected. Significant differences between groups ($p <$ 0.05) for each allergen are indicated by different letters; groups with the same letter were not significantly different.

(b)

induced a gastrointestinal response, which could be a result of the known relative lactase deficiency in adult dogs. Two, however, developed a yeast-associated otitis externa. None showed an increase in milk-specific IgE, although it should be pointed out that the milk was only fed on two single-dose occasions in four of five dogs, and only once in the remaining dog that manifested profuse vomiting. Thus, although there were dynamic changes in allergen-specific IgE in association with the diet change (albeit not with the milk challenge), these changes were not always antigen-specific.

The second report showed rather different results.[7] In this study, a greater number of dogs were included (14 vs 5 dogs). Institution of a diet of duck and rice actually resulted in a gradual rise of both corn- and soy-specific IgE, antigens that were supposedly absent from the diet. The authors suggested that this could have resulted from less IgE being complexed with IgG during times of lesser antigen exposure, but it is none-theless hard to reconcile the different response in the two trials. Further, although challenge with corn and soy often induced an increase in allergen-specific IgE,

Table 1.4.2 Levels of significance of allergen-specific IgG between groups (group with the higher level in parentheses)

Antigen	Group 1 vs group 2	Group 2 vs group 3	Group 1 vs group 3
Beef	0.015 (2)	NS	0.001 (3)
Lamb	0.021 (2)	NS	0.017 (3)
Chicken	NS	NS	0.010 (3)
Turkey	NS	NS	NS
Pork	NS	NS	0.001 (3)
Codfish	NS	NS	NS
Soybean	NS	NS	0.001 (3)
Potato	NS	NS	NS
Corn	NS	NS	0.005 (3)
Wheat	NS	NS	NS
Catfish	NS	0.006 (3)	NS
Casein	0.037 (2)	NS	0.003 (3)
Egg white	NS	0.035 (3)	0.006 (3)
Egg yolk	0.001 (2)	NS	0.001 (3)
Milk	NS	0.023 (3)	0.002 (3)
Lactoferrin	NS	NS	NS
β-Lactoglobulin A	0.003 (2)	NS	0.001 (3)
Bovine serum albumin	NS	0.010 (3)	0.046 (3)

NS, no significant difference; group 1, normal dogs; group 2, atopic dogs; group 3, dogs with confirmed adverse food reactions.

the increase was not always antigen-specific, i.e. when the dogs were fed corn, some had a corn-specific and/or soy-specific allergen response. Limited studies on this aspect have been conducted in our laboratory. In general, levels of allergen-specific IgE fall upon institution of a hypoallergenic diet. Indeed in one case that was the subject of a long-term study, institution of a hydrolysed protein diet led to a marked fall in the levels of allergen-specific IgE in the case of 15/18 allergens over a 3-month period. This included a dramatic fall in the level of peanut-specific IgE; peanuts were not fed to the dog, but peanut butter had been previously used to coat the anti-inflammatory tablets dosed to control the disease before the role of diet was recognised (data not shown).

The relevance of high levels of allergen-specific IgE or IgG was not assessed by allergen challenge studies, but then neither is this ordinarily undertaken in studies with atopic dogs, where the value of assaying for allergen-specific IgE is generally accepted. In considering whether such studies would be useful, or meaningful, one must also recognise that animals may be multisensitive, and that subclinical multisensitivity could also exist, as is believed to be the case in atopic dermatitis. Thus the patient could only become symptomatic when fed two or more of the offending antigens.

Surprisingly, the levels of IgG were generally a better predictor of an adverse food reaction than were the levels of IgE. Although it is generally assumed in man that food hypersensitivity usually results from IgE-, rather then IgG-mediated reactions,[14] there are no definitive data to support this contention. It is possible that the changes in both IgE and IgG are not causative of the disease, but merely reflections of it. It is certainly logical to conclude that if there is gastrointestinal disease, with resulting increased intestinal permeability, increased serum levels of any food antigen-specific antibody could result, either of the IgE and/or IgG class.

Correlation studies showed that, overall, the IgE and IgG antigen-specific responses were highly correlated. Significant correlations were also seen in respect of 7/18 antigens. Although to our knowledge there have been no previous studies that have addressed this issue, the results are not surprising. Examination of the correlation between anti-BSA and anti-beef were undertaken to ascertain a possible role for BSA as a major allergen to which the anti-beef response is directed. Paradoxical results were obtained with significant correlations in respect of IgG antibody, but none were evident for IgE. It is not therefore possible to draw any conclusions on this question.

It is possible that genetic or environmental differences might have contributed to the differences between the normal dogs and those with adverse food reactions. However, genetic differences are viewed as unlikely, in that among the 22 dogs with adverse food reactions, 10 breeds were represented, and there were six mixed-breed dogs. In the normal group, eight breeds were represented, and there were four mixed-breed dogs.

In conclusion, these studies have shown that populations of normal dogs and of dogs with confirmed adverse food reactions show different responses in respect of food allergen-specific IgE, and more particularly IgG. Although the levels of IgG antibody appeared to be the more discriminatory, multisensitivity in terms of the IgE response was seen more frequently among animals with adverse food reaction. It is thus suggested that, while not diagnostic, assays of food-specific IgE and IgG may be of value in identifying patients in which dietary trials are warranted, and in identifying suitable allergens for exclusion in any subsequent trials.

Funding

This study was funded by the Waltham Centre for Pet Nutrition.

References

1 Carlotti, D.N., Remy, I., Prost, C. Food allergy in dogs and cats: a review and report of 43 cases. *Veterinary Dermatology,* 1990; **1**: 55–62.

2 Loeffler, A., Lloyd, D.H., Bond, R., Kim, J.Y., Pfeiffer, D.U. Dietary trials with a commercial chicken hydrolysate diet in 63 pruritic dogs. *Veterinary Record,* 2004; **154**: 519–522.

3 Chesney, C.J. Food sensitivity in the dog: a quantitative study. *Journal of Small Animal Practice,* 2002; **43**: 203–207.

4 Patterson, S. Food hypersensitivity in 20 dogs with skin and gastrointestinal signs. *Journal of Small Animal Practice,* 1995; **36**: 529–534.

5 Leistra, H.G., Markwell, P.J., Willemse, T. Evaluation of selected-protein-source diets for management of dogs with adverse reactions to foods. *Journal of the American Veterinary Medical Association,* 2001; **219**: 1411–1414.

6 Jeffers, J.G., Meyer, E.K., Sosis, J. Responses of dogs with food allergies to single-ingredient dietary provocation. *Journal of the American Veterinary Medical Association,* 1996; **209**: 608–611.

7 Jackson H.A., Jackson, M.W., Coblentz, L., Hammerberg, B. Evaluation of the clinical and allergen-specific serum immunoglobulin E responses to oral challenge with cornstarch, corn, soy and a soy hydrolysate diet in dogs with spontaneous food allergy. *Veterinary Dermatology,* 2003; **14**:181–187.

8 Sampson, H.A. Utility of food-specific IgE concentrations in predicting symptomatic food allergy. *Journal of Allergy and Clinical Immunology,* 2001; **107**: 891–896.

9 Jeffers, J.G., Shanley, K.J., Meyer, E.K. Diagnostic testing of dogs for food hypersensitivity. *Journal of the American Veterinary Medical Association,* 1991; **198**: 245–250.

10 Mueller, R., Tsohalis, J. Evaluation of allergen-specific IgE for the diagnosis of adverse food reactions in the dog. *Veterinary Dermatology,* 1998; **9**: 167–171.

11 Rosser, E.J. Diagnosis of food allergy in the dog. *Journal of the American Veterinary Medical Association,* 1993; **203**: 259–262.

12 Lian, T.M., Halliwell, R.E.W. Allergen-specific IgE and IgGd antibodies in atopic dogs and normal dogs. *Veterinary Immunology and Immunopathology,* 1998; **66**: 203–223.

13 Jackson H.A., Hammerberg, B. Evaluation of a spontaneous canine model of immunoglobulin E-mediated food hypersensitivity: dynamic changes in serum and fecal allergen-specific IgE values relative to dietary change. *Comparative Medicine,* 2002; **52**: 318–324.

14 Sampson, H.A. Adverse reactions to food. In: Middleton, E., Reed, C., Ellis, E., Yunginger, J.W., Adkinson, N.F., Busse, W.W., eds. *Allergy Principles and Practice,* 5th edn, Vol II. Mosby, St Louis, MO, 1998: 1162–1182.

Evaluation of a rapid, qualitative, allergen-specific IgE screening immuno-assay in dogs with atopic dermatitis

E.J. Rosser Jr DVM

Department of Small Animal Clinical Sciences, College of Veterinary Medicine, Michigan State University, East Lansing, Michigan, USA

Summary

A rapid IgE screening immunoassay (E-Screen) was developed to detect the presence of aeroallergen-specific IgE in atopic dogs. The objective of this study was to compare the results of the E-Screen to the results of a 48-allergen-specific IgE immunoassay (ANRAS) and a 45-allergen intradermal test (IDT) in dogs with atopic dermatitis (AD). Forty-four dogs had an E-Screen, ANRAS and IDT performed. Only dogs with an IDT and ANRAS result compatible with the dog's history of pruritus were further evaluated and subsequently treated with allergen-specific immunotherapy (ASIT). The results of IDT and ANRAS were compatible with the dog's history of pruritus in 30 dogs, with the E-Screen test being negative in 17 dogs (57%) and positive in 13 dogs (43%). The E-Screen was negative in 5/6 dogs with warm weather seasonal pruritus and 10/15 dogs with non-seasonal pruritus but with exacerbation of disease in warm weather. The E-Screen was positive in 7/9 dogs with non-seasonal disease without seasonal exacerbation. Based on the results of this study, it is not recommended that the E-Screen be used to screen for the presence of allergen-specific IgE in the serum of potentially atopic dogs with a history of an exclusively warm weather seasonal pruritus, or dogs with a history of a non-seasonal pruritus which noticeably exacerbates in warm weather in the geographic region of the study. The E-Screen may be a useful tool for use in the screening of non-seasonally pruritic dogs with predominantly house dust and house dust mite reactions.

Introduction

Atopic dermatitis (AD) is becoming an increasingly important allergic skin disease and is reported to be one of the most common causes of pruritus in dogs.[1–3] It has been estimated to occur in 3–15% of the general canine population, with the incidence being much higher in dermatology referral practices.[2–7]

In support of a diagnosis of AD in the dog, intradermal testing (IDT) and allergen-specific IgE serum testing (ASIST) are considered important tests for demonstration of an IgE-mediated hypersensitivity component in this disease. However, false positive and false negative reactions can occur with either testing method for a variety of reasons .[8,9] Therefore the most important criteria used in the diagnosis of AD are the patient's history and the presence of typical clinical signs.[10–12] The criteria used in the evaluation of dogs suspected to have AD have recently been discussed.[11] The final step in considering a diagnosis of AD is to systematically rule out the other common causes of pruritus, especially (but not limited to) flea allergy dermatitis, cutaneous adverse food reactions (food allergy), scabies and other regional pruritic parasitic skin diseases (including so-called 'scabies incognito'), pruritic bacterial folliculitis and *Malassezia* dermatitis. Once these diseases have been excluded, and the history and clinical signs are compatible with a diagnosis of AD, the clinician should next discuss the various treatment options to be considered.

If the owner agrees to pursue allergen-specific immunotherapy (ASIT), it is then recommended that either IDT or ASIST be performed to aid the clinician in the selection of allergens for ASIT to attempt hyposensitisation of the atopic state.[1,2,13–24] It is important that these tests include all of the specific and relevant allergens for the geographical region where the IDT or ASIST is being performed. When the results of these tests are compatible with the patient's history, then each relevant and specific allergen is chosen for inclusion in the dog's ASIT protocol, as the response to this therapy is allergen-specific. Other treatment alternatives for AD include the use of a wide variety of antipruritic and anti-inflammatory topical and systemic drugs. As AD tends to be a lifelong skin disease in dogs, ASIT has become an increasingly valuable treatment for the long-term management of this disease.

Recently, an in-clinic IgE screening immunoassay (Allercept™ E-Screen™ [E-Screen]; Heska Corp., Fort Collins, CO, USA) has been developed to detect the presence of allergen-specific IgE in the serum of dogs with AD. The screening test was being developed to provide veterinarians with a rapid and inexpensive tool for screening clinically atopic dogs to predict the likelihood of the dog's serum testing positive to one or more allergens with the 48-allergen-specific IgE immunoassay (Allercept™ Northeast Regional Allergy Screen [ANRAS]; Heska Corp.) or with intradermal testing (IDT), to identify allergens for inclusion in allergen-specific immunotherapy (ASIT). A positive E-Screen test was to indicate a high probability that ASIT would be recommended based on the results of the ANRAS or IDT.

The working hypothesis of this study was that a positive E-Screen result will be an accurate indicator of the likelihood of a positive result on ANRAS and 45-allergen IDT in dogs with AD. The objective of the study was to compare the results of the E-Screen to the results of the ANRAS and IDT in dogs with AD.

Materials and methods

Forty-four dogs with a history suggestive of AD that were presented to the Veterinary Teaching Hospital's Dermatology Service were included in the study. The diagnosis of AD was based on history, physical findings and systematic ruling out of other causes of a primary pruritic skin disease. This included the use of home-cooked elimination diet trials for 8 weeks, and empirical treatment for scabies and other ectoparasites when appropriate. Dogs with a concurrent flea allergy dermatitis or cutaneous adverse reaction to foods were excluded from the study. All owners of the dogs in the study complied with the following drug withdrawal times prior to testing: 90 days for all repositol corticosteroids; 30 days for all other injectable, oral and topical corticosteroids; 14 days for all antihistamines, antibiotics, antifungals, cyclosporine and essential fatty acid supplements; 7 days for all non-steroidal anti-inflammatory drugs; no bathing for 7 days prior to examination. This was accomplished by mailing a letter that contained detailed information on withdrawal times for all drugs to each owner when the referral appointment was first scheduled.

The E-Screen, ANRAS and IDT were performed for each dog included in the study.[8,9] The allergens tested using the ANRAS and IDT are listed in Tables 1.5.1 and 1.5.2. All dogs were sedated using xylazine hydrochlo-

Table 1.5.1 Allergens used for intradermal testing at Michigan State University	Type of allergens	Allergens
	Indoor aeroallergens	House dust, *Dermatophagoides farinae*, *Dermatophagoides pteronyssinus*, mattress dust, tobacco, cotton linters, kapok, sheep wool, feather mix, cat epithelia
	Tree pollens	Chinese juniper, birch mix, box elder/maple, walnut, oak mix, cedar mix, tree mix no. 1 (white alder, aspen, American beech, American elm), tree mix no. 2 (American hazelnut, shagbark hickory, red mulberry, white poplar), tree mix no. 3 (American sycamore, black willow, green ash, white ash)
	Grass pollens	Kentucky blue grass, brome grass, rye grass, canary grass, quack/wheat grass mix, 7 grass mix (red top, meadow fescue, sweet vernal, Kentucky blue, orchard, perennial rye, timothy)
	Weed pollens	Common cocklebur, Russian thistle, yellow dock/sorrel, goldenrod, kochia, lamb's quarter, Mexican tea, marsh elder/burweed, nettle, giant and short ragweed mix, English plantain, Western water hemp, annual sagebrush, mugwort sagebrush, dandelion, spiny pigweed, rough redroot pigweed
	Moulds	Mould mix no. 1 (*Alternaria*, *Aspergillus*, *Cladosporium* (*Hormodendrum*), *Penicillium*, *Helminthosporium*), mould mix no. 2 (*Fusarium*, Curvularia, Rhizopus, Pullularia, Mucor), Michigan mould mix (*Stemphylium solani*, *Phoma herbarum*)

Type of allergen	Allergens
Indoor aeroallergens	*Dermatophagoides farinae, Dermatophagoides pteronyssinus*, cat epithelia
Tree pollens	Black birch, box elder, sugar maple, walnut, white oak, red cedar, quaking aspen, American elm, shagbark hickory, red mulberry, American sycamore, white ash, eastern cottonwood, yellow pine, bayberry wax myrtle
Grass pollens	June blue, brome, perennial rye, red top, sweet vernal, orchard, timothy, meadow fescue, Johnson, Bermuda
Weed pollens	Common cocklebur, Russian thistle, yellow dock, kochia, lamb's quarters, marsh elder/burweed, tall ragweed, short ragweed, English plantain, mugwort, rough redroot pigweed
Moulds	*Alternaria, Aspergillus, Cladosporium (Hormodendrum), Penicillium, Fusarium*

Table 1.5.2 Allergens used for allergen-specific IgE immunoassay (Allercept™ Northeast Regional Allergy Screen)

ride intravenously before performing each IDT. Reactions on IDT were recorded as 0, 1, 2, 3, or 4, where 0 is equal to the reaction of the negative control and 4 is equal to the reaction of the positive control. Any reaction of 2 or greater was regarded as positive. Reactions on ANRAS were measured in EA units with a range of 0–5000 EA units. Any reaction of 150 EA units or greater was regarded as positive.

The E-Screen is an enzyme-linked immunoassay (ELISA) that contains a canine-specific monoclonal anti-IgE antibody. The test kit includes a self-contained disposable square plastic housing in which a proprietary mixture of allergens is immobilised as a single test spot on a nitrocellulose membrane. A second control spot contains purified canine IgE. The patient's serum sample is then added to the test spots and passes through a nitrocellulose membrane into an absorbent material by capillary action. Allergen-specific canine IgE, if present in the serum sample, can then bind to the immobilised allergen mixture. A specific detection reagent, biotinylated anti-canine IgE monoclonal antibody, is then added to the membrane followed by an avidin–alkaline phosphatase conjugate. A precipitable substrate is then added to visualise the bound IgE in the control and test spots. This study was initiated during the early marketing stages of the E-Screen in our geographical location and it was agreed by the author and the company that a positive E-Screen result would be an effective indicator of the likelihood of a positive result on the ANRAS *and* IDT as performed by the Dermatology Service at Michigan State University's Veterinary Teaching Hospital.

The investigator was blinded as to the results of the E-Screen until the end of the study. Only dogs with an IDT and ANRAS result compatible with the dog's history of pruritus were considered for further evaluation .

Results

The results of IDT and ANRAS were compatible with the dog's history of pruritus in 30 dogs, with the E-Screen test being negative in 17 dogs (57%) and positive in 13 dogs (43%). Six of the dogs had a history of a warm weather seasonal pruritus only, with reactions to various combinations of trees, grasses, weeds and moulds on both IDT and ANRAS, with the E-Screen test being negative in five dogs, and positive in one dog (Table 1.5.3: case nos 1–6). Nine dogs had a history of non-seasonal pruritus that either did not exacerbate at any time of year, or that noticeably exacerbated in the winter months, with reactions to various combinations of primarily house dust and house dust mites. The E-Screen test was negative in two of these dogs and positive in seven dogs (Table 1.5.3: case nos 7–15). Fifteen of the dogs had a history of non-seasonal pruritus that noticeably exacerbated in warm weather with reactions to various combinations of house dust, house dust mites, trees, grasses, weeds and moulds on both IDT and ANRAS. The E-Screen test was negative in 10 dogs and positive in 5 dogs (Table 1.5.3: case nos 16–30).

Discussion

As AD has been reported to be the first or second most common cause of pruritus in dogs, being able to screen for the presence of circulating allergen-specific IgE in the serum of potentially atopic dogs in general practice would be a very useful diagnostic tool. Currently, the diagnosis of AD in dogs presents a challenge to the clinician, and involves a very time-consuming systematic approach. This initially involves a thorough prospective following, or retrospective re-

Table 1.5.3 Reactions to the E-Screen (Allercept™ E-Screen™), a 48-allergen-specific IgE immunoassay (Allercept™ Northeast Regional Allergy Screen) and 45-allergen intradermal testing

History	Case no.	E-Screen	Michigan State University Intradermal Test	Allercept™ NE Regional Allergy Screen
Dogs with seasonal warm weather pruritus	1	Negative	Positive (4 weeds, 1 mould)	Positive (3 weeds, 2 grasses)
	2	Negative	Positive (6 grasses, 2 weeds)	Positive (5 grasses, 3 weeds)
	3	Positive	Positive (8 trees, 6 grasses, 12 weeds, moulds)	Positive (15 trees, 10 grasses,11 weeds)
	4	Negative	Positive (2 trees, 3 grasses, 12 weeds)	Positive (1 tree, 4 grasses, 4 weeds)
	5	Negative	Positive (3 trees, 1 grass, 2 weed)	Positive (1 grass)
	6	Negative	Positive (4 trees, 4 weeds)	Positive (8 trees, 4 grasses, 5 weeds)
Dogs with non-seasonal pruritus	7	Negative	Positive (HD, DF)	Positive (DF)
	8	Negative	Positive (HD, DF, DP)	Positive (DF, DP)
	9	Positive	Positive (HD, DF, DP, moulds)	Positive (DF, moulds)
	10	Positive	Positive (HD, DF, DP, moulds)	Positive (DF, DP)
	11	Positive	Positive (HD, DF, DP, moulds, 2 trees, 5 grasses, 5 weeds)	Positive (DF, DP, moulds, 14 trees, 10 grasses, 11 weeds)
	12	Positive	Positive (HD, DF, DP, moulds)	Positive (DF, DP)
	13	Positive	Positive (HD, DF, DP)	Positive (DF, DP)
	14	Positive	Positive (HD, DP,DF)	Positive (DF, DP)
	15	Positive	Positive (HD, MD, kapok, cotton, DF, DP, 8 trees, 6 grasses, 17 weeds)	Positive (DF, DP, 15 trees,10 grasses, 12 weeds)
Dogs with non-seasonal pruritus and warm weather seasonal exacerbations	16	Negative	Positive (HD, DF, DP, 3 grasses)	Positive (DF, DP, 3 weeds, 9 grass)
	17	Negative	Positive (HD, DF, DP, 10 weeds, moulds)	Positive (DF, DP, 12 weeds, 8 trees, 10 grasses)
	18	Negative	Positive (HD, DF, DP, 8 weeds)	Positive (DF, DP, 4 weeds, 4 grass)
	19	Negative	Positive (HD, 9 trees, 6 grasses, 9 weeds)	Positive (Moulds, 13 trees, 10 grasses, 10 weeds)
	20	Negative	Positive (HD, DF, DP, 6 trees, 1 grass, 1 weed)	Positive (DP, 2 trees, 3 grasses)
	21	Positive	Positive (Moulds, 1 tree, 5 grasses, 5 weeds)	Positive (Moulds, 7 trees, 9 grasses, 9 weeds)
	22	Negative	Positive (HD, DF, 1 grass, 5 weeds)	Positive (DF, 1 weed, moulds)
	23	Negative	Positive (Moulds, HD, 6 trees, 1 weed)	Positive (Moulds, 1 tree, 2 grasses)
	24	Positive	Positive (HD, DF, DP, moulds)	Positive (DF, 6 grasses, 3 weeds)
	25	Positive	Positive (HD, DF, 1 weed, moulds)	Positive (DF, DP, 1 grass, 2 weeds, moulds)
	26	Negative	Positive (HD, DF, DP, 5 weeds)	Positive (DF, DP, 1 weed)
	27	Positive	Positive (HD, DF, DP, 1 weed, moulds)	Positive (DF, DP, 8 grasses, 2 weeds)
	28	Negative	Positive (Moulds, DF, 2 weeds)	Positive (Moulds, 1 weed)
	29	Positive	Positive (HD, DF, kapok, cat epithelia, 9 trees, 6 grasses, 17 weeds)	Positive (DF, 12 trees, 9 grasses, 8 weeds)
	30	Negative	Positive (HD, DF, DP, 6 grasses)	Positive (DF, DP, 10 grasses, 7 weeds)

Any allergen with ≥ 150 EA units of IgE on the immunoassay was regarded as positive. Any reaction of ≥ 2 (subjectively scored on a scale of 0–4) on the intradermal test was regarded as positive. HD, house dust; DF, *Dermatophagoides farinae*; DP, *Dermatophagoides pteronyssinus*.

view, of the patient's history over a period of at least 1 year. In addition, clinical signs recognised to be associated with the development of AD must be present. Lastly, the clinician needs to systematically rule out the other common causes of pruritus as previously mentioned. At this point it can be recommended to perform either IDT or *in vitro* allergen-specific IgE serum testing to aid the clinician in the selection of allergens for ASIT to attempt a hyposensitisation injection protocol. As to whether or not IDT or *in vitro* allergen-specific IgE serum testing should be the 'gold standard' for use in the selection of allergens for ASIT, is controversial.[13–20] The major problem with these

interpretations is that the allergenic extracts used, testing methodologies and test result interpretations have not been standardised for either method of testing. Until this has been accomplished, direct comparisons will remain problematic. For these reasons it was decided to evaluate the results of the E-Screen in dogs suspected of having AD only in instances when both the ANRAS and IDT were compatible with the dog's history of pruritus.

Using these criteria, the E-Screen had the poorest correlation with the patient's history and the results of the ANRAS and IDT in dogs with warm weather seasonal pruritus (negative in 5/6 dogs) and non-seasonal pruritus that exacerbates in warm weather (negative in 10/15 dogs). As the investigators were kept unaware as to the actual allergens included in the proprietary allergen mixture, the reasons for the high percentage of negative reactions overall can only be speculative. It seems reasonable that one of the most difficult components of such a screening immunoassay would be the use of a limited number of pollen allergens in the test kit, attempting to screen for approximately 30–40 pollens in our geographic location. In contrast, the E-Screen had the best correlation with the patient's history and the results of the ANRAS and IDT in dogs with non-seasonal pruritus (dogs primarily reacting to house dust and house dust mite) that either did not exacerbate at any time of year, or that noticeably exacerbated in the winter months (positive in 7/9 dogs). However, as the E-Screen was commonly negative in other dogs with both dust mite reactions and pollen reactions, this observation is difficult to interpret.

One of the recommended reasons for the use of the E-Screen was to identify dogs that should be further tested using ANRAS or IDT, with the ultimate goal of selecting allergens for use in ASIT. It is believed that the dogs used in this study were representative of dogs with AD that could benefit from ASIT. Based on the results of this study, it is not recommended that the E-Screen be used to screen for the presence of allergen-specific IgE in the serum of potentially atopic dogs with a history of an exclusively warm weather seasonal pruritus, or with a history of a non-seasonal pruritus which noticeably exacerbates in warm weather, in our geographic region. However, the E-Screen may be a very useful tool for use in the screening of non-seasonally pruritic dogs with predominantly house dust and house dust mite reactions.

Funding

The Allercept™ E-Screen™ test kits and the Allercept™ Northeast Regional Allergy Screen were provided free of charge by the Heska Corporation, Fort Collins, CO, USA.

References

1 Scott, D.W., Miller, W.H., Griffin, C.E. *Muller & Kirk's Small Animal Dermatology.* W.B. Saunders, Philadelphia, 2001: 574–601.

2 Reedy, L.M., Miller, W.H., Willemse, T. *Allergic Skin Diseases of Dogs and Cats.* W.B. Saunders, Philadelphia, 1997: 32–44.

3 DeBoer, D.J. Survey of intradermal skin testing practices in North America. *Journal of the American Veterinary Medical Association,* 1989; **195**: 1357–1363.

4 Hillier, A., Griffin, C.E. The ACVD task force on canine atopic dermatitis (I): incidence and prevalence. *Veterinary Immunology and Immunopathology,* 2001; **81**: 147–151.

5 Scott, D.W., Paradis, M. A survey of canine and feline skin disorders seen in a university practice: small animal clinic, University of Montreal, Saint-Hyacinthe, Quebec (1987–1988). *Canadian Veterinary Journal,* 1990; **31**: 830–835.

6 Carlotti, D.N., Costargent, F. Analysis of positive skin tests in 449 dogs with allergic dermatitis. *European Journal of Companion Animal Practice,* 1994; **4**: 42–59.

7 Saridomichelakis, M.N., Koutinas, A.F., Giolekas, D., Leontidis, L. Canine atopic dermatitis in Greece: clinical observations and the prevalence of positive intradermal test reactions in 91 spontaneous cases. *Veterinary Immunology and Immunopathology,* 1999; **69**: 61–73.

8 Hillier, A., DeBoer, D.J. The ACVD task force on canine atopic dermatitis (XVII): intradermal testing. *Veterinary Immunology and Immunopathology,* 2001; **81**: 289–304.

9 DeBoer, D.J., Hillier, A. The ACVD task force on canine atopic dermatitis (XVI): laboratory evaluation of dogs with atopic dermatitis with serum-based "allergy" tests. *Veterinary Immunology and Immunopathology,* 2001; **81**: 277–287.

10 Griffin, C.E., DeBoer, D.J. The ACVD task force on canine atopic dermatitis (XIV): clinical manifestations of canine atopic dermatitis. *Veterinary Immunology and Immunopathology,* 2001; **81**: 255–269.

11 DeBoer, D.J., Hillier, A. The ACVD task force on canine atopic dermatitis (XV): fundamental concepts in clinical diagnosis. *Veterinary Immunology and Immunopathology,* 2001; **81**: 271–276.

12 Hillier, A. Definitively diagnosing atopic dermatitis in dogs. *Veterinary Medicine,* 2002; **97**: 198–208.

13 Kleinbeck, M.L., Hites, M.J., Loker, J.L., Halliwell, R.E.W., Lee, K.W. Enzyme-linked immunosorbent assay for measurement of allergen-specific IgE antibodies in canine serum. *American Journal of Veterinary Research,* 1989; **50**:1831–1839.

14 Codner, E.C., Lessard, P. Comparison of intradermal allergy test and enzyme-linked immunosorbent assay in dogs with allergic skin disease. *Journal of the American Veterinary Medical Association,* 1993; **202**: 739–743.

15 Miller, W.H., Scott, D.W., Wellington, J.R., Scarlett, J.M., Panic, R. Evaluation of the performance of a serologic allergy system in atopic dogs. *Journal of the American Animal Hospital Association,* 1993; **29**: 545–550.

16 Bond, R., Thorogood, S.C., Lloyd, D.H. Evaluation of two enzyme-linked immunosorbent assays for the diagnosis of canine atopy. *Veterinary Record,* 1994; **135**: 130–133.

17 Mueller, R.S., Burrows, A., Tsohalis, J. Comparison of intradermal testing and serum testing for allergen-specific IgE using monoclonal IgE antibodies in 84 atopic dogs. *Australian Veterinary Journal,* 1999; **77**: 290–294.

18 Park, S., Ohya, F., Yamshita, K., Nishifuji, K., Iwasaki, T. Comparison of response to immunotherapy by intradermal skin test and antigen-specific IgE in canine atopy. *Journal of Veterinary Medical Science,* 2000; **62**: 983–988.

19 Hillier, A. Allergy testing and treatment for canine atopic dermatitis. *Veterinary Medicine,* 2002; **97**: 210–224.

20 Rosser, E.J. Aqueous hyposensitization in the treatment of canine atopic dermatitis: In: Kwochka, K.W., Willemse, T., von Tscharner, C., eds. *Advances in Veterinary Dermatology,* Vol. 3. Butterworth Heinemann, Oxford, 1998: 169–176.

21 Willemse, A., Van den Brom, W.E., Rijnberk, A. Effect of hypo-

sensitization on atopic dermatitis in dogs. *Journal of the American Veterinary Medical Association*, 1984; **184**: 1277–1280.

22 Scott, K.V., White, S.D., Rosychuk, R.A.W. A retrospective study of hyposensitization in atopic dogs in a flea-scarce environment. In: Ihrke, P.J., Mason, I.S., White, S.D., eds. *Advances in Veterinary Dermatology,* Vol. 2. Pergamon Press, Oxford, 1993: 79–87.

23 Griffin, C.E., Hillier, A. The ACVD task force on canine atopic dermatitis (XXIV): allergen specific immunotherapy. *Veterinary Immunology and Immunopathology*, 2001; **81**: 363–383.

24 Zur, G., White, S.W., Ihrke, P.J., Kass, P.H., Toebe, N. Canine atopic dermatitis: a retrospective study of 169 cases examined at the University of California, Davis, 1992–1998, Part II. Response to hyposensitization. *Veterinary Dermatology*, 2002; **13**: 89–102.

Comparison of intradermal testing and allergen-specific IgE serum testing in dogs with warm weather, seasonal atopic dermatitis

E.J. Rosser Jr DVM

Department of Small Animal Clinical Sciences, College of Veterinary Medicine, Michigan State University, East Lansing, Michigan, USA

Summary

Intradermal testing (IDT) and allergen-specific IgE serum testing (ASIST) are important tests for demonstration of IgE-mediated hypersensitivity in dogs with atopic dermatitis (AD). The purpose of this study was to compare results of IDT and ASIST to the history in 29 dogs with AD and a distinct warm weather seasonal component to their disease. Dogs were placed in one of three groups according to the seasonal onset/exacerbation of pruritus as follows: from April/May until killing frost (KF) in 15 dogs (group 1), June/July until KF in 9 dogs (group 2), and August until KF in 5 dogs (group 3).

For group 1, IDT and ASIST correlated well with the dog's history in 9/15 dogs (60%) and 12/15 dogs (80%), respectively. Combining results

of IDT and ASIST resulted in good correlations in 14/15 dogs (93%). For group 2, IDT and ASIST correlated well with the history in 3/9 dogs (33%) and 7/9 dogs (78%), respectively. Combining results of IDT and ASIST resulted in good correlations in 8/9 dogs (89%). For group 3, IDT and ASIST correlated well with the history in 5/5 dogs (100%) and 2/5 dogs (40%) respectively. Combining results of IDT and ASIST resulted in good correlations in 5/5 dogs (100%). In conclusion, IDT correlated well with the history of pruritus in 17/29 dogs (59%) for all groups, ASIST correlated well in 21/29 dogs (72%) for all groups, and combining IDT and ASIST correlated well in 27/29 dogs (93%) for all groups.

These results support the simultaneous use of IDT and ASIST for the selection of aeroallergens for allergen-specific immunotherapy in dogs with AD.

Introduction

Atopic dermatitis (AD) is becoming an increasingly important allergic skin disease and is reported to be one of the most common causes of pruritus in dogs.[1–3] It has been estimated to occur in 3–15% of the general canine population, with the incidence being even higher in dermatology referral practices.[2–7] In support of a diagnosis of AD in the dog, intradermal testing (IDT) and allergen-specific IgE serum testing (ASIST) are considered important tests for demonstration of an IgE-mediated hypersensitivity component in this disease. However, false positive and false negative reactions can occur using either testing method, for a variety of reasons.[8,9] Therefore the most important criteria

used in the diagnosis of AD are the patient's history and the presence of typical clinical signs.[10–12] The criteria used in the evaluation of dogs suspected to have AD have been discussed recently.[11] The final step in considering a diagnosis of AD is to systematically rule out the other common causes of pruritus, especially (but not limited to) flea allergy dermatitis, cutaneous adverse food reactions (food allergy), scabies and other regional pruritic parasitic skin diseases (including so-called 'scabies incognito'), pruritic bacterial folliculitis and *Malassezia* dermatitis. Once these diseases have been excluded, and the history and clinical signs are compatible with a diagnosis of AD, the clinician should next discuss the various treatment options to be considered.

If the owner agrees to pursue allergen-specific immunotherapy (ASIT), it is then recommended that either IDT or ASIST be performed to aid the clinician in the selection of allergens for ASIT to attempt hyposensitisation of the atopic state.[1,2,13–24] It is important that these tests include all of the specific and relevant allergens for the geographical region where the IDT or ASIST testing is being performed. When the results of these tests are compatible with the patient's history, then each relevant and specific allergen is chosen for inclusion in the dog's ASIT protocol, as the response to this therapy is quite allergen-specific. The other treatment alternatives include the use of a wide variety of anti-pruritic and anti-inflammatory topical and systemic drugs. As AD tends to be a lifelong skin disease in dogs, ASIT has become an increasingly valuable treatment for the long-term management of this disease.

The purpose of this study was to compare the results of IDT and ASIST to the history of dogs with AD and a distinct and specific warm weather seasonal pruritus component to their disease.

Materials and methods

Twenty-nine dogs with AD and a history of a warm weather seasonal pruritus or a year-round pruritus with distinct exacerbations during warm weather seasons were included in the study. Dogs were patients of the Dermatology Service at Michigan State University's Veterinary Teaching Hospital during the period April 2002 to October 2004. The diagnosis of AD was based on history, physical findings and the systematic ruling out of other causes of a primary pruritic skin disease. This included the use of home-cooked elimination diet trials for 8 weeks, and empirical treatment for scabies and other ectoparasites when appropriate. Dogs with a concurrent flea allergy dermatitis or cutaneous adverse reaction to foods were excluded from the study. The history of each dog was obtained by: (1) mailing a questionnaire to the owner for review when the appointment was first made, which the owner then brought to their scheduled appointment for review by the author; (2) review of the medical records from the referring veterinarian; (3) an initial interview by a veterinary student; and (4) a final interview and review of all information by the author.

The owners of the dogs in the study complied with the following drug withdrawal times prior to testing: 90 days for all repositol corticosteroids; 30 days for all other injectable, oral and topical corticosteroids; 14 days for all antihistamines, antibiotics, antifungals, cyclosporine and essential fatty acid supplements; 7 days for all non-steroidal anti-inflammatory drugs; and no bathing for 7 days prior to examination. This was accomplished by mailing a letter that contained detailed information on withdrawal times for all drugs to each owner when the referral appointment was first scheduled.

For each dog included in the study, a 45-allergen IDT and a 48-allergen-specific IgE immunoassay (Allercept™ Northeast Regional Allergy Screen [ANRAS], Heska Corp, Fort Collins, CO) were performed.[8,9] The allergens tested using the ANRAS and IDT are listed in

Table 1.6.1 Allergens used for intradermal testing at Michigan State University	Type of allergens	Allergens
	Indoor aeroallergens	House dust, *Dermatophagoides farinae*, *Dermatophagoides pteronyssinus*, mattress dust, tobacco, cotton linters, kapok, sheep wool, feather mix, cat epithelia
	Tree pollens	Chinese juniper, birch mix, box elder/maple, walnut, oak mix, cedar mix, tree mix no. 1 (white alder, aspen, American beech, American elm), tree mix no. 2 (American hazelnut, shagbark hickory, red mulberry, white poplar), tree mix no. 3 (American sycamore, black willow, green ash, white ash)
	Grass pollens	Kentucky blue grass, brome grass, rye grass, canary grass, quack/wheat grass mix, 7 grass mix (red top, meadow fescue, sweet vernal, Kentucky blue, orchard, perennial rye, timothy)
	Weed pollens	Common cocklebur, Russian thistle, yellow dock/sorrel, goldenrod, kochia, lamb's quarters, Mexican tea, marsh elder/burweed, nettle, giant and short ragweed mix, English plantain, Western water hemp, annual sagebrush, mugwort sagebrush, dandelion, spiny pigweed, rough redroot pigweed
	Moulds	Mould mix no. 1 (*Alternaria*, *Aspergillus*, *Cladosporium* (*Hormodendrum*), *Penicillium*, *Helminthosporium*), mould mix no. 2 (*Fusarium*, Curvularia, Rhizopus, Pullularia, Mucor), Michigan mould mix (*Stemphylium solani*, *Phoma herbarum*)

Type of allergen	Allergens
Indoor aeroallergens	*Dermatophagoides farinae*, *Dermatophagoides pteronyssinus*, cat epithelia
Tree pollens	Black birch, box elder, sugar maple, walnut, white oak, red cedar, quaking aspen, American elm, shagbark hickory, red mulberry, American sycamore, white ash, eastern cottonwood, yellow pine, bayberry wax myrtle
Grass pollens	June blue, brome, perennial rye, red top, sweet vernal, orchard, timothy, meadow fescue, Johnson, Bermuda
Weed pollens	Common cocklebur, Russian thistle, yellow dock, kochia, lamb's quarter, marsh elder/burweed, tall ragweed, short ragweed, English plantain, mugwort, rough redroot pigweed
Moulds	*Alternaria, Aspergillus, Cladosporium* (*Hormodendrum*), *Penicillium, Fusarium*

Table 1.6.2 Allergens used for allergen-specific IgE immunoassay (Allercept™ Northeast Regional Allergy Screen)

Tables 1.6.1 and 1.6.2. All dogs were sedated using xylazine hydrochloride intravenously, prior to performing each IDT. Reactions on IDT were recorded as 0, 1, 2, 3, or 4; where 0 is equal to the reaction of the negative control and 4 is equal to the reaction of the positive control. Any reaction of 2 or greater was regarded as positive. Reactions on ANRAS were measured in EA units with a range of 0–5000 EA units. Any reaction of 150 EA units or greater was regarded as positive.

In the geographical location where this study was performed (upper Midwest USA), the times of year for tree, grass and weed pollination are quite definite. Pollen levels for the period 2002–2004 were obtained for the state of Michigan from the American Academy of Allergy, Asthma, and Immunology, National Allergy Bureau Counting Stations (www.aaaai.org) for comparison with the dogs' histories and the grouping of dogs. A positive correlation of a dog's history with the result of an IDT or ANRAS was made if at least one specific allergen for that season was positive on either test.

Results

The mean age of the dogs at the time of presentation was 4 years (range 2–9 years), and the mean duration of pruritus was 2.5 years (range 0.5–7 years). The breeds affected included: Labrador retrievers (10 dogs), mixed breeds (6 dogs), golden retrievers (3 dogs), and 1 each of the following breeds: boxer, English bulldog, Jack Russell terrier, cairn terrier, great Dane, bull mastiff, beagle, English springer spaniel and bloodhound. The body sites with distribution pattern of pruritus for each patient is indicated in Table 1.6.3.

Each pollen group was reported as follows: tree pollens predominantly in April/May, grass pollens predominantly in June/July and weed pollens predominantly in August until 'killing frost' (KF) for the 2-year time period of this study. The owners of the 29 dogs reported their histories of seasonal onset or exacerbation of pruritus as follows: from April/May until KF (group 1) in 15 dogs (with 13/15 dogs in this group having non-seasonal pruritus that exacerbated in the spring and 2/15 dogs with only seasonal pruritus); June/July until KF (group 2) in 9 dogs (with 7/9 dogs in this group having non-seasonal pruritus that exacerbated in the early summer and 2/9 dogs with only seasonal pruritus); and August until KF (group 3) in 5 dogs (with 4/5 dogs in this group having non-seasonal pruritus that exacerbated in late summer and 1/5 dogs with only seasonal pruritus).

For group 1, IDT correlated well with positive reactions to tree, grass and weed pollens in 9/15 dogs (60%) and ANRAS correlated well in 12/15 dogs (80%) (Table 1.6.3, case nos 1–15). When combining the results of IDT and ANRAS for each dog, the correlation of the results with the history was 14/15 dogs (93%).

For group 2, IDT correlated well with positive reactions to grass and weed pollens in 3/9 dogs (33%) and ANRAS correlated well in 7/9 dogs (78%) (Table 1.6.3, case nos 16–24). When combining the results of IDT and ANRAS for each dog, the correlation of the results with the history was 8/9 dogs (89%).

For group 3, IDT correlated well with positive reactions to weed pollens in 5/5 dogs (100%) and ANRAS correlated well in 2/5 dogs (40%) (Table 1.6.3, case nos 25–29). When combining the results of IDT and ANRAS for each dog, the correlation of the results with the history was 5/5 dogs (100%).

Discussion

As AD has been reported to be one of the most com-

Table 1.6.3 Reactions to the 48-allergen IgE immunoassay (Allercept™ Northeast Regional Allergy Screen) and 45-allergen intradermal testing in 29 dogs with atopic dermatitis

Case	History	Michigan State University Intradermal Skin Test	Allercept™ NE Regional Allergy Screen
1	Non-seasonal pruritus, worsens in April to KF – head, axillae, forelegs	Positive (HD, DF, DP, 10 weeds, moulds)	Positive (DF, DP, 8 trees, 10 grasses, 12 weeds)
2	Non-seasonal pruritus, worsens in April to KF – feet, abdomen, ears (with otitis)	Positive (9 trees, 6 grasses, 9 weeds)	Positive (13 trees, 10 grasses, 10 weeds, mould)
3	Non-seasonal pruritus that worsens in April to KF – feet, ears	Positive (3 trees, 1 grass, 2 weeds)	Positive (1 grass)
4	Non-seasonal pruritus, worsens in April to KF – feet, forelegs, peri-orbital region	Positive (1 tree, 5 grasses, 5 weeds, mould)	Positive (7 trees, 9 grasses, 9 weeds, mould)
5	Non-seasonal pruritus, worsens in May to KF – ventral neck	Positive (HD, DF, DP, 1 tree, 4 weeds, moulds)	Positive (DF, DP, 11 trees, 8 grasses, 8 weeds)
6	Non-seasonal pruritus, worsens in April to KF – ears (with otitis), feet, peri-vulvar region	Positive (HD, DF, DP)	Positive (DF, DP, 2 trees, 10 grasses, 7 weeds)
7	Warm weather seasonal pruritus, April to KF – feet, inguinal region, medial thighs, abdomen, tail base	Positive (8 trees, 6 grasses, 12 weeds, moulds)	Positive (DF, cat epithelia, DP, 15 trees, 10 grasses, 11 weeds)
8	Warm weather seasonal pruritus, April to KF – face	Positive (2 trees, 3 grasses, 12 weeds)	Positive (DF, 1 tree, 4 grasses, 4 weeds)
9	Non-seasonal pruritus, worsens in April to KF – forelegs, face, axillae	Positive (HD, MD, kapok, cotton, DF, DP, 8 trees, 6 grasses, 17 weeds, moulds)	Positive (DF, DP, 15 trees, 10 grasses, 12 weeds)
10	Non-seasonal pruritus, worsens in April to KF – feet, ears (with otitis)	Positive (HD, DF, kapok, cat epithelia, 9 trees, 6 grasses, 17 weeds)	Positive (DF, 12 trees, 9 grasses, 8 weeds)
11	Non-seasonal pruritus, worsens in May to KF – generalized	Positive (HD, DF, cotton, kapok, 9 trees, 6 grasses, 17 weeds)	Positive (DF, 15 trees, 10 grasses, 12 weeds)
12	Non-seasonal pruritus, worsens in May to KF – hips, forelegs	Positive (HD, 1 tree, 2 weeds)	Negative
13	Non-seasonal pruritus, worsens in May to KF – ears (with otitis), face, feet, legs, ventrum	Positive (HD, DF, DP, moulds, 2 trees, 5 grasses, 5 weeds)	Positive (DP, DF, moulds, 14 trees, 10 grasses, 11 weeds)
14	Non-seasonal pruritus, worsens in April to KF – feet, ears	Positive (HD, 6 trees, 1 weed, mould)	Positive (1 tree, 2 grasses, mould)
15	Non-seasonal pruritus, worsens in April to KF – ears (with otitis), feet	Positive (4 trees, 4 weeds)	Positive (8 trees, 4 grasses, 5 weeds)
16	Warm weather seasonal pruritus, June to KF – inguinal/axillary regions, abdomen, chest	Positive (4 weeds, 1 mould)	Positive (3 weeds, 2 grasses)
17	Non-seasonal pruritus, worsens in June to KF – abdomen, neck, face, forelegs	Positive (HD, DF, DP, 1 weed, 3 grasses)	Positive (DF, DP, 3 weeds, 9 grasses)
18	Non-seasonal pruritus, worsens in June to KF – ears, axillae, face, forelegs	Positive (HD, DF, DP, 8 weeds)	Positive (DF, DP, 4 weeds, 4 grasses)
19	Non-seasonal pruritus, worsens in June to KF – ears (with otitis), feet, axillae, inguinal region	Positive (HD, DF, DP, 6 grasses)	Positive (DF, DP, 10 grasses, 7 weeds)
20	Non-seasonal pruritus, worsens in June to KF – abdomen, inguinal region, peri-orbital, head, feet	Positive (HD, DF, DP, 1 weed, moulds)	Positive (DF, DP, 8 grasses, 2 weeds)
21	Non-seasonal pruritus, worsens in June to KF – ears (with otitis), feet, face	Positive (HD, DF, 1 grass, 5 weeds)	Positive (DF, 1 weed, moulds)
22	Non-seasonal pruritus, worsens in June to KF – perianal, ears, feet, abdomen, inguinal region	Positive (HD, DF, DP, mould)	Positive (DF, 6 grasses, 3 weeds)
23	Non-seasonal pruritus, worsens in July to KF – ears (with otitis)	Positive (HD, DF, 1 weed, moulds)	Positive (DF, DP, 1 grass, 2 weeds, mould)

Table 1.6.3 (*Continued.*)

Case	History	Michigan State University Intradermal Skin Test	Allercept™ NE Regional Allergy Screen
24	Warm weather seasonal pruritus, June to KF – ears (with otitis) feet, face	Positive (6 grasses, 2 weeds, moulds)	Positive (DP, 5 grasses, 3 weeds)
25	Warm weather seasonal pruritus, August to KF – ears (with otitis), feet, face	Positive (5 weeds)	Positive (DF)
26	Non-seasonal pruritus, worsens in August to KF – ears (with otitis) feet, neck, inguinal region	Positive (DF, DP, 2 weeds, moulds)	Negative
27	Non-seasonal pruritus, worsens in August to KF – ears (with otitis), feet, hind/forelegs	Positive (4 weeds, moulds)	Positive (DF)
28	Non-seasonal pruritus, worsens in August to KF – ears (with otitis), feet, neck	Positive (DF, 2 weeds, moulds)	Positive (1 weed, mould)
29	Non-seasonal pruritus, worsens in August to KF – ears (with otitis)	Positive (HD, DF, DP, 5 weeds)	Positive (DF, DP, 1 weed)

Any allergen with ≥ 150 EA units of IgE on the Allercept screen immunoassay was regarded as positive. Any reaction of ≥ 2 (subjectively scored on a scale of 0–4) on the intradermal test was regarded as positive. KF, killing frost; HD, house dust; DF, *Dermatophagoides farinae*; DP, *Dermatophagoides pteronyssinus*.

mon causes of pruritus in dogs, and ASIT is one of the most common forms of therapy for the disease, being able to optimally select the allergens for ASIT on the initial presentation would be very useful, and in the long run more cost-effective for the client with an atopic dog. The question as to whether or not IDT or ASIST should be the gold standard for use in support of a diagnosis of atopic dermatitis is very controversial.[12–19] The major problem with these interpretations is that the allergenic extracts used, testing methodologies, and test result interpretations have not been standardised for either method of testing. Until this has been accomplished, direct comparisons will remain problematic.

Based on the results of this study, the simultaneous use of both IDT and ASIST (specifically ANRAS for this study) resulted in a superior correlation of the results when compared to each dog's history of pruritus versus use of either testing method alone. In theory, using this approach should result in an optimum response to ASIT. Subsequently, the initial cost to the client when using this approach would be significantly increased. However, in most cases (except IDT results for group 3 with 100% correlation) when either IDT or ANRAS were reviewed separately, there was always a percentage of cases (ranging from 20% to 67% of dogs in this study, depending on group and test) where it was apparent that either testing method did not yield results completely compatible with the dog's history of pruritus. In such instances it is often necessary to

re-evaluate such patients and consider repeating IDT and/or ANRAS at a future date, with a substantial increased cost to each client.

Unfortunately, these results are only applicable to the testing methods used in this study, as they were maintained as a constant for the 2-year duration of the study, and subsequent studies using different methods of IDT and ASIST may or may not yield comparable results. Whether improved response to ASIT based on results of IDT, ANRAS, or combined results of the tests is unknown and was not an objective of the present study.

Of interest were the poor correlations of test results to the dogs' history of pruritus for IDT in group 2, and ANRAS in group 3. In group 2, IDT only had a good correlation of 33% (3/9 dogs) compared with 78% (7/9 dogs) for ANRAS. Upon further examination of the six dogs with poor IDT correlations, in four of these six dogs the testing was performed from July to September. In these four cases, the consequences of the appropriate drug withdrawals during their 'peak' aeroallergen season resulted in very inflamed skin when attempting IDT. In the author's experience, this is one of several reasons for a 'false negative' IDT and many such cases in the past have been retested shortly after killing frost with subsequent IDT results with an improved correlation to the dog's history of pruritus. In contrast, the same six dogs evaluated using ANRAS correlated well during this time, and one would suspect the results of ASIST to be unaffected by very inflamed skin during testing. More importantly, one would expect that the circulating levels of allergen-specific IgE should be high and readily detected in such cases. In group 3, ANRAS only had a good correlation of 40% (2/5 dogs) compared with 100% (5/5 dogs) for IDT; however, no explanation could be suggested as related to the time of year that each dog was tested, as these dogs were all tested during a wide range of seasons. Most likely the small size of this group of dogs makes further evaluation difficult.

It is also interesting to note that only 5 of the dogs in the study had a strictly warm weather seasonal pruritic skin disease at the time of presentation, compared with 24 dogs having a history of a non-seasonal pruritus that exacerbated in warm weather. However, 11/24 of these non-seasonally pruritic dogs had an initial history of a strictly warm weather seasonal pruritic skin disease for at least 1 year before progressing into a non-seasonal problem that continued to exacerbate in warm weather. In summary, 16 dogs (55%) had an initial history of strictly seasonal pruritus and 13 dogs (45%) were non-seasonally pruritic with warm weather exacerbations from the onset of the dog's disease. The author's impression over the years has been that this increased incidence of non-seasonal AD from the onset, when compared to previous reports,[1] is mostly due to reactions to various non-seasonal moulds present in Michigan homes.

In conclusion, the results of this study support the recommendation for the simultaneous use of both IDT and ASIST in the selection of aeroallergens for ASIT in dogs suspected of having AD. In theory, using this approach should result in an optimum response to ASIT.

Funding

The cost of the concurrent testing of each dog with the 48-aeroallergen-specific IgE immunoassay (Allercept™ Northeast Regional Allergy Screen – ANRAS) was funded by the Michigan State University, College of Veterinary Medicine, Dermatology Research Account.

References

1 Scott, D.W., Miller, W.H., Griffin, C.E. *Muller & Kirk's Small Animal Dermatology*. W.B. Saunders, Philadelphia, 2001: 574–601.
2 Reedy, L.M., Miller, W.H., Willemse, T. *Allergic Skin Diseases of Dogs and Cats*. W.B. Saunders, Philadelphia, 1997: 32–44.
3 DeBoer, D.J. Survey of intradermal skin testing practices in North America. *Journal of the American Veterinary Medical Association*, 1989; **195**: 1357–1363.
4 Hillier, A., Griffin, C.E. The ACVD task force on canine atopic dermatitis (I): incidence and prevalence. *Veterinary Immunology and Immunopathology*, 2001; **81**: 147–151.
5 Scott, D.W., Paradis, M. A survey of canine and feline skin disorders seen in a university practice: small animal clinic, University of Montreal, Saint-Hyacinthe, Quebec (1987–1988). *Canadian Veterinary Journal*, 1990; **31**: 830–835.
6 Carlotti, D.N., Costargent, F. Analysis of positive skin tests in 449 dogs with allergic dermatitis. *European Journal of Companion Animal Practice*, 1994; **4**: 42–59.
7 Saridomichelakis, M.N., Koutinas, A.F., Giolekas, D., Leontidis, L. Canine atopic dermatitis in Greece: clinical observations and the prevalence of positive intradermal test reactions in 91 spontaneous cases. *Veterinary Immunology and Immunopathology*, 1999; **69**: 61–73.
8 Hillier, A., DeBoer, D.J. The ACVD task force on canine atopic dermatitis (XVII): intradermal testing. *Veterinary Immunology and Immunopathology*, 2001; **81**: 289–304.
9 DeBoer, D.J., Hillier, A. The ACVD task force on canine atopic dermatitis (XVI): laboratory evaluation of dogs with atopic dermatitis with serum-based "allergy" tests. *Veterinary Immunology and Immunopathology*, 2001; **81**: 277–287.
10 Griffin, C.E., DeBoer, D.J. The ACVD task force on canine atopic dermatitis (XIV): clinical manifestations of canine atopic dermatitis. *Veterinary Immunology and Immunopathology*, 2001; **81**: 255–269.
11 DeBoer, D.J., Hillier, A. The ACVD task force on canine atopic dermatitis (XV): fundamental concepts in clinical diagnosis. *Veterinary Immunology and Immunopathology*, 2001; **81**: 271–276.
12 Hillier, A. Definitively diagnosing atopic dermatitis in dogs. *Veterinary Medicine*, 2002; **97**: 198–208.
13 Kleinbeck, M.L., Hites, M.J., Loker, J.L., Halliwell, R.E., Lee, K.W. Enzyme-linked immunosorbent assay for measurement of allergen-specific IgE antibodies in canine serum. *American Journal of Veterinary Research*, 1989; **50**: 1831–1839.
14 Codner, E.C., Lessard, P. Comparison of intradermal allergy test and enzyme-linked immunosorbent assay in dogs with allergic skin disease. *Journal of the American Veterinary Medical Association*, 1993; **202**: 739–743.
15 Miller, W.H., Scott, D.W., Wellington, J.R., Scarlett, J.M., Panic, R. Evaluation of the performance of a serologic allergy system in atopic dogs. *Journal of the American Animal Hospital Association*, 1993; **29**: 545–550.
16 Bond, R., Thorogood, S.C., Lloyd, D.H. Evaluation of two enzyme-linked immunosorbent assays for the diagnosis of canine atopy. *Veterinary Record*, 1994; **135**: 130–133.
17 Mueller, R.S., Burrows, A., Tsohalis, J. Comparison of intradermal testing and serum testing for allergen-specific IgE using monoclonal IgE antibodies in 84 atopic dogs. *Australian Veterinary Journal*, 1999; **77**: 290–294.
18 Park, S., Ohya, F., Yamshita, K., Nishifuji, K., Iwasaki, T. Comparison of response to immunotherapy by intradermal skin test and antigen-specific IgE in canine atopy. *Journal of Veterinary Medical Science*, 2000; **62**: 983–988.
19 Hillier, A. Allergy testing and treatment for canine atopic dermatitis. *Veterinary Medicine*, 2002; **97**: 210–224.
20 Rosser, E.J. Aqueous hyposensitization in the treatment of canine atopic dermatitis: In: Kwochka, K.W., Willemse, T., von Tscharner, C., eds. *Advances in Veterinary Dermatology*, Vol. 3. Butterworth Heinemann, Oxford, 1998: 169–176.

21 Willemse, A., Van den Brom, W.E., Rijnberk, A. Effect of hypo-sensitization on atopic dermatitis in dogs. *Journal of the American Veterinary Medical Association*, 1984; **184**: 1277–1280.

22 Scott, K.V., White, S.D., Rosychuk, R.A.W. A retrospective study of hyposensitization in atopic dogs in a flea-scarce environment. In: Ihrke, P.J., Mason, I.S., White, S.D., eds. *Advances in Veterinary Dermatology*, Vol. 2. Pergamon Press, Oxford, 1993: 79–87.

23 Griffin, C.E., Hillier, A. The ACVD task force on canine atopic dermatitis (XXIV): allergen specific immunotherapy. *Veterinary Immunology and Immunopathology*, 2001; **81**: 363–383.

24 Zur, G., White, S.W., Ihrke, P.J., Kass, P.H., Toebe, N. Canine atopic dermatitis: a retrospective study of 169 cases examined at the University of California, Davis, 1992–1998, Part II. Response to hyposensitization. *Veterinary Dermatology*, 2002; **13**: 89–102.

Patch test reactions to house dust mites in dogs with atopic dermatitis

S.A.F. Nogueira DVM, MS, S.M.F. Torres DVM, MS, PhD, K. Horne, C. Jessen DVM

College of Veterinary Medicine, Department of Small Animal Clinical Sciences University of Minnesota, Saint Paul, Minnesota, USA

Summary

Environmental allergens are suspected to be absorbed through the skin and induce the typical skin lesions seen in atopic dermatitis (AD). Patch test (PT), whereby allergens are applied directly to the skin, has been shown to be a useful model of percutaneous allergen absorption in humans. The purpose of this study was to determine the percentage of dogs with spontaneous AD that show positive PT reactions to a commercially available 20% house dust mite (HDM) mixture. Further, we compared the clinical and histological features of HDM skin reactions on the PT with skin lesions of dogs with AD, and PT reactions induced by sodium lauryl sulfate (SLS).

The study included 12 dogs without AD, and 13 dogs with non-

seasonal AD. None of the dogs without AD reacted to HDM or white petrolatum (vehicle). Ten of the 13 dogs with AD reacted macroscopically and histopathologically to HDM. Macroscopic reactions to HDM were identical to lesional skin in 20% of the dogs, and identical to SLS reactions in 40% of the dogs.

Qualitative histological findings showed that HDM reactions were similar to lesional skin in 80% of the dogs and similar to SLS in 20% of the dogs. The proportion of neutrophils in SLS reactions was significantly higher compared to HDM reactions, which could be a differentiating factor between allergic and irritant reactions.

This study demonstrated that HDM penetrated the skin of dogs with AD and induced an inflammatory response that resembled a true allergic reaction.

Introduction

Atopic dermatitis (AD) is a common pruritic skin disorder of dogs and humans.[1–3] The pathogenesis of AD is complex, and not completely understood. However, an IgE-mediated hypersensitivity reaction to environmental allergens may play an important role in the development of skin lesions.[1–4] House dust mites (HDM), specifically *Dermatophagoides farinae* and *D. pteronyssinus*, are the most common environmental allergens inducing hypersensitivity in dogs and humans with AD.[1–4]

The mechanism of skin sensitisation in AD is still a topic of debate.[5–7] Two theories have been proposed to explain the route by which environmental allergens gain entry to the skin and trigger an inflammatory reaction. The first theory, as yet unsubstantiated, proposes that allergens are inhaled and once in the respiratory tract, they reach the skin via the circulation.[7] The second theory suggests that skin inflammation

occurs through epicutaneous contact with environmental allergens.[5,7] Studies have demonstrated that 16–100% of humans with AD develop eczematous skin lesions after patch test (PT) with environmental allergens.[5,6,8–17] The skin lesions induced after PT were shown to be clinically and microscopically similar to the natural disease.[6,9]

The theory of percutaneous penetration of environmental allergens and subsequent skin sensitisation in canine AD is supported by two key observations: the typical distribution of lesions in areas with a sparse hair coat (such as the face, feet and groin) and thus direct contact of skin with environmental surfaces; and the increased numbers of epidermal Langerhans cells expressing surface IgE found in lesional skin of dogs with AD, compared with non-lesional atopic skin.[2,7,18–20] Few studies have investigated the route of skin sensitisation in dogs,[21–24] and only one study has reported PT reactions to environmental allergens in dogs with spontaneous AD.[23] In that study, 27% of dogs with AD and 20% of healthy control dogs had positive PT reactions to environmental allergens.

The aims of the present study were: to determine the percentage of dogs with AD that showed positive PT reactions to HDM; to evaluate if the skin reactions induced after PT application of HDM were macroscopically and histologically similar to the natural skin lesions of dogs with AD; and to investigate if the HDM reactions were true allergic reactions.

Materials and methods

Study population

Privately owned dogs with year-round AD were recruited from patients of the Dermatology Service at the Veterinary Medical Center of the University of Minnesota. Inclusion criteria required: a diagnosis of AD based on compatible history and clinical signs; elimination of other pruritic disorders such as sarcoptic mange, cutaneous adverse food reaction and flea hypersensitivity; and at least one positive reaction on intradermal test (IDT) using a panel of 60 allergens.[18,25] Moreover, all dogs had to react to HDM on the IDT. The HDM mixture used for the IDT contained D. farinae and D. pteronyssinus at a concentration of 1:5000 w/v. Reactions were subjectively evaluated for erythema and induration using the negative control (saline) and the positive control (histamine 1:100 000) for comparison. Reactions were interpreted 15 minutes after the injections and a score of 0 to 4+ was assessed. Reactions mirroring the negative control received 0 scores and reactions mirroring the positive control received 4+ scores. Any reaction ≥ 2+ was considered positive. Dogs on allergen-specific immunotherapy were excluded from the study. Before entering the study, dogs received appropriate therapy for any existing secondary bacterial and yeast skin infections. Furthermore, antihistamines and essential fatty acids were withdrawn for 14 days, topical and oral glucocorticoids for 21 days, and injectable glucocorticoids for 60 days, before entry into the study. The clinical condition of the dogs was classified as mild, moderate or severe based on a previously described scoring system for erythema and pruritus.[26] Client consent was a requirement for participation in the study.

A group of dogs without a history or clinical signs of skin disorders was included to validate the test substances used in the AD dogs. These dogs were also subject to an IDT including the 10 most common environmental allergens present in the Minnesota metropolitan region (HDM mixture at 1:5000 w/v, house dust, dust mix, corn smut, corn pollen, cotton linters, grain mill dust, sheep epithelium, box elder, ragweed mix), in addition to flea antigen, and positive (histamine) and negative (saline) controls. No positive reactions were recorded in any of the dogs. This group comprised 12 clinically healthy, 20-month-old, intact female laboratory beagle dogs purchased for use in a terminal surgery laboratory course. The dogs were kept in a research facility until the end of the PT evaluation.

The study was approved by the Institutional Animal Care and Use Committee of the University of Minnesota.

Patch test design

The allergen consisted of a commercially available 20% HDM mixture containing equal parts of D. farinae and D. pteronyssinus in white petrolatum (WP) (Dormer Laboratories, Rexdale, Ontario, Canada).[27,28] A commercial WP preparation (Kendall Vaseline®, Tyco Healthcare Group LP, Mansfield, MA, USA) was used as negative control. A 10% sodium lauryl sulfate (SLS) solution (Sigma, St Louis, MO, USA) was used in each test as an irritant control.[29,30]

The test substances were placed on 8-mm diameter aluminium chambers adhered to a hypoallergenic tape (Finn Chambers on Scanpor®, Pharmacia & Upjohn, Kalamazoo, MI, USA). Approximately 25 mg of HDM and WP was applied per chamber. A volume of 0.05 ml SLS was added to a filter paper disc (Pharmacia & Upjohn) that was placed on the chamber to help retain the solution.

The chambers were placed on clinically uninvolved skin on the lateral thorax in duplicate parallel sets applied 1.5 cm apart, for 48 hours. Fifteen minutes prior to the PT application, the test area was shaved, but not cleaned or artificially prepared in any other way. To keep the chambers in place, another hypoallergenic tape (Bioclusive transparent dressing®, Johnson & Johnson, Arlington, TX, USA) was applied over the PT. In addition, the dogs also wore an elastic cotton vest for 72 hours (Quick Cover®, Four Flags Over Aspen Inc., St Clair, MN, USA).

Patch test evaluation

At 48 hours after PT application, the chambers were removed. Macroscopic and histologic evaluations were

Table 1.7.1 Visual grading system used for the macroscopic evaluation of the patch test reactions

Score	Visible lesions at test site
0	No visible reaction
1+	Mild reaction (erythema or papules)
2+	Moderate reaction (erythema and oedema with or without papules)
3+	Severe reaction (erythema, oedema, papules or vesicles, exudation and crust)

performed at 48 hours (upper set) and 72 hours (lower set). The HDM sites were compared to lesional skin and to SLS sites to evaluate if HDM reactions were allergic or irritant reactions. The WP sites were compared to non-lesional skin to ensure that the vehicle was not inducing an inflammatory response.

Macroscopic assessment

After allowing 10 minutes for non-specific reactions due to tape fixation or occlusion to subside, the test sites were evaluated using a scale adapted from a human study (Table 1.7.1).[28] The investigator interpreting the PT sites was not blinded.

Skin biopsies

Samples were collected from the centre of macroscopically positive and negative sites using a 6-mm punch biopsy (Miltex Instrument Company, Inc., Bethpage, NY, USA) under local anaesthetic (2% lidocaine hydrochloride®, Phoenix Pharmaceutical, Inc., St Joseph, MO, USA). In the AD group, samples were also collected from lesional and non-lesional skin areas used as controls.

Each sample was placed in 10% neutral buffered formalin for routine embedding in paraffin.

Histological staining

Sections (5 μm) were stained routinely with haematoxylin and eosin (H&E); for cell quantification, sec-

tions were stained with Giemsa and Luna's stain[31] for mast cells and eosinophils, respectively. Additionally, sections were processed for immunohistochemical staining of histiocytes and lymphocytes using mouse monoclonal and rabbit polyclonal antibodies that cross-react with canine leukocyte antigens (Table 1.7.2).[31–33] Plasma cell and neutrophil counts were determined on H&E stained sections.

Qualitative histological assessment

Epidermal changes and dermal inflammatory infiltrates were evaluated by an investigator who was blinded with regard to the origin of the sample. A reaction was considered positive when the epidermal changes and degree of inflammation in the PT reaction exceeded those in the non-lesional skin.

Quantitative histological assessment

Histiocytes, T and B lymphocytes, mast cells, eosinophils, neutrophils and plasma cells in the dermis of positive PT sites, lesional skin and non-lesional skin were quantified by an investigator who was blinded with regard to the origin of the sample. The area of greatest cellularity in the dermis was selected at ×4 magnification using a light microscope (BX45, Olympus, Tokyo, Japan). The microscopic field was then changed to ×40 magnification, encompassing an area of 2.98 mm^2, and all stained cells in this field were counted. In fields containing glands and hair follicles, only intervening dermal regions were counted. Intravascular and fibroblastic cells, and cells not completely within the microscopic field, were excluded from the count.

Statistical analysis

A chi-square test for homogenicity was used to compare the count of each dermal inflammatory cell type in relation to the total cell count among positive PT sites and lesional and non-lesional sites. This analysis was per-

Table 1.7.2 Antibody panel used for immunohistochemical staining

Antibody	Specificity	Clone	Dilution	Source
MAC 387*	Myeloid/histiocytic cells	MAC387	1:200	Dako
CD79a*	B lymphocytes	HM57	1:50	Dako
CD3†	T lymphocytes	–	1:50	Neomarkers

*Mouse monoclonal antibody. † Rabbit polyclonal antibody.

formed on each dog and the data were pooled to evaluate the cell counts from the sites in the entire sample of dogs. Data were reported as proportion of dermal cell types per ×40 microscopic field unless specified otherwise. A p value ≤ 0.05 was considered significant. Statistical analyses were performed using SPSS for Windows 11.5.1 (SPSS Inc., Chicago, IL, USA).

Results

None of the 12 dogs without AD showed macroscopically or histologically positive reactions to HDM and WP. Macroscopic and histological reactions to SLS were observed in seven (58%) and six (50%) of these dogs, respectively. Based on these results, the 20% HDM mixture was considered non-irritating to canine skin and SLS was considered irritant to canine skin.

The AD group comprised 13 dogs (4 spayed females and 9 neutered males) with a mean age of 5.2 years (range 1–10 years). Seven breeds were represented: Labrador retrievers (4), golden retrievers (4), greyhound (1), American Staffordshire terrier (1), Shetland sheepdog (1), Boston terrier (1) and blue heeler (1). The clinical condition was mild in six dogs, moderate in four dogs and severe in three dogs.

Macroscopic assessment

None of the dogs with AD had positive macroscopic reactions to WP when compared to non-lesional skin.

Positive macroscopic reactions to HDM and SLS were present in 10 (77%) of the 13 dogs with AD when both time points (48 and 72 hours) were considered (Table 1.7.3). Lesional skin was characterised by diffuse or macular erythema in 12 dogs, and diffuse erythema with papules in 1 dog. The HDM reactions were identical to lesional skin in 2/10 dogs that developed erythema. In 5/10 dogs, HDM reactions were similar to lesional skin: there was erythema and oedema in 4 dogs; and erythema, oedema and papules in 1 dog. In 3/10 dogs, HDM reactions were different from lesional skin, as HDM reactions were characterised by papules and lesional skin was characterised by erythema.

The HDM reactions were identical to SLS reactions in four dogs; there was erythema in one dog, while three dogs had erythema and oedema. In 5/10 dogs, HDM reactions were different from SLS reactions: HDM reactions were characterised by papules in 3 dogs, erythema and oedema in 1 dog, and erythema, oedema

Table 1.7.3 Macroscopic patch test reactions in dogs with atopic dermatitis according to a visual grading system

| Dogs with AD | Macroscopic PT reactions | | | |
| | HDM | | SLS | |
	48 h	72 h	48 h	72 h
1	2+	1+	3+	3+
2	0	0	0	0
3	1+	1+	3+	2+
4	2+	1+	2+	2+
5	2+	2+	2+	2+
6	1+	1+	3+	2+
7	1+	1+	3+	2+
8	1+	1+	1+	1+
9	2+	2+	2+	2+
10	0	0	0	0
11	0	0	1+	0
12	1+	1+	0	0
13	2+	1+	3+	2+

AD, atopic dermatitis; HDM, house dust mites; PT, patch test; SLS, sodium lauryl sulphate. Visual grade: see Table 1.7.1.

and papules in 1 dog; SLS reactions were characterised by erythema, oedema, vesicles, exudation and crust in 5 dogs. In 1/10 dogs, the comparison between HDM and SLS reactions was not possible due to the fact that that dog did not react to SLS.

Histological assessment

None of the dogs with AD had positive histological reactions to WP when compared to non-lesional skin.

Positive histological reactions to HDM and SLS were observed in 10 (77%) and 11 (85%) of the 13 dogs, respectively (Table 1.7.4) when both time points (48 and 72 hours) were considered.

Qualitative histological assessment

Epidermal changes in all positive HDM and SLS reactions and in lesional skin were characterised by variable degrees of orthokeratotic hyperkeratosis, hyperplasia, spongiosis and exocytosis of inflammatory cells (Table 1.7.5). These changes were more severe in HDM sites, compared with lesional skin in 6/10 dogs, and more severe in SLS sites compared to HDM sites, in all dogs with positive reactions. Focal parakeratotic hyperkeratosis (5/11 dogs), epidermal erosion or ulceration and necro-

Table 1.7.4 Histological patch test reactions in dogs with atopic dermatitis

Dogs with AD	Histological PT reactions			
	HDM		SLS	
	48 h	72 h	48 h	72 h
1	+	+	+	+
2	+	+	−	+
3	−	−	+	+
4	+	−	+	+
5	+	+	+	+
6	−	−	+	+
7	+	+	+	+
8	+	+	+	+
9	+	+	+	+
10	−	−	−	−
11	+	+	+	+
12	−	+	−	−
13	+	+	+	+

AD, atopic dermatitis; HDM, house dust mites; PT, patch test; SLS, sodium lauryl sulphate; +, positive reaction; −, negative reaction.

sis (7/11 dogs) (Fig. 1.7.1a), subcorneal or intracorneal microabscesses containing predominantly neutrophils (6/11 dogs) (Fig. 1.7.1b) and dermal-epidermal detachment (3/11 dogs) were observed only in SLS sites. Serocellular crusts were observed in SLS sites (7/11 dogs) and in HDM sites (4/10 dogs), but not in lesional skin. Epidermal eosinophilic exocytosis and focal intra-epidermal microabscess containing eosinophils were present in HDM sites of one dog (Fig. 1.7.2). The lesional skin of

one dog had a focal intracorneal microabscess containing neutrophils and few eosinophils.

The dermal inflammatory infiltrate in all positive HDM and SLS reactions, as well as in lesional skin, was arranged in a superficial perivascular to interstitial pattern. It extended to the periadnexae in HDM sites of 6/10 dogs, in lesional skin of 4/13 dogs, and to periadnexae and deep dermis in SLS sites of 8/11 dogs. The infiltration intensity in HDM sites was mild in 5/10 dogs, moderate in 2/10 dogs and severe in 3/10 dogs. In lesional skin, the infiltrate was mild in 9/13 dogs, moderate in 2/13 dogs and severe in 2/13 dogs. In contrast, in SLS sites, the infiltrate was mild in 3/11 dogs, moderate in 4/11 dogs and severe in 4/11 dogs. The dermal inflammatory infiltrate consisted predominantly of mast cells, lymphocytes and histiocytes in lesional skin of 12/13 dogs, in HDM sites of 8/10 dogs and in SLS sites of 2/11 dogs. Neutrophils, lymphocytes and histiocytes were the predominant cells in the lesional skin of 1 dog, while eosinophils, lymphocytes and histiocytes predominated in HDM sites of 2/10 dogs. In contrast, SLS reactions consisted predominantly of neutrophils, lymphocytes and histiocytes in 9/11 dogs. Eosinophils were present in HDM sites of all dogs, in lesional skin of 6/13 dogs and in SLS sites of 7/11 dogs. Neutrophils were present in HDM sites of 8/10 dogs, in lesional skin of 4/13 dogs and in SLS sites of all dogs. Very few plasma cells were seen in HDM sites, SLS sites and lesional skin. Dermal oedema was observed in HDM sites (4/10 dogs), in lesional skin (5/13 dogs) and in SLS sites (8/11 dogs).

Table 1.7.5 Number of dogs showing histological changes in lesional skin, house dust mite PT sites and sodium lauryl sulphate PT sites

Histological changes	LES (13 dogs)	HDM (10 dogs)	SLS (11 dogs)
Orthokeratotic hyperkeratosis	13	10	11
Focal parakeratotic hyperkeratosis	0	0	5
Serocellular crust	0	4	7
Intra-epidermal microabscess	0	1*	0
Subcorneal microabscess	0	0	3§
Intracorneal microabscess	1§	0	3§
Epidermal hyperplasia	13	10	11
Epidermal spongiosis	13	10	11
Epidermal exocytosis	13	10	11
Epidermal erosion/ulceration/necrosis	0	0	7
Dermal-epidermal detachment	0	0	3
Superficial perivascular to interstitial dermatitis	13	10	11
Periadnexal dermatitis	4	6	8
Dermal oedema	5	4	8

LES, lesional skin; HDM, house dust mites; SLS, sodium lauryl sulphate. *Microabscess with eosinophils.
§Microabscess with neutrophils.

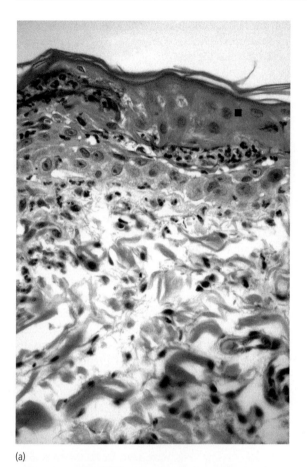

(a)

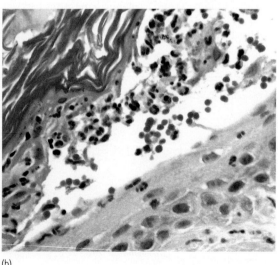

(b)

Fig. 1.7.1 Positive histological patch test reaction to sodium lauryl sulfate in a dog with atopic dermatitis showing (a) epidermal necrosis [■], and (b) subcorneal microabscess containing neutrophils (H&E stain; ×400 magnification).

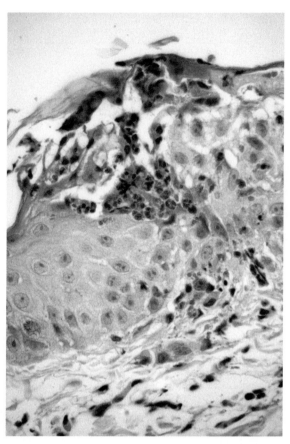

Fig. 1.7.2 Positive histological patch test reaction to house dust mites in a dog with atopic dermatitis showing spongiotic intra-epidermal microabscess containing eosinophils (H&E stain; ×400 magnification).

Quantitative histological assessment

Three dogs that did not react to HDM, and 1 dog that had excessive numbers of neutrophils in the lesional skin (suggestive of a secondary bacterial infection) were excluded from the quantitative analyses; therefore, quantitative comparison was performed in 9 of the 13 dogs included in the study.

The counts for B cells were excluded from the analysis due to lack of immunohistochemistry staining as a result of technical error. As there was a significant difference ($p < 0.05$) between HDM sites at 48 and 72 hours for all cells (except for eosinophils and plasma cells), the quantitative analyses were performed separately for each time point.

At 48 hours, the proportion of histiocytes ($p < 0.001$), eosinophils ($p < 0.001$) and plasma cells ($p <$

0.001) was significantly higher at HDM sites than lesional skin, but the proportion of mast cells ($p < 0.001$) and T lymphocytes ($p < 0.001$) was significantly lower. The proportion of neutrophils at HDM sites was not significantly different to that of lesional skin. Also at 48 hours, the proportion of eosinophils ($p = 0.025$) and plasma cells ($p = 0.042$) was significantly higher at HDM sites than SLS sites, but the proportion of histiocytes ($p < 0.001$) and neutrophils ($p < 0.001$) was significantly lower (Fig. 1.7.3). The proportion of mast cells and T lymphocytes at HDM sites was not significantly different to that at SLS sites.

At 72 hours, the proportion of histiocytes ($p < 0.001$) and eosinophils ($p < 0.001$) was significantly higher at HDM sites than lesional skin, but the proportion of mast cells ($p = 0.002$) was significantly lower. The

proportion of T lymphocytes, plasma cells and neutrophils at HDM sites was not significantly different compared to lesional skin. Also at 72 hours, the proportion of T lymphocytes ($p < 0.001$) and eosinophils ($p < 0.001$) was significantly higher at HDM sites than SLS sites, but the proportion of mast cells ($p = 0.036$) and neutrophils ($p < 0.001$) was significantly lower (Fig. 1.7.3). The proportion of histiocytes and plasma cells at HDM sites was not significantly different compared to SLS sites.

Discussion

The concept of environmental allergens penetrating the skin and initiating or exacerbating cutaneous inflammation in AD is still a matter of controversy. In the

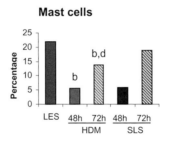

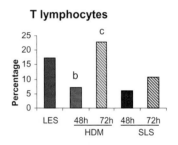

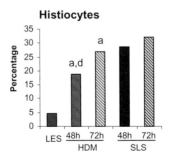

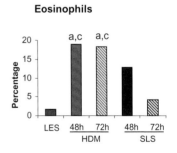

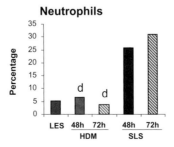

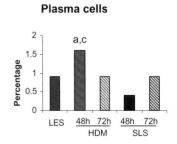

Fig. 1.7.3 Percentage of mast cells, T lymphocytes, histiocytes, eosinophils, neutrophils and plasma cells in lesional skin, house dust mite (HDM) sites at 48 and 72 hours, and sodium lauryl sulfate (SLS) sites at 48 and 72 hours, in nine dogs with atopic dermatitis. a = significantly higher than lesional skin; b = significantly lower than lesional skin; c = significantly higher than SLS; d = significantly lower than SLS.

present study, the PT with HDM allergens was macroscopically and histologically positive in 77% of the AD dogs, indicating that environmental allergens applied epicutaneously penetrate the skin and elicit skin inflammation in dogs with AD.

An earlier study reported a smaller percentage (27%) of AD dogs with positive PT reactions to environmental allergens.[24] This discrepancy may be explained in part by differences in allergenic material and biopsy site selection. In the previous study,[23] the investigators used allergen extracts in water solution, as commonly used in IDT, while in the present study, a commercially available standardised PT allergen extract mixed in WP was chosen.[27,28] As WP is a lipophilic vehicle, it may have promoted penetration and absorption of HDM.[34] Both positive and negative macroscopic reactions were biopsied in the present study, with two dogs having positive HDM reactions histologically despite negative macroscopic reactions. In contrast, in the previous study only macroscopically positive reactions were sampled, which may have underestimated the number of dogs that had positive histological PT reactions.[35]

It has been reported in humans with AD that the clinical and histopathological findings of PT reactions to environmental allergens reflect those observed in lesional skin.[6,9] Similar findings have also been reported at the site of allergen exposure in hyperresponsive IgE dogs.[21–24] In our study, the lesional skin of all AD dogs was characterised macroscopically by diffuse or macular erythema, with one dog also showing papules. However, only 20% of HDM sites were characterised by erythema alone, as seen in the lesional skin. This difference may be partially explained by the mild to moderate clinical condition of most dogs included in the study. In addition, oedema, often present at HDM sites in this study, can be difficult to assess macroscopically in lesional skin of dogs with AD. Further, the application of HDM allergen under occlusion on a small area possibly contributed to the development of stronger inflammatory reactions compared to lesional skin.

Anecdotal reports suggest that very small erythematous papules can be signs of an allergic response in a subset of dogs with AD. In the present study, one dog had erythematous papules in the lesional skin. Papules may be seen in the presence of a secondary bacterial infection.[2] However, the inflammatory infiltrate in the dog with papules was not neutrophilic, thus the lesions were unlikely to be associated with bacterial infection. Four dogs in our study showed papules at HDM sites. The development of an erythematous papular dermatitis was also reported in three of four experimentally sensitised beagle dogs and in human patients after epicutaneous HDM exposure.[9,24,36] Taken together, these findings indicate that the papular reactions seen at HDM sites and lesional skin of the AD dogs in the present study were associated with primary AD lesions. In contrast, papules were not present in any of the SLS reactions.

Little is known about the potential irritant effect of locally applied HDM allergens. Studies in humans have shown that healthy individuals have negative PT reactions to HDM.[8–17] Similarly, in this study, none of the dogs without AD had positive reactions to HDM. Moreover, mild macroscopically positive reactions to HDM were characterised by erythema only, identical to reactions at SLS sites in 40% of the dogs. This could imply that HDM caused an irritant reaction; however, it was previously reported that a weak irritant PT reaction cannot be morphologically differentiated from a weak allergic reaction.[36] Hence, in the present study, only severe SLS reactions could be differentiated from HDM reactions. Nevertheless, our results confirm that irritant and allergic reactions may not be differentiated on the basis of their macroscopic behaviour.

Intra-epidermal exocytosis of eosinophils and intra-epidermal eosinophilic microabscesses were observed in HDM sites of one dog but in none of the SLS sites. Other investigators have also reported eosinophil exocytosis and abscess formation after PT in IgE hyperresponsive beagle dogs.[24] Similarly, intra-epidermal eosinophilic pustules were seen in the HDM site in 1 of 11 AD dogs in a previous study and in human patients with AD after PT with environmental allergens.[23,37–39] In contrast, focal parakeratotic hyperkeratosis, neutrophilic microabscesses, epidermal necrosis and dermal-epidermal separation were observed only in SLS reactions. Similarly, a PT study performed in dogs using dinitrochlorobenzene to induce allergic and irritant reactions reported epidermal necrosis and dermal-epidermal separation only in the irritant reactions.[40] In studies in humans and mice, epidermal necrosis was also seen in reactions induced by lower concentrations of SLS.[41,42] These findings suggest that the epidermal changes induced by SLS, but not by HDM, are compatible with an irritant reaction.

Based on our qualitative analysis, HDM sites and lesional skin had similar dermal inflammatory infiltrates in 8 (80%) dogs. In contrast, HDM and SLS sites had similar inflammatory infiltrates in only 2 (20%) dogs. The inflammatory infiltrate in these reactions consisted predominantly of mast cells, lymphocytes and histiocytes. However, our quantitative results did not consistently agree with these findings where the proportion of mast cells, lymphocytes and histiocytes in HDM sites were, for the most part, significantly different from the lesional skin and SLS sites. Despite the fact that the qualitative results showed great similarity between HDM sites and lesional skin for mast cells, lymphocytes and histiocytes, the quantitative findings for these cells did not lead to any final conclusions that facilitated differentiation between allergic and irritant reactions.

Qualitative findings showed that lymphocytes were among the predominant cells in the majority of the lesional skin samples and HDM sites of the AD dogs. Moreover, the quantitative findings demonstrated that the proportion of T lymphocytes in HDM sites at 72 hours was comparable to that of lesional skin. The number of T lymphocytes in PT reactions and in lesional skin of humans and dogs with AD have previously been reported to be increased.[31,35] These findings confirm the presence of T cells in spontaneous AD and allergen PT reactions, and support the role of these cells in initiating and maintaining skin lesions in AD.[31]

Qualitative and quantitative findings showed that eosinophils were present in larger numbers in HDM sites compared with lesional skin and SLS sites. Eosinophilic dermatitis has been observed in two dogs and humans with AD after PT with environmental allergens.[15,23,37] The infiltration of eosinophils into atopic skin after PT with environmental allergens has been speculated to result from the release of chemotactic factors for eosinophils by keratinocytes and IgE-bound Langerhans cells following allergen challenge, thus supporting the theory of an immune response to epidermal allergen contact in AD.[31,37] It is tempting to suggest that the presence of eosinophils may allow the differentiation between allergic and irritant reactions. However, the large numbers of eosinophils in HDM sites in our study was due to two dogs with AD that had a higher proportion of eosinophils compared to the rest of the dogs. If the results of these two dogs were excluded from the quantitative analysis, the difference for eosinophils between HDM sites, lesional skin and

SLS sites was not significant. Thus, these data did not allow differentiation between allergic and irritant reactions.

Based on our qualitative and quantitative analyses, there were significantly more neutrophils in SLS reaction sites than in HDM sites. Histological investigations performed in humans, dogs and guinea-pigs also found a dermal neutrophilic infiltration in irritant contact reactions, as opposed to allergic reactions where a mononuclear infiltrate predominated.[40,42,43] Additionally, one study investigating the irritant effect of SLS reported that neutrophils were more pronounced in cases with focal necrosis, and interleukin-8, a chemotactant for neutrophils, was found in the reactions.[42] Based on our qualitative and quantitative analyses, it appears that a neutrophilic infiltrate could help in differentiating an allergic from an irritant reaction.

In the present study, qualitative and quantitative histological differences between HDM and SLS reactions, and the fact that none of the dogs without AD reacted to HDM, indicate that PT with HDM allergens on the skin of AD dogs does not induce an irritant response. Likewise, the qualitative histological similarities between HDM reactions and lesional skin suggest an allergic response to HDM.

Although our findings may not provide conclusive evidence that HDM induces an allergic reaction, our results do confirm the theory that HDM penetrate the skin of dogs with AD and induce an inflammatory reaction that likely contributes to the exacerbation or perpetuation of the clinical lesions seen in canine AD. Future studies need to be conducted that evaluate the interaction of HDM allergens and Langerhans cells in the epidermis and with T cells in the dermis, to prove the truly allergic nature of the inflammatory response induced by epicutaneous application of HDM.

Acknowlegements

The authors would like to thank Dr E. Warshaw for guidance in patch test technique and kind donation of patch test material, Drs S. Diaz and E. Kirzeder for technical assistance, and Drs S. Goyal and R. Koch for manuscript review.

Funding

Funding was provided by a CVM Small Companion Animal Grant, from the University of Minnesota.

References

1 Hillier, A., Kwochka, K.W., Pinchbeck, L.R. Reactivity to intradermal injection of extracts of *Dermatophagoides farinae*, *Dermatophagoides pteronyssinus*, house dust mite mix and house dust in dogs suspected to have atopic dermatitis: 115 cases (1996–1998). *Journal of the American Veterinary Medical Association*, 2000; **217**: 536–540.

2 Scott, D.W., Miller, W.H., Griffin, C.E. Skin immune system and allergic skin diseases. In: Scott, D.W., Miller, W.H., Griffin, C.E., eds. *Muller & Kirk's Small Animal Dermatology*, 6th edn. W.B. Saunders, Philadelphia, 2001: 543–666.

3 Leung, D.Y.M., Tharp, M., Boguniewicz, M. Atopic dermatitis (atopic eczema). In: Irwin M.F., Eisen, A.Z., Wolff, K., Austen, K.F., Goldsmith, L.A., Katz, S.I., Fitzpatrick, T.B. eds. *Fitzpatrick's Dermatology in General Medicine*, 5th edn, Vol. 2. McGraw-Hill, New York, 1999: 1464–1480.

4 Nuttal, T.J., Lamb, J.R., Hill, P.B. Peripheral blood mononuclear cell responses to *Dermatophagoides farinae* in canine atopic dermatitis. *Veterinary Immunology and Immunopathology*, 2001; **82**: 273–280.

5 Ring, J., Darsow, U., Gfesser, M., Vieluf, D. The "atopy patch test" in evaluating the role of aeroallergens in atopic eczema. *International Archives of Allergy and Immunology*, 1997; **113**: 379–383.

6 Darsow, U., Vieluf, D., Ring, J. Atopy patch test with different vehicles and allergen concentrations: an approach to standardization. *Journal of Allergy and Clinical Immunology*, 1995; **95**: 677–684.

7 Olivry, T., Hill, P.B. The ACVD task force on canine atopic dermatitis (IX): the controversy surrounding the route of allergen challenge in canine atopic dermatitis. *Veterinary Immunology and Immunopathology*, 2001; **81**: 219–225.

8 Van Voorst Vader, P.C., Lier, J.G., Woest, T.E., Coenraads, P.J., Nater, J.P. Patch tests with house dust mite antigens in atopic dermatitis patients: methodological problems. *Acta Dermato-Venereologica (Stockholm)*, 1991; **71**: 301–305.

9 Tanaka, Y., Tanaka, M., Anan, S., Yoshida, H. Immunohistochemical studies on dust mite antigen in positive reaction site of patch test. *Acta Dermato-Venereologica (Stockholm)*, 1989; **144** (Suppl.): 93–96.

10 Schopf, E., Baumgartner, A. Patch testing in atopic dermatitis. *Journal of the American Academy of Dermatology*, 1989; **21**: 860–862.

11 Langeveld-Wildschut, E.G., van Marion, A.M.W., Thepen, T., Mudde, G.C., Bruijnzeel, P.L.B., Bruijnzeel-Koomen, C.A.F.M. Evaluation of variables influencing the outcome of the atopy patch test. *Journal of Allergy and Clinical Immunology*, 1995; **96**: 66–73.

12 Langeveld-Wildschut, E.G., Bruijnzeel, P.L., Mudde, G.C., *et al.* Clinical and immunologic variables in skin of patients with atopic eczema and either positive or negative atopy patch test reactions. *Journal of Allergy and Clinical Immunology*, 2000; **105**: 1008–1016.

13 Darsow, U., Vieluf, D., Ring, J. Evaluating the relevance of aeroallergen sensitization in atopic eczema with the atopy patch test: a randomized, double-blind multicenter study. *Journal of the American Academy of Dermatology*, 1999; **40**: 187–93.

14 Darsow, U., Vieluf, D., Ring, J. The atopy patch test: an increased rate of reactivity in patients who have an air-exposed pattern of atopic eczema. *British Journal of Dermatology*, 1996; **135**: 182–186.

15 Mitchell, E.B., Crow, J., Chapman, M.D. Basophils in allergen-induced patch test sites in atopic dermatitis. *Lancet*, 1982; **1**:127–130.

16 Pigatto, P.D., Bigardi, A.S., Valsecchi, R.H., Di Landro, A. Mite patch testing in atopic eczema: a search for correct concentration. *Australian Journal of Dermatology*, 1997; **38**: 231–232.

17 Beltrani, V.S. The role of house dust mites and other aeroallergens in atopic dermatitis. *Clinics in Dermatology*, 2003; **21**: 177–182.

18 Marsella, A., Olivry, T. Animal models of atopic dermatitis. *Clinics in Dermatology*, 2003; **21**: 122–133.

19 Griffin, C.E., DeBoer, D.J. The ACVD task force on canine atopic dermatitis (XIV): clinical manifestations of atopic dermatitis. *Veterinary Immunology and Immunopathology*, 2001; **81**: 255–269.

20 Olivry, T., Moore, P.F., Affolter, V.K., Naydan, D.K. Langerhans cells hyperplasia and IgE expression in canine atopic dermatitis. *Archives of Dermatological Research*, 1996; **288**: 579–585.

21 McCall, C., Geoly, F., Clarke, C. Transdermal allergen exposure of genetically high IgE beagle puppies elicits allergen-specific IgE and dermatitis at the site of exposure (abstract). *Proceedings of the Annual Meeting of the American Academy of Veterinary Dermatology/American College of Veterinary Dermatology*, Norfolk, VA, 2001: 37.

22 Olivry, T., Buckler, K.E., Dunston, S.M., Clarke, K.B., McCall, C.A. Positive "atopy patch test" reactions in IgE-hyperresponsive beagle dogs are dependent upon elevated allergen-specific IgE serum levels and are associated with IgE-expressing dendritic cells (abstract). *Proceedings of the Annual Meeting of the American Academy of Veterinary Dermatology/American College of Veterinary Dermatology*, Norfolk, VA, 2001: 38.

23 Frank, L.A., McEntee, M.F. Demonstration of aeroallergen contact sensitivity in dogs. *Veterinary Allergy and Clinical Immunology*, 1995; **3**: 75–80.

24 Marsella, R., Olivry, T., Nicklin C.F., Saglio, S, Lopes, J., Dunstone, S.M. A model for canine atopic dermatitis: induction of dermatitis in IgE hyperresponsive Beagle dogs after house dust mite challenge (abstract). *Proceedings of the Annual Meeting of the American Academy of Veterinary Dermatology/American College of Veterinary Dermatology*, Monterey, CA, 2003: 206.

25 Willemse, T. Atopic skin disease: a review and a reconsideration of diagnostic criteria. *Journal of Small Animal Practice*, 1986; **27**: 771–778.

26 Marsella, R., Nicklin, C.F. Investigation on the use of 0.3% tacrolimus lotion for canine atopic dermatitis: a pilot study. *Veterinary Dermatology*, 2002; **13**: 203–210.

27 Mowad, C.M., Anderson, C.K. Commercial availability of a house dust mite patch test. *American Journal of Contact Dermatitis*, 2001; **12**: 115–118.

28 Jamora, M.J.J., Verallo-Rowell, V.M., Samson-Veneracion, M.T.Y. Patch testing with 20% *Dermatophagoides pteronyssinus/farinae* (Chemotechnique) antigen. *American Journal of Contact Dermatitis*, 2001; **12**: 67–71.

29 Elsner, P., Wigger-Alberti, W., Pantini, G. Perfluoropolyethers in the prevention of irritant and contact dermatitis. *International Journal for Clinical and Investigative Dermatology*, 1998; **197**: 141–145.

30 Wigger-Alberti, W., Caduff, L., Burg, G., Elsner, P. Experimentally induced chronic irritant contact dermatitis to evaluate the efficacy of protective creams in vivo. *Journal of the American Academy of Dermatology*, 1999; **40**: 590–596.

31 Olivry, T., Naydan, D.K., Moore, P.F. Characterization of the cutaneous inflammatory infiltrate in canine atopic dermatitis. *American Journal of Dermatopathology*, 1997; **19**: 477–486.

32 Pilozzi, E., Pulford, K., Jones, M., *et al.* Co-expression of CD79a (JBC117) and CD3 by lymphoblastic lymphoma. *Journal of Pathology*, 1998; **186**: 140–143.

33 Christgau, M., Caffesse, R.G., Newland, J.R., Schmalz, G., D'Souza, R.N. Characterization of immunocompetent cells in

the disease canine periodontium. *Journal of Histochemistry and Cytochemistry*, 1998; **46**:1443–1454.

34 Wahlberg, J.E. Vehicle role of petrolatum. *Acta Dermato-Venereologica (Stockholm)*, 1971; **51**: 129–134.

35 Buckley, C., Poulter, L.W., Rustin, M.H.A. Immunohistological analysis of "negative" patch test sites in atopic dermatitis. *Clinical and Experimental Allergy*, 1996; **26**: 1057–1063.

36 Reiche, L., Willis, C., Wilkinson, J., Shaw, S., de Lacharriere, O. Clinical morphology of sodium lauryl sulfate (SLS) and nonanionic acid (NNA) irritant patch test reactions at 48 and 96 h in 152 subjects. *Contact Dermatitis*, 1998; **39**: 240–243.

37 Bruynzeel-Koomen, C.A.F.M., van Wichen, D.F., Spry, C.J.F., Venge, P., Bruynzeel, P.L.B. Active participation of eosinophils in patch test reactions to inhalant allergens in patients with atopic dermatitis. *British Journal of Dermatology*, 1988; **118**: 229–238.

38 Bruijnzeel, P.L.B., Langeveld-Wildschut, A.G., Dubois, G.R., Bruijnzeel-Koomen, C.A.F.M. The involvement of eosinophils in the patch test reaction to aeroallergens in atopic dermatitis: its relevance for the pathogenesis of atopic dermatitis. *Environmental Dermatology*, 1997; **4**: 163–170.

39 Yamada, N., Wakugawa, M., Kuwata, S., Nakagawa, H., Tamaki, K. Changes in eosinophil and leukocyte infiltration and expression of IL-6 and IL-7 messenger RNA in mite allergen patch test reactions in atopic dermatitis. *Journal of Allergy and Clinical Immunology*, 1996; **98**: S201–S206.

40 Krawiec, D.R., Gaafar, S.M. A comparative study of allergic and primary irritant contact dermatitis with dinitrochlorobenzene (DNCB) in dogs. *Journal of Investigative Dermatology*, 1975; **65**: 248–251.

41 Moon, S.H., Seo, K.I., Han, W.S., *et al.* Pathological findings in cumulative irritation induced by SLS and croton oil in hairless mice. *Contact Dermatitis*, 2001; **44**: 240–245.

42 Flier, J., Boorsma, D.M., Bruynzeel, D.P., *et al.* The CXCR3 activating chemokines IP-10, Mig, and IP-9 are expressed in allergic but not in irritant patch test reactions. *Journal of Investigative Dermatology*, 1999; **113**: 574–578.

43 Karl, H., Burg, G., Braun-Falco, O. Quantitative and qualitative dynamics of the epidermal and cellular inflammatory reaction in primary toxic and allergic dinitrochlorobenzene contact dermatitis in guinea pigs. *Archives of Dermatology*, 1974; **249**: 207–226.

Conventional and rush allergen-specific immunotherapy in the treatment of canine atopic dermatitis

R.S. Mueller Dr med vet, Dr habil, K.V. Fieseler DVM, S. Zabel TÄ, MS, R.A.W. Rosychuk DVM

College of Veterinary Medicine and Biomedical Sciences, Colorado State University, Fort Collins, Colorado, USA

Summary

The purpose of this double-blinded, randomised study was to compare the results of treatment with rush allergen-specific immunotherapy (ASIT) and conventional ASIT in dogs with atopic dermatitis (AD). Twenty-four dogs with AD were included in the study (12 dogs in each group). All dogs were premedicated for 3 days with an antihistamine, and then hospitalised for 1 day. Injections with prepared treatment sets were administered every 30 minutes subcutaneously for 7 hours. Dogs were then discharged and continued with ASIT for 12 months. All dogs were evaluated for pruritus, clinical lesions and administration of concurrent medications. After 12 months of rush ASIT, significant decreases in pruritus, lesion, medication and total scores were detected with repeated measures of ANOVA as well as with the Tukey-Kramer multiple comparison test, except there was no significant decrease in the pruritus score when analysed by the Tukey-Kramer test. An improvement of >50% was observed: for pruritus in 6/11 dogs receiving rush ASIT, and 5/11 dogs receiving conventional ASIT; for lesion scores in 7/11 dogs receiving rush ASIT, and 7/11 dogs receiving conventional ASIT; and for total scores in 5/11 dogs receiving rush ASIT, and 4/11 dogs receiving conventional ASIT, respectively. The mean percentage decrease in pruritus was 36% in dogs receiving rush ASIT and 15% in dogs receiving conventional ASIT. There was no significant difference between groups in the time to 50% improvement or to maximal improvement in pruritus or lesion scores. No adverse effects were noted during the induction phase in any dogs. The results of this study suggest that rush ASIT with subcutaneous allergen injection is safe and shows promise as an efficacious treatment for canine AD.

Introduction

Canine atopic dermatitis (AD) is a common disease in small animal practice.[1] Symptomatic treatments include antihistamines, fatty acid supplementation, immunophilin-binding macrolides and glucocorticoids.[2–4] The only specific treatment presently known is allergen-specific immunotherapy (ASIT).[5–7]

Typically, conventional ASIT is initiated with a low dose of the allergen extract with gradually increasing doses over a period of weeks to months (induction period), followed by long-term administration of high doses of allergen extract at specific regular intervals (maintenance period). Conventional ASIT has been reported to have significant beneficial effects in 45–100% of dogs with AD.[5–9] The efficacy of conventional ASIT is greater than that seen with antihistamines or fatty acid supplementation, and adverse effects occur less frequently than with glucocorticoid administration.[5–7] However, the majority of patients do not show significant improvement in the first few months of conventional ASIT.[5] Thus, pruritus persists during this time, causing significant distress for the affected dog and concern for their owners. At the commencement of conventional ASIT, there is a potential for misunderstanding due to the changing dosages of allergens and the multiple vials of allergens of increasing concentration that form part of the induction period. A more ideal regimen would circumvent these potential problems in the induction period, as well as provide a more rapid clinical response than is currently experienced with conventional ASIT.

Rush ASIT has been extensively used in allergic human patients with good success.[10–12] Rush ASIT is characterised by a dramatically reduced time interval between injections of increasing quantities of allergen, with a consequent decrease in the induction period to 1–3 days. Rush ASIT has been described in veterinary medicine[13] and its safety has been established,[14] although its clinical efficacy in the treatment of canine AD has not previously been reported.

The aims of this study were to determine the efficacy of rush ASIT in the treatment of canine AD, to compare the efficacy of rush ASIT with the efficacy of conventional ASIT, and to assess whether rush ASIT leads to a more rapid reduction in clinical signs than conventional ASIT.

Materials and methods

Dogs included in this study were patients of the Dermatology Service of the Veterinary Teaching Hospital, Colorado State University. AD was diagnosed based on history, clinical examination and exclusion of differential diagnoses, such as cutaneous adverse food reaction or scabies, with appropriate tests or treatments, as described previously.[2,5]

Offending allergens were identified with a routine intradermal test (IDT).[15] Reactions were graded from 0 to 4 compared to a negative control (graded 0) (a solution of 0.04% potassium phosphate, 0.11% sodium phosphate, 0.50% sodium chloride and 0.40% phenol; Sterile diluent for allergenic extracts [Greer Laboratories, Lenoir, NC, USA]) and a positive control (graded 4) (histamine phosphate 0.275 mg/ml; Histatrol [Center Laboratories, Port Washington, NY, USA]). Reactions graded 2 or higher were considered to be positive.

Owners of dogs with AD who elected to pursue ASIT as the treatment of choice for their pet's disease were offered the opportunity to participate in this study, and signed a consent form prior to their inclusion. Allergens that were positive on the IDT, and where exposure to these allergens correlated well with the clinical history, were included in the allergen extract for ASIT. Allergen extracts were prepared as reported previously.[5] All owners volunteering their pet for the study were given identical extensive education (irrespective of the type of ASIT their pet was to receive) about conventional and rush ASIT prior to inclusion in the study. They were informed of the possible adverse effects of ASIT in general (e.g. anaphylactic reactions, increased pruritus and local injection reactions) and the possibility of an increased chance of such adverse effects during the rush induction period on day 1. All dogs were evaluated by a clinician prior to commencement of therapy. Both the clinicians and the owners were blinded as to which form of ASIT was to be administered. The study was approved by the Animal Care and Use Committee of Colorado State University.

ASIT protocols

Two sets of syringes were prepared by a veterinary technician for each dog. The first set contained syringes labelled from no. 1 to no. 12 to be used on day 1. The second set contained syringes labelled from no. 1 to no. 13 and was sent home with the owner together with a vial of the most concentrated allergen extract for maintenance therapy.

Dogs were assigned to one of two groups using a table of random numbers and simple randomisation. Dogs in group A were to receive rush ASIT, while dogs in group B received conventional ASIT. In group A, the first set of syringes contained increasing concentrations of allergen extract (Table 1.8.1). Based on the results of an unpublished pilot study, the final injection of the induction regimen for rush ASIT was 0.4

Table 1.8.1 Allergen set for dogs in group A (rush ASIT) used on day 1

Time	Syringe no.	Total allergen content (PNU)	Time	Syringe no.	Total allergen content (PNU)	Time	Syringe no.	Total allergen content (PNU)
8.30	1	40	11.00	6	400	13.30	11	4000
9.00	2	80	11.30	7	800	14.00	12	8000
9.30	3	120	12.00	8	1200			
10.00	4	160	12.30	9	1600			
10.30	5	200	13.00	10	2000			

PNU, protein nitrogen units.

Table 1.8.2 Allergen set for dogs in group A (rush ASIT) sent home with the owner

Day	Syringe no.	Total allergen content (PNU)	Day	Syringe no.	Total allergen content (PNU)	Day	Syringe no.	Total allergen content (PNU)
3	1	0	13	6	0	23	11	0
5	2	0	15	7	20 000	25	12	0
7	3	12 000	17	8	0	27	13	20 000
9	4	0	19	9	0	35	Maintenance vial	20 000
11	5	16 000	21	10	20 000	Every 7 days		20 000

PNU, protein nitrogen units.

ml of the most concentrated allergen extract (20 000 protein nitrogen units [PNU]/ml) to minimise the number of dogs having adverse reactions to the allergens.

The second set of syringes for dogs in group A contained 1 ml saline in most syringes, except that syringe no. 3 was filled with 0.6 ml of allergen extract (12 000 PNU); syringe no. 5 with 0.8 ml of allergen extract (16 000 PNU); and syringe nos 7, 10 and 13 with 1 ml of allergen extract (20 000 PNU) (Table 1.8.2).

In group B, the first set of syringes contained saline solution with the exception of syringe no. 1 that contained 40 PNU of allergen extract (Table 1.8.3). The second set of syringes for dogs of group B contained increasing quantities of allergen extract as described previously;[7] saline solution was added to fill each syringe to provide a total volume of 1 ml (Table 1.8.4).

The quantity of allergen (in PNU) for each injection was the combined total of all allergens included in the extract. Thus, the quantity of each individual allergen in each injection varied between dogs depending on the number of allergens included in the extract for the individual dog.

All allergen injections in both groups were administered subcutaneously.

Induction phase

All dogs were premedicated with an antihistamine at the recommended dose[2,3,16] for 3 days before the commencement of the induction phase, irrespective of their previous or concurrent medications. Dogs were then hospitalised at 8.00 a.m. on day 1 of the study. Day 1 was always in the first half of the week to ensure availability of a clinician as well as a local veterinarian during the first 2–3 days post treatment.

An intravenous catheter was placed in the cephalic vein and bandaged in place. Epinephrine 1:1000 (1 mg/ml [Amphastar IMS, Rancho Cucamonga, CA, USA]) was drawn up in a labelled syringe at a dose of 0.02 mg/kg and was available for immediate use during the day. Injections with prepared treatment sets were administered every 30 minutes subcutaneously. Prior to each injection, dogs were examined and the pulse, respiratory rate, temperature and capillary refill time were recorded, along with any changes identified on physical examination. If any of these parameters were recorded to be outside of the normal range, or if abnormalities were detected on physical examination, the next injection was not administered and the dog was re-evaluated 30 minutes later. If the abnormal parameters had normalised after 30 minutes, the next

Table 1.8.3 Allergen set for dogs in group B (conventional ASIT) used on day 1

Time	Syringe no.	Total allergen content (PNU)	Time	Syringe no.	Total allergen content (PNU)	Time	Syringe no.	Total allergen content (PNU)
8.30	1	40	11.00	6	0	13.30	11	0
9.00	2	0	11.30	7	0	14.00	12	0
9.30	3	0	12.00	8	0			
10.00	4	0	12.30	9	0			
10.30	5	0	13.00	10	0			

PNU, protein nitrogen units.

Table 1.8.4 Allergen set for dogs in group B (conventional ASIT) sent home with the owner

Day	Syringe no.	Total allergen content (PNU)	Day	Syringe no.	Total allergen content (PNU)	Day	Syringe no.	Total allergen content (PNU)
3	1	80	13	6	800	23	11	8000
5	2	120	15	7	1200	25	12	12 000
7	3	160	17	8	1600	27	13	16 000
9	4	200	19	9	2000	35	Maintenance vial	20 000
11	5	400	21	10	4000	Every 7 days		20 000

PNU, protein nitrogen units.

injection was administered. If not, the induction phase was discontinued and the dog was discharged and prescribed conventional ASIT as described previously.[7]

Dogs were monitored closely by a veterinary technician at all times during the first day of treatment until at least 2 hours after the last injection was administered. In case of anaphylactic shock, epinephrine was to be administered intravenously[17] and the dog was to be transferred to the intensive care unit of the Veterinary Teaching Hospital at Colorado State University to receive further treatment as determined by the emergency care clinician. All dogs that successfully completed the rush induction on day 1 were discharged with an injection protocol as outlined in Tables 1.8.2 and 1.8.4, depending on group assignment.

Follow-up evaluations

Each dog was presented to the clinician for evaluation after 3, 6, 9 and 12 months of ASIT. With few exceptions, the same clinician evaluated each patient at each revisit.

Pruritus score

The owner was asked at each revisit to mark the average pruritus as observed during the last month on a visual analogue scale ranging from 0 to 30.

Lesion score

Lesions evaluated by the clinician included alopecia, erythema, papules, crusts, hyperpigmentation and greasiness. Each lesion was described as mild (only found on thorough examination, score 1.5 points), moderate (affecting < 20% of the body, score 3 points) and severe (affecting > 20% of the body, score 4.5 points).

Medication score

The medication score was determined based on the medications given during the 2 weeks prior to the examination. No concurrent medication was scored 0 points, topical therapy alone was scored 5 points, and antihistamines and/or fatty acid supplementation were scored 10 points. The score for glucocorticoids was determined by calculating the average daily dose of glucocorticoid being administered. A dose of >1 mg/kg of prednisone or prednisolone scored 40 points, a dose of 0.5–1 mg/kg scored 30 points, a dose of 0.2–0.5 mg/kg scored 20 points, and a dose <0.2 mg/kg scored 10 points.

Total scores

Total scores were calculated by adding the medication and lesion score at the time of examination and the owner's pruritus score over the last month.

Evaluation of time until 50% improvement

As a mean reduction in lesion and pruritus score of > 50% is perceived as satisfactory by owners,[18] the number of dogs improving by > 50% in lesion and pruritus scores was determined. In addition, the time to 50% improvement of lesion, pruritus and total scores, as well as the time to maximal improvement of pruritus scores was compared between dogs receiving rush ASIT and dogs receiving conventional ASIT.

Statistical analysis

Pruritus, lesion and medication scores were compared by repeated measures ANOVA. Subjective evaluations of pruritus, performed by continuous scale plotting, were quantitated, and the scale distances were evaluated as continuous data for normality of distribution by a Kolmogorov-Smirnov test. Normally distributed data were compared over time by repeated measures ANOVA. With significance measured by ANOVA, a multiple comparison post test was conducted and group means were compared by a Tukey-Kramer multiple comparison test. The time to 50% improvement of pruritus, lesion and total scores and to maximal improvement of pruritus for each type of ASIT were compared with an unpaired Student t-test. Patients not completing the study were recorded and included as 'intention to treat' analysis with last measured values carried forward. Age, duration of disease and the number of allergens included in the extracts were compared between groups using an unpaired t-test with confirmed normality of distribution, otherwise a Mann–Whitney test was used. In addition, the percentage improvement in lesion, medication, pruritus, and total scores after 12 months of treatment were calculated, and differences between the groups were compared with an unpaired t-test. A p value of < 0.05 was considered significant.

Results

Twenty-four dogs were included in the study. Twelve dogs were treated with rush ASIT (group A) and 12 dogs with conventional ASIT (group B). The mean age of the dogs in group A was 3.6 years (range 1.5–8 years) and 4.8 years (range 1.5–9 years) for dogs in group B. The mean duration of disease for dogs in group A was 2.4 years (range 1–6 years), and 2.1 years (range 1–4 years) for dogs in group B. The mean number of allergens included in the extract was 19 (range 4–44) for dogs in group A, and 16 (range 4–41) for dogs in group B. There was no significant difference between groups for the age of dogs, duration of disease or the number of allergens included in the extract.

Dogs in group A included: Labrador retriever (n = 3), mixed breed (3), Boston terrier (1), cocker spaniel (1), golden retriever (1), pug (1), Shih Tzu (1) and Staffordshire terrier (1). Dogs in group B included: Labrador retriever (5), golden retriever (2), dalmatian (2), Maltese (1), Saint Bernard (1) and mixed breed (1). In each group, 10 dogs had non-seasonal AD. In group A, one dog had clinical signs in spring and summer, and in group B, one dog had clinical signs in summer and fall. One dog from each group did not complete the study: the dog in group A was euthanased due to severe AD; the owner of the dog in group B refused to return for re-evaluations.

There was no significant difference in medication scores, pruritus scores and lesion scores between the groups at the beginning of the study. None of the dogs showed any adverse effects during the rush ASIT induction day (day 1). The scores for pruritus, lesions, medication and total scores prior to ASIT and after 12 months of ASIT for each group of dogs are presented in Fig. 1.8.1. There was a significant decrease in the median pruritus scores (p = 0.0333), lesion scores (p = 0.0001), medication scores (p = 0.0001) and total scores (p = 0.0001) after 12 months in dogs receiving rush ASIT. There were no significant differences for any of the evaluated scores after 12 months in dogs receiving conventional ASIT.

Using a Tukey-Kramer multiple comparison test, the mean medication score and mean total score of dogs receiving rush ASIT were significantly decreased after 3 months of therapy, and the mean lesion score of dogs receiving rush ASIT was significantly decreased after 6 months of therapy (Table 1.8.5). These significant decreases from baseline values (day 1) were maintained throughout the course of rush ASIT. There was no significant difference in pruritus scores in the rush ASIT group at any time point (compared to baseline) with the Tukey-Kramer multiple comparison test.

There was no significant difference in any of the scores at any time point (compared to baseline) in dogs receiving conventional ASIT with the Tukey-Kramer multiple comparison test.

Although the average time to achieve 50% improvement in pruritus scores was shorter in dogs receiving rush ASIT compared with those receiving conventional ASIT (5.4 and 7.6 months, respectively), this difference was not significant. Similarly, the time to maximal improvement of pruritus was shorter in dogs receiving rush ASIT than in dogs receiving conventional ASIT (6.8 and 9.2 months, respectively), but the difference was also not significant. There was no significant difference between groups in the time taken to achieve 50% reduction, or maximal reduction, in lesion and total scores.

An improvement of >50% was recorded after 12 months of therapy for each scoring parameter in individual dogs as follows: for pruritus score in 6/11 dogs receiving rush ASIT and 5/11 dogs receiving conventional ASIT; for lesion scores in 7/11 dogs in both groups; for medication scores in 7/11 dogs receiving rush ASIT and 2/11 receiving conventional ASIT; and for total scores in 5/11 dogs receiving rush ASIT and 4/11 dogs receiving conventional ASIT.

The mean percentage decrease for each scoring parameter in each group after 12 months of therapy was

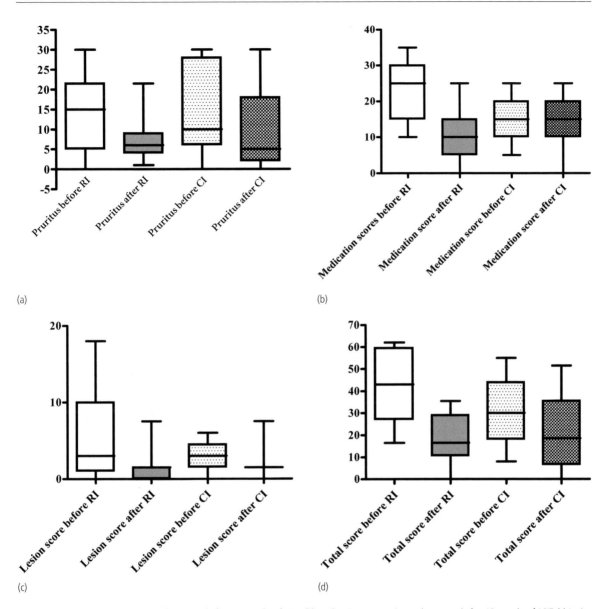

Fig. 1.8.1 (a) Pruritus scores prior to therapy and after 12 months of ASIT. (b) Medication scores prior to therapy and after 12 months of ASIT. (c) Lesion scores prior to therapy and after 12 months of ASIT. (d) Total scores prior to therapy and after 12 months of ASIT. The line represents the median value for all dogs in the group. The box indicates the 25th to 75th percentile for all dogs in the group. The bars indicate the range of scores for all dogs in the group. ☐ Dogs receiving rush ASIT: prior to therapy. ■ Dogs receiving rush ASIT: 12 months of therapy. ▨ Dogs receiving conventional ASIT: prior to therapy. ▨ Dogs receiving conventional ASIT: 12 months of therapy. CI, conventional immunotherapy. RI, rush immunotherapy.

recorded as follows: for pruritus scores there was a 36% decrease in the dogs receiving rush ASIT compared with a 15% decrease in those receiving conventional ASIT; for medication scores there was a 41% decrease in dogs receiving rush ASIT compared with a 5% decrease in those receiving conventional ASIT; for lesional scores there was a 54% decrease in dogs receiving rush ASIT compared with a 27% decrease in those receiving conventional ASIT; and for total scores there was a 48% decrease for dogs receiving rush ASIT compared with a 31% decrease in those receiving conventional ASIT. There was no significant difference in the mean

Table 1.8.5 Pruritus, medication, lesion and total scores of dogs undergoing ASIT (mean ± standard deviation) at 0, 3, 6, 9 and 12 months

Parameter	Rush ASIT	Conventional ASIT
Pruritus		
0 months	13.5 ± 9.4	13.9 ± 10.8
3 months	9.5 ± 8.1	9.9 ± 8.8
6 months	6.4 ± 4.0	7.1 ± 7.3
9 months	6.2 ± 3.3	13.0 ± 9.6
12 months	6.7 ± 5.6	10.3 ± 11.0
Medication score		
0 months	23.6 ± 8.4	14.1 ± 6.6
3 months	11.4 ± 9.5*	13.6 ± 10.7
6 months	14.1 ± 10.7*	10.5 ± 6.9
9 months	10.9 ± 10.0*	8.1 ± 8.2
12 months	10.0 ± 7.1*	13.6 ± 7.1
Lesion score		
0 months	5.9 ± 5.9	3.0 ± 2.0
3 months	2.6 ± 3.0	2.2 ± 3.6
6 months	1.6 ± 1.6*	1.9 ± 2.1
9 months	1.5 ± 1.3*	1.6 ± 1.1
12 months	1.9 ± 2.5*	1.9 ± 2.0
Total score		
0 months	42.0 ± 15.9	30.6 ± 14.7
3 months	26.7 ± 14.7*	25.7 ± 19.8
6 months	23.6 ± 13.1*	19.5 ± 11.8
9 months	15.6 ± 13.8*	24.9 ± 15.4
12 months	18.1 ± 11.1*	21.5 ± 16.7

*Significant difference from value at 0 months (Tukey-Kramer multiple comparison test).

percentage decrease in any of the scoring parameters between treatment groups.

No adverse reactions to ASIT were reported in any of the dogs at any time throughout the course of the study.

Discussion

This double-blinded, randomised study provides supportive evidence for the safety and efficacy of rush ASIT as a treatment for canine AD.

In conventional ASIT, allergens are injected subcutaneously in gradually increasing concentrations (typically starting at 200–400 PNU/ml) during the induction period of several weeks or months, and increasing to a maintenance dose of allergen (typically 20 000–40 000 PNU/ml).[2,5,7,18] Maintenance therapy is usually continued lifelong; some patients stay in remission after discontinuing ASIT.[5] Conventional ASIT has been reported to be successful in 45–100% of ca-

nine patients,[5–9] reflecting differences between studies regarding the parameters used to determine success, injection protocols, allergen sources, allergen concentration, numbers of patients included and follow-up periods.

Rush ASIT aims to avoid the problems inherent in an extended induction period. It has been used extensively in human medicine when there is a need to achieve rapid clinical improvement in patients with severe (and sometimes life-threatening) conditions. This has been predominantly in patients with hypersensitivity to wasps or bees,[10–12,10–12] but also in patients allergic to house dust mite,[19,20] grass pollen[21] and moulds.[22]

MacDonald administered rush ASIT to six laboratory dogs with atopy and five client-owned atopic dogs; however, the efficacy of the therapy was not reported.[13] A successful outcome of rush ASIT was reported in one dog with severe ragweed and grass pollen allergy.[23] In an unpublished rush ASIT pilot study, the authors observed a rapid resolution in pruritus within the first weeks of therapy in some of the animals. Furthermore, two dogs that had deteriorated during conventional ASIT and discontinued this therapy subsequently responded to the same allergen extract when administered according to a rush ASIT protocol.

The goal of this study was to provide evidence for the efficacy of rush ASIT following a double-blinded, randomised design. Due to the long duration of the study, a placebo control was considered unethical. Instead, the control group consisted of dogs treated with the currently accepted standard conventional ASIT.

We found that rush ASIT was associated with a significant improvement in all scoring parameters after 12 months of therapy when analysed by repeated measures of ANOVA. There was also significant improvement in medication, lesion and total scores (but not pruritus scores) when analysed by the Tukey-Kramer multiple comparison test. In contrast, there was no significant improvement for any of the scoring parameters in dogs receiving conventional ASIT. These results suggest that rush ASIT may have the potential to be more efficacious than conventional ASIT.

However, there was no significant difference in the mean percentage decrease in any of the scoring parameters between dogs that received rush ASIT and those that received conventional ASIT, and neither was there a significant decrease in pruritus in either group when the pruritus scores were analysed by the Tukey-Kramer multiple comparison test. Furthermore, at least 50%

improvement in pruritus and lesion scores were recorded in a similar number of dogs in each treatment group (7/11 in each group for lesion score, and 6/11 for pruritus score in the rush ASIT group and 5/11 in pruritus score for the conventional ASIT group). These results suggest that rush ASIT and conventional ASIT have similar efficacy.

There are several possible reasons for these conflicting results. Foremost, the number of patients included in this study was small. Future studies that include a larger sample size (where variables such as patient characteristics and differences in allergen content of ASIT, for example, would be minimised) may provide significant findings. In studies with a small sample size, a severe deterioration in a few patients impacts mean scores more than global assessment scores.

Secondly, most reports of clinical response to ASIT have considered only global assessments without performance of specific medication and clinical scores.[5,7–9] In only one report were lesions and pruritus scored by investigators and owners respectively, but improvement in pruritus and lesion score was not separated and only total scores were subsequently reported.[6] Detailed scoring systems to assess treatment responses have only recently become internationally accepted in veterinary dermatology. Assessment of 50% improvement seems to be the closest outcome measure to previously reported global assessments. Thus, in our study, the number of patients with at least 50% improvement in pruritus and lesion scores was similar to the previously reported response to conventional ASIT. Comparison of mean clinical and treatment scores is not possible as these have not been previously performed and statistical analysis has not been applied to the data in any of the previous studies, except one which was the only blinded trial.[6]

Thirdly, it is known that assessment of efficacy in open studies is in general much better than that of corresponding blinded, randomised, controlled trials.[4] Only one previous study of ASIT in canine AD was blinded,[6] and the lack of significant changes in clinical and treatment scores in dogs receiving conventional ASIT in our study emphasises the need for randomised, controlled trials (with appropriate scoring systems and clear outcome measures) when evaluating treatments of canine AD.

Finally, dogs in this study remained on the predetermined protocol of ASIT injections, irrespective of individual response. Variation and adjustment of the quantity of allergen injected, and the frequency of injections is considered to increase the success rate, and may have improved the results seen in this study as well.

Improvement of clinical signs may occur as early as 4 weeks after the commencement of ASIT, typically only occurs after 4–6 months of ASIT, and may take even longer in some cases.[5,7] This delay in response can cause significant distress for the pruritic animals and be of great concern to their owners. In addition, the induction period with conventional ASIT is characterised by constantly changing allergen dose and concentration (usually utilising multiple vials of allergen), thus increasing the risk of incorrect treatment or discontinuation of therapy. Circumventing the longer induction period of conventional ASIT, and the potential for a more rapid clinical response with rush ASIT, could have a significant impact on the well-being of the animal. In the study reported here, although the mean time to 50% improvement of pruritus and the mean time to maximal improvement of pruritus were more rapid in dogs receiving rush ASIT compared with dogs receiving conventional ASIT, these differences were not significant. As previously stated, this may be due to the small number of patients included in the study. It is also possible that more frequent patient evaluation and scoring (for example, monthly instead of every 3 months) may have allowed more accurate assessment of the time taken until 50% improvement was detected.

Studies in humans provide some insight into reasons why rush ASIT may be efficacious and clinical response may be seen more rapidly. In oral tolerance, high doses of antigen induce an antigen-specific anergic state in the peripheral immune system.[24] Similarly, IL-4 production of T cells derived from allergic individuals is down-regulated with high doses of antigen.[25] Furthermore, a rapid increase in allergen-specific IgG4 concentrations was demonstrated in human house dust mite allergic patients in contrast to the slow increase seen with conventional ASIT.[26] The immunologic mechanisms activated during the rapid induction phase with rush ASIT in canine AD, and how these mechanisms may differ from those induced by conventional ASIT, are currently unknown.

Several studies have evaluated the safety of rush ASIT in humans.[12,27,28] Adverse effects included mild exacerbation of clinical symptoms and, less commonly, anaphylactic shock. However, no patients had to be admitted to an intensive care unit and rush ASIT was considered a safe therapy to administer in an ambulatory setting. In two previous studies, the incidence of adverse effects was significantly reduced when patients were premedicated with antihistamines[28] or glucocorticoids.[27] In another study, reactions occurred more commonly during the induction period and were rare during maintenance therapy. Adverse effects were seen within the first 45 minutes.[19]

In a pilot study to assess safety in veterinary medicine, rush ASIT was administered to 30 dogs and found to be a safe treatment.[14] The safety of rush ASIT was confirmed in the study reported here. None of the 12 dogs receiving rush ASIT showed any adverse effects during the induction phase. In the previously performed pilot study, increased pruritus was seen in 32% of the dogs with intradermal injections of allergen extract and local irritation was seen in some dogs. The protocol for the current study was subsequently modified whereby allergens were injected subcutaneously; this modification appears to have eliminated the adverse effects described previously.

In summary, this study provides evidence that rush ASIT shows promise as an efficacious treatment for canine AD. As adverse effects appear to be minimal when allergens are administered subcutaneously, rush ASIT may be useful in overcoming the potential for misunderstanding, and deviation from the intended protocol, that are inherent in the longer induction phase of conventional ASIT. Further controlled studies, with larger numbers of dogs, are necessary to confirm the efficacy of rush ASIT and whether rush ASIT is associated with a more rapid clinical response than conventional ASIT.

Acknowledgements

The authors would like to thank Tracey Greenwalt for her organisational skills and expert technical help, Dr Sonya Bettenay for technical assistance, and the owners of the dogs included in the study for their dedication.

Funding

This study was supported by a grant from the Morris Animal Foundation.

References

1 Scott, D.W., Paradis, M. A survey of canine and feline skin disorders seen in a university practice: small animal clinic, University of Montreal, St Hyacinthe, Quebec (1987–1988). *Canadian Veterinary Journal,* 1990; **31**: 830–835.
2 Scott, D.W., Miller, W.H., Griffin, C.E. *Small Animal Dermatology,* 6th edn. W.B. Saunders, Philadelphia, 2001: 547–601.
3 Mueller, R.S. Diagnosis and management of canine atopic disease. *Australian Veterinary Practitioner,* 1993; **23**: 20–27.
4 Olivry, T., Mueller, R.S. Evidence-based veterinary dermatology: a systematic review on the pharmacotherapy of canine atopic dermatitis. *Veterinary Dermatology,* 2003; **14**: 121–146.
5 Mueller, R.S., Bettenay, S.V. Long-term immunotherapy of 146 dogs with atopic dermatitis – a retrospective study. *Australian Veterinary Practitioner,* 1996; **26**: 128–132.
6 Willemse, A., Van den Brom, W.E., Rijnberk, A. Effect of hyposensitisation on atopic dermatitis in dogs. *Journal of the American Veterinary Medical Association,* 1984; **184**: 1277–1280.
7 Scott, K.V., White, S.D., Rosychuk, R.A.W. A retrospective study of hyposensitization in atopic dogs in a flea-scarce environment. In: Ihrke, P.J., Mason, I.S., White, S.D., eds. *Advances in Veterinary Dermatology.* Pergamon Press, New York, 1993: 79–87.
8 Walton Angarano, D., MacDonald, J.M. Immunotherapy in canine atopy. In: Kirk, R.W., ed. *Current Veterinary Therapy XI.* W.B. Saunders, Philadelphia, 1992: 505–508.
9 Scott, D.W. Observations on canine atopy. *Journal of the American Animal Hospital Association,* 1981; **17**: 91–100.
10 Prinz, J.C., Bieber, T., Ring, J., Rieber, E.P. Influence of rush immunotherapy with bee venom on allergen induced lymphocyte proliferation and FcepsilonRII/CD23-expression on T-lymphocytes. *Allergologie,* 1990; **13**: S35–S38.
11 Antonicelli, L., Pucci, S., Bilo, M.B., Garritani, M.S., Bonifazi, F. Early decrease in skin reactivity after rush venom immunotherapy. *Journal of Allergy and Clinical Immunology,* 1994; **4**: 57–60.
12 Bernstein, J.A., Kagen, S.L., Bernstein, D.I., Bernstein, I.L. Rapid venom immunotherapy is safe for routine use in the treatment of patients with Hymenoptera anaphylaxis. *Annals of Allergy,* 1994; **73**: 423–428.
13 MacDonald, J.M. Rush hyposensitization in the treatment of canine atopy (abstract). *Proceedings of the 15th Annual Meeting of the American Academy of Veterinary Dermatology/American College of Veterinary Dermatology,* Maui, HI, 1999: 95–97.
14 Mueller, R.S., Bettenay, S.V., Tan, W. Evaluation of the safety of an abbreviated course of injections of allergen extracts (rush immunotherapy) for the treatment of dogs with atopic dermatitis. *American Journal of Veterinary Research,* 2001; **62**: 307–311.
15 Mueller, R.S., Bettenay, S.V., Tideman, L. Aero-allergens in canine atopic dermatitis in south-eastern Australia based on 1000 intradermal skin tests. *Australian Veterinary Journal,* 2000; **78**: 392–399.
16 Paterson, S. Use of antihistamines to control pruritus in atopic dogs. *Journal of Small Animal Practice,* 1994; **35**: 412–419.
17 Cohen, R.D. Systemic anaphylaxis. In: Bonagura, J.D., ed. *Kirk's Current Veterinary Therapy XII.* W.B. Saunders, Philadelphia, 1995: 150–152.
18 Olivry, T., Steffan, J., Fisch, R.D. Randomized controlled trial of the efficacy of cyclosporine in the treatment of atopic dermatitis in dogs. *Journal of the American Veterinary Medical Association,* 2002; **221**: 370–377.
19 Bousquet, J., Hejjaoui, A., Dhivert, H., Clauzel, A.M., Michel, F.B. Immunotherapy with a standardized *Dermatophagoides pteronyssinus* extract. III. Systemic reactions during the rush protocol in patients suffering from asthma. *Journal of Allergy and Clinical Immunology,* 1989; **83**: 797–802.
20 Leynadier, F., Nissen, A.F., Halpern, G.M., Murrieta, M., Garcia-Duarte, C., Dry, J. Blocking IgG antibodies after rush immunotherapy with mites. *Annals of Allergy,* 1986; **57**: 325–329.
21 Bousquet, J., Guerin, B., Dotte, A., *et al.* Comparison between

rush immunotherapy with a standardized allergen and an alum adjuved pyridine extracted material in grass pollen allergy. *Clinical Allergy,* 1985; **15**: 179–193.

22 Horst, M., Hejjaoui, A., Horst, V., Michel, F.B., Bousquet, J. Double-blind, placebo-controlled rush immunotherapy with a standardized Alternaria extract. *Journal of Allergy and Clinical Immunology,* 1990; **85**: 460–472.

23 Patterson, R., Harris, K.E. Rush immunotherapy in a dog with severe ragweed and grass pollen allergy. *Annals of Allergy, Asthma and Immunology,* 1999; **83**: 213–216.

24 Xiao, B.G., Link, H. Mucosal tolerance: a two-edged sword to prevent and treat auto-immune diseases. *Clinical Immunology and Immunopathology,* 1997; **85**: 119–128.

25 Secrist, H., DeKryuff, R.H., Umetsu, D.T. Interleukin 4 production by CD4+ T cells from allergic individuals is modulated by antigen concentration and allergen presenting cell type. *Journal of Experimental Medicine,* 1995; **181**: 1081–1089.

26 Lack, G., Nelson, H.S., Amran, D., *et al.* Rush immunotherapy results in allergen-specific alterations in lymphocyte function and interferon-gamma production in CD4+ T cells. *Journal of Allergy and Clinical Immunology,* 1997; **99**: 530–538.

27 Hejjaoui, A., Dhivert, H., Michel, F.B., Bousquet, J. Immunotherapy with a standardized *Dermatophagoides pteronyssinus* extract. IV. Systemic reactions according to the immunotherapy schedule. *Journal of Allergy and Clinical Immunology,* 1990; **85**: 473–479.

28 Berchtold, E., Maibach, R., Muller, U. Reduction of side effects from rush immunotherapy with honey bee venom pretreatment with terfenadine. *Clinical and Experimental Allergy,* 1992; **22**: 59–65.

Dermatophagoides farinae-specific IgG subclass responses in atopic dogs undergoing allergen-specific immunotherapy

C. Hou BVM[1], T.J. Nuttall BSc, BVSc, PhD[2], M.J. Day BSc, BVMS (Hons), PhD[3], P.B. Hill BVSc, PhD, DVD[1]

[1] Royal (Dick) School of Veterinary Studies, University of Edinburgh, Roslin, Midlothian, UK
[2] Faculty of Veterinary Science, University of Liverpool, Liverpool, UK
[3] School of Clinical Veterinary Science, University of Bristol, Langford, North Somerset, UK

Summary

The molecular and immunologic mechanisms involved in successful allergen-specific immunotherapy (ASIT) have not been completely elucidated. The aim of this study was to characterise the changes in *Dermatophagoides farinae*-specific total IgG and IgG subclasses during ASIT of dogs with atopic dermatitis.

Twenty-one dogs with *D. farinae* hypersensitivity were treated with alum-precipitated vaccines for 9 months. Serum samples were collected before and after 3, 6 and 9 months of therapy and used to probe Western blots containing separated proteins of *D. farinae*. IgG responses were detected using a polyclonal antibody and a colorimetric substrate, whereas IgG subclasses were detected using a panel of monoclonal anti-IgG antibodies and chemiluminescence. The blots were analysed using a semi-quantitative digital image analysis system that provided the number and molecular weight of bands, as well as their intensity, which was related to IgG concentration. Prior to ASIT, all dogs showed an IgG, IgG1 and IgG4 response to multiple proteins of different molecular weights, the most common being 98 kDa and 44 kDa. There was virtually no detectable IgG2 or IgG3 response. During ASIT, the total IgG, IgG1 and IgG4 response to *D. farinae* antigens varied widely between dogs and could increase, decrease, fluctuate or remain the same, but there was no induction of IgG2 or IgG3 antibodies. There were no significant increases in total IgG or IgG subclass responses in dogs showing a complete or partial response to ASIT. However, dogs showing no response to ASIT had significantly higher *D. farinae*-specific total IgG levels prior to the start of therapy, compared to dogs that responded to ASIT.

Introduction

Allergen-specific immunotherapy (ASIT) is the practice of administering gradually increasing quantities of an allergen extract to an allergic subject to ameliorate the symptoms associated with subsequent exposure to the causative allergen.[1,2] Since the first reports of ASIT in humans[3,4] and in the dog,[5] many studies, and a large body of clinical observations by veterinary dermatologists, have suggested that ASIT can be effective in controlling the signs of atopic dermatitis (AD) in dogs.[2,6,7] Most of these data are either anecdotal or originate from questionnaire-based studies and, to date, there has been only one placebo-controlled study that has investigated this form of treatment in dogs.[8] Collectively, this body of information and literature has resulted in efficacy claims ranging from 50% to 100%, with a response usually being defined as an improvement in clinical signs of at least 50%.[2]

Two main forms of ASIT vaccines are currently used in dogs: aqueous vaccines are favoured in North America whereas aluminium-adsorbed vaccines are commonly used in Europe. A comparison between these vaccine types of their true efficacy is not possible because different studies quote differences in allergen extracts, the number of allergens used, the concentration of allergens, the frequency of administration, as well as symptom scores which are easily influenced by other factors such as infections. However, one potential advantage of aluminium-adjuvanted vaccines is the more rapid development of high titre, and long-lasting, antibody responses after primary immunisation.[9] The mechanism of action of aluminium adjuvants likely involves the formation of a depot, increasing targeting of antigens to antigen-presenting cells, and non-specific activation of the immune response.[10]

Although the clinical efficacy of ASIT is well documented in humans and dogs, the molecular and immunological mechanisms involved are incompletely understood. Current evidence from rodent and human studies suggests that ASIT exerts effects on several aspects of the immune system, including modulation of allergen-specific B cells as well as T-cell responses. Studies on the effect of ASIT have demonstrated reduced basophil reactivity to allergens,[11] deviation of Th2-cytokine responses to allergens in favour of a Th1 response,[12–15] and the induction of IL-10-producing regulatory T cells.[16–18] In addition, changes in serum antibody titres in response to ASIT have been described, mostly as increases in allergen-specific IgG antibodies, particularly of the IgG1 and IgG4 isotypes.[19,20] Allergen-specific IgG produced in response to ASIT has been termed 'blocking antibody' because it has been proposed that competition with IgE may prevent successful activation of mast cells.

To the authors' knowledge, only two studies investigating changes in IgG concentrations have been reported in dogs.[21,22] In the first of these reports, increases in allergen-specific IgG antibodies to various pollens were reported during ASIT with aqueous allergens.[21] The second report showed that concentrations of total IgG1 (i.e. not allergen-specific) could increase following ASIT using adjuvanted vaccines.[22] However, no studies have reported changes in IgG antibodies specific for antigens derived from the house dust mite *Dermatophagoides farinae*, a major cause of AD in dogs.[23–26]

The aim of this study was to use a semi-quantitative blot analysis system[27] (C. Hou, M.J. Day, T.J. Nuttall, P.B. Hill, unpublished data) to investigate the changes in total IgG, and the subclasses IgG1, IgG2, IgG3 and IgG4, to separated antigens from *D. farinae*, during ASIT with aluminium-adsorbed vaccines. Our hypothesis was that allergen-specific IgG antibodies would increase after the administration of allergen-specific immunotherapy in dogs with AD.

Materials and methods

Study population

Serum samples used in this study were obtained from 21 dogs with AD taking part in another study to evaluate the efficacy of two different allergen-specific immunotherapy (ASIT) protocols. Details of the inclusion and exclusion criteria, study design, clinical assessment and scoring, use of concurrent medications and analysis of treatment efficacy, will be reported elsewhere.[28] Briefly, the diagnosis of AD was based on a combination of a compatible history and clinical signs,[29] exclusion of other pruritic skin diseases (e.g. ectoparasite infestation and adverse food reaction), and the presence of at least one positive reaction either in an intradermal test or a commercially available allergen-specific IgE assay (Allercept™, Heska Corporation, Fort Collins, CO, USA). All dogs included in the present study had a positive reaction to *D. farinae* at a dilution of 1/1000 w/v on an intradermal test; test sites were scored from 0 to 4 compared to the positive (1/100 000 w/v histamine) control and the negative (diluent) control, with reactions ≥ 2 being considered positive. Multiple coat brushings and skin scrapings were used to eliminate the possibility of an ectoparasite infestation. All dogs were also placed on a rigorous flea and sarcoptic mange control programme using selamectin (Stronghold® spot-on, Pfizer Animal Health, Sandwich, UK) for 6 weeks before the start of the study and at monthly intervals throughout the study. Dogs that experienced complete resolution of clinical signs after treatment were excluded. A 6-week novel ingredient home-cooked diet trial was conducted to eliminate the possibility of adverse food reactions. Concurrent staphylococcal pyoderma was managed with oral cephalexin and topical treatment with either benzoyl peroxide (Paxcutol®, Virbac, UK) or 10% ethyl lactate (Etiderm®, Virbac). Concurrent *Malassezia* infection was treated with 2% miconazole/2% chlorhexidine shampoo (Malaseb®, Leo Animal Health, UK). No glucocorticoids were given for 3 months prior to the initiation of ASIT.

Ten dogs received a standard immunotherapy protocol (Artuvetrin® Therapy, ARTU, The Netherlands), as used in the dermatology clinic at the Royal (Dick) School of Veterinary Studies in Edinburgh (Table 1.9.1). This involved administration of an allergen mixture comprising up to eight allergens, at least one of which was *D. farinae* which accounted for 2.5–10%

Table 1.9.1 Standard-dose and low-dose protocols for allergen-specific immunotherapy using aluminium-adsorbed allergens administered by subcutaneous injection

Week	Dose of allergen extract (ml)	
	Standard-dose ASIT	Low-dose ASIT
0	0.2	0.1
2	0.4	0.1
4	0.6	0.1
6	0.8	0.1
9	1.0	0.1
12	1.0	0.1
16	1.0	0.1
20	1.0	0.1
Every 4 weeks	1.0	0.1

v/v of the allergen mixture. Eleven dogs received an alternative protocol in which the frequency of injections was identical but the maintenance dose of allergen was only 1/10 that of the standard protocol (Table 1.9.1). The precise concentration of allergens is not provided by the manufacturer.

Dogs were assessed for pruritus by the owners using a 0–5 point behaviour-based scale and for skin lesions by a single investigator using a modified canine atopic dermatitis extent and severity index (CADESI).[28] Assessments took place on the day the ASIT was started and after 3, 6 and 9 months (90, 180 and 270 days) of ASIT. A complete response to ASIT was defined as a dog whose pruritus score had fallen to zero by the end of the study without the need for additional anti-pruritic medication. A partial response to ASIT was defined as a dog whose pruritus score was lower at the end of the 9-month treatment period compared to the beginning. No response to ASIT was defined as a dog whose pruritus score was the same or higher after 9 months of treatment compared to the beginning. Glucocorticoid therapy was permitted for the first 6 months of the study, but not during the final 3 months of ASIT.

Serum samples

Serum samples were to be collected from each dog before and after 3, 6 and 9 months of ASIT. However, due to unavoidable logistical and technical circumstances, serum samples could not be collected at every time point in every dog. All dogs were sampled prior to the start of ASIT but some only had serum samples taken at one or two of the remaining three time points. There

were 4/24 missing data points in the complete response group, 5/20 in the partial response group and 5/40 in the no response group.

All samples were obtained with the owner's consent. As the samples were to be used for measurement of allergen-specific antibody responses, which represented diagnostically and therapeutically useful information; UK Home Office approval was not required. After collection, serum was separated by centrifugation and stored in aliquots at −20°C until used.

D. farinae *extract*

Lyophilised whole-body *D. farinae* crude extract (Greer Laboratories, Lenoir, NC, USA) was reconstituted to 1 mg/ml in sterile phosphate-buffered saline (PBS, pH 7.5) and 200-μl aliquots were stored at −20°C until used.

Sodium dodecyl sulphate-polyacrylamide gel electrophoresis (SDS-PAGE)

SDS-PAGE was performed according to the method of Laemmli[30] using a 10% Tris-glycine polyacrylamide (ProtoGel®, National Diagnostics, UK) separating gel and 4% stacking gel in a discontinuous buffer system containing 25 mM Tris-HCl (Trizma® hydrochloride; Sigma-Aldrich, Dorset, UK), 0.2 M glycine (Fisher Scientific, Loughborough, UK) and 0.1% SDS (Fisher Scientific), pH 8.3. A total of 50 μl (for total IgG colorimetric blots) or 100 μl (for IgG subclass chemiluminescent blots) of *D. farinae* extract, and 0.5 μl of the molecular weight markers, were diluted 1:1 and 1:20, respectively, with reducing sample buffer containing 125 mM Tris-HCl, 4% SDS, 20% glycerol (BDH Chemicals, Poole, UK), 0.005% bromophenol blue (BDH) and 10% 2-mercaptoethanol (Sigma-Aldrich) and heated at 95°C for 5 minutes. The extract was then loaded into one broad well across the top of the gel alongside a lane containing the molecular weight markers and the electrophoresis was run at 200 V for 40 minutes according to the manufacturer's recommendations (Mini-Protean II®; Biorad, Hercules, USA).

Western blots

Separated *D. farinae* proteins were transferred to polyvinylidene fluoride (PVDF) microporous membranes (Millipore Immobilon™-P Transfer Membrane, Millipore Corporation, Bedford, MA, USA) in a semi-dry electrophoretic transfer cell (Trans-Blot® SD, Biorad) using 0.3 M Tris-HCl/10% methanol (pH 10.4) on the lower anode, 25 mM Tris-HCl/10% methanol (pH 10.4) on the upper anode and 25 mM Tris-HCl/40 mM 6-amino-n-hexonic acid/10% methanol (pH 9.4) on the cathode according to the manufacturer's instructions. The transfer was run at 80 mA per minigel for 1 hour, after which the membranes were dried and stored at 4°C. The quality of transfer was checked by staining gels and molecular weight standards blotted onto the membrane with Coomassie brilliant blue R-250 (BDH).

Antibodies

To assess total IgG responses to separated antigens from *D. farinae*, a polyclonal horseradish peroxidase-conjugated goat anti-dog IgG (Bethyl Laboratories Inc., Montgomery, TX, USA) was used. The specificity of this reagent for IgG is verified by the manufacturer and has been documented in previous studies.[27,31] Potential cross-reactivity of the reagent with canine IgE is not relevant in colorimetric immunoblots because the method is not sensitive enough to detect the low concentrations of IgE present, even if specific anti-IgE reagents are used.[31]

To assess IgG subclass responses to separated antigens from *D. farinae*, a panel of four mouse monoclonal antibodies (mAbs) specific for the subclasses of canine IgG were used. The preparation and characterisation of these mAbs has been described.[32–35] mAb B6 has restricted specificity for canine IgG1 and IgG3, but reacts specifically with IgG1 in serological and immunohistochemical assays. mAb E5 is specific for canine IgG2 and antibody A3G4 is specific for canine IgG3. mAb A5 has restricted specificity for canine IgG2 and IgG4 but reacts specifically with IgG4 in serological and immunohistochemical assays. The specific activity of the subclass-restricted mAbs B6 and A5 is probably due to conformational differences between the target IgG subclasses in solid-phase assays versus other serological and immunohistochemical techniques.[33,35] mAbs A5, E5 and B6 were used as 45% ammonium sulphate precipitates of tissue culture supernatants, and A3G4 was used as a tissue culture supernatant. The applicability of these mAbs in Western blotting was confirmed by probing a commercial preparation of canine IgG purified by ion-exchange chromatography (Sigma-Aldrich).

Immunoblotting

Blotting membranes with transferred separated *D. farinae* proteins were cut longitudinally into 4-mm wide strips to allow probing by individual dog sera. Strips were placed in individual lanes of an eight-channel incubation tray (Biorad), blocked with 5% skimmed milk in Tris-buffered saline (TBS, pH 7.5) containing 20 mM Tris-HCl and 0.5 M NaCl (Sigma-Aldrich) for 1 hour at room temperature, and washed with 0.1% Tween 20 (Fisher Scientific)/TBS (TTBS) three times for 5 minutes. All sera and primary and secondary reagents were diluted with dilution buffer (1% skimmed milk/TTBS) to a final volume of 1 ml and to concentrations that had been determined in previous studies to yield strong bands against a clear background[27] (C. Hou, M.J. Day, T.J. Nuttall, P.B. Hill, unpublished data).

For total IgG immunoblots, duplicate strips were probed with individual dog sera at 1/100 for 1 hour, followed by a 1-hour incubation with the horseradish peroxidase-conjugated goat anti-dog IgG at 1/1000. After further washing with washing buffer, the strips were developed for 1 minute with 3,3'-diaminobenzidine (DAB) peroxidase substrate (Vector Laboratories Inc., Burlingame, CA, USA), prepared according to the manufacturer's recommendations. The strips were air-dried overnight prior to analysis.

For detection of IgG subclass responses, duplicate strips were probed for 1 hour with dog sera diluted to 1/20, followed by a 1-hour incubation with one of the four IgG subclass-specific mAbs diluted to 1/500. After washing, a horseradish peroxidase-conjugated bovine anti-mouse IgG (Bethyl Laboratories) diluted to 1/1000 was added for another hour followed by thorough washing. The surface of each strip containing the detected proteins was then covered for 1 minute with a chemiluminescent luminal solution (ECL, Amersham-Pharmacia Biotech, Little Chalfont, UK), used for its higher sensitivity. The excess liquid was then drained off prior to immediate image acquisition as described below.

Digital image acquisition and semi-quantitative analysis

Strips probed with the polyclonal anti-canine IgG and developed with the colorimetric substrate DAB, along with the molecular weight standards, were aligned and digitally scanned using a flatbed scanner (Epson Perfection 1650, Hemel Hempstead, UK) set at 16-bit grey scale. For IgG subclass-specific blots, developed with the chemiluminescent substrate ECL, the strips were wrapped in cling film and placed protein side down on a Kodak Digital Science™ Image Station 440CF (Kodak, Rochester, NY, USA) along with the Coomassie blue-stained molecular weight standards. In this system, the images are acquired with a charge coupled device (CCD) camera. Three exposures, each lasting 5 minutes, were used to eliminate the possibility of image saturation.

The scanned and acquired images were then imported into image analysis software (Kodak Digital Science™ 1D Image Analysis Software, Kodak, USA) to detect the bands on the blots. This software can determine, without operator bias, the molecular weight of bands by analysing their positions relative to the molecular weight standards as well as the signal magnitude of individual bands. We have shown in previous studies that this system can be used for semi-quantitative analysis of antibody concentrations because a linear standard curve is obtained when band intensity is plotted against log serum dilutions[27] (C. Hou, M.J. Day, T.J. Nuttall, P.B. Hill, unpublished data). Furthermore, the coefficients of variation obtained from repeated assay of samples are approximately 10–20%, and the conditions used do not lead to saturation effects[27] (C. Hou, M.J. Day, T.J. Nuttall, P.B. Hill, unpublished data). The sum of the band intensities on each strip therefore provides an indication of the antibody response to D. farinae as a whole, whereas the intensity of each band provides an indication of the antibody response to individual antigens. For each dog, the final band intensity was derived from an average of each set of duplicate strips.

Statistical analysis

Numerical data derived from the image analysis software were exported to Graphpad Prism, Version 3.0 for Windows (Graphpad software, San Diego, USA). As antibody concentrations in dogs are not normally distributed,[36] the Kruskal–Wallis non-parametric ANOVA was used to compare antibody responses at multiple time points. If significant differences were detected by Kruskal–Wallis, comparisons between two individual time points were made by the Mann–Whitney test. The following comparisons were made: data from four time points (days 0, 90, 180 and 270) when all the dogs were combined as a single group; data from corresponding time points when dogs were divided into two groups based on those that showed no response to ASIT versus dogs that showed some response (complete or partial); data from corresponding time points when dogs were divided into three groups comprising those that showed a complete, partial or no response to ASIT; data from the four time points within each response group; and data from eight time points when dogs were divided into two groups based on those that received the standard ASIT protocol versus those that received the low-dose ASIT protocol. A p value of < 0.05 was considered to be significant.

Results

All the dogs had detectable levels of D. farinae-specific total IgG, IgG1 and IgG4 prior to the start of, and during, ASIT (Figure 1.9.1). There was no detectable response by IgG2 and IgG3 antibodies, despite attempts to increase the sensitivity of the assay by increasing reagent concentrations and incubation times (data not shown). Both total IgG, and the subclasses IgG1 and IgG4, recognised multiple proteins from D. farinae with the most visually obvious bands having molecular weights of approximately 98 kDa and 44 kDa, both of which have been identified as major allergens[26] (Fig. 1.9.1). The 66-kDa protein was often detected in samples and it has also been classified as a minor allergen for dogs.[26]

Visual analysis of the strips from individual dogs showed that the strength of the bands varied during ASIT. However, there was no clearly obvious trend for the band intensity to increase or decrease with time. Over the course of 9 months of ASIT, individual dogs could show an obvious increase in band strength (Fig. 1.9.1a), a decrease (Fig. 1.9.1b), remain relatively static (Fig. 1.9.1c), or fluctuate. For each dog, the changes seen with total D. farinae-specific IgG were approximately mirrored by similar changes in IgG1 and IgG4. No consistent induction or disappearance of specific bands at any molecular weight was observed.

This visual impression was confirmed by the numerical data from the image analysis software which showed that, during ASIT, there was no consistent increase in the total antibody response (the sum of all the band intensities on each strip) for IgG, IgG1 or IgG4 (Fig. 1.9.2a). There was also no con-

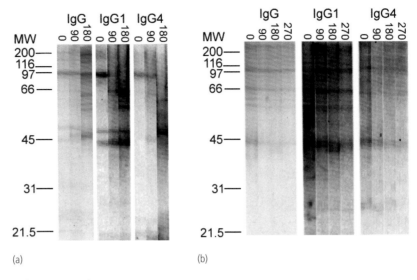

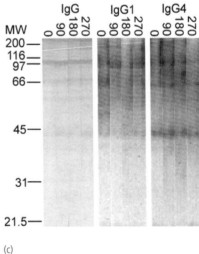

Fig. 1.9.1 Examples of immunoblots showing total IgG-, IgG1- and IgG4-binding profiles to *Dermatophagoides farinae* extract in dogs undergoing allergen-specific immunotherapy. Serum samples were collected before and after immunotherapy for 90, 180 and 270 days. The IgG responses to *D. farinae* allergens varied widely between dogs and could increase (a), decrease (b), remain the same (c) or fluctuate. Changes in total *D. farinae*-specific IgG were usually paralleled by equivalent changes in IgG1 and IgG4. MW, molecular weight in kilodaltons (kDa).

sistent change in the response to the 98-kDa band (Fig.1.9.2b) or the 44-kDa band (Fig. 1.9.2c) for any of the antibodies.

When all the dogs were considered as a single group, there was no significant difference in the total antibody response to *D. farinae* (sum of the band intensities on each strip) or the response to the 98-kDa and 44-kDa proteins at any of the four time points during ASIT for IgG, IgG1 or IgG4 ($p > 0.05$ for all nine analyses). However, when dogs that showed no response to ASIT were compared to dogs that showed a response (partial and complete response groups combined), there was a significant difference among the time points for total IgG. This difference was attributable to a significantly greater total IgG response to *D. farinae*, and the 98-kDa and 44-kDa proteins, in the group that was non-responsive to ASIT at day 0, compared to the response group at day 0. In the case of the 44-kDa band, there was also a significantly greater total IgG response in the non-responsive group at day 90 compared to the response group at day 90.

When the dogs were divided into three response groups and compared separately, there was a significant difference among time points for total IgG responses to *D. farinae*. This was due to a significantly higher IgG response in the non-responsive group at day 0, compared to the partial ($p = 0.019$) and the complete ($p = 0.011$) response groups . The total IgG responses to the 98-kDa and 44-kDa proteins were also significantly higher at day 0 in the non-responsive group compared with the complete response groups ($p = 0.023$ and $p = 0.042$, respectively).

In addition, there was also significant variation among the time points in the standard- and low-dose ASIT protocols for IgG1 against total *D. farinae* antigens. This was attributable to significantly lower IgG1

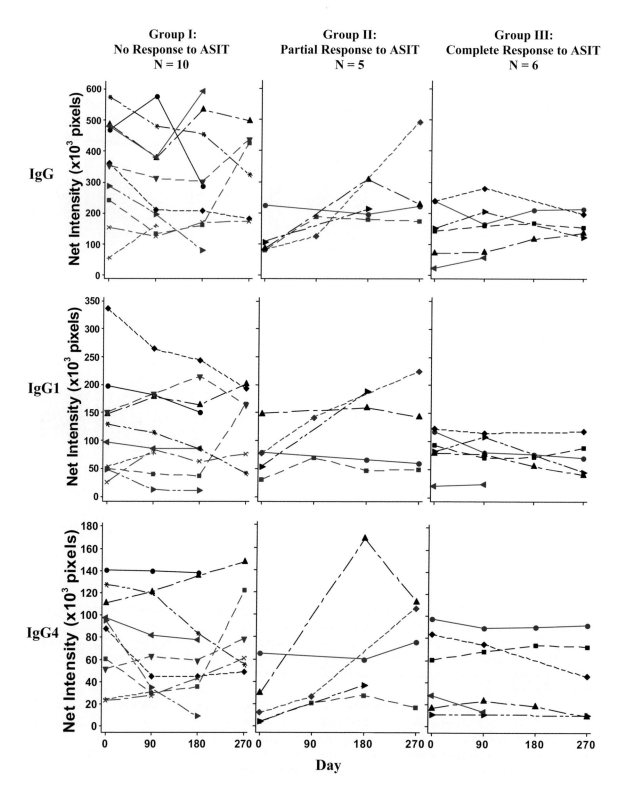

Fig. 1.9.2 *Dermatophagoides farinae*-specific total IgG, IgG1 and IgG4 antibody responses during 9 months of allergen-specific immunotherapy. (a) The total antibody response to *D. farinae* antigens (calculated as the sum of all band intensities on each immunoblot strip). The dogs are divided into three groups categorized by clinical outcome. Dogs that received the standard-dose immunotherapy protocol are plotted in black. Dogs that received the low-dose immunotherapy protocol are plotted in red.

(a)

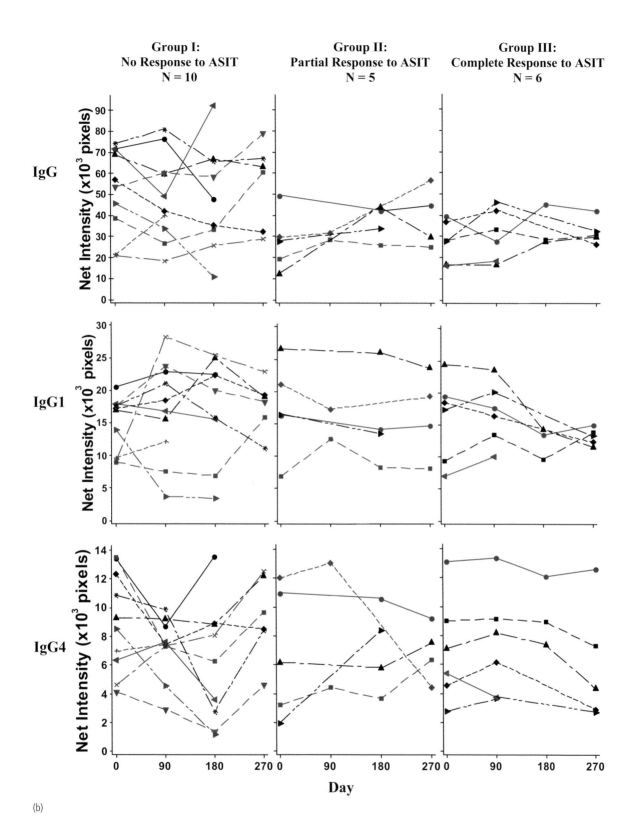

Fig. 1.9.2 *Dermatophagoides farinae*-specific total IgG, IgG1 and IgG4 antibody responses during 9 months of allergen-specific immunotherapy. (b) Antibody responses to the 98-kDa band. Dogs that received the standard-dose immunotherapy protocol are plotted in black. Dogs that received the low-dose immunotherapy protocol are plotted in red.

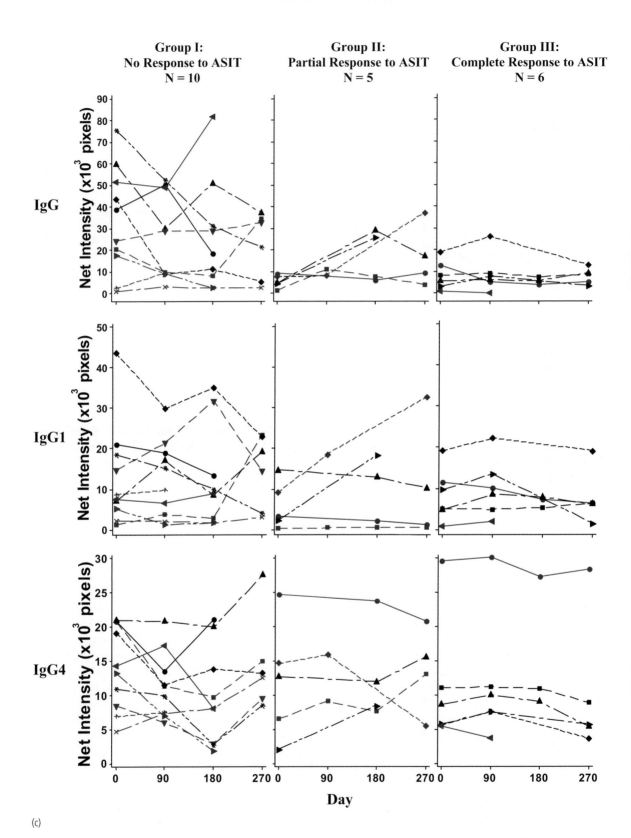

(c)

Fig. 1.9.2 *Dermatophagoides farinae*-specific total IgG, IgG1 and IgG4 antibody responses during 9 months of allergen-specific immunotherapy. (c) Antibody responses to the 44-kDa band. The dogs are divided into three groups categorized by clinical outcome. Dogs that received the standard-dose immunotherapy protocol are plotted in black. Dogs that received the low-dose immunotherapy protocol are plotted in red.

levels to *D. farinae* at day 0 in the dogs receiving the low-dose protocol compared with those receiving the standard dose ($p = 0.01$). There were no other significant differences for *D. farinae* or the 98-kDa or 44-kDa proteins at any time point for any other antibody between the standard-dose and low-dose protocol groups.

Discussion

In this study, we documented allergen-specific total IgG, IgG1 and IgG4 responses to various antigens of the house dust mite *D. farinae* in dogs with AD. No IgG2 or IgG3 antibodies were detected with specificity for *D. farinae*. These findings were in accordance with previous studies recently conducted in our laboratory[27] (C. Hou, M.J. Day, T.J. Nuttall, P.B. Hill, unpublished data). During ASIT, there was no consistent augmentation of the total quantity of *D. farinae*-specific IgG or IgG subclass antibodies to antigens from the mite. Levels of the antibodies could increase or fall but there was no significant increase by day 270 compared to day 0. This was the case for the total response to all the *D. farinae* proteins (measured by summing all the band intensities on each strip) as well as the response to the 98-kDa and 44-kDa proteins. These latter proteins were chosen for specific analysis because they were the strongest and most visually obvious bands on the strips. The 98-kDa band is likely to be the high molecular weight chitinase recently designated Der f 15, a major *D. farinae* allergen for dogs with AD.[23,24,26] The identity of the 44-kDa protein is currently unknown, but it may be a fragment of a larger antigen because it only appeared on blots performed with reducing buffers and not on blots performed with non-reducing buffers in an earlier study.[26]

Although not exactly parallel, the changes in IgG1 and IgG4 tended to mirror the changes seen with total IgG. The lack of significant increases in levels of allergen-specific IgG, IgG1 and IgG4 is surprising. Previous studies have demonstrated that increases in allergen-specific IgG1 and IgG4 are seen following ASIT in man.[19,20,37] In atopic dogs, concentrations of pollen-specific IgG were shown to increase following at least 6 months of ASIT using aqueous allergens.[21] An increase in total (non-allergen-specific) IgG1 was also observed in most dogs that were given ASIT using alum-precipitated vaccines.[22] The reason for the difference in the findings between our study and previous studies is not clear, but there are a number of possible explanations.

First, although administration of adjuvanted proteins should lead to a marked IgG response, some studies in humans have shown poor clinical efficacy to alum-precipitated vaccines as well as a lack of alteration in immune responses.[38,39] It is possible that the vaccines used in this study did not contain sufficient protein to induce an allergen-specific IgG response, even though they were shown to elicit an increase in total IgG1 in most of the dogs in a prior study.[22] The allergen manufacturer used in this study does not provide the specific protein content of allergens within vaccines, so it is not possible to know the precise amount of *D. farinae* that is present. Further, the quantity of *D. farinae* in each vaccine is likely to be different depending on the number of other allergens included. It is also possible that the amount of *D. farinae* antigens may vary from batch to batch, leading to further variation in specific immune responses. Evidence for the above possibility is provided by the lack of significant differences in IgG, IgG1 and IgG4 levels in dogs receiving either the standard ASIT protocol or the low-dose protocol, which involved administering 1/10 of the recommended dose. It would have been expected that dogs receiving the higher doses would have mounted a greater antibody response, as long as sufficient protein was present initially. To resolve some of these issues, further studies are required to compare the total and allergen-specific IgG responses in dogs receiving different aqueous allergen and alum-precipitated ASIT protocols. It is also important that allergen manufacturers work towards standardisation of allergens so that the precise protein concentrations can be included in vaccines, allowing direct comparison.

A second possibility for the discrepancy may relate to the different methods employed in the various studies. In this study we used a validated semi-quantitative blot analysis system in which the net intensity of bands shows a linear relationship to log antibody concentrations[27] (C. Hou, M.J. Day, T.J. Nuttall, P.B. Hill, unpublished data). This system allows a whole range of separated proteins from *D. farinae* to be studied simultaneously. This is a major advantage compared with ELISA assays, which can only measure a single protein at a time. However, ELISA assays can provide a more accurate measurement of a protein's concentration in mg/ml and they tend to have lower coefficients of variation, indicating superior repeatability. Hence, in future studies, we intend to directly compare the results obtained by blot analysis to ELISA.

Thirdly, the increase in total IgG1 documented in the earlier study[26] was quantified using a radial-immuno-diffusion technique. This method measured the total quantity of IgG1 present and did not relate to specific allergens. Hence, the increase seen in that study could have been due to other allergens or non-specific IgG activation and not directly related to *D. farinae* proteins.

Finally, it is possible that production of *D. farinae*-specific IgG antibodies is not induced in dogs with AD undergoing ASIT. This has not previously been studied and it is not known whether the formulation of the allergens, or the expression of the epitopes of major allergens in ASIT, are appropriate or sufficient to stimulate this arm of the immune system. If not, clinical efficacy may be related to some other mechanism such as down-regulation of cellular function or changes in cytokine profiles.

An interesting finding arising from this study was that dogs showing no response to ASIT had significantly higher *D. farinae*-specific total IgG levels on day 0 compared with dogs showing a partial or complete response. This was the case both for total *D. farinae* antigens, and the 98-kDa and 44-kDa proteins. This suggested that if a dog with AD had a pre-existing high level of IgG antibodies to *D. farinae* prior to the onset of ASIT, it was less likely to respond. This is a potentially exciting finding, as it may suggest a means by which dogs could be screened prior to initiation of ASIT. Dogs with a low level of IgG antibodies could be given a better prognosis than those with high levels. Alternatively, this might allow alterations in dosage schedule to be predicted in advance. This finding clearly needs to be substantiated using additional methods and in a larger group of dogs to ensure that it is a repeatable phenomenon. If so, the discriminatory power of the measurement would have to be carefully determined.

A statistical quirk that arose in this study was the finding that dogs receiving the standard-dose ASIT protocol had significantly higher levels of IgG1 to total *D. farinae* proteins at day 0 compared with those receiving the low-dose protocol. This can only have arisen by chance, as the dogs were assigned to their relative groups using block randomisation. This chance occurrence did not seem to have any bearing on the subsequent efficacy of the ASIT because there were no significant differences in response rates between the two groups.[28]

In summary, this study did not demonstrate the production of *D. farinae*-specific IgG blocking antibodies in atopic dogs undergoing ASIT based on alum-precipitated vaccines. However, a high pre-existing level of total IgG to *D. farinae* antigens, including the 98-kDa and 44-kDa proteins, suggested that dogs were less likely to respond to ASIT.

References

1 Bousquet, J., Lockey, R., Malling, H.-J. Allergen immunotherapy: therapeutic vaccines for allergic diseases. A WHO position paper. *Journal of Allergy and Clinical Immunology*, 1998; **102**: 558–562.

2 Griffin, C.E., Hillier, A. The ACVD task force on canine atopic dermatitis (XXIV): allergen-specific immunotherapy. *Veterinary Immunology and Immunopathology*, 2001; **81**: 363–383.

3 Noon, L. Prophylactic inoculation against hay fever. *Lancet*, 1911; **1**: 1572–1573.

4 Freeman, J. Further observation on the treatment of hay fever by hypodermic inoculation of pollen vaccine. *Lancet*, 1911; **2**: 814–817.

5 Wittich, F.W. Spontaneous allergy (atopy) in the lower animal. *Journal of Allergy*, 1941; **12**: 247–251.

6 Mueller, R.S., Bettenay, S.V. Long-term immunotherapy of 146 dogs with atopic dermatitis – a retrospective study. *Australian Veterinary Practitioner*, 1996; **26**: 128–132.

7 Nuttall, T.J., Thoday, K.L., van den Broek, A.H.M., Jackson, H.A., Sture, G.H., Halliwell, R.E.W. Retrospective survey of allergen immunotherapy in canine atopy. *Veterinary Record*, 1998; **143**: 139–142.

8 Willemse, A., van den Brom, W.E., Rijnberk, A. Effect of hypo-sensitization on atopic dermatitis in dogs. *Journal of the American Veterinary Medical Association*, 1984; **184**: 1277–1280.

9 Volk, V.K., Bunney, W.E. Diphtheria immunization with fluid toxoid and alum precipitated toxoid. *American Journal of Public Health*, 1942; **32**: 690–699.

10 Gupta, R.K. Aluminum compounds as vaccine adjuvants. *Advanced Drug Delivery Reviews*, 1998; **32**: 155–172.

11 Kimura, I., Tanizaki, Y., Goda, Y., Komagoe, H., Kitani, H. Decrease in reactivity of basophils by immunotherapy with house-dust extract. *Clinical Allergy*, 1985; **15**: 1–7.

12 Secrist, H., Chelen, C.J., Wen, Y., Marshall, J.D., Umetsu, D.T. Allergen immunotherapy decreases interleukin 4 production in CD4+ T cells from allergic individuals. *Journal of Experimental Medicine*, 1993; **178**: 2123–2130.

13 Jutel, M., Pichler, W.J., Skrbic, D., Urwyler, A., Dahinden, C., Muller, U.R. Bee venom immunotherapy results in decrease of IL-4 and IL-5 and increase of IFN-gamma secretion in specific allergen-stimulated T cell cultures. *Journal of Immunology*, 1995; **154**: 4187–4194.

14 McHugh, S.M., Deighton, J., Stewart, A.G., Lachmann, P.J., Ewan, P.W. Bee venom immunotherapy induces a shift in cytokine responses from a TH-2 to a TH-1 dominant pattern: comparison of rush and conventional immunotherapy. *Clinical and Experimental Allergy*, 1995; **25**: 828–838.

15 Akoum, H., Tsicopoulos, A., Vorng, H., *et al.* Venom immunotherapy modulates interleukin-4 and interferon-gamma messenger RNA expression of peripheral T lymphocytes. *Immunology*, 1996; **87**: 593–598.

16 Bellinghausen, I., Metz, G., Enk, A.H., Christmann, S., Knop, J., Saloga, J. Insect venom immunotherapy induces interleukin-10 production and a Th2-to-Th1 shift, and changes surface marker expression in venom-allergic subjects. *European Journal of Immunology*, 1997; **27**: 1131–1139.

17 Akdis, C.A., Blesken, T., Akdis, M., Wuthrich, B., Blaser, K. Role of interleukin 10 in specific immunotherapy. *Journal of Clinical Investigation*, 1998; **102**: 98–106.

18 Francis, J.N., Till, S.J., Durham, S.R. Induction of IL-10+CD4+CD25+ T cells by grass pollen immunotherapy. *Journal of Allergy and Clinical Immunology*, 2003; **111**: 1255–1261.

19 Muller, U., Helbling, A., Bischof, M. Predictive value of venom-specific IgE, IgG and IgG subclass antibodies in patients on immunotherapy with honey bee venom. *Allergy*, 1989; **44**: 412–418.

20 McHugh, S.M., Lavelle, B., Kemeny, D.M., Patel, S., Ewan, P.W. A placebo-controlled trial of immunotherapy with two extracts of *Dermatophagoides pteronyssinus* in allergic rhinitis, comparing clinical outcome with changes in antigen-specific IgE, IgG, and IgG subclasses. *Journal of Allergy and Clinical Immunology*, 1990; **86**: 521–531.

21 Hites, M.J., Kleinbeck, M.L., Loker, J.L., Lee, K.W. Effect of immunotherapy on the serum concentrations of allergen-specific IgG antibodies in dog sera. *Veterinary Immunology and Immunopathology*, 1989; **22**: 39–51.

22 Fraser, M.A., McNeil, P.E., Gettinby, G. Examination of serum total IgG1 concentration in atopic and non-atopic dogs. *Journal of Small Animal Practice*, 2004; **45**: 186–190.

23 Noli, C., Bernadina, W.E., Willemse, T. The significance of reactions to purified fractions of *Dermatophagoides pteronyssinus* and *Dermatophagoides farinae* in canine atopic dermatitis. *Veterinary Immunology and Immunopathology*, 1996; **52**: 147–157.

24 McCall, C., Hunter, S., Stedman, K., *et al.* Characterization and cloning of a major high molecular weight house dust mite allergen (Der f 15) for dogs. *Veterinary Immunology and Immunopathology*, 2001; **78**: 231–247.

25 Hill, P.B., DeBoer, D.J. The ACVD task force on canine atopic dermatitis (IV): environmental allergens. *Veterinary Immunology and Immunopathology*, 2001; **81**: 169–186.

26 Nuttall, T.J., Lamb, J.R., Hill, P.B. Characterisation of major and minor *Dermatophagoides* allergens in canine atopic dermatitis. *Research in Veterinary Science*, 2001; **71**: 51–57.

27 Hou, C., Pemberton, A., Nuttall, T.J., Hill, P.B. IgG responses to antigens from *Dermatophagoides farinae* in healthy and atopic dogs. *Veterinary Immunology and Immunopathology*, 2005 (in press).

28 Colombo, S., Hill, P.B., Shaw, D.J., Thoday, K.L. Effectiveness of low dose immunotherapy in the treatment of canine atopic der-matitis: a prospective, double-blinded study. *Veterinary Dermatology*, 2004; **15** (Suppl.): 38.

29 Willemse, T. Atopic skin disease – a review and a reconsideration of diagnostic criteria. *Journal of Small Animal Practice*, 1986; **27**: 771–778.

30 Laemmli, U.K. Cleavage of structural proteins during the assembly of the head of bacteriophage T4. *Nature*, 1970; **227**: 680–685.

31 Chen, T.A., Halliwell, R.E.W., Hill, P.B. Immunoglobulin G responses to *Malassezia pachydermatis* antigens in atopic and normal dogs. In: Thoday, K.L., Foil, C.S., Bond, R., eds. *Advances in Veterinary Dermatology*, Vol. 4. Blackwell Publishing, Oxford, 2002: 202–209.

32 Mazza, G., Duffus, W.P.H., Elson, C.J., Stokes, C.R., Wilson, A.D., Whiting, A.H. The separation and identification by monoclonal antibodies of dog IgG fractions. *Journal of Immunological Methods*, 1993; **161**: 193–203.

33 Mazza, G., Whiting, A.H., Day, M.J., Duffus, W.P. Development of an enzyme-linked immunosorbent assay for the detection of IgG subclasses in the serum of normal and diseased dogs. *Research in Veterinary Science*, 1994; **57**: 133–139.

34 Mazza, G., Whiting, A.H., Day, M.J., Duffus, W.P. Preparation of monoclonal antibodies specific for the subclasses of canine IgG. *Research in Veterinary Science*, 1994; **57**: 140–145.

35 Day, M.J., Mazza, G. Tissue immunoglobulin G subclasses observed in immune-mediated dermatopathy, deep pyoderma and hypersensitivity dermatitis in dogs. *Research in Veterinary Science*, 1995; **58**: 82–89.

36 Hill, P.B., Moriello, K.A., DeBoer, D.J. Concentrations of total serum IgE, IgA, and IgG in atopic and parasitized dogs. *Veterinary Immunology and Immunopathology*, 1995; **44**: 105–113.

37 van Neerven, R.J., Wikborg, T., Lund, *et al.* Blocking antibodies induced by specific allergy vaccination prevent the activation of CD4+ T cells by inhibiting serum-IgE-facilitated allergen presentation. *Journal of Immunology*, 1999; **163**: 2944–2952.

38 Lichtenstein, L.M., Norman, P.S., Winkenwerder, W.L. Antibody response following immunotherapy in ragweed hay fever: allpyral vs. whole ragweed extract. *Clinical Allergy*, 1968; **41**: 49–57.

39 Bousquet, J., Guerin, B., Dotte, A., *et al.* Comparison between rush immunotherapy with a standardized allergen and an alum adjuved pyridine extracted material in grass pollen allergy. *Clinical Allergy*, 1985; **15**: 179–193.

Effect of treatment with recombinant canine IFN-γ on the clinical signs, histopathology and Th1/Th2-cytokine mRNA profiles in Shih Tzu dogs and a Basset hound with atopic dermatitis

T. Iwasaki DVM, PhD[1], S.J. Park DVM, PhD[1], N. Kagawa DVM[2], N. Kanazawa DVM[1], T. Mori DVM[2], T. Kubo DVM[2], Y. Momoi DVM, PhD[1], H. Tanikawa DVM, PhD[3]

[1] Department of Veterinary Internal Medicine, Tokyo University of Agriculture & Technology, Fuchu, Tokyo, Japan
[2] Hokuai Animal Hospital, Sapporo, Japan
[3] Department of Veterinary Pathology, Rakuno Gakuen University, Ebetsu, Hokkaido, Japan

Summary

Atopic dermatitis (AD) is caused by immunologic abnormalities induced by Th1/Th2-cytokine imbalance. Several studies focusing on the therapeutic effects of interferon-γ (IFN-γ) in human AD have met with success; however, the mechanism of action of IFN-γ is not completely understood. This study investigated the effects of recombinant canine IFN-γ (rCaIFN-γ) in ten dogs with AD (nine Shih Tzus and one Basset hound) and evaluated the ratio of IL-4 mRNA to IFN-γ mRNA in peripheral blood mononuclear cells, the serum total IgE level and histological changes in the skin. After six injections of rCaIFN-γ, seven of the ten dogs showed clinical improvement, and six of the seven exhibited decreases in the IL-4/IFN-γ mRNA ratios over a span of 2 weeks. In contrast, two of the three dogs that were not clinically improved exhibited increased IL-4/IFN-γ mRNA ratios. The serum total IgE levels were significantly decreased in nine of the ten dogs. The number of IgE-positive cells detected by immunostaining and the number of mast cells were decreased. The results of this small pilot study indicate that rCaIFN-γ may be a novel, safe and effective therapeutic option for the treatment of canine AD, although follow-up long-term studies in a larger group of dogs will be necessary to validate these preliminary findings. The rCaIFN-γ may act by modulating the Th2/Th1-cytokine balance and a reduction of serum total IgE production.

Introduction

Atopic dermatitis (AD) is defined as a hereditary, IgE- and/or IgGd-mediated hypersensitivity to environmental allergens. It is clinically characterised by pruritus, with or without accompanying skin lesions.[1,2] AD is one of the most common allergic skin diseases in dogs, affecting between 3 and 15% of the canine population.[3] The disease is associated with multiple abnormalities in IgE regulation, as well as defective cutaneous cell-mediated immunity.[2]

AD is characterised by a Th1/Th2-cytokine imbalance, which results in increased IL-4 expression and reduced IFN-γ production. Human AD patients exhibit increased levels of IL-4 and low levels of IFN-γ.[4,5] In the skin of dogs with AD, IL-4-cytokine gene transcripts were detected more commonly than Th1-cytokine gene transcripts.[6,7] In mice, the over-expression of IL-4 results in marked increases in serum total IgE levels, and the appearance of inflammatory lesions with histopathological features that are characteristic of allergic reactions.[8] This cytokine imbalance may promote the increase in IgE production, and the reduction of cellular immune responses as observed in AD patients.[5]

IFN-γ is a cytokine that plays an important role as an immune modulator, and is anticipated to be useful as a therapeutic agent for immune disorders. A few clinical trials have indicated that recombinant human IFN-γ (rhIFN-γ) has therapeutic efficacy against AD in humans.[4,9–14] However, the mechanism by which rhIFN-γ acts to decrease skin inflammation in AD is currently unknown.

Recently, the cloning and expression of the cDNA for canine IFN-γ has been reported, as well as the production of recombinant canine IFN-γ (rCaIFN-γ).[15] The aim of this study was to investigate the therapeutic efficacy of rCaIFN-γ in the treatment of canine AD by monitoring clinical signs, histopathological and immunohistochemical findings, and evaluating changes in the Th1/Th2-cytokine balance and serum total IgE levels following treatment.

Materials and methods

Animals and inclusion criteria

Ten dogs with AD were enrolled in the study. The diagnosis of AD was based on case histories, typical clinical signs and exclusion of other dermatologic disorders. *Sarcoptes scabiei* and other ectoparasitic infestations (such as flea infestation) were ruled out on the basis of negative multiple skin scrapings and lack of response to appropriate parasiticidal therapy (including 300 µg/kg of ivermectin by subcutaneous injections and fipronil applications when scabies or flea allergy dermatitis were suspected, respectively). Cutaneous adverse food reactions were ruled out by lack of response to feeding of a commercial hypoallergenic diet for a minimum of 4 weeks. Prior to entry into the study, dogs with bacterial or yeast infections of the skin were treated with antimicrobial agents to resolution of the infection. Intradermal testing (IDT) was performed under local or general anaesthesia. Eighteen allergens were used in the IDT panel and included house dust mite mix (equal parts *Dermatophagoides farinae* and *D. pteronyssinus*) (Greer Laboratories, Lenoir NC, USA) and Japanese cedar (Hitachi Chemical, Ibaragi, Japan). No medications were administered for at least 4 weeks prior to entry into the study. Erythema, wheal formation and induration at injected sites were evaluated 15 minutes after the intradermal injection. The same investigator performed IDT on all patients on the same day. All patients were hospitalised at the same time (11–23 June 2000) at the University Hospital of Rakunou Gakuen University, for the duration of the study.

Treatment

Each dog was injected subcutaneously with 20 000 units/kg rCaIFN-γ three times weekly for 2 weeks (days 1, 2, 3, 8, 9 and 10). The dosing regimen was selected on the basis of the results of a preliminary study (data not shown). The rCaIFN-γ was dissolved in 1.2 ml of physiological saline and injected by the investigator.

A full physical examination was performed on each patient on each day of the study. Further, complete blood counts (CBC) and serum chemistry profiles were performed on each patient prior to entry into the study, and on day 14 of the study.

Scoring of clinical signs

Evaluation of clinical signs was performed by a single investigator throughout the study. Pruritus and the clinical signs of erythema, lichenification and alopecia were evaluated on a scale of 0 (absent) to 3 (severe) (Table 1.10.1) on days 0, 7 and 14. Scores for each individual parameter were combined to provide a total clinical score for each time point. The percentage change in total clinical score was categorised as mild improvement if there was a 0–25% decrease in the score, moderate improvement if there was a 25–50% decrease in the score, and good improvement if there was > 50% decrease in the score.

Table 1.10.1 Clinical scoring parameters and scheme

Clinical sign/lesion	Score	Parameters
Pruritus	0	No visible scratching
	1	Sporadic scratching by hind legs
	2	Frequent scratching by hind legs
	3	Incessant scratching by hind legs and licking
Erythema	0	No visible erythema
	1	Mild erythema
	2	Severe erythema
	3	Multifocal erythema with fever
Lichenification	0	Normal thickness of skin
	1	Mild increase in skin thickness by palpation
	2	Moderate increase in skin thickness by palpation
	3	Severe increase in skin thickness with wrinkles
Alopecia	0	No hair loss
	1	Scarce hair at lesions
	2	Complete hair loss at lesions
	3	Extensive hair loss

Collection of peripheral blood mononuclear cells and cell culture

Peripheral blood mononuclear cells (PBMCs) were obtained by drawing 20 ml of heparinised peripheral venous blood from the jugular vein on day 0, day 7 and day 14. The PBMCs were collected by density-gradient centrifugation using 1.119 Ficoll-Hypaque (HISTOPAQUE-1119, Sigma, St Louis MI, USA) and 1.077 Ficoll-Hypaque (HISTOPAQUE-1077, Sigma). Cells were cultured in RPMI 1640 medium (Gibco BRL, Langley, OK, USA) containing 10% FCS at 2×10^2 cells/ml and stimulated with 10 mg/ml ConA in 5% CO_2 for 8 hours. By this method, the percentage of PBMCs recovered from whole blood cells is estimated to be 50–60% in our laboratory.

Serum total IgE levels

Blood was collected on day 0 and day 14 for measurement of serum total IgE levels. Quantification of serum total IgE level was performed by means of a commercial enzyme-linked immunosorbent assay (ELISA) with a goat anti-dog IgE ELISA Quantitation Kit (Bethyl Laboratories Inc., Montgomery, TX, USA).

RNA extraction and semi-quantitative reverse transcription-polymerase chain reaction (RT-PCR)

Total RNA was extracted from PBMCs on day 0, day 7 and day 14 with Trizole LS reagent (Gibco-BRL, Rockville, USA) according to a previous study.[4] The RNA content was quantified at an optical density (OD) of 260 nm measured on a Life Science UV spectrophotometer (Beckman, Fullerton, CA, USA). Specific dog oligonucleotide primers for amplification of canine IFN-γ and IL-4 and G3PDH were designed based on the published nucleic acid sequences of these genes (Table 1.10.2). Samples were amplified for 40 or 35 cycles with denaturation at 94°C for 2 minutes, annealing at 55°C (IL-4, G3PDH), 52°C (IFN-γ) for 1 minute, and extension at 72°C for 1 minute. The final extension involved incubation at 72°C for 1 minute. Following amplification, products of each triplicate reaction series were separated on 2% TAE agarose gels, stained with ethidium bromide and photographed with a digital camera. The relative levels of cytokine expression were compared with that of the housekeeping protein

Table 1.10.2 Sequences of the oligonucleotide primers used to amplify dog cytokines and G3PDH cDNA by RT-PCR

Gene	Primer sequence
IFN-γ	Forward 5'ATTTTGAAGAAATGGAGAGAGG3'
	Reverse 5'AAAATTCAAATAGTGCTGGCAGG3'
IL-4	Forward 5'ACTGATTCCAACTCTGGTCTG3'
	Reverse 5'TGCTGCTGAGGTTCCTGTAGA3'
G3PDH	Forward 5'ACCACAGTCCATGCCATCAC3'
	Reverse 5'TCCACCACCCTGTTGCTGTA3'

G3PDH and expressed as the ratio of the band intensity of the cytokine RT-PCR amplification product to that of the corresponding G3PDH RT-PCR product.

Histology and immunohistochemistry

Skin samples were obtained from lesional skin on the lateral neck (a predilection site for AD in the Shih Tzu breed – personal observation) of three dogs using an 8-mm biopsy trephine punch on day 0. A second biopsy was performed on day 14 at the same site as the first biopsy. Biopsy specimens were fixed in 10% formalin prior to routine embedding in paraffin and sliced into 4-μm thick sections. The sections were stained with haematoxylin and eosin (H&E) and toluidine blue.

Immunohistochemical staining was conducted for canine IgE as follows. The tissue sections were deparaffinised, rehydrated and immersed in 0.01% periodic acid for 10 minutes to block endogenous peroxidase activity. Non-specific staining was eliminated by incubation for 30 minutes with normal rabbit serum. Excess normal serum was removed and replaced by the primary antibodies and incubated overnight at 4°C. Primary antibody was a mouse anti-canine IgE antibody (1:50 dilution) (ICN Biomedicals Inc., OH, USA). After washing the slides, the sections were incubated with secondary biotin-labelled anti-mouse antibody for 30 minutes and followed by avidin-biotin complex (ABC) (Vectastain Elite ABC kit, Vector Laboratories, Burlingame, CA, USA) for 30 minutes. Subsequently, the colour was developed with 3,3'-diaminobenzidine tetrahydrochloride with hydrogen peroxide in PBS buffer for 10 minutes. Slides were counterstained with Mayer's haematoxylin. Positive cells were counted in ten randomly chosen fields in the superficial dermis.

Table 1.10.3 Clinical data and intradermal test results of dogs with atopic dermatitis entered into the study

Case no.	Sex	Breed	Age (years)	Age at onset (years)	IDT-positive allergens
1	M	Shih Tzu	4	2	HDM, MC, HW
2	F	Shih Tzu	6	1	HDM, CE, MC, HW, JC
3	F	Shih Tzu	3	1	HDM, CE, MC, HW, JC, WM
4	F	Shih Tzu	6	1	HDM, MC, HW
5	F	Shih Tzu	6	1	HDM, MC
6	F	Shih Tzu	8	5	HDM, CE, MC, HW
7	F	Shih Tzu	9	1	HDM, MC, HW
8	F	Shih Tzu	5	4	HDM, CE, MC, HW
9	M	Shih Tzu	6	2	HDM, CE, MC, HW, JC
10	F	Basset hound	1	1	HDM, CE, MC, HW, JC

IDT, intradermal test; M, male; F, female; HDM, house dust mite; CE, cat epithelia; MC, mugwort (common); HW, hogweed; JC, Japanese cedar; WM, grass mixes.

Statistics

The serum total IgE levels were analysed by the two-tailed Student's t-test. The results of histopathology and immunohistochemistry were statistically analysed by the two-tailed Student's t-test. A p value < 0.05 was considered significant.

Results

Ten dogs (nine Shih Tzus and one Basset hound) were included in the study: clinical data are presented in Table 1.10.3.

Clinical signs

The total clinical scores at each time point and percentage change in total clinical scores from day 0 to day 7, and day 0 to day 14, are shown in Table 1.10.4 and Fig. 1.10.1. On day 7, the total clinical scores showed good improvement in two dogs (nos 6 and 7), mild to moderate improvement in four dogs (nos 3, 4, 8 and 9), and no improvement in four dogs (nos 1, 2, 5 and 10). On day 14, total clinical scores showed good improvement in two dogs (nos 6 and 7), mild to moderate improvement in five dogs (nos 4, 5, 8, 9 and 10), and no improvement in three dogs (nos 1, 2 and 3). Aside from cutaneous lesions associated with AD, no other clinical abnormalities were detected on physical examination throughout the course of the study. In addition, no abnormal findings were recorded on CBC and serum chemistry profiles either before or after treatment.

Changes in cytokine mRNA expression

The IL-4 mRNA levels were decreased in four dogs on day 7, and were near the lower limits of detection on day 14 (Fig. 1.10.2a). On day 14 of the study, the IL-4 mRNA levels were decreased in seven dogs and increased in three.

On the other hand, the IFN-γ mRNA levels were increased in seven dogs and decreased in three dogs on day 14, compared with those on day 0 (Fig. 1.10.2b). The latter three dogs had high levels of IFN-γ mRNA on day 0, compared with the other dogs in the study.

The IL-4/IFN-γ mRNA ratios were increased in four dogs and decreased in six dogs on day 14 (Fig. 1.10.2c). The IL-4/IFN-γ mRNA ratio on day 14 was decreased in both dogs with good improvement of total clinical score. The ratio was decreased by 50% in five dogs showing improvement, whereas it was increased in

Table 1.10.4 Total clinical scores of dogs with atopic dermatitis prior to administration of rCaIFN-γ (day 0) and after 7 and 14 days of treatment

Patient no.	Day 0	Day 7	Day 14
1	17	18	22
2	8	16	14
3	4	3	4
4	10	7	7
5	8	8	7
6	5	2	0
7	6	2	0
8	10	7	6
9	24	20	22
10	11	11	9

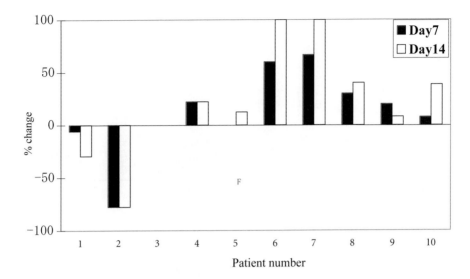

Figure 1.10.1 Percentage improvement of total clinical severity scores (from baseline before treatment). Total clinical severity scores were improved in seven dogs with AD on day 14 after the start of rCaIFN-γ injection.

all three dogs with no improvement in total clinical score.

Serum total IgE

The total IgE (mean ± SD) was 1089 ± 187 ng/ml on day 0, 815 ± 148 ng/ml on day 7 and 878 ± 197 ng/ml on day 14. As the serum total IgE levels of the dogs varied markedly on day 0, the serum total IgE levels were expressed in terms of percentage, assuming that the serum total IgE level on day 0 was 100. After six injections of rCa IFN-γ, the serum total IgE levels were decreased by 10–40% in all the patients on day 14, with a significant difference ($p = 0.024$) between day 0 and day 14.

Histopathological findings

In the biopsy specimens obtained on day 0, all the samples showed moderate to severe irregular hyperplasia with prominent rete ridges. The epithelial hyperplasia was composed of severe acanthosis and mild spongiosis of the epidermis. There was mild dermal oedema and superficial perivascular infiltration composed mainly of lymphocytes, mast cells and a few eosinophils. Mast cells contained purple granules in their cytoplasm in toluidine blue stain. There were scattered anti-IgE-positive cells in the superficial dermis.

The biopsy specimens sampled on day 14 showed decreased epidermal thickness and a decreased number of epidermal layers, compared with day 0.

The mean number of mast cells in the dermis was significantly decreased on day 14 ($p = 0.0236$), and the mean number of IgE-positive cells in the dermis was also decreased on day 14 ($p = 0.001$).

Discussion

The administration of six subcutaneous injections of rCaIFN-γ to ten dogs with AD over a period of 2 weeks led to an improvement in the total clinical scores in six of the dogs. The IL-4/IFN-γ mRNA ratios were decreased in most of the patients that showed improved total clinical scores, whereas the IL-4/IFN-γ mRNA ratios were increased in patients that showed no improvement in the total clinical scores.

A human *ex vivo* study of human atopic patients reported similar results where the serum IgE level is negatively correlated with the ability of PBMCs to produce IFN-γ.[16] The modulation of the Th1/Th2-cytokine ratio was suggested to be caused by the reduction of IL-4 mRNA expression.

In dogs with AD, IL-4-cytokine gene transcripts were detected in PBMCs and skin,[6,7] and IL-4 mRNA was overexpressed in skin lesions.[17] In contrast, a low percentage of IFN-γ mRNA was transcribed in the skin ex-

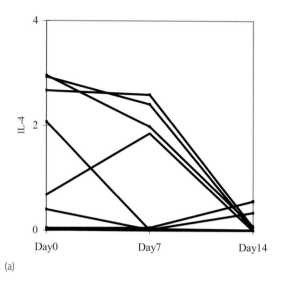

(a)

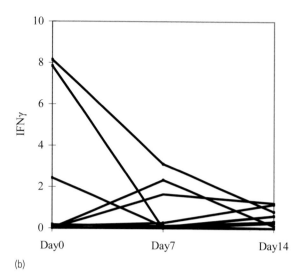

(b)

Figure 1.10.2 Time course of IL-4 mRNA expression (a), IFN-γ mRNA expression (b), IL-4: IFN-γ mRNA expression ratio (c) in dogs with atopic dermatitis.

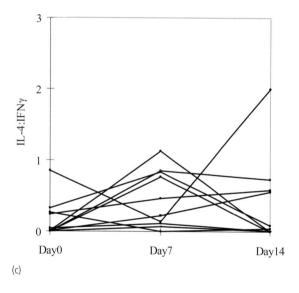

(c)

tract from dogs with AD, and IFN-γ mRNA expression in PBMCs of dogs with AD was significantly lower than that of control dogs.[7] Those findings imply that canine AD has characteristics similar to those of human and mouse AD. Therefore, rCaIFN-γ is suggested to modulate the Th1/Th2-cytokine imbalance towards Th1 dominance, from Th2 dominance, in dogs with AD.

One study of rIFN-γ therapy in human AD patients has revealed an increase in IFN-γ mRNA expression in PBMCs, but no increase in IL-4 mRNA expression.[10] Our results are similar in that IL-4 mRNA expression was decreased in our dogs that showed improvement in total clinical scores, but was increased in those showing no improvement.

IFN-γ has been reported to inhibit the production of IL-4 by helper T lymphocytes, and to inhibit the production of IgE antibodies by B lymphocytes.[17] The modulation of the cytokine balance in canine AD by IFN-γ may be due to the suppression of IL-4 expression *in vivo*. In addition, the decrease in the IL-4/IFN-γ-mRNA ratio is accompanied by a decrease in the serum total IgE level. However, the serum total IgE levels are not significantly different between healthy and atopic dogs,[18,19] whereas the allergen-specific IgE levels are higher in most AD dogs. The number of IgE-positive cells in skin lesions seen on immunohistochemistry also seemed to have decreased, as the numbers of

dermal IgE-positive cells and mast cells were decreased 2 weeks after the administration of rCaIFN-γ.

When rhIFN-γ was administered to human AD patients, the clinical symptoms were improved markedly without any decrease in serum total IgE levels.[11,12,20] However, in dogs, it has been reported that the serum total IgE level was not significantly different between normal and atopic dogs.[21] In our study, the IgE level before and after rCaIFN-γ injection was evaluated. The injection of rCaINF-γ was associated with a decrease in total serum IgE level.

One study has suggested that a major mechanism of action of rIFN-γ therapy in humans may be related to the inhibition of Th2 cytokines in local skin lesions, and that IFN-γ does not affect the production of serum total IgE.[13] The injection frequency and the dosage of IFN-γ in this study, and the difference in the minimum IFN-γ concentration between dog and human required for the inhibition IgE production, may contribute to the reduction of circulating serum total IgE levels. From these results, a series of injections of rCaIFN-γ may be effective for the treatment of canine AD, and its mechanism of action may be correlated with the suppression of IgE production through the modulation of Th1/Th2-cytokine expression.

Although the results of this pilot study are encouraging, we recognise the limitations of the study, which include: only a small number of patients were treated; the treatment was for a very short period of time; patients were removed from their home environment during the course of treatment; the patients were mostly of one breed (Shih Tzu); and most patients were of the female gender. Nevertheless, the apparent efficacy of rCaIFN-γ in the patients in this study with AD does raise the possibility of reducing the use of corticosteroids in canine AD. Further studies are needed to evaluate the long-term effects and possible adverse reactions, and to determine whether these results can be translated into a larger and more diverse group of dogs with AD.

Acknowledgement

rCaIFN-γ was a gift from Toray Company (Tokyo, Japan).

References

1 Willemse, T. Atopic skin disease: a review and reconsideration of diagnostic criteria. *Journal of Small Animal Practice*, 1986; **27**: 771–778.

2 Willemse, T. Comparative aspects of the immunopathogenesis and treatment of atopic dermatitis in dogs and humans. *Japanese Journal of Dermatoallergology*, 2001; **9**: 1–8.

3 Scott, D.W., Miller, W.H., Griffin, C.E. *Small Animal Dermatology*, 6th edn. W.B. Saunders, Philadelphia, 2000: 574–661.

4 Chang, T.T., Stevens, S.R. Atopic dermatitis: the role of recombinant interferon-gamma therapy. *American Journal of Clinical Dermatology*, 2002; **3**: 175–183.

5 Jujo, K., Renz, H., Abe, J., Gelfand, E.W., Leung, D.Y. Decreased interferon gamma and increased interleukin-4 production in atopic dermatitis promotes IgE synthesis. *Journal of Allergy and Clinical Immunology*, 1992; **90**: 323–331.

6 Nuttall, T.J., Knight, P.A., McAleese, S.M., Lamb, J.R., Hill, P.B. T-helper 1, T-helper 2 and immunosuppressive cytokines in canine atopic dermatitis. *Veterinary Immunology and Immunopathology*, 2002; **87**: 379–384.

7 Olivry, T., Dean, G.A., Tompkins, M.B., Dow, J.L., Moore, P.F. Toward a canine model of atopic dermatitis: amplification of cytokine-gene transcripts in the skin of atopic dogs. *Experimental Dermatology*, 1999; **8**: 204–211.

8 Trautmann, A., Akdis, M., Schmid-Grendelmeier, P., *et al.* Targeting keratinocyte apoptosis in the treatment of atopic dermatitis and allergic contact dermatitis. *Journal of Allergy and Clinical Immunology*, 2001; **108**: 839–846.

9 Boguniewicz, M., Jafee, H.S., Izu, A., *et al.* Recombinant gamma interferon in treatment of patients with atopic dermatitis and elevated IgE levels. *American Journal of Medicine*, 1990; **88**: 365–370.

10 Hanifin, J.M., Schnieder, L.C., Leung, D.Y., *et al.* Recombinant interferon gamma therapy for atopic dermatitis. *Journal of American Academy of Dermatology*, 1993; **28**: 189–197.

11 Noh, G.W., Lee, K.Y. Blood eosinophils and serum IgE as predictors for prognosis of interferon-gamma therapy in atopic dermatitis. *Allergy*, 1998; **53**: 1202–1207.

12 Reinwald, U., Wehrmann, W., Kukel, S., Kreysel, H.W. Recombinant interferon-gamma in severe atopic dermatitis. *Lancet*, 1990; **335**: 1282.

13 Schneider, L.C., Baz, Z., Zarcone, C., Zurakowski, D. Long-term therapy with recombinant interferon-gamma (rIFN-gamma) for atopic dermatitis. *Annals of Allergy, Asthma and Immunology*, 1998; **80**: 263–268.

14 Sinke, J.D., Thepen, T., Bihari, I.C., Rutten, V.P., Willemse, T. Immunophenotyping of skin-infiltrating T-cell subsets in dogs with atopic dermatitis. *Veterinary Quarterly*, 1998; **20**: S107.

15 Okano, F., Satoh, M., Ido, T., Okamoto, N., Yamada, K. Production of canine IFN-gamma in silkworm by recombinant baculovirus and characterization of the product. *Journal of Interferon and Cytokine Research*, 2000; **20**: 1015–1022.

16 Teramoto, T., Fukao, T., Tashita, H., *et al.* Serum IgE level is negatively correlated with the ability of peripheral mononuclear cells to produce interferon gamma (IFN-γ): evidence of reduced expression of IFN-γ mRNA in atopic patients. *Clinical and Experimental Allergy*, 1998; **28**: 74–82.

17 Hayashiya, S., Tani, K., Morimoto, M., *et al.* Expression of T helper 1 and T helper 2 cytokine mRNAs in freshly isolated peripheral blood mononuclear cells from dogs with atopic dermatitis. *Journal of Veterinary Medicine Series A*, 2002; **49**: 27–31.

18 Del Prete, G.F., De Carli, M., Ricci, M., Romagnani, S. Helper activity for immunoglobulin synthesis of T helper type I (Th1) and Th2 human T cell clones: the help of Th1 clones is limited by their cytolytic capacity. *Journal of Experimental Medicine*, 1994; **174**: 809–813.

19 Griot-Wenk, M.E., Busato, A., Welle, M., *et al.* Total serum IgE and IgA antibody levels in healthy dogs of different breeds and exposed to different environments. *Research in Veterinary Science*, 1999; **67**: 239–243.

20 Racine, B.P., Marti, E., Busato, A., Weilenmann, R., Lazary, S., Griot-Wenk, M.E. Influence of sex and age on serum total immunoglobulin E concentration in Beagles. *American Journal of Veterinary Research*, 1999; **60**: 93–97.

21 Hill, P.B., Moriello, K.A., DeBoer D.J. Concentrations of total serum IgE, IgA and IgG in atopic and parasitized dogs. *Veterinary Immunology and Immunopathology*, 1995; **44**: 105–113.

Effects of the immunomodulatory drugs tacrolimus, rapamycin and cilomilast on dendritic cell function in a rodent model of allergic contact dermatitis

W. Bäumer Dr med vet[1], B. Sülzle Dr med vet[1], H. Weigt Dr rer nat[2], M. Hecht Dr rer nat[3], M. Kietzmann Dr med vet[1]

[1] Department of Pharmacology, Toxicology and Pharmacy, University of Veterinary Medicine Hannover Foundation, Hannover, Germany
[2] LipoNova GmbH, Hannover, Germany
[3] Fraunhofer Institute of Toxicology and Experimental Medicine, Hannover, Germany

Summary

The *in vitro* and *in vivo* immunomodulatory effects of the phosphodiesterase-4 inhibitor cilomilast were compared to tacrolimus and rapamycin, immunosuppressive drugs for use in organ transplantation. Tacrolimus is also registered for treatment of human atopic dermatitis. *In vitro*, the effect of these agents on the mixed leukocyte reaction (dendritic cell-mediated T-cell activation) was tested. Cilomilast and tacrolimus, as well as rapamycin, were able to inhibit proliferation in a dose-dependent manner.

In vivo, the inhibitory action of the immunomodulatory drugs was compared in the toluene-2,4-diisocyanate (TDI)-induced allergic inflammatory response. After topical administration, cilomilast and tacrolimus, but not rapamycin, inhibited the inflammatory response. Only combined topical and systemic administration of rapamycin caused a distinct inhibition of the allergic reaction. Cilomilast (20 mg/kg) and rapamycin (20 mg/kg) as well as tacrolimus (2.5 mg/kg) were administered intraperitoneally at 16 and 0.5 hours before challenge, and topically onto mouse ears (cilomilast 3%, rapamycin 1%, tacrolimus 0.5%) 2 hours before challenge. All substances induced a significant inhibition of the ear swelling measured 16 hours after TDI challenge, accompanied by a reduction of the draining auricular lymph node weight and lymphocyte cell count. Corresponding to this, the density of Langerhans cells in the epidermis was higher in cilomilast-, tacrolimus- and rapamycin-treated mice compared with vehicle-treated mice. Dendritic cell migration, as measured in a skin dendritic cell migration assay on cultivated ears, was also significantly inhibited by all agents.

Introduction

The launch of cyclosporin A for the treatment of canine atopic dermatitis (AD) provides a promising alternative to classical glucocorticoid therapy and has focused attention on new immunomodulatory therapeutics. The immunosuppressive agents tacrolimus and rapamycin are macrolide antibiotics in clinical use as immunosuppressive drugs for the treatment of transplant rejection and autoimmune diseases. Tacrolimus is also registered for the topical treatment of human AD. The inhibitory action of rapamycin and tacrolimus in models of allergic contact dermatitis is controversial. Both agents showed inhibitory activity in a murine contact sensitivity reaction provoked by trinitrochlorobenzene.[1] Tacrolimus was also effective in dinitrofluorobenzene-induced contact sensitivity in domestic pigs, whereas rapamycin was ineffective when administered by either topical or systemic routes.[2] Similar results were obtained by Duncan[3] in a comparable model of delayed-type hypersensitivity in guinea-pigs.

The phosphodiesterase-4 inhibitor cilomilast, currently available for the treatment of asthma and chronic obstructive pulmonary disease,[4] has demonstrated inhibitory effects in models of allergic contact dermatitis.[5–7]

Langerhans cells, as well as dermal dendritic cells (DCs), carry haptens (such as toluene-2,4-diisocyanate [TDI]) from the skin through afferent lymphatic vessels to draining lymph nodes. There, haptens (bound to peptides) are presented to T cells which subsequently become specific T cells (induction phase). When the hapten is applied for a second time, Langerhans cells or dermal DCs present it to specific T cells, which are then activated, produce cytokines, and activate further inflammatory cells (elicitation phase).[8]

The aim of this study was to compare the anti-inflammatory and immunomodulatory activity of cilomilast, tacrolimus and rapamycin in a model of TDI-induced allergic contact dermatitis with particular focus on DC migration and activation.

Materials and methods

Mice

Female BALB/c mice were purchased from Charles River GmbH (Sulzfeld, Germany) at the age of 8 weeks (20 g body weight). The mice were housed in groups of six mice per cage at 22°C with a 12-hour light/dark cycle. Water and a standard diet (Altromin, Lage/Lippe, Germany) were available *ad libitum*. The animal experiments were approved by Bezirksregierung Hannover, Germany (Az. 509.6-42502-03/711).

DC generation from bone marrow cultures

Bone marrow-derived DCs were generated in high purity according to the protocol of Lutz *et al.*[9] with slight modifications as described previously.[10] Briefly, bone marrow was cultivated with RPMI 1640 (Biochrom, Berlin, Germany), 10% fetal calf serum (Biochrom) and 50 µmol/L 2-mercaptoethanol (Sigma, Deisenhofen, Germany). The medium contained 20 ng/ml granulocyte-macrophage colony-stimulating factor (GM-CSF) (Sigma). On days 3, 6 and 8, fresh medium supplemented with GM-CSF was added. FACS analysis of the 10-day-old cell suspension demonstrated a high yield of CD11c and major histocompatibility complex (MHC) class II-positive cells.[10]

Incubation with cilomilast, tacrolimus and rapamycin

After cultivation for 9 days, the cells were incubated with 10 µmol/L cilomilast (Elbion AG, Radebeul, Germany), 100 nmol/L tacrolimus (Calbiochem, Darmstadt, Germany) or 1 µmol/L rapamycin (Wyeth-Ayerst, Princeton, NJ, USA) for 24 hours. The selected concentrations were high, but did not influence the cell viability as determined by CellTiter© AQueous One Solution cell proliferation assay (Promega, Mannheim, Germany) (data not shown).

At day 10 the cells were again incubated with the agents as indicated above and stimulated by addition of 1 µg/ml lipopolysaccharide (*Escherichia coli*, O127: B8, Sigma) working solution. The supernatant was collected 24 hours later and tumour necrosis factor alpha (TNF-α) and interleukin (IL)-12p70 were analysed by enzyme-linked immunosorbent assay (ELISA) (DuoSet and Quantikine respectively, R&D Systems, Wiesbaden, Germany). Three independent experiments were performed.

Mixed leukocyte reaction

T cells were isolated from the spleen of female NMRI mice (an outbred strain) by a plastic adherence method.[11] The cells (1×10^5/well) were seeded in a 96-well U-bottomed plate. DCs derived from BALB/c mice (day 10 of culture) were added in doubling quantities (Table 1.11.1) and incubated with cilomilast (10 µmol/L), tacrolimus (100 nmol/L) and rapamycin (1 µmol/L). After 6 days, proliferation of T cells was determined by incorporation of ^{3}H-thymidine (1 µCi/well) (Hartmann Analytics, Braunschweig, Germany) during the last 18 hours of culture. The cells were subsequently harvested on filtermats (Canberra-Packard, Dreieich, Germany). After drying, 20 µl of liquid scintillator (Canberra-Packard) were added and the plates were sealed. Counts per minute were determined on a Topcount Microplate Scintillation Counter (Canberra-Packard). Three independent experiments were performed with each agent.

Mouse ear swelling test

Sensitisation was performed as described previously.[6] After 1 week of acclimitisation, the abdominal skin of the mice was shaved and depilated with Veet® (Reckitt

Table 1.11.1 Inhibitory action (% inhibition of ^{3}H-thymidine incorporation) of cilomilast (10 µmol/L), tacrolimus (100 nmol/L) and rapamycin (1 µmol/L) in the mixed leukocyte reaction

Agent	DCs					
	312	625	1250	2500	5000	100 000
Cilomilast	61 ± 4	57 ± 6	80 ± 5	74 ± 9	69 ± 20	75 ± 12
Tacrolimus	96 ± 2	93 ± 1	93 ± 2	93 ± 2	92 ± 2	90 ± 3
Rapamycin	85 ± 7	90 ± 1	88 ± 5	94 ± 1	89 ± 5	81 ± 10

The indicated amounts of dendritic cells (DCs) were added to 1×10^5 T cells. Mean ± standard deviation (SD) of five single values per concentration is given for one representative of three independent experiments. The inhibition is highly significant for all agents ($p < 0.01$) compared with the untreated control (set at 100%).

& Colman, Hamburg, Germany). The abdominal skin was stripped with adhesive tapes (Tesafilm, Beiersdorf, Germany). For active sensitisation, 100 µl TDI (5% in acetone) were administered to the stripped epidermis on 3 consecutive days.

The allergic reaction was evaluated 21 days later by administration of 20 µl TDI (0.5% in acetone) on both the inner and outer surface of the left ear to examine the sensitisation status. Ear thickness was measured with a cutimeter (Mitutoyo, Neuss, Germany) and the swelling was calculated by comparison of the ear thickness before challenge and 24 hours after challenge. Animals with a mean increase in ear thickness of < 20% at 24 hours after challenge were excluded as being not sensitised (< 5% of all sensitised mice). The included mice were, according to their swelling intensity, equally distributed to the treatment groups ($n = 6$), so that each group contained animals with various degrees of swelling. The swelling was allowed to abate until the ear thickness had reached an almost normal level after 7 days. To exclude contamination by residues of the allergen on the ears, the untreated right ears were used for the main experiment.

Drug administration

Cilomilast (20 mg/kg), tacrolimus (2.5 mg/kg) (a kind gift from Prof. Dr G. Wozel, Dresden, Germany) and rapamycin (20 mg/kg) were administered intraperitoneally in 50% polyethylene glycol 300, 2.5% Tween 80 (Sigma) and 10% ethanol (VWR, Darmstadt, Germany) at the same doses and times as indicated above.[12] For topical administration, the agents were dissolved in acetone/DMSO (1:9) with addition of ethanol (10%). The concentrations were: cilomilast 3% (600 µg/ear), rapamycin 1% (200 µg/ear) and tacrolimus 0.5% (100 µg/ear); 20-µl amounts were applied to each ear.

This combination of topical and intraperitoneal administration was performed for each substance at least twice ($n = 6$ for each group and each experiment) with similar results.

Skin DC migration assay

At 16 hours after challenge and determination of ear thickness, mice were sacrificed by cervical dislocation. The cartilage-free dorsal halves of split mouse ear skin were cultured in 24-well microtitration plates based on the method described by Ortner et al.[13] Directly before cultivation, the ear halves were treated again with cilomilast, tacrolimus, rapamycin or vehicle (10 µl). The ear halves were laid epidermal side up on tables made of sieves.[10] As a chemotactic factor for DCs, macrophage inflammatory protein-3β was added (50 ng/ml; R&D Systems, Wiesbaden, Germany). The tables were changed daily, with new wells and new media (including macrophage inflammatory protein-3β). Migrated cells from each ear (days 2 and 3) were pooled and counted with a haemocytometer (Neubauer, VWR). The viability of the cells was assessed by trypan blue exclusion.

Determination of cell count in lymph nodes

The auricular lymph nodes were sampled and weighed and single cell suspensions were prepared in PBS by means of a glass potter (VWR). The cells were counted (Casy plus, Schärfe System GmbH, Reutlingen, Germany).

Preparation of epidermal sheets for immunohistochemistry

The preparation and the evaluation of epidermal sheets was performed as described previously.[10] In short, skin was floated on 0.5 M ammonium thiocyanate (Riedel de Haën, Hannover, Germany) for 10 minutes at 37°C. The epidermis was separated from the dermis and immediately fixed in cold acetone. The DCs were detected with monoclonal anti-mouse MHC class II (I-A/I-E, rat IgG2b; Beckton Dickinson, Heidelberg, Germany). Labelling of the antibodies was visualised using biotinylated rabbit anti-rat immunoglobulin G (DAKO, Hamburg, Germany) and streptavidin-fluorochrome (carbocyanin 3; Jackson Immunoresearch Laboratories, PA, USA). Analyses were performed by using Kontron KS 400 image analysis system. The density of Langerhans cells was analysed (×40 magnifications, calibrated grid). Sixteen randomly chosen fields were counted per ear. Six each of the vehicle-, rapamycin-, cilomilast- and tacrolimus-treated ears were analysed.

Statistical evaluation

Figures are presented as mean (± SEM). Significant differences between the drug treatments and controls were assessed by a one-way ANOVA followed by a post hoc test (Dunnett's test).

Results

Mixed leukocyte reaction

The inhibitory potential of the substances was evaluated as the percentage of inhibition of proliferation calculated by division of the untreated control by the respective treatment group times 100. Incubation of the MLR with tacrolimus (100 nmol/L), rapamycin (1 µmol/L) as well as cilomilast (10 µmol/L) inhibited the

DC-induced T-cell proliferation (Table 1.11.1). A dose-response experiment revealed a significant inhibition of T-cell proliferation by cilomilast only at 10 µmol/L, whereas tacrolimus and rapamycin inhibited the proliferation even at the lowest tested dose of 10 pmol/L and 100 pmol/L, respectively (data not shown). To discriminate between inhibitory action of cilomilast on T cells and DCs, an additional study was performed, where only DCs or T cells were preincubated with 10 µmol/L cilomilast and then washed thoroughly before the MLR. A preincubation of T cells resulted in comparable results to co-incubation. A preincubation of DCs resulted only in a moderate to slightly significant inhibition of the MLR (data not shown).

LPS-induced cytokine secretion

The secretion of TNF-α and IL-12 is significantly induced by LPS in BM-derived DCs. Cilomilast significantly inhibited the production of TNF-α as well as IL-12 in each experiment. In contrast, tacrolimus significantly inhibited TNF-α production and IL-12 production in only one of three experiments each. Further, rapamycin significantly inhibited TNF-α production in two of three experiments and IL-12 production in one of three experiments. The effects of tacrolimus and rapamycin were less pronounced than cilomilast in all experiments (Table 1.11.2).

Mouse ear swelling test, skin DC migration assay

TDI induced a strong increase in ear thickness (mean 130 µm) which was nearly totally inhibited by cilomilast and also significantly reduced by rapamycin and tac-

	Control	LPS	LPS + cilomilast	LPS + tacrolimus	LPS + rapamycin
TNF-α (pg/ml)					
Expt 1	97 ± 20	3819 ± 228	1561 ± 196*	3435 ± 192	2366 ± 196*
Expt 2	766 ± 76	5908 ± 576	2164 ± 360*	5126 ± 468	4060 ± 148
Expt 3	305 ± 30	2475 ± 120	1585 ± 85*	1900 ± 85*	1595 ± 105*
IL-12p70 (pg/ml)					
Expt 1	< 4	121 ± 9	38 ± 9*	62 ± 19*	156 ± 18
Expt 2	< 4	18 ± 4	4 ± 1*	42 ± 15	8 ± 3
Expt 3	< 4	208 ± 17	51 ± 3*	181 ± 9	135 ± 7*

Table 1.11.2 Effect of cilomilast, tacrolimus and rapamycin on LPS-induced TNF-α and IL-12 release in murine BM-derived dendritic cells (DCs)

DCs were treated with cilomilast (10 µM), tacrolimus (100 nM) and rapamycin (1 µM) 24 and 0.5 hours before lipopolysaccharide (LPS) stimulation (1 µg/ml). Supernatants were taken 24 hours after LPS challenge. *n* = 5 per group, *p < 0.01.

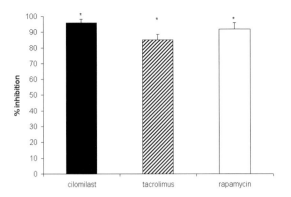

Fig. 1.11.1 Inhibition of the ear swelling 16 hours after TDI challenge. The induced ear swelling by TDI (mean swelling 130 μm) was significantly reduced by a combined topical and systemic treatment with cilomilast (black bar), rapamycin (white bar) and tacrolimus (cross-hatched bar) $n = 6$ mice per group, *$p < 0.01$.

rolimus (Fig. 1.11.1). Compared with vehicle-treated mouse ears, significantly less DCs migrated from ears treated with cilomilast, rapamycin or tacrolimus (Fig. 1.11.2). As the DC migration is induced by cytokines like TNF-α and IL-1β, we measured these cytokines in the skin of TDI-treated mice 30 minutes after challenge. However, we did not detect an increase of these two cytokines in TDI-challenged ear skin at this early time point (data not shown). Further studies need to be done at later time points. First results reveal a vast

increase of IL-1β but an unchanged TNF-α concentration 4 hours after TDI challenge.

Lymph node weight and cell count

Draining lymph nodes of TDI-treated mice were significantly increased in weight and cell count. Pretreatment with cilomilast caused a slight reduction while tacrolimus as well as rapamycin induced a significant reduction of lymph node weight. Tacrolimus also significantly reduced the cell count (Fig. 1.11.3).

MHC II-positive cells in the epidermis

Compared with vehicle (1352 ± 78 cells/mm²), the treatment with cilomilast (2246 ± 148 cells/mm²), rapamycin (1781 ± 168 cells/mm²) and tacrolimus (1960 ± 111 cells/mm²) resulted in a significantly higher cell count of MHC II-positive cells in the epidermis of TDI-challenged mice 16 hours after treatment (Fig. 1.11.4).

Discussion

As cyclosporin A has recently been registered for the treatment of canine AD, increased attention in veterinary dermatology has focused on various compounds with similar modes of action. Therefore, we tested the

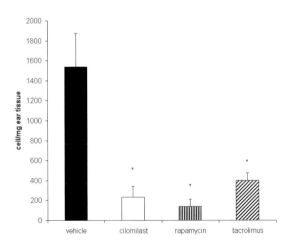

Fig. 1.11.2 Skin dendritic cell (DC) migration from mouse ear explants. Ears were cultivated 16 hours after TDI challenge: the ears were again treated topically with the agents directly before cultivation as indicated in Materials and methods. The DC migration was significantly inhibited by cilomilast, rapamycin and tacrolimus. $n = 6$ mice per group, *$p < 0.01$.

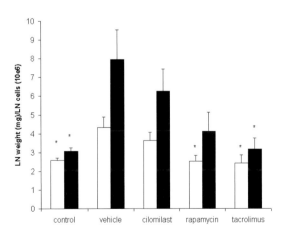

Fig. 1.11.3 Lymph node (LN) weight (white bars) and cell count (black bars) from the draining lymph nodes 16 hours after TDI challenge. TDI induced a significant increase in weight and cell count compared with untreated controls. Cilomilast, rapamycin and tacrolimus inhibited the TDI-induced increase to different extents. $n = 6$ mice per group, *$p < 0.01$.

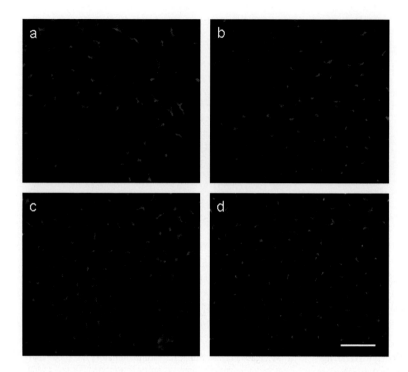

Fig. 1.11.4 Effect of rapamycin, tacrolimus and cilomilast on Langerhans cell density in murine skin 16 hours after TDI challenge. There are fewer cells in vehicle-treated mouse ears than in those treated with cilomilast, rapamycin and tacrolimus. (a) vehicle; (b) rapamycin; (c) tacrolimus; (d) cilomilast. Bar represents 50 μm.

macrolides tacrolimus and rapamycin in a model of TDI-induced allergic contact dermatitis. This model displays some similarities to atopic diseases as far as cell influx and induced cytokines are concerned.[14] We compared the effects of these agents with the highly selective phosphodiesterase-4 inhibitor cilomilast, a promising agent for the treatment of allergic diseases like asthma and AD in humans.[15,16] The immunosuppressant cyclosporine A has previously demonstrated reliable inhibitory actions in the model of allergic dermatitis in our laboratory.[17]

Furthermore, the described study was performed to compare the anti-inflammatory and immunomodulatory action of cilomilast, tacrolimus and rapamycin, with particular focus on migration and activation of DCs. As DCs are the most potent antigen-presenting cells in the induction phase, as well as the elicitation phase, of allergic contact dermatitis, it can be postulated that the inhibition of DC migration may explain, at least in part, the inhibitory action of these immunosuppressive agents. Their influence on T-cell activation has been widely examined.[18–20] The inhibitory action of cilomilast, tacrolimus and rapamycin in the MLR experiment in our study may also be explained by the inhibition of the T-cell response. However, due

to the treatment of both cell types (T cells and DCs) during the co-incubation, we cannot exclude the possibility that DC function is also affected, as demonstrated for cilomilast. Essayan et al.[21] obtained similar results for the PDE4 inhibitor rolipram in a model of antigen-driven proliferation. The influence of tacrolimus, rapamycin and cilomilast on DC function is still controversial.[22–26] Similar to our results, it was also demonstrated by Heystek et al.[25] that cilomilast (10 μM) did not influence the LPS-induced up-regulation of surface expression of CD80 and CD86 in human monocyte-derived DCs. However, they also observed an inhibitory action of cilomilast on LPS-induced TNF-α and IL-12 secretion. From the IL-12 results it was concluded that PDE4 inhibitors may also diminish Th1 responses in vivo. An earlier study from our laboratory showed that PDE4 inhibitors also diminish secretion of typical Th2 cytokines (such as IL-4) in inflamed skin.[6] Thus, it is likely that PDE4 inhibitors like cilomilast can modulate inflammatory reactions characterised by both Th1 and Th2 cytokines.

Matsue et al.[24] could not detect inhibition of IL-12p40 by rapamycin or tacrolimus in LPS-stimulated bone marrow-derived DCs. Tacrolimus, on the other hand, inhibited the IL-12p70 secretion during antigen presentation in a co-culture of DCs and ovalbumin-specific T cells (DO11.10) in the presence of ovalbumin, whereas rapamycin caused only slight inhibitory action.[24] A recent study revealed that LPS-stimulated bone marrow-derived DCs expressed high levels of IL-12, which was not influenced by rapamycin (20 ng/ml) either at the mRNA or the protein level.[26]

The influence of cilomilast on DC migration in non-inflamed skin has been demonstrated.[10] Additionally, a recent study demonstrated the inhibitory effect of cyclosporine A on DC migration through skin.[27] Analysis of epidermal sheets in the study reported here demonstrated that all substances caused an inhibition of Langerhans cell migration compared with vehicle-treated mouse ears. This was confirmed by the skin DC migration assay. It has to be stressed that the ear halves were cultivated 16 hours after TDI challenge, which provides some time for Langerhans cell migration to commence. On the other hand, this time point (16 hours) allowed a determination of the status quo in the epidermis (Fig. 1.11.4). Interestingly, cilomilast induced only a slight reduction of draining lymph node weight and cell count after TDI challenge (Fig. 1.11.3). As seen in the MLR, cilomilast can inhibit T-cell proliferation only at the high concentration of 10 μmol/L. It is questionable whether these high concentrations will be achieved *in vivo* in the lymph node. Therefore, the distinct inhibition of ear swelling (Fig. 1.11.1) and Langerhans cell migration (Fig. 1.11.4) might be due to the direct action of topically administered agents on keratinocytes and Langerhans cells. Thus, it may be speculated that PDE4 inhibitors with a much lower IC_{50} for PDE4 (e.g. roflumilast) could also induce inhibition of the T-cell response.

It is well established that proinflammatory signals like TNF-α and IL-1β, secreted by keratinocytes for example, play a crucial role as early signals for Langerhans cell migration.[28,29] Nevertheless, for cilomilast, significant inhibition of IL-1β secretion in ear skin 4, 8 and 16 hours after TDI challenge has already been demonstrated.[7] Thus, it can be concluded that all tested agents may have only moderate direct effects on DC function *in vitro*, but that they display an inhibitory effect on Langerhans cell migration. This may be orchestrated by an interaction between keratinocytes and Langerhans cells in a way that the secretion of proinflammatory mediators like TNF-α and IL-1β is modulated. These signals are crucial in the early migration phase of Langerhans cells.[28,29] An inhibition of Langerhans cell migration could at least partly explain the anti-inflammatory and immunomodulatory action of cilomilast, tacrolimus and rapamycin in allergic dermatitis.

Acknowledgements

We would like to thank Elbion AG for supplying cilomilast and Prof. Dr G. Wozel for supplying tacrolimus. Our thanks go to Ulrike Seegers, Olaf Macke and Sabine Schild for their valuable assistance in the laboratory.

Funding

This study was self-funded.

References

1 Salerno, A., Bonanno, C.T., Caccamo, N., *et al*. The effect of cyclosporin A, FK506 and rapamycin on the murine contact sensitivity reaction. *Clinical and Experimental Immunology*, 1998; **112**: 112–119.

2 Meingassner, J.G., Stutz, A. Antiinflammatory effects of macrophilin-interacting drugs in animal-models of irritant and allergic contact-dermatitis. *International Archives of Allergy and Immunology*, 1992; **99**: 486–489.

3 Duncan, J.I. Differential inhibition of cutaneous T-cell-mediated reactions and epidermal cell proliferation by cyclosporin A, FK-506, and rapamycin. *Journal of Investigative Dermatology*, 1994; **102**: 84–88.

4 Giembycz, M.A. Cilomilast: a second generation phosphodiesterase 4 inhibitor for asthma and chronic obstructive pulmonary disease. *Expert Opinion on Investigational Drugs*, 2001; **10**: 1361–1379.

5 Griswold, D.E., Webb, E.F., Badger, A.M., *et al*. SB 207499 (Ariflo), a second generation phosphodiesterase 4 inhibitor, reduces tumor necrosis factor alpha and interleukin-4 production in vivo. *Journal of Pharmacology and Experimental Therapeutics*, 1998; **287**: 705–711.

6 Baumer, W., Gorr, G., Hoppmann, J., Ehinger, A.M., Rundfeldt, C., Kietzmann, M. AWD 12-281, a highly selective phosphodiesterase 4 inhibitor, is effective in the prevention and treatment of inflammatory reactions in a model of allergic dermatitis. *Journal of Pharmacy and Pharmacology*, 2003; **55**: 1107–1114.

7 Baumer, W., Gorr, G., Hoppmann, J., Ehinger, A.M., Ehinger, B., Kietzmann, M. Effects of the phosphodiesterase 4 inhibitors SB 207499 and AWD 12-281 on the inflammatory reaction in a model of allergic dermatitis. *Euopean Journal of Pharmacology*, 2002; **446**: 195–200.

8 Kimber, I., Dearman, R.J. Allergic contact dermatitis: the cellular effectors. *Contact Dermatitis*, 2002; **46**: 1–5.

9 Lutz, M.B., Kukutsch, N., Ogilvie, A.L., *et al*. An advanced culture method for generating large quantities of highly pure dendritic cells from mouse bone marrow. *Journal of Immunological Methods*, 1999; **223**: 77–92.

10 Baumer, W., Tschernig, T., Sulzle, B., Seegers, U., Luhrmann, A., Kietzmann, M. Effects of cilomilast on dendritic cell function in contact sensitivity and dendritic cell migration through skin. *Euopean Journal of Pharmacology*, 2003; **481**: 271–279.

11 Gunzer, M., Weishaupt, C., Planelles, L., Grabbe, S. Two-step negative enrichment of CD4+ and CD8+ T cells from murine spleen via nylon wool adherence and an optimized antibody cocktail. *Journal of Immunological Methods*, 2001; **258**: 55–63.

12 Hackstein, H., Taner, T., Logar, A.J., Thomson, A.W. Rapamycin inhibits macropinocytosis and mannose receptor-mediated endocytosis by bone marrow-derived dendritic cells. *Blood*, 2002; **100**: 1084–1087.

13 Ortner, U., Inaba, K., Koch, F., *et al.* An improved isolation method for murine migratory cutaneous dendritic cells. *Journal of Immunological Methods*, 1996; **193**: 71–79.

14 Nuttall, T.J., Knight, P.A., McAleese, S.M., Lamb, J.R., Hill, P.B. T-helper 1, T-helper 2 and immunosuppressive cytokines in canine atopic dermatitis. *Veterinary Immunology and Immunopathology*, 2002; **87**: 379–384.

15 Hanifin, J.M., Chan, S.C., Cheng, J.B., *et al.* Type 4 phosphodiesterase inhibitors have clinical and in vitro anti-inflammatory effects in atopic dermatitis. *Journal of Investigative Dermatology*, 1996; **107**: 51–56.

16 Griffiths, C.E., Van Leent, E.J., Gilbert, M., Traulsen, J. Randomized comparison of the type 4 phosphodiesterase inhibitor cipamfylline cream, cream vehicle and hydrocortisone 17-butyrate cream for the treatment of atopic dermatitis. *British Journal of Dermatology*, 2002; **147**: 299–307.

17 Ehinger, A.M., Gorr, G., Hoppmann, J., Telser, E., Ehinger, B., Kietzmann, M. Effects of the phosphodiesterase 4 inhibitor RPR 73401 in a model of immunological inflammation. *European Journal of Pharmacology*, 2000; **392**: 93–99.

18 Tocci, M.J., Matkovich, D.A., Collier, K.A., *et al.* The immunosuppressant FK506 selectively inhibits expression of early T cell activation genes. *Journal of Immunology*, 1989; **143**: 718–726.

19 Dumont, F.J., Melino, M.R., Staruch, M.J., Koprak, S.L., Fischer, P.A., Sigal, N.H. The immunosuppressive macrolides FK-506 and rapamycin act as reciprocal antagonists in murine T cells. *Journal of Immunology*, 1990; **144**: 1418–1424.

20 Barnette, M.S., Christensen, S.B., Essayan, D.M., *et al.* SB 207499 (Ariflo), a potent and selective second-generation phosphodiesterase 4 inhibitor: in vitro anti-inflammatory actions. *Journal of Pharmacology and Experimental Therapeutics*, 1998; **284**: 420–426.

21 Essayan, D.M., Huang, S.K., Kagey-Sobotka, A., Lichtenstein, L.M. Differential efficacy of lymphocyte- and monocyte-selective pretreatment with a type 4 phosphodiesterase inhibitor on antigen-driven proliferation and cytokine gene expression. *Journal of Allergy and Clinical Immunology*, 1997; **99**: 28–37.

22 Gantner, F., Schudt, C., Wendel, A., Hatzelmann, A. Characterization of the phosphodiesterase (PDE) pattern of in vitro-generated human dendritic cells (DC) and the influence of PDE inhibitors on DC function. *Pulmonary Pharmacology and Therapeutics*, 1999; **12**: 377–386.

23 Hatzelmann, A., Schudt, C. Anti-inflammatory and immunomodulatory potential of the novel PDE4 inhibitor roflumilast in vitro. *Journal of Pharmacology and Experimental Therapeutics*, 2001; **297**: 267–279.

24 Matsue, H., Yang, C., Matsue, K., Edelbaum, D., Mummert, M., Takashima, A. Contrasting impacts of immunosuppressive agents (rapamycin, FK506, cyclosporin A, and dexamethasone) on bidirectional dendritic cell-T cell interaction during antigen presentation. *Journal of Immunology*, 2002; **169**: 3555–3564.

25 Heystek, H.C., Thierry, A.C., Soulard, P., Moulon, C. Phosphodiesterase 4 inhibitors reduce human dendritic cell inflammatory cytokine production and Th1-polarizing capacity. *International Immunology*, 2003; **15**: 827–835.

26 Chiang, P.H., Wang, L., Bonham, C.A., *et al.* Mechanistic insights into impaired dendritic cell function by rapamycin: inhibition of Jak2/Stat4 signaling pathway. *Journal of Immunology*, 2004; **172**: 1355–1363.

27 Chen, T., Guo, J., Yang, M., *et al.* Cyclosporin A impairs dendritic cell migration by regulating chemokine receptor expression and inhibiting cyclooxygenase-2 expression. *Blood*, 2004; **103**: 413–421.

28 Cumberbatch, M., Dearman, R.J., Kimber, I. Inhibition by dexamethasone of Langerhans cell migration: influence of epidermal cytokine signals. *Immunopharmacology*, 1999; **41**: 235–243.

29 Stoitzner, P., Zanella, M., Ortner, U., *et al.* Migration of Langerhans cells and dermal dendritic cells in skin organ cultures: augmentation by TNF-alpha and IL-1beta. *Journal of Leukocyte Biology*, 1999; **66**: 462–470.

Temporal development of ovine cutaneous hypersensitivity responses to *Psoroptes ovis* (sheep scab mite)

A.H.M. van den Broek BVSc, PhD, DVR[1], J.F. Huntley MSc, PhD, MIBiol[2], R.E.W. Halliwell MA, VetMB, PhD[1],
A. Mackellar[2], M.A. Taylor BVMS, PhD, CBiol, MIBiol[3], H.R.P. Miller BVMS, PhD[1]

[1] Department of Veterinary Clinical Studies, Royal (Dick) School of Veterinary Studies, University of Edinburgh, Easter Bush Veterinary Centre, Easter Bush, Roslin, United Kingdom
[2] Division of Parasitology, Moredun Research Institute, Pentlands Science Park, Bush Loan, Penicuik, United Kingdom
[3] Central Science Laboratory, Sand Hutton, York, United Kingdom

Summary

Wheal reactions to repeated bites of several haematophagous arthropods develop in an orderly sequence; a delayed response, both immediate and delayed responses, and an immediate response. *Psoroptes ovis* infestations of sheep elicit immediate (IH) and a delayed-type (DTH) hypersensitivity responses; however, the temporal development of these reactions has not been reported.

In the study described here, clinical and histological examination of responses provoked by intradermal injection of *P. ovis* whole-mite extract (WME) were employed to investigate the temporal development of hypersensitivity responses of sheep to *P. ovis*. In addition, the relationship between the numbers of eosinophils and CD4+ T cells in the DTH was examined. In contrast to the classical response pattern, IH wheal reactions occurred first and were observed at 7 weeks, relatively late in the course of the infestation. Although none of the sheep had developed a delayed wheal reaction by 9 weeks after infestation, histology at this time demonstrated that *P. ovis* WME provoked an eosinophil-rich DTH. There was a strong correlation between numbers of CD4+ T cells and eosinophils at sites of intradermal challenge with *P. ovis* WME, suggesting that CD4+ T cells may be involved in the genesis of the eosinophil-rich DTH response to *P. ovis*.

Introduction

Host responses to ectoparasitic arthropods commonly include immediate (IH) and delayed-type (DTH) cutaneous hypersensitivity responses.[1,2] Several studies have demonstrated a definite sequence in the pattern of IH and DTH wheal reactions elicited by repeated exposure of hosts to the bites of haematophagous arthropods.[2–5] However, histopathology accompanying these responses has been examined in only a limited number of studies.[6–8] Although this typical sequence of hypersensitivity reactions also has been demonstrated in pigs infested with the burrowing mite *Sarcoptes scabiei*, the temporal development of responses to other ectoparasitic mites has not been reported.[9]

Wheal reactions to intradermal injection of *Psoroptes* spp. extract in infested rabbits, cattle and sheep have demonstrated that *Psoroptes* spp. infestations

provoke IH, DTH, and possibly a late-phase response (LPR) or Arthus-type reaction.[1,10–13] In addition, histopathology has indicated that, in sheep, the LPR and DTH elicited by intradermal injection of *P. ovis* whole-mite extract (WME) are characterised by an eosinophil-rich infiltrate.[13] However, the pattern of IH and DTH development in the course of infestation has not been reported.

This study employed clinical and histological examination of the responses elicited by intradermal injection of *P. ovis* WME to investigate the temporal development of hypersensitivity responses of sheep infested with *P. ovis*. In addition, as the T-cell dependence of the eosinophil-rich DTH response to *S. mansoni* cercariae and eggs has been demonstrated,[14,15] this study also examined the relationship between eosinophils and CD+ T cells at a limited number of intradermal test sites.

Materials and methods

Animals

Suffolk-cross sheep, between 1 and 2 years of age, and with no previous exposure to *P. ovis*, were used in these experiments.

Five sheep were infested to the left of the withers with a cluster of 25–50 ovigerous *P. ovis* mites as described previously.[16] Throughout the experiment the fleece over the right lateral thorax and abdomen was kept closely clipped, exposing the skin, and petroleum jelly (Vaseline®, Leverfaberge, GmbH, 21614 Buxtehude, Germany) was applied daily at the perimeter of this area. This preserved a lesion-free area for intradermal tests (IDTs). In one animal the infestation failed to become established, consequently it was omitted from the results. Five sheep were used as naive (uninfested) controls.

Allergen extracts

P. ovis WME was prepared as follows: *P. ovis* mites (adults, nymphs and larvae) were collected from infested sheep. The live mites were washed by vortex mixing for 5 minutes in ice-cold phosphate-buffered saline (PBS; pH 7.2), followed by 1% sodium dodecyl sulphate at room temperature, and finally 10 washes in ice-cold PBS. Mites were then homogenised and sonicated in ice-cold PBS. The final homogenate was centrifuged at 10 000 g for 10 minutes and the supernatant (WME) was harvested, aliquoted and stored at –70°C. Protein content of the supernatant was determined, in accordance with the manufacturer's instructions, with a BCA™ Protein Assay Kit (Pierce Biotechnology Inc., Rockford, IL, USA). Fresh solutions of sterile PBS containing *P. ovis* WME were prepared immediately before each skin test.

Performance of IDTs

IDTs were carried out 1, 3, 5, 7 and 9 weeks after infestation and at the same intervals in the case of the naive controls. Sheep were restrained in lateral recumbency and a 3 × 2 grid was marked on the clipped flank, with a minimum of 2.5 cm between each point. Intradermal injections were made with a 25-gauge needle, bevelled edge rotated toward the epidermis, and an insulin syringe. Intradermal injections of 0.05 ml of *P. ovis* WME (10 μg protein/ml) and 0.05 ml of the diluent (PBS) control were performed at three randomised sites on the flank. At 0.5, 6, 24 and 48 hours after challenge, reactions were graded on a scale of 1–4 on which the reaction to the negative control (diluent) at 0.5 hours scored 0 and that to the positive control (histamine) scored 4. Reactions were graded on the basis of wheal diameter and/or induration (DTH). Those occurring at 0.5 hours were classified as IH, at 6 hours as LPR, and at 24–48 hours as DTH.

Histology and immunohistochemistry

At 6 hours after challenge, a 6-mm punch biopsy was used to collect a skin sample from one of the antigen sites and one of the diluent control sites, following subcutaneous injection of a local anaesthetic (Lignol, Arnolds Veterinary Products) beneath each site. The remaining antigen and diluent control sites were biopsied at 24 and 48 hours in a similar fashion. At 9 weeks, two additional sites were injected, one with *P. ovis* WME and the other with the diluent control. These sites were biopsied, following the same protocol, 72 hours later. Immediately after collection, the skin samples were bisected. Half of the sample was fixed in 4% paraformaldehyde in PBS for 6 hours,[17] then stored in 70% ethanol at 4°C,[18] processed and embedded in paraffin wax. Serial 5-μm tissue sections were cut for mounting. Eosinophils were stained with Lendrum's carbol chromotrope solution for 1 hour[19] and counterstained for 10 seconds with haematoxylin. Dermal eosinophils in a minimum of 20 successive graticule fields (1.25 mm^2) were counted using an Olympus BX 50 microscope at ×400 magnification.

The other half of the skin sample was fixed in a non-aldehyde, zinc salts fixative (ZSF) as described by Gonzalez *et al.*[20] Briefly, the sample was immersed in ZSF solution (0.1 M Tris buffer with calcium acetate 0.05% [pH 7–7.4], containing zinc acetate 0.5% and zinc chloride 0.05%) for 72 hours at room temperature. The sample was then placed in plastic cassettes and transferred to 78% ethanol, 30 minutes before processing in paraffin wax. Five-μm thick sections were cut, placed on treated glass slides (Superfrost Plus; Menzel-Glazer, Germany) and dried overnight at 37°C.

Sections were dewaxed and then submitted to two blocking procedures; quenching endogenous peroxidase activity with 0.03% hydrogen peroxide for 5 minutes at room temperature followed by removal of non-specific tissue antigens with 25% normal goat serum in Tris-buffered saline (TBS: 0.05 M Tris HCl, 0.015 M

NaCl, pH 7.2–7.6) for 30 minutes at room temperature. The EnVision Plus HRP System (Dako, Ely, UK) was used to amplify monoclonal antibody-labelling of $CD4^+$ T cells. Sections were incubated overnight at 4°C with $CD4^+$ T-cell-specific mAb, 17D[21] (Basel Institute of Immunology, Basel, Switzerland), prepared at a dilution of 1/50 in TBS. This was followed by incubation with the secondary antibody (peroxidase-labelled polymer conjugated to goat anti-mouse immunoglobulins) for 30 minutes at room temperature. Conjugate binding was detected by incubating with the substrate chromogen, 3,3'-diaminobenzidine (DAB), for 7–8 minutes at room temperature. Sections were washed in TBS between each stage of the labelling procedure. After a final wash with distilled water they were counter-stained with haematoxylin, rinsed, dehydrated in graded alcohols, cleared and mounted. A negative control was provided by omission of the primary antibody.

$CD4^+$ T cells were identified in skin samples collected from infested sheep 48 hours after intradermal injection of diluent and antigen at 1 and 9 weeks. Labelled cells were counted in a minimum area of 0.2 mm².

Statistics

Eosinophil counts were logarithmically (log_{10}) transformed prior to analysis in order to normalise the residuals. Twenty-five samples where no eosinophils were observed were excluded from the analysis, as their inclusion prevented normalisation of the residuals. This exclusion made no qualitative difference to the analysis as 24/25 samples were in the diluent (control) group where eosinophil counts were expected to be low (see Fig 1.12.1B).

Analysis of log_{10} eosinophil counts was carried out using linear mixed effect models (GenStat release 6.1; Lawes Agricultural Trust, Numerical Alogrithms Group Ltd, Oxford, UK) where sheep identification was entered as a random effect to account for the repeated sampling of the same sheep. Whether sheep were infested or naive, challenged with *P. ovis* WME or diluent, how many hours after challenge they were sampled, and the week of challenge were entered, in that order, into the various models as fixed effects.

The correlation between log_{10} eosinophils and $CD4^+$ lymphocytes 48 hours after intradermal challenge with *P. ovis* WME was investigated using Pearson product moment correlation tests in Minitab (Release 13.1).

Results

Wheal reactions in infested and naïve sheep

Immediate wheal reactions were first recorded at 7 weeks after infestation when three of the four successfully infested sheep scored 3 (Table 1.12.1). No delayed wheal reactions were detected in any of the infested sheep and no immediate or delayed reactions were observed in the naive controls.

Eosinophil counts at sites of intradermal challenge

Analysis of the complete data set indicated that log_{10} eosinophil counts were significantly greater in infested than naive sheep ($p < 0.001$), greater at sites of intradermal challenge with *P. ovis* WME than diluent challenge ($p < 0.001$), varied at the different hours post-challenge ($p = 0.004$), and were different with respect to week of challenge ($p < 0.001$) (Fig. 1.12.1a and b).

The eosinophil count provoked by the diluent control was significantly greater ($p < 0.001$) in infested than naive sheep (Fig. 1.12.1a and b) and probably reflected the development of a circulating eosinophilia in infested, but not naive, sheep. However, the counts observed in naive sheep were not significantly different at 6, 24 and 48 hours after challenge, or at different weeks of challenge ($p = 0.381$ and $p = 0.09$, respectively). The eosinophil counts elicited at sites challenged with *P. ovis* WME were also significantly higher ($p = 0.002$) in infested than naïve sheep and, in contrast to naïve sheep, were significantly different at different hours after challenge ($p < 0.001$) and at different weeks of challenge ($p < 0.001$). At 9 weeks, intradermal challenge of infested sheep with *P. ovis* WME elicited a dramatic influx of eosinophils that persisted from 24 to 72 hours and was significantly greater ($p < 0.001$) than that present at 1, 3, 5 and 7 weeks after infestation (Fig. 1.12.1A). Further analysis demonstrated that eosinophil counts present at 24 and 48 hours after challenge with *P. ovis* WME were significantly greater ($p < 0.001$ and $p = 0.012$, respectively) at 9 weeks than 7 weeks (Fig. 1.12.1A). In addition, at 9 weeks, but not before, eosinophil counts 24 and 48 hours after challenge of infested sheep with *P. ovis* WME were significantly greater ($p < 0.001$) than those at 6 hours (Fig. 1.12.1A).

In naïve sheep, challenge with *P. ovis* WME provoked significantly greater eosinophil counts at 24 and 48 hours than at 6 hours ($p = 0.011$ and $p = 0.004$,

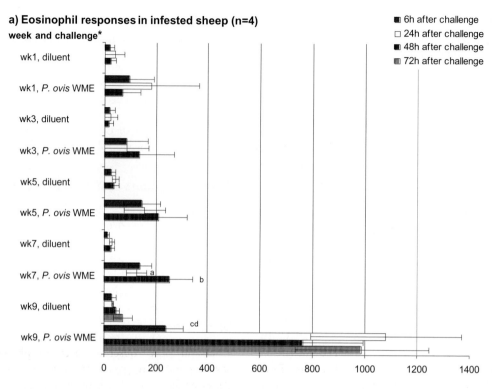

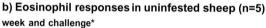

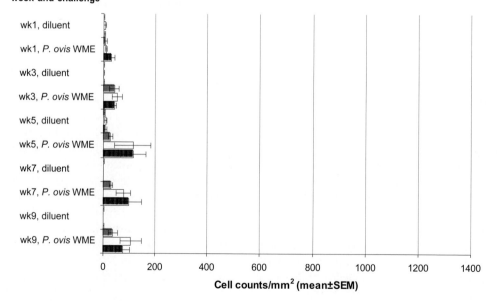

Fig. 1.12.1 Temporal development of eosinophil responses of (a) infested and (b) naive sheep to intradermal injection of *P. ovis* WME (whole-mite extract). *50 µl diluent and *P. ovis* WME (10 µg/ml) injected intradermally. Eosinophil responses marked with the same letter are significantly different: a, c and d: $p < 0.001$; b: $p = 0.012$).

Table 1.12.1 Temporal development of wheal reactions to intradermal challenge of infested sheep with *P. ovis* extract

Sheep no.	Weeks 1, 3 and 5		Week 7		Week 9	
	Immediate	Delayed	Immediate	Delayed	Immediate	Delayed
1	0	0	3	0	3	0
2	0	0	3	0	3	0
3	0	0	1	0	0	0
4	0	0	3	0	3	0

Immediate, wheal reaction at 0.5 hours after intradermal injection; delayed, wheal/induration at 24–48 hours after intradermal injection. Graded on a scale of 1–4 where diluent was scored as 0 and histamine was scored as 4.

respectively), but counts were not significantly different at different weeks (Fig. 1.12.2B).

CD4⁺ T lymphocytes and eosinophils

At 1 and 9 weeks after infestation, mean counts of CD4$^+$ helper T cells were significantly greater ($p = 0.035$ and $p = 0.028$ respectively) at sites challenged with *P. ovis* WME, than at sites injected with the diluent control (Fig. 1.12.2). Comparison of mean cell counts elicited by challenge with *P. ovis* WME indicated CD4$^+$ T-cell counts were greater at 9 weeks than at 1 week after infestation, but this increase was not statistically significant. There was a strong correlation between CD4$^+$ T

cells and $\log_{10}$ eosinophil counts for the combined data of weeks 1 and 9 ($\rho = 0.750$; $p = 0.001$). There was also a significant correlation between CD4$^+$ T cells and $\log_{10}$ eosinophil counts 48 hours after challenge with *P. ovis* WME ($\rho = 0.858$; $p = 0.006$) but not after injection of diluent ($\rho = 0.219$; $p = 0.603$).

Discussion

Jones and Mote[22] observed successive phases in the development of responses of human patients to intradermal injection of foreign proteins: induction (no response); only a delayed response; both immediate and delayed responses; only an immediate response.

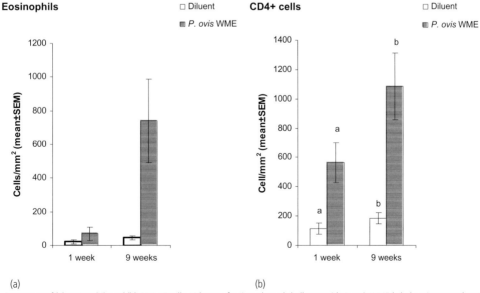

(a)   (b)

Fig. 1.12.2 Responses of (a) eosinophils and (b) CD4+ T cells 48 hours after intradermal challenge with *P. ovis* WME (whole-mite extract) at 1 and 9 weeks after infestation ($n = 4$). *50 μl diluent and *P. ovis* WME (10 μg/ml) injected intradermally. Counts with the same letter are significantly different: a: $p = 0.035$; b: $p = 0.028$.

Subsequently, clinical observations have indicated that this temporal pattern of cutaneous hypersensitivity reactions, plus a final phase of desensitisation, is typical of host responses to several haematophagous arthropods, such as mosquitoes (*Aedes aegypti* and *A. albopictus*), fleas (*Ctenocephalides felis*), sucking lice and bedbugs.[2–6,23]

In the majority of previous studies, the occurrence of hypersensitivity reactions was determined solely on the basis of clinical evidence of wheal reactions without reference to the accompanying histopathology. In the present investigation, histopathology proved more reliable than wheal reactions in revealing the presence of the DTH reaction and also demonstrated the non-classical eosinophil-rich nature of this response in sheep. It is clear from the evidence provided by wheal reactions and histopathology that, in three of the four sheep, *P. ovis* first elicited an immediate response that was succeeded by a phase when both IH and DTH reactions occurred, in contrast to the classical response pattern. In a further animal, a weak IH reaction was followed by a phase when only a marked DTH response was detected.

Deviation from the classical response has been recorded in a number of instances. Jones and Mote[22] recorded immediate reactions before delayed reactions in 4% of patients and, contrary to classical response pattern elicited by fleas (*C. felis*) in guinea-pigs, no consistent sequence was found in the development of hypersensitivity reactions of dogs to *C. felis*.[7] Similarly, contrary to the observations in man, *A. aegypti* provoked only immediate and late-phase hypersensitivity reactions in rabbits.[24] Furthermore, in contrast to the classic response seen in pigs, only immediate hypersensitivity reactions were elicited in the course of *S. scabiei* infestation of foxes,[25] while immediate and 6-hour, but not delayed reactions, were observed in cats infested with *Otodectes cynotis*.[26,27] It is clear from these examples that a given ectoparasite, such as *C. felis*, *A. aegypti* or *S. scabiei*, can deposit antigens at the same site in different species and individuals and elicit dissimilar response patterns. These observations, and the diversity of response patterns exhibited by different individuals and species, suggest that the host genotype plays a critical role in determining the pattern of hypersensitivity responses. The sheep employed in this study were unrelated, but further studies need to be carried out to determine whether the Suffolk breed is predisposed to the development of hypersensitivity responses to *P. ovis*.

The present study has also demonstrated that IH and non-classical DTH responses are not detected until relatively late (approximately 7 and 9 weeks, respectively) in the course of *P. ovis* infestation. This temporal occurrence of an immediate wheal reaction is consistent with the detection of a significant increase in the serum level of *P. ovis* antigen-specific IgE 7 weeks after infestation.[16] In protracted primary infestations and in challenge infestations that provoke an amnestic response, immediate and, more importantly, the non-classical delayed hypersensitivity response may have a significant role in recruitment of eosinophils to lesional sites. Both of these responses may participate in host defence mechanisms and may be associated with the failure of challenge infestations to become established.[16]

The observation in the present investigation, of a distinct temporal separation in the occurrence of IgE-mediated type I hypersensitivity and delayed hypersensitivity reactions suggests that different mechanisms are involved in the immunopathogenesis of these reactions. In murine models, T-cell dependence of the eosinophil-rich, delayed-type hypersensitivity reaction to *S. mansoni* cercariae has been demonstrated by transfer of the response to naive mice by T cells harvested from sensitised mice, and by abolition of the same response to *S. mansoni* eggs by depletion of CD4$^+$ cells with anti-CD4$^+$ monoclonal antibody.[14,15] In the present investigation, the strong correlation between numbers of CD4$^+$ T cells and eosinophils at sites of *P. ovis* WME challenge may indicate the involvement of CD4$^+$ cells in the genesis of the eosinophil-rich delayed hypersensitivity response to *P. ovis*. However, CD4$^+$ cell counts at other times, particularly when the immediate response first occurs, also need to be examined.

The present study has demonstrated the occurrence of immediate and eosinophil-rich delayed hypersensitivity responses in *P. ovis* infestations and shown that their temporal development does not follow the classical response pattern to arthropod infestations. These hypersensitivity responses developed relatively late in the course of infestation and their contribution to lesional pathology in primary infestations is therefore of questionable significance. However, they may be more important in heavy infestations when responses appear to develop more rapidly and in protracted and challenge infestations. Distinct temporal separation of the first manifestation of immediate and delayed responses has evidence that they are mediated by different mechanisms. Further investigations need to be carried out to determine whether or not the delayed response is mediated by CD4+ cells.

Acknowledgements

The advice of Dr Darren J. Shaw as regards statistical analysis of the data is gratefully acknowledged. This work was funded by MAFF (Contract CSA 3503). Dr J.F. Huntley received funding from the Scottish Executive, Environment and Rural Affairs Department.

References

1 Wikel, S.K. Immune responses to arthropods and their products. *Annual Review of Entomology*, 1982; **27**: 21–48.

2 Allen, J.R. Host resistance to ectoparasites. *Revue Scientifique et Technique Office International des Epizooties*, 1994; **13**: 1287–1303.

3 Mellanby, K. Man's reaction to mosquito bites. *Nature*, 1946; **158**: 554.

4 Benjamini, E., Feingold, B.F., Kartman, L. Skin reactivity in guinea pigs sensitised to flea bites: the sequence of reactions. *Proceedings of the Society for Experimental Biology and Medicine*, 1961; **108**: 700–702.

5 Jones, C.J. Immune responses to fleas, bugs and sucking lice. In: Wikel, S.K., ed. *The Immunology of Host–Ectoparasite Arthropod Relationships*. Oxon: CAB International, 1996: 150–174.

6 Larrivee, D.H., Benjamini, E., Feingold, B.F., Shimizu, M. Histological studies of guinea pig skin: different stages of allergic reactivity to flea bites. *Experimental Parasitology*, 1964; **15**: 491–502.

7 Gross, T.L., Halliwell, R.E. Lesions of experimental flea bite hypersensitivity in the dog. *Veterinary Pathology*, 1985; **22**: 78–81.

8 Foster, A.P., Lees, P., Cunningham, F.M. Actions of PAF receptor antagonists in horses with the allergic skin disease sweet itch. *Inflammation Research*, 1995; **44**: 412–417.

9 Davis, D.P., Moon, R.D. Density of itch mite, *Sarcoptes scabiei* (Acari: Sarcoptidae) and temporal development of cutaneous hypersensitivity in swine mange. *Veterinary Parasitology*, 1990; **36**: 285–293.

10 Weisbroth, S.H., Wang, R., Scher, S., Spohr, B., Luft, B. Immunopathology of psoroptic otitis in laboratory rabbits. A model for allergic mechanisms in acariasis. *Federation Proceedings*, 1972; **31**: 614.

11 Losson, B., Detry-Pouplard, M., Pouplard, L. Haematological and immunological response of unrestrained cattle to *Psoroptes ovis*, the sheep scab mite. *Research in Veterinary Science*, 1988; **44**: 197–201.

12 Ravindran, R., Jayaprakasan, V., Subramanian, H. Cellular response to *Psoroptes cuniculi*. *Journal of Veterinary Parasitology*, 2000; **14**: 175–176.

13 van den Broek, A.H., Huntley, J.F., Halliwell, R.E., Machell, J., Taylor, M., Miller, H.R. Cutaneous hypersensitivity reactions to *Psoroptes ovis* and Der p 1 in sheep previously infested with *P. ovis* – the sheep scab mite. *Veterinary Immunology and Immunopathology*, 2003; **91**: 105–117.

14 Ch'ang, L.Y., Colley, D.G. Cutaneous sensitivity induced by immunization with irradiated *Schistosoma mansoni* cercariae. I. Induction, elicitation, and adoptive transfer analysis of cell-mediated cutaneous sensitivity. *Cell Immunology*, 1986; **100**: 119–128.

15 Teixeira, M.M., Talvani, A., Tafuri, W.L., Lukacs, N.W., Hellewell, P.G. Eosinophil recruitment into sites of delayed-type hypersensitivity reactions in mice. *Journal of Leukocyte Biology*, 2001; **69**: 353–360.

16 van den Broek, A.H., Huntley, J.F., Machell, J., *et al.* Cutaneous and systemic responses during primary and challenge infestations of sheep with the sheep scab mite, *Psoroptes ovis*. *Parasite Immunology*, 2000; **22**: 407–414.

17 Newlands, G.F., Huntley, J.F., Miller, H.R. Concomitant detection of mucosal mast cells and eosinophils in the intestines of normal and *Nippostrongylus*-immune rats. A re-evaluation of histochemical and immunocytochemical techniques. *Histochemistry*, 1984; **81**: 585–589.

18 Miller, H.R., Jackson, F., Newlands, G., Appleyard, W.T. Immune exclusion, a mechanism of protection against the ovine nematode *Haemonchus contortus*. *Research in Veterinary Science*, 1983; **35**: 357–363.

19 Lendrum, A.C. The staining of eosinophil polymorphs and enterochromaffin cells in histological sections. *Journal of Pathology and Bacteriology*, 1944; **56**: 441.

20 Gonzalez, L., Anderson, I., Deane, D., Summers, C., Buxton, D. Detection of immune system cells in paraffin wax-embedded ovine tissues. *Journal of Comparative Pathology*, 2001; **125**: 41–47.

21 Maddox, J.F., Mackay, C.R., Brandon, M.R. Surface antigens, SBU-T4 and SBU-T8, of sheep T lymphocyte subsets defined by monoclonal antibodies. *Immunology*, 1985; **55**: 739–748.

22 Jones, T.D., Mote, J.R. The phases of foreign protein sensitisation in human beings. *New England Journal of Medicine*, 1934; **210**: 120–123.

23 Oka, K., Ohtaki, N. Clinical observations of mosquito bite reactions in man: a survey of the relationship between age and bite reaction. *Journal of Dermatology*, 1989; **16**: 212–219.

24 Hudson, A., McKiel, J.A., West, A.S., Bourns, T.K.R. Reactions to mosquito bites. *Mosquito News*, 1958; **18**: 249–252.

25 Little, S.E., Davidson, W.R., Rakich, P.M., Nixon, T.L., Bounous, D.I., Nettles, V.F. Responses of red foxes to first and second infection with *Sarcoptes scabiei*. *Journal of Wildlife Diseases*, 1998; **34**: 600–611.

26 Weisbroth, S.H., Powell, M.B., Roth, L., Scher, S. Immunopathology of naturally occurring otodectic otoacariasis in the domestic cat. *Journal of the American Veterinary Medical Association*, 1974; **165**: 1088–1093.

27 Powell, M.B., Weisbroth, S.H., Roth, L., Wilhelmsen, C. Reaginic hypersensitivity in *Otodectes cynotis* infestation of cats and mode of mite feeding. *American Journal of Veterinary Research*, 1980; **41**: 877–882.

Part 2

Therapy

Immunomodulatory therapy

M.J. Day BSc, BVMS (Hons), PhD

Division of Veterinary Pathology, Infection and Immunity, School of Clinical Veterinary Science, University of Bristol, Langford, North Somerset, United Kingdom

Summary

This review examines the current and future practice of immunomodulatory therapy in companion animal medicine. At this time, we are experienced in the art of medical immunosuppression, but the drugs that are used for this purpose are decades old, non-specific in their immunological effects, and carry a relatively high risk of adverse events. By contrast, the options for immunostimulation in current practice are limited, and available products often lie in the 'grey area' of therapeutics. Although we presently employ some novel immunomodulatory procedures (e.g. allergen-specific immunotherapy, autogenous vaccination, or intravenous gammaglobulin therapy), these too are relatively crude procedures for which we lack knowledge of mechanisms by which they are effective.

Over the past two decades, our knowledge of basic immune function has expanded dramatically. We are now aware of the key roles played by the multiple different effector and regulatory subsets of CD4+ T lymphocytes and the cytokines elaborated by these cells. A further focus has been on the recognition of the importance of the innate immune system, and knowledge that the initial encounter between antigen and antigen-presenting cells can direct the nature of the subsequent adaptive immune response. The complex network of new immunological pathways has paved the way for the development of approaches to either inhibit or enhance the key cells and molecules that comprise them. Therefore, we now have a wide range of monoclonal antibody therapy, recombinant cytokine therapy, mucosal tolerance and gene therapy that is already entrenched or undergoing clinical trials in human medicine. These approaches are relatively safe and exquisitely specific for particular components of the immune system, even to the level of particular clones of antigen-specific lymphocytes that mediate immunopathology. This chapter reviews the recent advances in basic immunology and gives examples of these new therapeutic approaches to immunomodulation. Despite these strides forward, we should not necessarily expect these advances to become available in veterinary medicine in the immediate future.

Introduction

In veterinary medicine, the therapeutic approach to numerous disease states centres on suppression of an over-active immune system (e.g. hypersensitivity, autoimmunity). By contrast, in other situations it may be desirable to enhance an ineffective immune response (e.g. infectious disease, cancer). Currently available methods of such immunomodulation are relatively crude, but advances in knowledge of basic immune responses and immunoregulation have already led to the development of a new generation of immunotherapeutics for human use. The relatively small market and high developmental and licensing costs for veterinary therapeutics mean that these products will not rapidly translate to our day-to-day clinical practice; however, we should be aware of these new approaches and their potential applications to treatment of animal disease.

Current immunomodulatory therapy

Medical immunosuppression

Immunosuppression for the management of hypersensitivity or autoimmune diseases in veterinary medicine is generally achieved by systemic administration of glucocorticoids, with or without concurrent cytotoxic agents such as azathioprine or cyclophosphamide (or chlorambucil in cats).[1–3] The use of these agents in human medicine is firmly rooted in the 1960s, and the protocols for dosage and tapering that veterinary medicine adapted for use of such immunosuppressive drugs are largely empirical and have not changed for many years. These drugs affect the function of a wide range of immune cells, and produce a 'blanket immunosuppression' that inhibits the desired immune response, but which may also non-specifically inhibit protective responses to potential pathogens. In addition, these drugs carry a range of well-recognised side effects (e.g. iatrogenic hyperadrenocorticism, bone marrow suppression), which means that there is a 'risk-benefit ratio' to their use for management of immune-mediated disease. In this respect, one recent study has evaluated the relative efficacy of prednisone compared to prednisone in combination with cyclophosphamide for the management of canine immune-mediated haemolytic anaemia. The combination therapy was less efficacious than prednisone monotherapy, and dogs treated with the combination had a worse clinical outcome.[4] On this basis, cyclophosphamide can no longer be recommended as a part of the therapeutic management of this disease.

In addition to the cytotoxic agents listed above, a range of other drugs have at various times been used (at least in part) for their immunosuppressive effect. These include danazol,[1] gold salts (chrysotherapy),[3] leflunomide,[5] megestrol acetate, pentoxifylline,[6] mycophenolate mofetil,[3] and the combination of tetracycline (or doxycycline[7]) and niacinamide.[8] A number of these agents are used as glucocorticoid-sparing drugs and thus given in combination with oral prednisolone.[3] Other antimicrobial drugs (e.g. metronidazole) are known to have immunomodulatory effects in other species,[9] but the action of these agents on the immune system of companion animals has not been characterised.

There is a distinct lack of 'evidence-based' application of traditional immunosuppressive agents. Few studies have addressed the way in which these drugs are administered, their precise mode of action in veterinary species, and the outcome of therapy in sufficiently large, multicentre trials. The catalogue of effects that glucocorticoids and cytotoxic agents supposedly have on the canine or feline immune system is largely derived by extrapolation from experimental studies in humans or laboratory rodents.[10]

Some studies of the effect of administration of oral prednisolone on canine immune and inflammatory parameters have been conducted. Short-term (2 or 3 weeks) daily dosing with 1 mg/kg prednisolone did not affect the concentration of complement C3 within the serum[11] but did enhance a range of *in vitro* neutrophil functions.[12]

One very informative study was that published by Rinkardt and others.[13] In this experimental study, three groups of six beagle dogs were treated by different im-

munosuppressive protocols, and the effect on a series of immune parameters was measured. The first group of dogs were treated with azathioprine at 2 mg/kg once daily for 14 days but this did not result in alterations in blood lymphocyte subsets or serum immunoglobulin concentration. This result might simply reflect the relatively short duration of the experiment and the known delayed onset of efficacy of this drug. The second group of dogs received oral prednisone monotherapy (2 mg/kg once daily for 14 days). In these dogs there was a reduction in serum IgG, IgM and IgA concentrations and decreases in blood CD4[+] and CD8[+] T lymphocytes and B lymphocytes. The final group was treated with both prednisone and azathioprine (both at 2 mg/kg once daily for 14 days) which caused selective decreases in serum IgG concentration and the number of CD8[+] T lymphocytes (thereby elevating the CD4:CD8 ratio).

A major recent advance in veterinary therapeutics has been the licensing of the microemulsion form of cyclosporin A for the treatment of canine atopic dermatitis.[14–16] This drug is a potent immunosuppressive agent that derives from human transplantation medicine and clearly has application to companion animal renal transplantation,[17,18] in addition to treatment of a wide range of immune-mediated diseases.[19] One surprise with this agent was the apparent efficacy it has in the management of anal furunculosis,[20] although long-term studies do suggest that the rapid immediate effects of this drug may not be sustained, and that surgical approaches to disease relapse are sometimes required.

Cyclosporin A takes veterinary immunosuppressive therapy one step further in refinement. The precise mode of action of this drug is well characterised and the end effect is selective paralysis of T lymphocytes via inhibition of cytokine secretion (Fig. 2.1.1). The *in vitro* inhibition of feline lymphocyte proliferation by cyclosporin A (and a range of other immunosuppressive agents) has recently been demonstrated.[21] However, although cyclosporin A might be heralded as an advance, this is a relatively old agent in human medicine, and there are now newer and more potent variants (tacrolimus and rapamycin). Moreover, cyclosporin A still has broad immunosuppressive effects on T lymphocytes of a wide range of antigenic specificity, in addition to those particular T cells that might be responsible for mediating the signs of disease in an animal. Blanket inhibition of T cells results in loss of B-

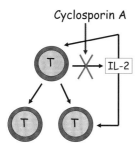

Fig. 2.1.1 Mode of action of cyclosporin A. Upon antigen-specific activation, the T lymphocyte releases stimulatory cytokines (e.g. IL-2) and up-regulates expression of membrane receptors for these cytokines. These cytokines drive cellular division (clonal proliferation). Cyclosporin A blocks production of these stimulatory cytokines and thus selectively inhibits T-cell proliferation. The humoral immune response (B lymphocytes) will be secondarily suppressed due to failure of T-cell 'help'. T, T cells; IL-2, interleukin-2.

cell function (removal of T-cell help) and reduced immunoglobulin synthesis, thus a state of generalised immune inhibition results, similar to that induced by the older immunosuppressive agents. Cyclosporin A also carries a catalogue of potential side effects, although these may not be as extreme as those potentially triggered by glucocorticoid and cytotoxic agents. Finally, the related topical immunosuppressive, tacrolimus, has also been evaluated for efficacy in the treatment of canine atopic dermatitis.[22]

Medical immunostimulation

Albeit with the weaknesses described above, when medical immunosuppression is required for our animal patients we have a selection of agents and protocols to choose from. In contrast, when we might wish to stimulate, rather than suppress, the immune system the cupboard appears relatively bare. The current immunomodulatory drugs are relatively crude agents with poorly characterised modes of action and poor clinical efficacy.

Historically, the anthelmintic agent levamisole has been used as a non-specific immune stimulant, and the use of this drug has also been described for the treatment of canine systemic lupus erythematosus.[23] Although levamisole is also used as a vaccine adjuvant for large animal species, there is little evidence to support a mechanism for an immunomodulatory effect in companion animals. Moreover, the known association of this drug with adverse effects, such as erythema multiforme, weigh heavily on the 'risk' side of risk-benefit analysis.

One study has examined the potential immunomodulatory application of the anthelmintic ivermectin, but administration of this drug did not affect blood lymphocyte subsets or the proliferative responses of these cells.[24] A range of crude bacterial, yeast or plant derivatives are also commercially available (e.g. Immunoregulin, Staphage Lysate, Staphoid A-B, muramyl tripeptide, Regressin V, *Serratia* extract, acemannan) and these have found widest application in the management of canine staphylococcal pyoderma or as adjunct immune stimulants in cancer therapy.[25–27] The effects of these preparations on the canine or feline immune systems have not been well characterised.[28–31]

A range of other means of potentially modulating the immune system of animals has been described, but again the precise effects are not well understood. Several studies have shown that stimulation of acupuncture points whilst administering vaccine to animals can have an adjuvant-like effect on vaccine efficacy.[32] In the world of nutrition, numerous studies suggest the benefits to 'gastrointestinal health' and possible systemic immune effects of incorporating dietary prebiotics or probiotics,[33] fermentable fibre[34] or altering the n3:n6 polyunsaturated fatty acid ratio in the diet.[35] Similar approaches have potential for the adjunct therapy of inflammatory bowel diseases[36] or atopy.[37]

Immunomodulation

There are some exceptions to the current broad-spectrum approach to immunomodulation, which involve manipulations that probably have a more selective effect on either suppressing or enhancing specific portions of the immune system. The classical example of this would be allergen-specific immunotherapy (ASIT) for the management of atopic dermatitis. Although this has been widely practised in human medicine since early last century, and is increasingly undertaken in companion animal dermatology,[38,39] there is still debate as to the precise nature of the beneficial immunological effects that result from repeated subcutaneous injection with increasing concentrations of allergen. There are limited data to suggest that dogs undergoing ASIT have alteration in concentration of serum allergen-specific IgE and IgG (including IgG subclasses) akin to observations in humans.[40,41] The possibility that ASIT induces a 'blocking' IgG antibody that competes with mast cell-bound IgE for allergen has not been entirely discounted. More recent theories suggesting that the process induces a 'switch' from Th1- to Th2-dominated immunity have been extended to encompass the possibility that the process induces expansion of regulatory T cells (see below) that in turn suppress the Th2 effectors (see below).[42]

A second example of a more directed immunotherapy would be the use of autogenous vaccination for the management of canine staphylococcal pyoderma.[43] As for ASIT, this process has variable efficacy in individual cases, but is likely to work via an antigen-specific or bacterial superantigen-mediated enhancement of relevant immune cell populations.

A further example is the use of intravenous immunoglobulin therapy (IVIG), that has now been shown to be valuable for the treatment of autoimmune haemolytic anaemia and thrombocytopenia in the dog and diseases within the erythema multiforme-toxic epidermal necrolysis spectrum in the dog and cat.[44–46] The administration of this immunoglobulin concentrate is likely to work at different levels (Fig. 2.1.2). It has been shown that the human immunoglobulin is able to occupy Fc receptors on canine macrophages, suggesting that 'receptor blockade' underlies much of the efficacy in treatment of immune-mediated cytopenias. However, it is also known that some immunoglobulin binds to the surface of T and B lymphocytes and may cause

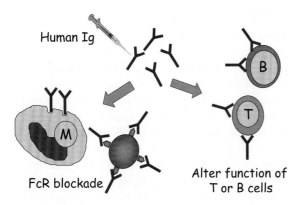

Fig. 2.1.2 High-dose intravenous human immunoglobulin therapy. Administration of human immunoglobulin probably acts at several levels. The human immunoglobulin binds Fc receptors on the surface of macrophages, thus inhibiting uptake of target cells (e.g. erythrocytes or platelets) coated with endogenous (e.g. canine) immunoglobulin. Human immunoglobulin also likely binds to a range of molecules expressed by T and B lymphocytes, resulting in functional inhibition of these populations. Ig, immunoglobulin; B, B cell; T, T cell; M, macrophage; FcR, immunoglobulin receptor.

down-regulation of the function of these cells.[47] Recent human studies have shown that this therapy has a plethora of effects, including down-regulation of T-cell proliferation, reduced adhesion molecule expression and production of interleukin-1 (IL-1), inhibition of Fas-Fas ligand (CD95-CD95L) interaction, and inhibition of complement deposition.[48] In humans, IVIG has been used successfully in the treatment of a range of haematological, rheumatological, neurological and dermatological disorders including atopic dermatitis, pemphigus foliaceus and pemphigus vulgaris.[49]

A final novel approach to immunotherapy is plasmapheresis, which aims to reduce the concentration of antibody and circulating immune complexes in the blood. The special equipment required limits widespread application of this methodology, but the technique has been applied to the treatment of dogs with systemic lupus erythematosus, myasthenia gravis and immune-mediated haemolytic anaemia.[50,51]

The immunological basis for development of novel immunotherapy

Future approaches to the treatment of numerous diseases will involve novel immunomodulatory agents. Such therapies derive from rapid progress in our understanding of basic immunological mechanisms, particularly the concept that most immune responses are regulated by cytokines released by specific populations of lymphocytes. As this understanding is pivotal to the design and application of such therapies, the immunological background will be briefly reviewed here.

In the mid-1980s it was recognised that there were functional subpopulations of CD4[+] T lymphocytes that were (and remain) difficult to define by phenotypic means (Fig. 2.1.3). The two most important subpopulations are the Th1 and Th2 lymphocytes.[52] The Th1 cells are characterised by the preferential production of the cytokines IL-2 and interferon gamma (IFN-γ). As such, these cells are active in the enhancement of cell-mediated and cytotoxic immune responses driven by antigens derived from intracellular pathogens and neoplastic cells. Th1 cells (at least in mice) have limited ability to provide 'help' for B cells that undergo terminal differentiation to plasma cells that secrete a restricted subclass of IgG (IgG2a in mice).

By contrast, Th2 lymphocytes preferentially produce the cytokines IL-4, IL-5, IL-6, IL-10 and IL-13. These cells are most active in humoral immune re-

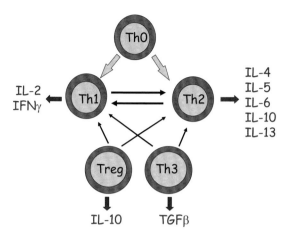

IL-2
IFNγ

IL-4
IL-5
IL-6
IL-10
IL-13

IL-10   TGFβ

Fig. 2.1.3 Functional subsets of CD4+ T lymphocytes. There are now known to be several functional subsets of CD4+ T cells that are defined by cytokine production, rather than the expression of particular surface molecules. Th0 cells are the precursors of the two major effector subsets (Th1 and Th2) and the molecular nature of the initial encounter between Th0 and antigen-expressing dendritic cells determines which effector subset is preferentially activated. Th1 cells preferentially release IL-2 and IFN-γ and drive cell-mediated (cytotoxic) immune responses. Th2 cells release a range of interleukins and selectively activate the humoral immune response (B-cell activation, plasma cell differentiation, and antibody production). The Th1 and Th2 subsets are cross-regulatory, such that the cytokines produced by one subset are inhibitory of the other, and vice versa. In addition, both subsets may be down-regulated by the action of other populations of CD4+ T-regulatory (suppressor) cells such as the induced Treg cells (that produce IL-10) or the induced Th3 cells (that produce TGF-β).

sponses involving the terminal differentiation of plasma cells capable of producing IgG (the IgG1 subclass in mice), IgA and IgE. These two lymphocyte subsets have a tendency to be mutually antagonistic by virtue of their non-overlapping cytokine profiles. The IL-10 produced by Th2 cells is inhibitory of the Th1 population, and the Th1-derived IFN-γ is inhibitory of the Th2 population. In some circumstances, this effect results in polarisation of immune responses, a situation known as 'immune deviation'. The genesis of Th1 and Th2 cells is thought to be via a common precursor (Th0) cell that produces an overlapping cytokine panel, and is driven to differentiate to become a Th1 or Th2 effector by a range of signals, in particular the nature of the driving antigen.[53]

This strand of contemporary immunological thinking resulted from the rediscovery of the importance of the innate immune system in directing the subsequent nature of the adaptive immune response. It is now recognised that the antigen-presenting cells (APCs) (e.g.

dendritic cells and macrophages) that process and present antigen for activation of T cells via the T-cell receptor and other co-stimulatory molecular interactions, express on their surface a selection of molecules that are collectively known as pattern recognition receptors (PRR; or Toll-like receptors). The ligands for these receptors are highly conserved epitopes expressed by microbes ('pathogen associated molecular patterns', PAMPs). The interaction of a specific PAMP with the cognate PRR initiates signalling to the T cell that is in turn activated by processed antigen displayed by the APCs.[54] The nature of this signalling determines the outcome of the type of immunity generated (Th1 or Th2). It has been suggested that the 'default pathway' for such signalling is generation of a Th2 response, but that many microbial PRRs can switch this towards Th1 immunity.

In reality, it has been more difficult to define these Th1 and Th2 populations, and the phenomenon of immune deviation, in outbred species such as humans, dogs and cats.[55,56] Whilst these cell populations undoubtedly exist, and preferential cytokine expression has been clearly demonstrated in many situations, in most spontaneously arising diseases there is a mixed Th1/Th2 response, or a temporal progression from one to another at different stages of disease. It has been further suggested that a similar dichotomy in functional lymphocyte subpopulations occurs within the CD8+ T lymphocytes (Tc1 and Tc2) and even among those T cells that express the specialised γδT-cell receptor.

This model of T-cell-regulated immunity was further expanded in the 1990s with the rediscovery of 'suppressor' T lymphocytes, rechristened for the new era as 'regulatory cells'. These too would appear to come in different flavours, and the type of suppression may vary depending upon the nature of the immune response. Fundamentally, these regulatory cells are now considered to be either spontaneously arising and a constitutive part of the immune system ('natural' regulators), or to be induced as part of a specific immune response ('induced' regulators).[57] In most species, natural regulatory cells are characterised by surface expression of the molecule CD25 (for example, CD25+CD4+) and by expression of a range of other molecules including CTLA-4 and some Toll-like receptors, and expression of GITR (glucocorticoid-induced TNF receptor-related gene) and the regulatory gene Foxp3.[58] In most model systems, these cells appear to mediate their suppressive function by direct physical contact with the cell that they wish to inhibit ('cognate interaction'). By contrast, the induced regulatory cells probably come in different forms. The two best characterised are the Treg cells and Th3 cells. Induced regulators tend to mediate inhibition, not by cognate interaction, but via the secretion of inhibitory cytokines. Treg cells are characterised by the secretion of IL-10 and Th3 cells by transforming growth factor-β (TGF-β) production.[59] Again, the definition of these populations in our animal species is at an early stage, although feline Treg cells have recently been clearly defined in an FIV infection model.[60]

Future immunotherapeutic approaches

Modulation of cytokines

Armed with this knowledge, it is easy to appreciate the crucial role that the interplay between these populations has in the initiation and suppression of immune responses. Key to the function of all of these subsets are the cytokines that they secrete. Therefore, there is therapeutic potential in being able to manipulate immune responses by delivering high concentrations of specific regulatory cytokines, or by interfering with the secretion of cytokines, or the binding of cytokines to their receptors. There are various practical approaches to achieving this aim, including: (1) administration of recombinant cytokine, (2) administration of monoclonal antibody that can neutralise specific cytokines, and (3) administration of genes encoding cytokines.

Recombinant cytokine therapy

There is experimental evidence in murine model systems that the nature of an immune response to a particular antigen can be altered by exposing the immune system to high concentrations of recombinant cytokine of a specific type. For example, delivery of recombinant IFN-γ to a patient would be likely to enhance Th1 immunity and suppress the function of Th2 cells. This type of recombinant cytokine therapy is now firmly entrenched in human medicine, where intravenous infusion of IFN-γ is a valuable adjunct therapy for patients with severe infection, immunodeficiency or neoplastic disease. Trials of administration of recombinant IL-4 and IL-10 for psoriasis,[61] and of recombinant IL-10 for Crohn's disease,[62] have been undertaken. Similarly, treatment with recombinant IFN-β is now an established part of the management

of relapsing multiple sclerosis.[63] Cytokines generally have a relatively short half-life, thus systemic administration of these products is not always a viable option. However, local intralesional injection of cytokine can have profound effects on the recruitment of 'appropriate' lymphocytes to the site of infection or neoplasia. Intralesional IFN-γ is efficacious in the management of the cutaneous manifestations of human leishmaniasis or leprosy. Other Th1-associated cytokines such as IL-12 and IL-18 are also candidates for this effect, or may be used in combination for additive effect[64] (Fig. 2.1.4). Recombinant canine IFN-γ and IL-12, and feline IFN-γ, IL-12 and IL-18 have all been produced,[65,66] and stimulation of blood mononuclear cells from dogs with leishmaniasis with recombinant IL-12 induces up-regulation of expression of mRNA encoding IFN-γ.[67]

Recombinant cytokine therapy at a different level has been investigated in companion animal medicine. The colony stimulating factors (CSF) such as granulocyte-CSF (G-CSF) and granulocyte-monocyte CSF (GM-CSF) are involved in the release of neutrophils and monocytes from the bone marrow. Administration of these cytokines would therefore be of benefit in situations where an animal was neutropenic (e.g. cyclic haematopoiesis of grey collie dogs, following chemotherapy, or following parvoviral infection). As the biochemical composition of some (but not all) cytokines is relatively conserved across species, it has proven possible to use some human recombinant cytokines

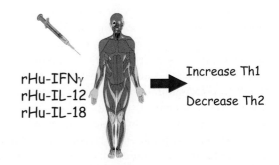

rHu-IFNγ
rHu-IL-12
rHu-IL-18

Increase Th1

Decrease Th2

Leprosy, leishmaniasis, cancer, immunodeficiency

Fig. 2.1.4 Recombinant cytokine therapy. Systemic administration of recombinant Th1-associated cytokines results in 'skewing' of the patient's immune system towards Th1 immunity. Such an effect would be desirable in a range of disease states. rHu-IFNγ, recombinant human interferon-γ; rHu-IL-12, recombinant human interleukin-12; rHu-IL-18, recombinant human interleukin-18.

in companion animals. For example, recombinant human G-CSF is able to induce neutrophil release in both dogs and cats but the effect is only transient as the animal immune system recognises the human molecule as immunologically 'foreign' and mounts an immune (antibody) response that eventually neutralises not only the human molecule, but the endogenous canine or feline homologue (Fig. 2.1.5). This problem does not arise when recombinant molecules of the appropriate species are used; canine G-CSF and GM-CSF have been produced and used in this manner, but are not commercially available.[68,69] In experimental studies, normal dogs or dogs with neoplasia have also been administered recombinant human IL-2 (intravenously, subcutaneously or by inhalation of IL-2-containing liposomes) and this resulted in lymphocytosis and enhanced *in vitro* lymphocyte proliferation and target cell cytotoxicity.[70] Similar studies have evaluated the potential for recombinant human IL-12 therapy in canine cancer patients.

Recently, the first companion animal recombinant cytokine product has been licensed. Feline omega-interferon (Virbagen Omega™) is one of several 'type I' (non-immune or antiviral) interferons in the cat and has been produced in recombinant form. Although this product clearly has a role for the adjunct treatment of feline viral disease (where recombinant human products are currently widely used), the initial marketing authorisation for the product is for the adjunct therapy of dogs with parvovirus infection.[71]

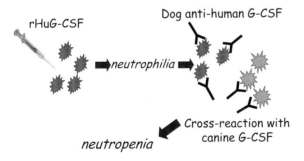

Fig. 2.1.5 Administration of recombinant human G-CSF to dogs. Recombinant human G-CSF is able to markedly elevate blood neutrophil numbers in severely neutropenic dogs. However, in time the dog's immune system recognises the human recombinant as a foreign antigen and mounts an antibody response to the protein. This not only neutralises any further human recombinant G-CSF, but can prevent activity of any endogenous canine G-CSF that may be produced due to antigenic cross-reactivity between the human recombinant and canine endogenous molecules. rHuG-CSF, recombinant human granulocyte colony stimulating factor.

Neutralisation of cytokines

If administration of recombinant cytokine can have beneficial therapeutic effect, then so too should neutralisation of cytokines that mediate undesirable outcomes in a patient. To this end, a growing range of therapeutic monoclonal antibodies specific for particular cytokines that may be injected into a patient to target and neutralise the effect of that cytokine, are now available in human medicine. One potential problem with the use of monoclonal antibody therapy is that the antibodies are often generated in a rodent species. To that end, the ability to 'humanise' such reagents by manufacturing chimeric rodent-human antibodies (e.g. rodent antigen-binding sites with a human Fc portion) has proven valuable.[72] One of the most widely used such products is infliximab, a monoclonal antibody specific for human tumour necrosis factor-α (TNF-α), a proinflammatory cytokine implicated in many disease states. Infliximab has been used effectively in patients with rheumatoid arthritis, psoriasis and refractory Crohn's disease.[73] Although generally considered relatively safe, side effects to monoclonal antibody therapy are reported. In one recent review of 500 patients treated with infliximab for Crohn's disease, a range of side effects (serum sickness-like reaction, opportunist infection, autoimmunity) was reported in a small proportion of patients.[74] Another example of this type of therapy is in the use of humanised monoclonal antibody to cytokines (e.g. IL-5) and chemokines (e.g. eotaxin) involved in the recruitment of eosinophils to sites of allergic disease (e.g. the lung in asthma).[75]

An alternative approach to cytokine neutralisation is to administer soluble forms of the appropriate cytokine receptor to neutralise the cytokine. Such 'cytokine traps' may take a variety of forms. For example, one approach is to develop a fusion protein comprising a human immunoglobulin Fc region linked to cytokine receptors. The combination of human IgG1 heavy chain and recombinant TNF receptor molecules has a more profound effect on neutralisation of TNF than infliximab, with less risk of developing neutralising antibodies to the therapeutic agent.[63] A similar construct of canine IL-13 receptor linked to canine IgG heavy chain has been produced and shown to inhibit the *in vitro* production of flea-specific IgE by blood mononuclear cells from flea allergic dogs.[76] Finally, monoclonal antibodies specific for cytokine receptors (e.g. humanised anti-IL-2 receptor), or cytokine receptor antagonist molecules (e.g. IL-1 receptor antagonist) may be administered to block the receptor and inhibit the action of endogenous cytokine. Similar approaches may be taken to inhibit the function of a wide range of chemokines, soluble molecules that are largely involved in the recruitment of leukocytes to sites of inflammation. Chemokines bind specific chemokine receptors, and therapeutic use of antagonists for these receptors would have benefit in a wide range of inflammatory diseases.[77]

Yet another approach to inhibition of cytokine activity is medical therapy. Recent studies have evaluated the use of the drug thalidomide for its anti-TNF-α activity in human inflammatory bowel disease,[36] and part of the activity of the prostaglandin E_1 analogue misoprostol is thought to be via inhibition of monocyte/macrophage production of IL-1β and TNF-α. Misoprostol has been shown to be of benefit in the treatment of canine atopic dermatitis and to lower cutaneous TNF-α concentration as assessed immunohistochemically.[78]

Administration of cytokine genes

Administration of recombinant cytokine protein clearly shows clinical benefit in many circumstances, but the process of producing the recombinants and the problems of limited half-life are maintained. It would be more refined to deliver the gene encoding a specific cytokine (or group of cytokines) so that there was local expression of protein at the site where it was required (Fig. 2.1.6). Proof of this concept is widely available, and cytokine genes within plasmids have been delivered to various body sites within 'carrier' micro-organisms (e.g. adenovirus or attenuated *Salmonella*). Even more exciting is the use of 'naked DNA' technology, whereby plasmids incorporating cytokine genes (and often also genes encoding specific antigens) are directly delivered to a specific tissue (often muscle) by needle injection, or are delivered transepidermally via the use of a 'gene gun' (high speed propulsion of DNA-coated particles) into or through the epidermis, or even by passive absorption across the epidermal barrier. These genes transfect local tissue cells (particularly APCs such as macrophages or dendritic cells) with eventual secretion of cytokine product. Locally transfected APCs migrate to regional lymphoid tissue where the effects of cytokines on initiation of immune responses may be pivotal in determining the nature of that response.

An example of cytokine gene therapy is the inhibition of adjuvant-induced arthritis in a rat model by

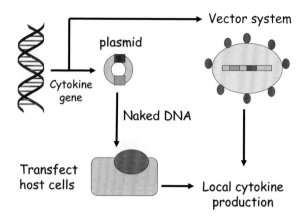

Fig. 2.1.6 Cytokine gene therapy. A gene sequence encoding a specific cytokine can be incorporated into a microbial vector which is delivered into the patient. The vector might also be used to deliver other genes, such as those encoding the immunogenic molecules of infectious agents. In the situation depicted, the vector organism has been used to carry two genes: one encoding a target microbial antigen that is expressed on the surface of the vector, and one encoding a mammalian cytokine that is released from the vector to modulate the nature of the immune response generated to the antigenic molecule. Alternatively, in 'naked DNA' therapy, a bacterial plasmid is used to deliver target antigen and cytokine genes. Dendritic antigen-presenting cells at the site of delivery are transfected, resulting in intracellular expression of target antigen that is subsequently processed and presented for interaction with T cells. Local expression of the cytokine gene results in similar polarisation of the ensuing immune response.

intra-articular administration of adenovirus containing the IL-4 gene,[79] or suppression of collagen-induced arthritis in mice by local injection of adenovirus carrying a viral homologue of the IL-10 gene.[80] On the basis of this type of study, phase I clinical trials of cytokine gene therapy have commenced in human rheumatoid arthritis patients,[81] and preliminary studies have been performed to investigate the potential application of this modality to canine arthritis. A contrasting use of cytokine gene therapy is the delivery of virus vectored IL-12 or IL-18 genes to the airways of ovalbumin-sensitised mice to inhibit Th2-driven eosinophilic respiratory disease.[82,83]

This process has experimentally been further refined via the use of 'dendritic cell therapy'. In this procedure, purified immature dendritic cells are manipulated *in vitro* and then administered intravenously to congenic rodents. For example, when cultured dendritic cells infected with adenovirus containing the murine IL-4 gene were injected into mice with established collagen-induced arthritis, there was significant inhibition of disease.[84]

This type of molecular manipulation also has relevance to cancer therapy. Experimentally, neoplastic cells can be removed from a tumour and transfected with genes encoding cytokines or chemokines, or genes allowing expression of particular molecules on the surface of the cell (e.g. major histocompatibility molecules for tumour-antigen presentation). When such modified cells are then re-injected into the periphery of the tumour, they may initiate and enhance local antitumour immune responses.[85] This approach is under investigation in veterinary medicine where transfection of tumour cells with the GM-CSF gene has been reported.[86] Alternatively, plasmids (or vectors containing plasmids) incorporating cytokine genes may be directly injected into the tumour; this approach has been attempted using the IL-2 gene in canine oncology.[30] Incorporation of 'molecular adjuvants' such as bacterial DNA CpG motifs (see below) can further enhance the polarisation of the local immune response that is generated. Experimentally, this technology has now been widely investigated in companion animal vaccine production. Microbial genes encoding structural antigens have been successfully delivered within vector organisms (e.g. the use of canarypox to deliver FeLV, canine distemper antigens or rabies virus antigens) or as naked plasmids, and cytokine genes have been incorporated into such plasmids for the adjuvant effect of the encoded cytokine.[87,88] However, adjuvant cytokine genes do not always deliver the expected effect. In one study where the IL-12 gene was co-administered with plasmids containing coronavirus genes to cats, the vaccine did not protect the cats but enhanced their susceptibility to challenge with feline infectious peritonitis virus.[89]

Blockade of immunological molecules

The application of monoclonal antibody therapy is not simply limited to interference with cytokine pathways. Numerous other immunological molecules involved in many stages of the immune response lend themselves to this form of targeted immunotherapy. Already, there is a range of such products for use in human immune-mediated disease. One of the earliest such therapeutic antibodies was CamPath-1™, which targets the CD52 molecule on the surface of lymphocytes and monocytes and is given to cause depletion of the T-cell population to prevent their activity in T-cell-mediated disease. CamPath-1 has application to transplantation

medicine and to the therapy of immune-mediated diseases such as rheumatoid arthritis and multiple sclerosis, and a humanised version of CamPath-1 (CamPath-1H) is now used. Recent studies have shown potential side effects of CamPath-1 therapy, sounding a note of caution that the rapid development of these novel immunomodulators requires strict pharmacovigilance when they are introduced into the market. When the antibody was used to treat 27 patients with multiple sclerosis, 9 of them developed thyroid autoimmune disease secondary to therapy.[90]

A second example of this form of immunotherapy is natalizumab, a monoclonal antibody that binds to the α_4 component of the $\alpha_4\beta_7$ molecule found on the surface of circulating T lymphocytes. This molecule binds to the vascular addressin MAdCAM, an interaction which is crucial in the recruitment of circulating T cells into the intestinal lamina propria. Blockade of this interaction results in inhibition of lymphocyte infiltration of the gut mucosa, and use of the product has shown clinical benefit in patients with inflammatory bowel disease.[91]

Monoclonal antibody therapy has widespread potential for the treatment of numerous diseases. The ability to conjugate toxins, cytokines or pro-drugs to monoclonal antibodies specific for tumour cells has relevance to the 'magic bullet' targeting of neoplastic tissue. Similarly, bi-specific monoclonal antibodies that permit linkage of cytotoxic lymphocytes to tumour cell targets have been developed (Fig. 2.1.7). Monoclonal antibodies might also be designed for therapy of infectious disease; for example, to block the binding of microbes to host cellular receptors.

Blockade of immunological processes may also be achieved by the administration of recombinant molecules, or the genes encoding them. For example, one molecular interaction between APCs and T lymphocytes involved in lymphocyte interaction is that between the CD2 molecule on the T cell and its ligand LFA-3 on the APC. A recombinant form of LFA-3 fused to human IgG1 (alefacept, Amevive®) effectively blocks this interaction by binding CD2, but can additionally activate adjacent natural killer (NK) cells via interaction of the NK FcγRIII with the IgG1 component of the molecule. This potentially results in the induction of apoptosis within the T cell. Alefacept has been used in the treatment of psoriasis in humans.[92] Another approach to down-regulating T cells involves the interaction between the molecules CD28 and

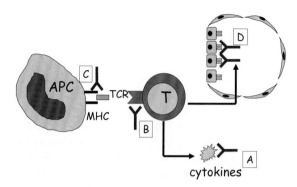

Fig. 2.1.7 Monoclonal antibody therapy. Monoclonal antibodies administered systemically will target and bind to the specific molecule to which they have been raised. This results in inhibition of function by either neutralising the target (e.g. cytokines [A]), disrupting molecular interactions (e.g. between T-cell receptor and antigenic peptide presented by MHC molecules [B & C]) or by causing destruction ('depletion') of the cell expressing the target molecule by fixing complement leading to cytolysis (D). APC, antigen-presenting cell; TCR, T-cell receptor.

CTLA-4 (CD152) expressed by CD4[+] T cells, and the shared ligand for these molecules, CD80/86, expressed by APCs. Engagement of CD80/86 by CD28 results in T-cell activation, whereas binding of CTLA-4 inhibits the T cell. Use of a CTLA-4-IgG fusion protein, or vectored genes for this molecule, has been able to similarly ameliorate experimental autoimmune disease.[93] Feline CD28 and CTLA-4 have been cloned and sequenced and there is increased expression of mRNA encoding both molecules in mitogen-stimulated lymphocytes.[94]

Inhibition of immunological activity might also be induced by 'vaccination' such that the host animal mounts an endogenous inhibitory immune response. This approach is exemplified by the canine studies in which dogs were immunised with a synthetic peptide derived from the region of the IgE ε heavy chain that interacts with the high-affinity FcεRI. The peptide was linked to a T-cell epitope derived from measles virus as a means of breaking the normal 'tolerance' towards endogenous IgE, and mounting an anti-IgE humoral immune response. Vaccinated dogs had reduced concentration of serum IgE.[95]

Certain non-immunological molecules may also have profound immunoregulatory effects, in particular bacterially derived products such as the B-subunit of *Escherichia coli* heat-labile enterotoxin. The latter molecule is able to bind to numerous cell surface glycoproteins and, when injected into mice developing collagen-induced arthritis, was able to inhibit clinical disease and joint pathology and switch the immune response from Th1- to Th2-dominated.[96] Much current interest focuses on synthetic oligodeoxynucleotides containing CpG motifs designed to mimic the high frequency of unmethylated CpG motifs in bacterial DNA. These CpG motifs are microbial PAMPs that preferentially interact with the PRR Toll-like receptor 9 expressed by dendritic cells, resulting in induction of a Th1-immune response. Such potent Th1 stimulants have obvious therapeutic application, and human phase I clinical trials have already examined their utility as vaccine adjuvants, adjunct cancer therapeutics, and as a means of redirecting the aberrant Th2 responses of allergic rhinitis and asthma.[97] CpG motifs have been shown to be capable of stimulating canine and feline lymphocytes *in vitro* and likely have similar potential application in veterinary medicine.[98] Finally, ovalbumin-sensitised mice treated intranasally with mycobacterial antigen (BCG) were protected from allergic respiratory changes on antigen challenge, suggesting that the bacterial antigen had modified the immune response from Th2 to Th1.[99]

Immunological tolerance

Although many of the methods described above are vastly more selective than the blanket medical immunomodulation currently utilised in veterinary medicine, they still influence lymphocytes of many antigen specificities, both relevant and irrelevant to a specific disease process. The 'holy grail' for immunotherapy is to develop means to selectively inhibit or stimulate the function of particular clones of lymphocytes relevant to a selected antigen. Such approaches have now been developed for inhibition of antigen-specific immune responses, and rely on the phenomenon of immunological tolerance.

Tolerance is the failure to mount an immune response when exposed to an antigen and comes in several different experimentally induced and spontaneously arising forms. Neonatal tolerance results when an animal is exposed to an antigen in the neonatal period and fails to react to that antigen when it is administered in an immunogenic form later in life. Tolerance may also be induced experimentally in adult animals by exposure to antigen via either repeated injections of low-dose antigen or a single injection of high-dose antigen. The mechanisms underlying these effects are not completely understood, but are known to differ in the type of lymphocyte that is 'tolerised'. Oral tolerance represents a classical experimental tolerance whereby an animal fed a particular antigen fails to respond to the same antigen that is subsequently administered systemically.[100] Oral tolerance to ovalbumin has been demonstrated experimentally in dogs.[101]

Important forms of spontaneously arising tolerance are self-tolerance to autoantigens, and mucosal tolerance to innocuous environmental allergens or dietary components. Failure of these forms of tolerance results in the onset of autoimmune disease or allergy. Numerous immunological mechanisms underlie these forms of tolerance. Self-tolerance relies primarily on deletion of autoreactive T cells during their intrathymic development, but this mechanism is not fail-safe, as self-reactive T cells do 'escape' from the thymus and have the potential to mediate autoimmune disease. Further mechanisms control these extra-thymic autoreactive lymphocytes, including deletion in the peripheral tissues, failure to fully activate these cells (anergy), failure to expose them to relevant autoantigen (immunological ignorance), and active suppression by regulatory cells (e.g. Treg).[102] Tolerance in T lymphocytes generally results in tolerance in B cells that fail to receive appropriate T-cell help. A range of similar mechanisms is likely to be involved in maintaining tolerance of the respiratory mucosa to inhaled environmental allergens, and tolerance of the gastrointestinal mucosa to dietary antigen and endogenous microflora.

The therapeutic potential of the phenomenon of oral (and more recently nasal) tolerance has recently been recognised. If an individual has lost tolerance to an autoantigen or allergen, then tolerance might be restored by administering that antigen across a mucosal surface in a classical oral tolerance protocol. A careful balance must be achieved in such an approach, because mucosal delivery of antigen may also stimulate immune responses, and there is active research into 'mucosal vaccination' with 'mucosal adjuvants' such as cholera toxin or *E. coli* heat-labile enterotoxin (see above for an alternative effect of this latter product).[103] To add further complication, cholera toxin conjugated with low-dose antigen has also been used to induce oral tolerance, suggesting that the protocol by which mucosal adjuvants are used is critical.[104]

One of the more radical approaches to therapeutic restoration of tolerance (e.g. to aeroallergens in atopic patients, or intestinal microbial flora in patients with inflammatory bowel disease) arises from the observation that helminth parasites are potent inducers of regulatory cells.[105] Establishment of a therapeutic intestinal infection with *Trichuris suis* has proven to have clinical benefit in humans with atopic disease or inflammatory enteropathy.[106] This concept also underlies the modification of the 'hygiene hypothesis' that explains the negative association between allergy and intestinal parasitism in underdeveloped countries, and suggests that a natural level of endoparasitism may be protective for immune-mediated disease. It is interesting to ponder whether any rise in prevalence of immune-mediated disease in companion animals might similarly relate to rigorous worming programmes that are generally practised in our pet population.

Oral tolerance

Numerous rodent experimental studies have shown that oral exposure to a specific autoantigen can either prevent the induction of an autoimmune disease, or ameliorate the clinical course of ongoing autoimmune disease. For example, mice fed collagen remain refractory to the subsequent induction of collagen-induced arthritis when collagen in adjuvant is injected subcutaneously.[107] The same principle has been adopted for clinical trials in humans with autoimmune disease. Patients have been fed a variety of autoantigens (e.g. collagen, retinal antigen, myelin, insulin) in attempts to modulate autoimmune diseases such as rheumatoid arthritis, uveoretinitis or multiple sclerosis.[108,109] However, although clinical improvement in individual patients is documented, this approach has proven less than spectacular overall. Oral tolerance has also been utilised in clinical veterinary medicine, where one commercially available product (C_2Collaplex™) incorporates fed type II collagen in an attempt to ameliorate the pathology associated with canine joint disease.

A similar exploitation of oral tolerance has been applied to experimental studies of aeroallergen or dietary hypersensitivity. Mice can be sensitised to allergen (e.g. ovalbumin, dust mite or peanut) by repeated intraperitoneal injection of allergen followed by challenge. Mice fed dust mite,[110] or genes encoding the major dust mite,[111] or peanut allergens (coupled to protective chitosan microparticles) developed Th1-dominated immune responses, rather than Th2-dominated immune responses, and failed to produce an anaphylactic response on challenge (in the case of peanut allergen). One similar study has been reported in a canine model. High-IgE responder beagle dogs were orally tolerised to ovalbumin and subsequently sensitised by repeated injection to both ovalbumin or recombinant Timothy grass pollen allergen. A control group was sensitised without prior oral tolerisation. Tolerised dogs had reduced allergic conjunctivitis following ocular challenge with ovalbumin and reduced features of allergic airway disease following challenge by nebulisation. These protective effects were associated with elevation of levels of mRNA expressing the regulatory cytokines IL-10 and TGF-β in cells derived from the bronchoalveolar lavage fluid.[112]

Nasal tolerance

Oral tolerance has been recognised for many years, but only recently it was discovered that similar, and indeed more potent, effects could be induced when antigen was delivered across the nasal mucosa. It was further discovered that entire antigens were not required for induction of this selective tolerance. Small peptide sequences derived from disease-inducing polypeptides were also capable of inducing very potent and antigentargeted tolerance. The proof of concept for so-called 'intranasal peptide therapy' lies in the numerous studies in rodent model systems. Instillation of peptides derived from autoantigens (e.g. myelin, collagen type II) or allergens (e.g. dust mites) onto the nasal mucosa can inhibit the induction of experimental disease, or ameliorate the clinical signs of ongoing disease.[113,114] Intranasal peptide therapy for treatment of human multiple sclerosis is now currently in phase I clinical trial.

Gene therapy

The final application of molecular biology to disease management is in 'gene replacement therapy' for animals with absent or mutated genes. Gene therapy is applicable to monogenic disorders and involves delivery of functional normal genes, generally via a microbial vector.[115] Early clinical trials have recently been performed in humans, specifically in children with severe combined immunodeficiency.[116] However, in 2003 these trials were halted in Europe when it was discovered that a proportion of the children developed leukaemia subsequent to the therapy. The trials have only recently recommenced.

This methodology has already been experimentally applied to dogs with factor IX deficiency (haemophilia B). Delivery of the gene encoding factor IX within a retroviral vector by injection into the portal vein following partial hepatectomy resulted in production of factor IX and improvement in coagulation for a 9-month period following treatment.[117] Similar production of factor IX was obtained with the use of an adenoviral vector[118] (Figure 2.1.8). One problem with this approach was the development of an immune response to factor IX in the genetically reconstituted dogs. Clearly a dog that had never produced this protein perceived the presence of the molecule as a foreign antigen and immunological tolerance had never been induced. Further application of this gene therapy would therefore require a means of establishing tolerance to the protein.[119] Alternatively, gene transfer in neonatal haemophiliac dogs has proven successful, as a form of neonatal tolerance must be induced.[120]

Although numerous candidate monogenic diseases are recognised in the dog (e.g. canine leukocyte adhesion deficiency, CLAD), in reality, gene replacement is likely to be considered less important than the elimination of the traits from animals by genetic testing. In fact, for the CLAD mutation such a testing programme has already proven successful within Irish setters in Australia.[121] The next such issue to arise will be with respect to cloned animals. Already, the technology for cloning cats has been reported and similar ethical discussions to those surrounding human cloning will no doubt take place.

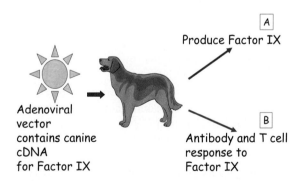

Fig. 2.1.8 Gene therapy. Gene replacement therapy for monogenic disorders has already been applied to canine models of human disease. For example, dogs congenitally deficient in factor IX of the coagulation cascade have been administered viral vector containing a functional canine factor IX gene. This treatment restores factor IX production (A) and clinically resolves the bleeding tendency in these animals. However, as these dogs have never been exposed to the factor IX molecule, they perceive it as immunologically foreign and mount an antibody response that in time neutralises the factor IX and reverses the clinical benefits (B).

Conclusion

It is clear that the current medical approach to immunomodulation in companion animal medicine is dated, relatively crude in conception, and fraught with the risks of adverse events. Despite this, our current pharmacological approach is, in many cases, clinically efficacious and priced within the means of our clients. Recent developments in basic immunology have led to a plethora of new and exciting approaches to manipulation of the immune system in patients. Future immunotherapy is likely to be safer and specifically targeted to particular cells or molecules of the immune system, or indeed to specific lymphocytes carrying an antigen-specific receptor that characterises them as directly involved in disease pathogenesis. Although these newer approaches are already available, or in clinical trial for human medicine, it is likely to be some time before any translate into veterinary practice. We require further basic knowledge of the canine and feline immune systems, together with studies demonstrating that these novel approaches are also valid for companion animals. Even when these criteria are satisfied, the developmental and licensing costs may be prohibitive of such products entering the relatively small veterinary marketplace.

References

1 Miller, E. Immunosuppressive therapy in the treatment of immune-mediated disease. *Journal of Veterinary Internal Medicine*, 1992; **6**: 206–213.
2 Dunn, J. Therapy of immune-mediated disease in small animals. *In Practice*, 1998; **20**: 147–153.
3 Rosenkrantz, W.R. Pemphigus: current therapy. *Veterinary Dermatology*, 2004; **15**: 90–98.
4 Mason, N., Duval, D., Shofer, F.S., Giger, U. Cyclophosphamide exerts no beneficial effect over prednisone alone in the initial treatment of acute immune-mediated hemolytic anemia in dogs: a randomized controlled clinical trial. *Journal of Veterinary Internal Medicine*, 2003; **17**: 206–212.
5 Gregory, C.R., Stewart, A., Sturges, B., *et al.* Leflunomide effectively treats naturally occurring immune-mediated and inflammatory diseases of dogs that are unresponsive to conventional therapy. *Transplantation Proceedings*, 1998; **30**: 4143–4148.
6 Marsella, R., Kunkle, G.A., Lewis, D.T. Use of pentoxifylline in the treatment of allergic contact reactions to plants of the *Commelinceae* family in dogs. *Veterinary Dermatology*, 1997; **8**: 121–126.
7 Patel, R.N., Attur, M.G., Dave, *et al.* A novel mechanism of action of chemically modified tetracyclines: inhibition of cox-2-mediated prostaglandin E$_2$ production. *Journal of Immunology*, 1999; **163**: 3459–3467.
8 Mueller, R.S., Fieseler, K.V., Bettenay, S.V., Rosychuk, R.A.W. Influence of long-term treatment with tetracycline and niacinamide on antibody production in dogs with discoid lupus ery-

thematosus. *American Journal of Veterinary Research*, 2002; **63**: 491–494.
9 Arndt, H., Palitzsch, K.D., Grisham, M.B., Granger, D.N. Metronidazole inhibits leukocyte-endothelial cell adhesion in rat mesenteric venules. *Gastroenterology*, 1994; **106**: 1271.
10 Cohn, L.A. The influence of corticosteroids on host defense mechanisms. *Journal of Veterinary Internal Medicine*, 1991; **5**: 95–104.
11 Lucena, R., Ginel, P.J., Hernandez, E., Novales, M. Effects of short courses of different doses of prednisone and dexamethasone on serum third component of complement (C3) levels in dogs. *Veterinary Immunology and Immunopathology*, 1999; **68**: 187–192.
12 Trowald-Wigh, G., Hakansson, L., Johannisson, A., Edqvist, L.E. The effect of prednisolone on canine neutrophil function: in vivo and in vitro studies. *Acta Veterinaria Scandinavica*, 1998; **39**: 201–213.
13 Rinkardt, N.E., Kruth, S.A., Kaushik, A. The effects of prednisone and azathioprine on circulating immunoglobulin levels and lymphocyte subpopulations in normal dogs. *Canadian Journal of Veterinary Research*, 1999; **63**: 18–24.
14 Olivry, T., Rivierre, C., Jackson, H.A., Marcy Murphy, K., Davidson, G., Sousa, C.A. Cyclosporine decreases skin lesions and pruritus in dogs with atopic dermatitis: a blinded randomized prednisolone-controlled trial. *Veterinary Dermatology*, 2002; **13**: 77–87.
15 Steffan, J., Alexander, D., Brovedani, F., Fisch, R. Comparison of cyclosporine A with methylprednisolone for treatment of canine atopic dermatitis: a parallel, blinded, randomized controlled trial. *Veterinary Dermatology*, 2003; **14**: 11–22.
16 Guaguere, E., Steffan, J., Olivry, T. Cyclosporin A: a new drug in the field of canine dermatology. *Veterinary Dermatology*, 2004; **15**: 61–74.
17 Mathews, K.G., Gregory, C.R. Renal transplants in cats: 66 cases (1987–1996). *Journal of the American Veterinary Medical Association*, 1997; **211**: 1432–1436.
18 Mathews, K.A., Holmberg, D.L., Miller, C.W. Kidney transplantation in dogs with naturally occurring end-stage renal disease. *Journal of the American Animal Hospital Association*, 2000; **36**: 294–301.
19 Robson, D.C., Burton, G.G. Cyclosporin: applications in small animal dermatology. *Veterinary Dermatology*, 2003; **14**: 1–9.
20 Mathews, K.A., Sukhiani, H.R. Randomized controlled trial of cyclosporine for treatment of perianal fistulas in dogs. *Journal of the American Veterinary Medical Association*, 1997; **211**: 1249–1253.
21 Kyles, A.E., Gregory, C.E., Craigmill, A.L. Comparison of the *in vitro* antiproliferative effects of five immunosuppressive drugs on lymphocytes in whole blood from cats. *American Journal of Veterinary Research*, 2000; **61**: 906–909.
22 Marsella, R., Nicklin, C.F. Investigation of the use of 0.3% tacrolimus lotion for canine atopic dermatitis: a pilot study. *Veterinary Dermatology*, 2002; **13**: 203–210.
23 Chabanne, L., Fournel, C., Rigal, D., Monier, J-C. Canine systemic lupus erythematosus. Part II. Diagnosis and treatment. *Compendium of Continuing Education for the Practising Veterinarian*, 1999; **21**: 402–410.
24 Frank, L.A., Kania, S.A. The effect of ivermectin on lymphocyte blastogenesis and T-cell subset ratios in healthy dogs. *Veterinary Allergy and Clinical Immunology*, 1997; **5**: 27–30.
25 Becker, A.M., Janik, T.A., Smith, E.K. *Propionibacterium acnes* immunotherapy in chronic recurrent canine pyoderma. *Journal of Veterinary Internal Medicine*, 1989; **3**: 26–30.
26 DeBoer, D.J., Moriello, K.A., Thomas, C.B. Evaluation of a commercial staphylococcal bacterin for management of idiopathic

recurrent superficial pyoderma in dogs. *American Journal of Veterinary Research*, 1990; **51**: 636–639.

27 Day, M.J. Immunomodulatory therapy. In: Maddison, J.E., Page, S.W., Church, D., eds. *Small Animal Clinical Pharmacology*. W.B. Saunders, London, 2002: 233–249.

28 Shi, F., Kurzman, I.D., MacEwan, E.G. In-vitro and in-vivo production of interleukin-6 induced by muramyl peptides and lipopolysaccharide in normal dogs. *Cancer Biotherapy*, 1995; **10**: 317–325.

29 King, G.K., Yates, K.M., Greenlee, P.G., *et al.* The effect of acemannan immunostimulant in combination with surgery and radiation therapy on spontaneous canine and feline fibrosarcomas. *Journal of the American Animal Hospital Association*, 1995; **31**: 439–447.

30 Kruth, S.A. Biological response modifiers: interferons, interleukins, recombinant products, liposomal products. *Veterinary Clinics of North America: Small Animal Practice*, 1998; **28**: 269–295.

31 McCaw, D.L., Boon, G.D., Jergens, A.E., Kern, M.R., Bowles, M.H., Johnson, J.C. Immunomodulation therapy for feline leukemia virus infection. *Journal of the American Animal Hospital Association*, 2001; **37**: 356–363.

32 Hu, S. Acupuncture stimulation to enhance immune responses: research and clinical application. *Proceedings of the North American Veterinary Conference*, 2004; **18**: 31–33.

33 Campieri, M., Gionchetti, P. Probiotics in inflammatory bowel disease: new insight to pathogenesis or a possible therapeutic alternative? *Gastroenterology*, 1999; **116**: 1246–1260.

34 Field, C.J., McBurney, M.I., Massimino, S., Hayek, M.G., Sunvold, G.D. The fermentable fiber content of the diet alters the function and composition of canine gut associated lymphoid tissue. *Veterinary Immunology and Immunopathology*, 1999; **72**: 325–341.

35 Hall, J.A., Tooley, K.A., Gradin, J.L., Jewell, D.E., Wander, R.C. Effects of dietary n-6 and n-3 fatty acids and vitamin E on the immune response of healthy geriatric dogs. *American Journal of Veterinary Research*, 2003; **64**: 762–772.

36 Shanahan, F. Inflammatory bowel disease: immunodiagnostics, immunotherapeutics, and ecotherapeutics. *Gastroenterology*, 2001; **120**: 622–635.

37 Kalliomaki, M., Salminen, S., Arvilommi, H., Kero, P., Koskinen, P., Isolauri, E. Probiotics in primary prevention of atopic disease: a randomised placebo-controlled trial. *Lancet*, 2001; **357**: 1076–1079.

38 Zur, G., White, S.D., Ihrke, P.J., Kass, P.H., Toebe, N. Canine atopic dermatitis: a retrospective study of 169 cases examined at the University of California, Davis, 1992–1998. Part II. Response to hyposensitization. *Veterinary Dermatology*, 2002; **13**: 103–111.

39 Nuttall, T.J., Thoday, K.L., van den Broek, A.H.M., Jackson, H.A., Sture, G.H., Halliwell, R.E.W. Retrospective survey of allergen immunotherapy in canine atopy. *Veterinary Record*, 1998; **143**: 139–142.

40 Hites, M.J., Kleinbeck, M.L., Loker, J.L., Lee, K.W. Effect of immunotherapy on the serum concentrations of allergen-specific IgG antibodies in dog sera. *Veterinary Immunology and Immunopathology*, 1989; **22**: 39–51.

41 Hou, C-C., Nuttall, T.J., Day, M.J., Hill, P.B. *Dermatophagoides farinae*-specific IgG subclass responses in atopic dogs undergoing allergen-specific immunotherapy. In: Hillier, A., Foster, A.P., Kwochka, K.W., eds. *Advances in Veterinary Dermatology*, Vol. 5. Blackwell Publishing, Oxford, 2005: 70–81.

42 Nouri-Aria, K.T., Wachholz, P.A., Francis, J.N., *et al.* Grass pollen immunotherapy induces mucosal and peripheral IL-10 responses and blocking IgG activity. *Journal of Immunology*, 2004;

172: 3252–3259.

43 Curtis, C.F., Lamport, A.I., Lloyd, D.H. Blinded, controlled study to investigate the efficacy of a staphylococcal autogenous bacterin for the control of canine idiopathic recurrent pyoderma (abstract). *Proceedings of the 16th Annual Congress of European Society of Veterinary Dermatology/European College of Veterinary Dermatology, Helsinki*, 1999: 148.

44 Scott-Moncrieff, J.C., Reagan, W.J., Synder, P.W., Glickman, L.T. Intravenous administration of human immune globulin in dogs with immune-mediated hemolytic anemia. *Journal of the American Veterinary Medical Association*, 1997; **210**: 1623–1627.

45 Byrne, K.P., Giger, U. Use of human immunoglobulin for the treatment of severe erythema multiforme in a cat. *Journal of the American Veterinary Medical Association*, 2002; **220**: 197–201.

46 Nuttall, T.J., Malham, T. Successful intravenous human immunoglobulin treatment of drug-induced Stevens-Johnson syndrome in a dog. *Journal of Small Animal Practice*, 2004; **45**: 357–361.

47 Reagan, W.J., Scott-Moncrieff, C., Christian, J., Snyder, P., Kelly, K., Glickman, L. Effects of human intravenous immunoglobulin on canine monocytes and lymphocytes. *American Journal of Veterinary Research*, 1998; **59**: 1568–1574.

48 Sewell, W.A.C., Jolles, S. Immunomodulatory action of intravenous immunoglobulin. *Immunology*, 2002; **107**: 387–393.

49 Ahmad, A.R. Intravenous immunoglobulin therapy results in long-term remission in pemphigus vulgaris patients non-responsive to conventional immunosuppressive treatment. *Clinical Immunology*, 2001; **99**: 169.

50 Matus, R.E., Schrader, L.A., Leifer, C.E., Gordon, B.R., Hurvitz, A.I. Plasmapheresis as adjuvant therapy for autoimmune hemolytic anemia in two dogs. *Journal of the American Veterinary Medical Association*, 1985; **186**: 691–693.

51 Matus, R.E., Gordon, B.R., Leifer, C.E., Saal, S., Hurvitz, A.I. Plasmapheresis in five dogs with systemic immune-mediated disease. *Journal of the American Veterinary Medical Association*, 1985; **187**: 595–599.

52 Murphy, K.M., Reiner, S.L. The lineage decisions of helper T cells. *Nature Reviews Immunology*, 2002; **2**: 933–944.

53 Bellinghausen, I., Brand, U., Enk, A.H., Knop, J., Saloga, J. Signals involved in the early Th1/Th2 polarization of an immune response depending on the type of antigen. *Journal of Allergy and Clinical Immunology*, 1999; **103**: 298–306.

54 Kapsenberg, M.L. Dendritic-cell control of pathogen-driven T-cell polarization. *Nature Reviews Immunology*, 2003; **3**: 984–993.

55 Sukura, A., Higgins, J., Pedersen, N.C. Compartmentalization of Th1/Th2 cytokine response to experimental *Yersinia pseudotuberculosis* infection in cats. *Veterinary Immunology and Immunopathology*, 1998; **65**: 139–150.

56 Fujiwara, S., Yasunaga, S., Iwabuchi, S., Masuda, K., Ohno, K., Tsujimoto, H. Cytokine profiles of peripheral blood mononuclear cells from dogs experimentally sensitized to Japanese cedar pollen. *Veterinary Immunology and Immunopathology*, 2003; **93**: 9–20.

57 Bach, J.F. Regulatory T cells under scrutiny. *Nature Reviews Immunology*, 2003; **3**: 189–198.

58 Sakaguchi, S. Control of immune responses by naturally arising CD4+ regulatory T cells that express Toll-like receptors. *Journal of Experimental Medicine*, 2003; **197**: 397–401.

59 Romagnani, S. The increased prevalence of allergy and the hygiene hypothesis: missing immune deviation, reduced immune suppression, or both? *Immunology*, 2004; **112**: 352–363.

60 Vahlenkamp, T.W., Tompkins, M.B., Tompkins, W.A.F. Feline immunodeficiency virus infection phenotypically and func-

tionally activates immunosuppressive CD4⁺CD25⁺ T regulatory cells. *Journal of Immunology*, 2004; **172**: 4752–4761.

61 Asudullah, K., Volk, H-D., Sterry, W. Novel immunotherapies for psoriasis. *Trends in Immunology*, 2002; **23**: 47–53.

62 Colombel, J-F., Rutgeerts, P., Malchow, H., *et al.* Interleukin 10 (Tenovil) in the prevention of postoperative recurrence of Crohn's disease. *Gut*, 2001; **49**: 42–46.

63 Adorini, L. Cytokine-based immunointervention in the treatment of autoimmune diseases. *Clinical and Experimental Immunology*, 2003; **132**: 185–192.

64 Modlin, R.L. Th1-Th2 paradigm: insights from leprosy. *Journal of Investigative Dermatology*, 1994; **102**: 828–832.

65 Zucker, K., Lu, P., Asthana, D. Production and characterization of recombinant canine interferon-γ from *Eschericia coli*. *Journal of Interferon Research*, 1993; **13**: 91.

66 Argyle, D.J., Harris, M., Lawrence, C., *et al.* Expression of feline recombinant interferon-γ in Baculovirus and demonstration of biological activity. *Veterinary Immunology and Immunopathology*, 1998; **64**: 97–105.

67 Ramires dos Santos, L., Barrouin-Melo, S.M., Chang, Y-F., *et al.* Recombinant single-chain interleukin 12 induces interferon gamma mRNA expression in peripheral blood mononuclear cells of dogs with visceral leishmaniasis. *Veterinary Immunology and Immunopathology*, 2004; **98**: 43–48.

68 Henry, C.J., Buss, M.S., Lothrop, C.D. Veterinary uses of recombinant human granulocyte colony-stimulating factor. Part I. Oncology. *Compendium of Continuing Education for the Practising Veterinarian*, 1998; **20**: 728–734.

69 Rewerts, J.M., Henry, C.J. Veterinary uses of recombinant human granulocyte colony-stimulating factor. Part II. Infectious diseases. *Compendium of Continuing Education for the Practising Veterinarian*, 1998; **20**: 823–827.

70 Helfand, S.C., Soergel, S.A., MacWilliams, P.S., Hank, J.A., Sondel, P.M. Clinical and immunological effects of human recombinant interleukin-2 given by repetitive weekly infusion to normal dogs. *Cancer Immunology and Immunotherapy*, 1994; **39**: 84–92.

71 DeMari, K., Maynard, L., Eun, H.M., Lebreux, B. Treatment of canine parvoviral enteritis with interferon-omega in a placebo-controlled field trial. *Veterinary Record*, 2003; **152**: 105–108.

72 Sanz, L., Blanco, B., Alvarez-Vallina, L. Antibodies and gene therapy: teaching old 'magic bullets' new tricks. *Trends in Immunology*, 2004; **25**: 85–91.

73 Chaudari, U., Romano, P., Mulchay, L.D., Dooley, L.T., Baker, D.G., Gottlieb, A.B. Efficacy and safety of infliximab monotherapy for plaque-type psoriasis: a randomised trial. *Lancet*, 2001; **357**: 1842–1847.

74 Colombel, J-F., Loftus, E.V., Tremaine, W.J., *et al.* The safety profile of infliximab in patients with Crohn's disease: the Mayo Clinic experience in 500 patients. *Gastroenterology*, 2004; **126**: 19–31.

75 Leckie, M.J., ten Brinke, A., Khan, J. Effects of an interleukin-5 (IL-5) blocking monoclonal antibody on eosinophils, airway hyperresponsiveness, and the response to allergen in patients with asthma. *Lancet*, 2000; **356**: 2144–2148.

76 Tang, L., Boroughs, K.L., Morales, T., *et al.* Recombinant canine IL-13 receptor α2-Fc fusion protein inhibits canine allergen-specific-IgE production in vitro by peripheral blood mononuclear cells from allergic dogs. *Veterinary Immunology and Immunopathology*, 2001; **83**: 115–122.

77 Proudfoot, A.E.I. Chemokine receptors: multifaceted therapeutic targets. *Nature Reviews Immunology*, 2002; **2**: 106–115.

78 Olivry, T., Dunston, S.M., Rivierre, C., *et al.* A randomized controlled trial of misoprostol monotherapy for canine atopic dermatitis: effects on dermal cellularity and cutaneous tumour

necrosis factor-alpha. *Veterinary Dermatology*, 2003; **14**: 37–46.

79 Woods, J.M., Katschke, K.J., Volin, M.V., *et al.* IL-4 adenoviral gene therapy reduces inflammation, proinflammatory cytokines, vascularisation, and bony destruction in rat adjuvant-induced arthritis. *Journal of Immunology*, 2001; **166**: 1214–1222.

80 Whalen, J.D., Lechman, E.L., Carlos, C.A., *et al.* Adenoviral transfer of the viral IL-10 gene periarticularly to mouse paws suppresses development of collagen-induced arthritis in both injected and uninjected paws. *Journal of Immunology*, 1999; **162**: 3625–3632.

81 Tarner, I.H., Garrison Fathman, C. Gene therapy in autoimmune disease. *Current Opinions in Immunology*, 2001; **13**: 676–682.

82 Stampfli, M.R., Neigh, G.S., Wiley, R.E., *et al.* Regulation of allergic mucosal sensitization by interleukin-12 gene transfer to the airway. *American Journal of Respiratory Cellular and Molecular Biology*, 1999; **21**: 317–326.

83 Walter, D.M., Wong, C.P., DeKruyff, R.H., Berry, G.J., Levy, S., Umetsu, D.T. IL-18 gene transfer by adenovirus prevents the development of and reverses established allergen-induced airway hyperreactivity. *Journal of Immunology*, 2001; **166**: 6392–6398.

84 Kim, S.H., Kim, S., Evans, C.H., Ghivizzani, S.C., Oligino, T., Robbins, P.D. Effective treatment of established murine collagen-induced arthritis by systemic administration of dendritic cells genetically modified to express IL-4. *Journal of Immunology*, 2001; **166**: 3499–3505.

85 Finn, O.J. Cancer vaccines: between the idea and reality. *Nature Reviews Immunology*, 2003; **3**: 630–641.

86 Modiano, J.F., Ritt, M.G., Wojcieszyn, J. The molecular basis of canine melanoma: pathogenesis and trends in diagnosis and therapy. *Journal of Veterinary Internal Medicine*, 1999; **13**: 163–174.

87 Lodmell, D.L., Parnell, M.J., Weyhrich, J.T., Ewalt, L.C. Canine rabies DNA vaccination: a single-dose intradermal injection into ear pinnae elicits elevated and persistent levels of neutralizing antibody. *Vaccine*, 2003; **21**: 3998–4002.

88 Hanlon, L., Argyle, D., Bain, D., *et al.* Feline leukemia virus DNA vaccine efficacy is enhanced by coadministration with interleukin-12 (IL-12) and IL-18 expression vectors. *Journal of Virology*, 2001; **75**: 8424–8433.

89 Glansbeek, H.L., Haagmans, B.L., te Lintelo, E.G., *et al.* Adverse effects of feline IL-12 during DNA vaccination against feline peritonitis virus. *Journal of General Virology*, 2002; **83**: 1–10.

90 Coles, A.J., Wing, M., Smith, S., *et al.* Pulsed monoclonal antibody treatment and autoimmune thyroid disease in multiple sclerosis. *Lancet*, 1999; **354**: 1691–1695.

91 Gordon, F.H., Lai, C.W.Y., Hamilton, M.I., *et al.* A randomized placebo-controlled trial of humanized monoclonal antibody to α4 integrin in active Crohn's disease. *Gastroenterology*, 2001; **121**: 268–274.

92 Ellis, C.N., Krueger, M.D. Treatment of chronic plaque psoriasis by selective targeting of memory effector T lymphocytes. *New England Journal of Medicine*, 2001; **345**: 248–255.

93 Quattrocchi, E., Dallman, M.J., Feldmann, M. Adenovirus-mediated gene transfer of CTLA-4-4Ig fusion protein in the suppression of experimental autoimmune arthritis. *Arthritis and Rheumatism*, 2000; **43**: 1688–1697.

94 Choi, I-S., Hash, S.M., Collisson, E.W. Molecular cloning and expression of feline CD28 and CTLA-4 cDNA. *Veterinary Immunology and Immunopathology*, 2000; **76**: 45–59.

95 Wang, C.Y., Walfield, A.M., Fang, X., *et al.* Synthetic IgE peptide vaccine for immunotherapy of allergy. *Vaccine*, 2003; **21**: 1580–1590.

96 Williams, N.A., Stasiuk, L., Nashar, T.O., *et al.* Prevention of au-

toimmune disease by GM1-induced modulation of lymphocyte responses. *Proceedings of the National Academy of Sciences USA*, 1997; **94**: 5290–5295.

97 Klinman, D.M. Immunotherapeutic uses of CpG oligodeoxynucleotides. *Nature Reviews Immunology*, 2004; **4**: 249–258.

98 Wernette, C.M., Smith, B.F., Barksdale, Z.L., Hecker, R., Baker, H.J. CpG oligodeoxynucleotides stimulate canine and feline immune cell proliferation. *Veterinary Immunology and Immunopathology*, 2002; **84**: 223–236.

99 Hopfenspirger, M.T., Agrawal, D.K. Airway hyperresponsiveness, late allergic response, and eosinophilia are reversed with mycobacterial antigens in ovalbumin-presensitized mice. *Journal of Immunology*, 2002; **168**: 2516–2522.

100 Mowat, A.McI. Anatomical basis of tolerance and immunity to intestinal antigens. *Nature Reviews Immunology*, 2003; **3**: 331–341.

101 Deplazes, P., Penhale, W.J., Greene, W.K., Thompson, R.C.A. Effect on humoral tolerance (IgG and IgE) in dogs by oral administration of ovalbumin and Der pI. *Veterinary Immunology and Immunopathology*, 1995; **45**: 361–367.

102 Walker, L.S.K., Abbas, A.K. The enemy within: keeping self-reactive T cells at bay in the periphery. *Nature Reviews Immunology*, 2002; **2**: 11–19.

103 Bouvet, J-P., Decroix, N., Pamonsinlapatham, P. Stimulation of local antibody production: parenteral or mucosal vaccination? *Trends in Immunology*, 2002; **23**: 209–213.

104 Sun, J-B., Rask, C., Olsson, T., Holmgren, J., Czerkinsky, C. Treatment of experimental autoimmune encephalomyelitis by feeding myelin basic protein conjugated to cholera toxin B subunit. *Proceedings of the National Academy of Sciences USA*, 1996; **93**: 7196–7201.

105 Maizels, R.M., Yazdanbakhsh, M. Immune regulation by helminth parasites: cellular and molecular mechanisms. *Nature Reviews Immunology*, 2003; **3**: 733–744.

106 Weinstock, J.V., Summers, R., Elliott, D.E. Helminths and harmony. *Gut*, 2004; **53**: 7–9.

107 Thompson, S.J., Thompson, H.S.G., Harper, N., *et al.* Prevention of pristane-induced arthritis by the oral administration of type II collagen. *Immunology*, 1993; **79**: 152–157.

108 Barnett, M.L., Kremer, J.M., St Clair, E.W., *et al.* Treatment of rheumatoid arthritis with oral type II collagen. Results of a multicentre, double-blinded, placebo-controlled trial. *Arthritis and Rheumatism*, 1998; **41**: 290–297.

109 Mayer, L., Shao, L. Therapeutic potential of oral tolerance. *Nature Reviews Immunology*, 2004; **4**: 407–419.

110 Sato, M.N., Carvalho, A.F., Silva, A.O., Maciel, M., Fusaro, A.E., Duarte, J.S. Low dose of orally administered antigen down-regulates the T helper type 2-response in a murine model of dust mite hypersensitivity. *Immunology*, 1999; **98**: 338–344.

111 Chew, J.L., Wolfowicz, C.B., Mao, H-Q., Leong, K.W., Chua, K.Y. Chitosan nanoparticles containing plasmid DNA encoding house dust mite allergen, Der pI for oral vaccination in mice. *Vaccine*, 2003; **21**: 2720–2729.

112 Zemann, B., Schwaerzler, C., Griot-Wenk, M., *et al.* Oral administration of specific antigens to allergy-prone infant dogs induces IL-10 and TGFβ expression and prevents allergy in adult life. *Journal of Allergy and Clinical Immunology*, 2003; **111**: 1069–1075.

113 Staines, N.A., Harper, N., Ward, F.J., Malmstrom, V., Holmdahl, R., Bansal, S. Mucosal tolerance and suppression of collagen-induced arthritis (CIA) induced by nasal inhalation of synthetic peptide 184–198 of bovine type II collagen (CII) expressing a dominant T-cell epitope. *Clinical and Experimental Immunology*, 1996; **103**: 368–375.

114 Wraith, D.C. Antigen-specific immunotherapy of autoimmune disease: a commentary. *Clinical and Experimental Immunology*, 1996; **103**: 349–352.

115 Argyle, D.J. Gene therapy in veterinary medicine. *Veterinary Record*, 1999; **144**: 369–376.

116 Fischer, A., Hacein-Bey, S., Cavazzana-Calvo, M. Gene therapy of severe combined immunodeficiencies. *Nature Reviews Immunology*, 2002; **2**: 615–621.

117 Kay, M.A., Rothenberg, S., Landen, C.N., *et al.* In-vivo gene-therapy of hemophilia-B: sustained partial correction in factor-IX deficient dogs. *Science*, 1993; **262**: 117–119.

118 Ehrhardt, A., Xu, H., Dillow, A.M., Bellinger, D.A., Nichols, T.C., Kay, M.A. A gene-deleted adenoviral vector results in phenotypic correction of canine hemophilia B without liver toxicity or thrombocytopenia. *Blood*, 2003; **102**: 2403–2411.

119 Opdenakker, G., Van den Steen, P.E., Laureys, G., Hunninck, K., Arnold, B. Neutralizing antibodies in gene-defective hosts. *Trends in Immunology*, 2003; **24**: 94–100.

120 Xu, L.F., Gao, C.H., Sands, M.S., *et al.* Neonatal or hepatocyte growth factor-potentiated adult gene therapy with a retroviral vector results in therapeutic levels of canine factor IX for hemophilia B. *Blood*, 2003; **101**: 3924–3932.

121 Jobling, A.I., Ryan, J., Augusteyn, R.C. The frequency of the canine leukocyte adhesion deficiency (CLAD) allele within the Irish setter population of Australia. *Australian Veterinary Journal*, 2003; **81**: 763–765.

Lufenuron does not augment effectiveness of terbinafine for treatment of *Microsporum canis* infections in a feline model

D.J. DeBoer DVM[1], K.A. Moriello DVM[1], L.M. Volk BS[1], R. Schenker PhD[2], J. Steffan MS[2]

[1] Department of Medical Sciences, School of Veterinary Medicine, University of Wisconsin, Madison, Wisconsin, USA
[2] Novartis Animal Health, Basel, Switzerland

Summary

Evidence suggests that lufenuron may have antifungal properties with application for treatment of dermatophytosis in animals. The objectives of the current study were to evaluate lufenuron as: (1) a *primary treatment* for experimental *Microsporum canis* infections in cats; and (2) an *adjuvant treatment* for such infections, in combination with the antifungal drug terbinafine. Groups of five or six experimentally infected juvenile cats were treated with either: (1) lufenuron suspension (Program®), 133 mg orally once every 2 weeks; (2) terbinafine, 15–30 mg/kg orally once daily; (3) lufenuron plus terbinafine, both given at the above dosages; or (4) itraconazole 8 mg/kg orally once daily. A fifth group was left untreated as controls. Cats were scored weekly for clinical signs of dermatophytosis, and cultured for fungi once weekly, until the cat was deemed to be cured. Cats in the following treatment groups had the quickest cure of their infections: itraconazole (7.8 ± 1.3 weeks to cure), terbinafine (8.6 ± 1.8 weeks), and lufenuron and terbinafine (8.7 ± 1.2 weeks). These values were significantly ($p \leq 0.05$) less than untreated control cats (11.3 ± 2.2 weeks). Mean time to cure in cats treated with lufenuron alone was 9.3 ± 1.6 weeks, a lower mean, but not significantly less, than untreated control cats. Itraconazole and terbinafine performed equivalently with regard to reduction in fungal culture scores and in time-to-cure, yet differently with regard to reduction in clinical signs during infection. The results of this study showed no evidence for a synergistic effect of lufenuron when used in combination with terbinafine.

Introduction

Lufenuron is a drug marketed worldwide for control of fleas on cats and dogs. This drug works via interference with the synthesis of chitin, a critical component of the insect exoskeleton.[1] As the cell walls of fungi also contain chitin, there arose speculation that lufenuron may have antifungal properties as well. Early trials of antifungal activity against *Coccidioides immitis* yielded conflicting results.[2,3] A case report suggested that the drug might have value in treating fungal endometritis in mares.[4]

Several studies have examined a possible role for lufenuron in the treatment of dermatophytosis. Treatment of dogs or cats with lufenuron was strongly associated with recovery from dermatophytosis in one retrospective study,[5] and this report provided the grounds for further controlled study of potential antifungal properties of the drug. In an initial controlled study where the challenge infection was induced by application of fungal spores to the skin,[6] lufenuron treatment of cats did not prevent establishment of *Microsporum canis* infection. A second study[7] examined the effects of lufenuron treatment on the establishment and course of experimental *M. canis* infections in cats, where the challenge was accomplished by exposure to an infected cat, as would occur in a typical field case. In the latter study, lufenuron did not prevent infection, nor significantly reduce the time it took for the infection to resolve. However, in both of these controlled studies, a slight delay was noted in establishment of the infection in the lufenuron-treated cats, as compared with control cats. This suggested a possible inhibitory effect of lufenuron on the growth of *M. canis* in feline skin, but not sufficient to prevent development of infection, nor significantly affect its course. We speculated that this potential slight inhibitory effect of lufenuron on establishment of dermatophyte infection, even if not effective as a sole treatment, may be therapeutically valuable as an adjuvant in combination with conventional antifungal therapy. The goals of the present study were to evaluate: (1) lufenuron and terbinafine as a primary treatment for already established *M. canis* infections in cats; and (2) any possible synergism of these drugs given in combination, in comparison with itraconazole, a conventional antifungal drug which has demonstrated activity in feline fungal infections.

Materials and methods

Animals

This study was performed using 30 barrier-reared domestic short-haired juvenile cats (14 males and 16 females), of varying coat colours and 8 weeks of age at the beginning of the study (Liberty Research, Waverly, NY, USA). The cats were housed in biohazard containment rooms for the duration of the study; they were housed individually in stainless steel cages, 15 per room. The 30 cats were divided into 5 experimental groups of 6 cats each, and cats from all 5 groups were equally represented in each of the two housing rooms. Within experimental groups, cats were distributed approximately evenly according to sex, weight and coat colour. Cats were fed standard dry feline growth ration and water *ad libitum* during the study. The protocol for animal use was approved by the Animal Care Committee of the School of Veterinary Medicine, University of Wisconsin-Madison.

Infection protocol

All animals were infected by topical inoculation with *M. canis* in accordance with previously published procedures.[8,9] Briefly, cats were sedated with ketamine and the lateral flank on both sides was clipped closely with a no. 40 blade. A 3.5-cm diameter circle was drawn on the clipped skin at the inoculation sites. Fungal macroconidia (spores of *M. canis*, strain UW-8, in 200 µl PBS-glycerol) were applied to the marked area and distributed with a glass rod. An inoculum of 10^5 spores was applied to each side. An occlusive bandage was ap-

plied over the areas, and secured around the trunk with stretch gauze and adhesive tape, with care taken not to interfere with respiratory motions. Cats were fitted with plastic Elizabethan collars to prevent grooming and disturbance of the bandage. Bandages were removed after 72 hours. Elizabethan collars remained on the cats for a total of 4 weeks after inoculation.

Monitoring schedule

After inoculation with fungal spores, cats were examined and scored once weekly for signs and severity of dermatophytosis, using criteria and a scoring system similar to those published previously.[9] Cats were examined by close direct examination and by examination under a Wood's lamp. Only one side of each cat was scored for lesion severity; the side with the largest initial lesion size was chosen for each cat, and this same lesion was scored for the duration of the study. Lesion areas were traced on clear acetate tape, and the total affected area was determined (in cm²) using image analysis software (SigmaScan, SPSS Science, Chicago, IL, USA). For the purposes of computation of the total infection score, the lesion size was also expressed semi-quantitatively as a size score, as follows: score of 0 (no lesion), 1 (< 10 cm² total area), 2 (10–19.9 cm²), 3 (20–29.9 cm²), or 4 (≥ 30 cm²).

Each week, scores for the following subjective infection criteria were assigned on a 0–3 point scale; induration, scale/crust, erythema and fluorescence under Wood's lamp.[9] The presence of any satellite lesions, i.e. lesions distant from the area of inoculation, was assessed by assigning a score of 0–6, with one point given for lesions found on each of the following body regions: muzzle, head/ears, forelimbs, hindlimbs, dorsal aspect of trunk and ventral aspect of trunk.

Dermatophyte culture was performed weekly, according to standard techniques, using a toothbrush method and a selective fungal culture agar medium (Mycosel agar, Becton Dickinson, Cockeysville, MD, USA).[10] A toothbrush was passed 20 times over the lateral aspect of the thorax and abdomen, including the lesion area. The toothbrush was used to inoculate an agar plate by pressing the bristles to the agar 10 times. Plates were incubated at room temperature for 3 weeks, and examined daily for growth. Results were recorded as no growth, contaminant growth, or positive for *M. canis*. The number of colonies per plate was recorded for cultures that were positive for *M.*

canis. For purposes of computation of the total infection score, the culture result also was expressed semi-quantitatively as a culture score, as follows: score of 0 (no colonies), 1 (1–5 colonies), 2 (6–10 colonies), or 3 (> 10 colonies).

A total infection score was computed weekly, as the sum of the erythema score, induration score, scaling/crusting score, satellite lesion score, Wood's lamp score, size score and culture score (total score possible, 25 points).

Treatment protocol

Treatment began for each cat 4–6 weeks after inoculation, at the first week for which each cat's lesions attained an induration score of at least 2, plus a scaling score of at least 2, plus a lesion size > 5 cm². A total of 28/30 cats progressed to the treatment phase; one cat died of unrelated causes during the infection phase, and one cat could not be infected despite repeated attempts, and was excluded from the study. The 28 cats were divided into groups and treated as follows: group L (*n* = 6) received lufenuron (Program® oral suspension, Novartis Animal Health, Basel, Switzerland) as currently marketed for feline use, in accordance with the actual label use instructions, i.e. 1 ampoule (133 mg) per cat, but given once every 2 weeks. Mean cat weight in this group was 1.36 kg at the beginning of the study, and approximately 3.3 kg at the end of the study, thus, the dose achieved was initially ~100 mg/kg and finally ~40 mg/kg. Dosing was continued once every 2 weeks for the duration of the study. Group T (*n* = 5) received terbinafine orally, at a dosage between 15 and 30 mg/kg once daily, adjusted weekly according to body weight as follows: up to 1.0 kg, 15.6 mg daily; 1.1–2.0 kg, 31.3 mg daily; 2.1–4.0 kg, 62.5 mg daily, for the duration of the study (Lamisil® 125 mg tablets, Novartis, Basel, Switzerland). Group LT (*n* = 6) received a combination of both drugs. Lufenuron was administered exactly as specified for the lufenuron-only group; terbinafine was administered exactly as specified for the terbinafine-only group. Group I received itraconazole oral solution (Sporanox® Oral Solution, 10 mg/ml, Janssen Pharmaceutica, Titusville, NJ, USA) at a dosage of 8 mg/kg once daily for the duration of the study; dose was adjusted once weekly based upon body weight. Group C, the control group (*n* = 6), received no treatment; the infection was allowed to progress without drug therapy.

Statistical methods

The area under the curve (AUC) on a graph of response vs treatment time was calculated for each cat and each response criterion (i.e. using graphs similar to those presented in Figs 2.2.1 to 2.2.8). The AUC was thus a composite representation of both the time and severity of infection over its total course in each cat. In addition, a time-to-cure (TTC) was determined for each cat, defined as the number of weeks of treatment necessary to result in a combination of no visible lesions, negative Wood's lamp examination, and two successive culture scores of 0 or 1. To define differences between cat groups, AUC and TTC data were evaluated using the Mann-Whitney test. Results were deemed significantly different with $p < 0.05$.

Results

Clinical scoring and culture data on infected, treated cats over the time course of the study are presented in Figs 2.2.1–2.2.8. In examining the AUC data, there was no significant difference ($p > 0.05$) between treatment groups for lesion size (Fig. 2.2.1), erythema (Fig. 2.2.2), or satellite lesion score (Fig. 2.2.3). Induration score, scaling/crusting scores and total infection scores (Figs 2.2.4–2.2.6) were significantly lower in itraconazole-treated cats than in all other groups. Wood's lamp scores (Fig. 2.2.7) were significantly lower in the itraconazole- and lufenuron/terbinafine-treated groups than in control cats, but not significantly different from other groups. Culture scores (Fig. 2.2.8) were significantly lower than control cats in the itraconazole-, terbinafine-, and lufenuron/terbinafine-treated groups. Culture scores were also significantly lower than lufenuron-treated cats in those groups treated with itraconazole or lufenuron/terbinafine.

TTC data are presented in Table 2.2.1. Cats in the following treatment groups had the quickest cure of their infections: itraconazole, terbinafine alone, and lufenuron-terbinafine. These values were significantly less than untreated control cats. Mean TTC in cats treated with lufenuron alone was lower than that in untreated controls, but not significantly so.

Thus, clinical sign scores during the course of active infection were most consistently significantly lower in itraconazole-treated cats. Terbinafine and terbinafine/lufenuron treatment reduced clinical scores as well, but generally not significantly. However, both itraconazole

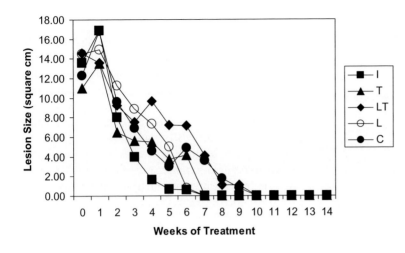

Fig. 2.2.1 Dermatophytosis lesion size in groups of infected, treated cats. Treatment groups are depicted in the key. I, itraconazole; T, terbinafine; LT, lufenuron and terbinafine; L, lufenuron; C, no treatment.

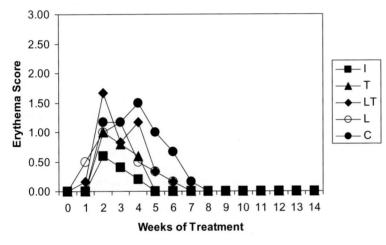

Fig. 2.2.2 Dermatophytosis lesion erythema in groups of infected, treated cats. I, itraconazole; T, terbinafine; LT, lufenuron and terbinafine; L, lufenuron; C, no treatment.

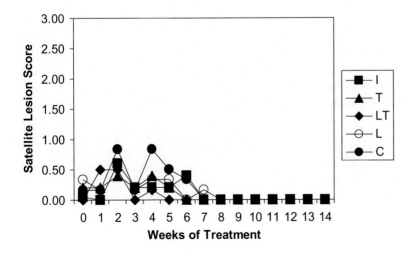

Fig. 2.2.3 Dermatophytosis satellite lesion scores in groups of infected, treated cats. I, itraconazole; T, terbinafine; LT, lufenuron and terbinafine; L, lufenuron; C, no treatment.

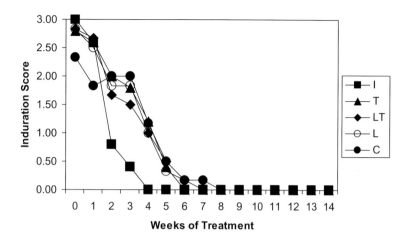

Fig. 2.2.4 Dermatophytosis lesion induration in groups of infected, treated cats. I, itraconazole; T, terbinafine; LT, lufenuron and terbinafine; L, lufenuron; C, no treatment.

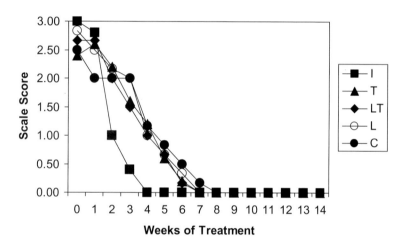

Fig. 2.2.5 Dermatophytosis lesion scaling/crusting in groups of infected, treated cats. I, itraconazole; T, terbinafine; LT, lufenuron and terbinafine; L, lufenuron; C, no treatment.

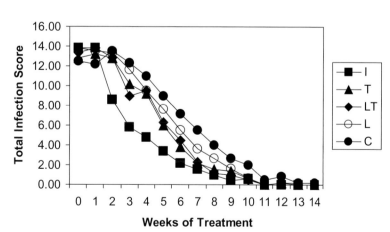

Fig. 2.2.6 Dermatophytosis lesion total infection scores in groups of infected, treated cats. I, itraconazole; T, terbinafine; LT, lufenuron and terbinafine; L, lufenuron; C, no treatment.

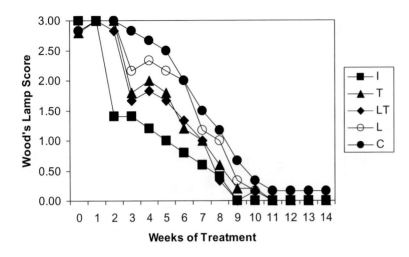

Fig. 2.2.7 Dermatophytosis lesion Wood's lamp scores in groups of infected, treated cats. I, itraconazole; T, terbinafine; LT, lufenuron and terbinafine; L, lufenuron; C, no treatment.

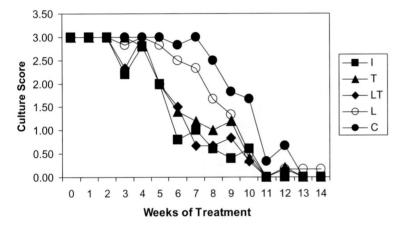

Fig. 2.2.8 Dermatophyte culture scores in groups of infected, treated cats. I, itraconazole; T, terbinafine; LT, lufenuron and terbinafine; L, lufenuron; C, no treatment.

and terbinafine performed equivalently with regard to reduction in fungal culture scores and in TTC. Lufenuron treatment did not result in significantly lower clinical scores, fungal culture scores, or TTC.

Discussion

Both itraconazole and terbinafine have been used for treatment of dermatophytosis in cats, although itraconazole has a longer history of use, and seems to be used by many veterinary dermatologists as a primary 'drug-of-choice treatment' for this disease. Terbinafine has been less extensively studied for feline use. One uncontrolled study reported clearing of *M. canis* infection from a laboratory cat colony, with mycologic cure, at a dose of 8.25 mg/kg for 3 weeks.[11] A later controlled study with experimentally infected cats found that

Table 2.2.1 Time-to-cure (TTC) data in groups of *Microsporum canis*-infected cats treated with various antifungal drugs or left untreated

Group	Treatment	Time-to-cure (weeks, mean ± SD)	p (control vs treated)
C	Untreated control	11.3 ± 2.2	–
I	Itraconazole	7.8 ± 1.3	0.009*
T	Terbinafine	8.6 ± 1.8	0.039*
L	Lufenuron	9.3 ± 1.6	0.15
LT	Lufenuron plus terbinafine	8.7 ± 1.2	0.015*

p values in the right-hand column were determined using the Mann–Whitney test. *$p < 0.05$ was significant.

cats treated at 10–20 mg/kg once daily improved no faster than untreated controls; however, dose levels of 30–40 mg/kg once daily were found to be more effective. The higher doses resulted in significantly greater terbinafine levels in hair (but not in plasma).[12] The dose of terbinafine used in the current study (15–30 mg/kg once daily) was approximately in-between these two dose ranges. At this dose, we found that terbinafine treatment resulted in mycologic cure in approximately the same time as with itraconazole treatment. We found no evidence that addition of lufenuron to the treatment regimen resulted in faster cure.

Interestingly, in general the antifungal drugs appeared to have their greatest effect on fungal culture results rather than on clinical observation criteria. All three groups treated with a conventional antifungal drug (groups I, T or LT) had lower culture scores than control cats, whereas only itraconazole-treated cats had lower scores for clinical criteria such as induration and scaling. This discrepancy between the clinical scores and the culture scores could have occurred if the dose of terbinafine used was suboptimal, i.e. use of a higher terbinafine dose might also have produced lower clinical scores. However, culture scores were not significantly different from itraconazole, suggesting that the dose is sufficient for curing the infection. Alternatively, this discrepancy might occur if itraconazole has, in addition to its antifungal properties, some anti-inflammatory effect that would reduce clinical signs of infection. There is, in fact, limited *in vitro* evidence that itraconazole could have an anti-inflammatory effect by virtue of its ability to inhibit 5-lipoxygenase.[13]

In summary, the present study provided little or no evidence for effectiveness of lufenuron as a primary treatment for experimental *M. canis* dermatophytosis in cats. Likewise, we found no evidence for a synergistic or adjuvant effect of lufenuron when used along with terbinafine, at the dosages used in the present study. It should be noted that our study was conducted using a single strain of *M. canis*, and that there may be variation in susceptibility of different strains of this organism to any antifungal drug. Likewise, clinicians have used a variety of lufenuron doses in attempting to treat field cases, including doses even higher than those in the present study. These points may, in part, explain the apparent benefit of lufenuron in some field cases, despite lack of evidence of efficacy in controlled laboratory studies.

Acknowledgements

The authors thank Jennifer Cyborski and Darin Flaska for their assistance in care and treatment of the cat colony, and Dr Wolfgang Seewald for statistical analysis. This study was funded by Novartis Animal Health.

References

1 Dean, S.R., Meola, R.W., Meola, S.M., Sitterz-Bhatkar, H., Schenker, R. Mode of action of lufenuron on larval cat fleas (Siphonaptera: Pulicidae). *Journal of Medical Entomology*, 1998; **35**: 720–724.

2 Bartsch, R., Greene, R. New treatment of coccidioidomycosis. *Veterinary Forum*, 1997; **4**: 50–52.

3 Johnson, S.M., Zimmermann, C.R., Kerekes, K.M., Davidson, A., Pappagianis, D. Evaluation of the susceptibility of *Coccidioides immitis* to lufenuron, a chitin synthase inhibitor. *Medical Mycology*, 1997; **37**: 441–444.

4 Hess, M.B., Parker, N.A., Purswell, B.J., Dascanio, J.D. Use of lufenuron as a treatment for fungal endometritis in four mares. *Journal of the American Veterinary Medical Association*, 2002; **221**: 266–267.

5 Ben-Ziony, Y., Arzi, B. Use of lufenuron for treating fungal infections of dogs and cats: 297 cases (1997–1999). *Journal of the American Veterinary Medical Association*, 2000; **217**: 1510–1513.

6 Moriello, K.A., DeBoer, D.J., Volk, L.M., Blum, J. Prevention of *Microsporum canis* infection in a cat challenge model (abstract). *Veterinary Dermatology*, 2002; **13**: 225.

7 DeBoer, D.J., Moriello, K.A., Blum, J.L., Volk, L.M. Effects of lufenuron treatment in cats on the establishment and course of *Microsporum canis* infection following exposure to infected cats. *Journal of the American Veterinary Medical Association*, 2004; **222**: 1216–1220.

8 DeBoer, D.J., Moriello, K.A.. Development of an experimental model of *Microsporum canis* infection in cats. *Veterinary Microbiology*, 1994; **42**: 289–295.

9 Moriello, K.A., DeBoer, D.J. Efficacy of griseofulvin and itraconazole in the treatment of experimentally induced dermatophytosis in cats. *Journal of the American Veterinary Medical Association*, 1995; **207**: 439–444.

10 Moriello, K.A., DeBoer, D.J. Fungal flora of the coat of pet cats. *American Journal of Veterinary Research*, 1991; **52**: 602–606.

11 Castanon-Olicares, L.R., Manzano-Gayosso, P., Lopez-Martinez, R., De la Rosa-Velazquez, I.A., Soto-Reyes-Solis, E. Effectiveness of terbinafine in the eradication of *Microsporum canis* from laboratory cats. *Mycoses*, 2001; **44**: 95–97.

12 Kotnik, T., Kozuh Erzen, N., Kuzner, J., Drobnic-Kosorok, M. Terbinafine hydrochloride treatment of *Microsporum canis* experimentally-induced ringworm in cats. *Veterinary Microbiology*, 2001; **83**: 161–168.

13 Steinhilber, D., Jaschonek, K., Knospe, J., Morof, O., Roth, H.J. Effects of novel antifungal azole derivatives on the 5-lipoxygenase and cyclooxygenase pathway. *Arzneimittel-Forschung*, 1990; **40**: 1260–1263.

An overview of pharmacokinetic and pharmacodynamic studies in the development of itraconazole for feline *Microsporum canis* dermatophytosis

K.M.J.A. Vlaminck DVM, M.A.C.M. Engelen DVM

Janssen Animal Health, Beerse, Belgium

Summary

Itraconazole is commercially available as an oral solution (Itrafungol,™ 10 mg/ml) in most countries within the European Union. It is approved for treatment of *Microsporum canis* dermatophytosis in cats. The treatment schedule consists of once daily oral administration of 5 mg/kg body weight for three 1-week periods, with each week of treatment followed by a week without treatment. This schedule was determined on the basis of *in vitro* data (= MIC_{90}), pharmacodynamic and pharmacokinetic data from pilot trials, and data from two specific trials in naturally infected cats.

Initially, antifungal concentrations of itraconazole in hair samples were determined by means of a bioassay. Later, plasma and hair concentrations of itraconazole and its active metabolite, hydroxy-itraconazole, were determined in a pivotal trial, according to Good Laboratory Practices (GLP). Plasma and hair samples were then analysed by high pressure liquid chromatography (HPLC). The correlation between the HPLC assay and the bioassay was established prior to conducting this pivotal trial. Median concentration of itraconazole in cat hair samples was 0.168 µg/g at 24 hours after the first dose. There was an increase after 1 week of treatment to 1.17 µg/g. At the end of the second 1-week dosing period, the median concentration was 2.00 µg/g, and was 2.99 µg/g at the end of the third dosing period. At the end of each of the 1-week intermittent periods without treatment, hair concentrations of itraconazole dropped 25–30% to median values of 0.8–1.5 µg/g. Two weeks after the last dose of the full treatment schedule, median hair concentrations were still 1.5 µg/g. Concentrations were well above the minimum inhibitory concentration for 90% of the strains (MIC_{90}) for *M. canis* (0.1 µg/ml in various broth media) shortly after the first dose and for up to 2 weeks after the last dose. This illustrates that based on reported MIC_{90} values for *M. canis*, the recommended treatment schedule provides adequate concentrations of itraconazole in the hairs to effectively treat the infection for at least 7 weeks after start of treatment.

Introduction

Itraconazole is commercially available as a 10 mg/ml oral solution (Itrafungol™, Janssen Animal Health, Beerse, Belgium) for treatment of *Microsporum canis* dermatophytosis in cats in most countries in the European Union. Itraconazole is a very lipophilic and keratinophilic compound. It is readily distributed from the plasma to the adipose tissue, sebaceous glands and stratum corneum of the skin and hairs and accumulates in these tissues.[1] This characteristic makes itraconazole readily available at the site of infection in cases of dermatophytosis. The treatment schedule for Itrafungol™ consists of once-daily oral administration of 5 mg/kg body weight for three 1-week periods, with each week of treatment followed by a week without treatment. The purpose of this review was to demonstrate the value of generating data on efficacy and safety of itraconazole in cats in parallel with pharmacokinetic studies in order to determine the optimal dose and treatment schedule for this drug. Subsequently, the selected dose and treatment schedule were evaluated in a pivotal pharmacokinetic trial in order to confirm the plasma and, more importantly, the hair levels that can be expected with this treatment.

In vitro pharmacodynamic data

The developmental activities focused on the treatment of *M. canis* infections, as this is the predominant dermatophyte species in cats. *In vitro* data on itraconazole, generated in brain heart infusion (BHI) broth, indicated that a complete inhibition of > 90% of all dermatophyte species and strains ($= MIC_{90}$) occurred from concentrations of ≥ 0.1 µg/ml.[2] However, *M. canis* strains are inhibited at ≥ 0.01 µg/ml.[3] The MIC values of azole derivatives have to be interpreted within the context of a given laboratory, as they can be affected by technical variables such as the choice and pH of the test medium, the inoculum size and the incubation time. Given the fact that all mycological assays during the whole development of Itrafungol™ were performed in the same laboratory, the MIC_{90} values mentioned above were relevant in further developmental activities.[4] The MIC_{90} values were considered to reflect the minimal concentrations needed in hairs in order to predict mycological cure of *M. canis* infection.

Dose determination

European short-haired cats were artificially infected with *M. canis*.[5] Doses of itraconazole at 0, 1.25, 2.5, 5 and 10 mg/kg were administered orally, once daily for 2 consecutive weeks. Clinical and mycological evaluations were performed before treatment, and at weekly intervals up to 4 weeks after the end of treatment. Cats were considered to be cured whenever clinical lesions were absent, microscopic examination of hair and squame samples were negative, and mycological culture was negative. Concurrently, itraconazole concentrations in hairs (root, middle and tip) were determined by a bioassay method with a detection limit of 0.005 µg/ml. Thus, the combined antifungal activity of itraconazole and its active metabolite was assessed. This study demonstrated that a daily dose of 2.5 mg/kg resulted in an improvement of the condition but no cure, whereas the doses of 5 and 10 mg/kg were very effective, especially from a clinical (lesion score) and microscopic point of

view. In these dosing groups, mycological cultures were negative in at least half of the cats, or contained a largely reduced number of colonies. At 2.5 mg/kg and above, dose-related concentrations of itraconazole were observed in the hairs.[6] Only in the 5 and 10 mg/kg groups did these concentrations remain above the MIC_{90} for *M. canis* 4 weeks after the end of treatment. Based on this observation and the fact that the dose of 5 mg/kg was the lowest effective dose from a clinical and microscopic point of view, this dose was selected as the one on which to focus further development. Fine-tuning of the treatment schedule was considered useful to further increase the rate of mycological cure, as determined by mycological cultures. This approach was supported by the fact that morphological studies of yeast and fungal cultures exposed to itraconazole demonstrated that alterations induced by this compound are both dose- and time-dependent.[7] Target animal safety (TAS) as well as pharmacokinetic data were generated for the final selection of the recommended dose.

Determination of treatment schedule

Dermatophytosis in long-haired breeds of cats usually requires more thorough and prolonged treatment with antifungal agents than that needed for short-haired breeds. Therefore, the dose-schedule determination was performed in field circumstances in long-haired Persian cats naturally infected with *M. canis*. In the first trial, daily oral treatment at 5 mg/kg was prolonged from 2 to either 3 or 4 consecutive weeks.[8] Culture results clearly demonstrated that prolonged treatment improved the rate of mycological cure. However, no significant difference in mycological cure between the 3- and 4-week administration schedule was noted 2 weeks after the end of treatment. Consequently, a 21-day treatment was selected as the optimal treatment schedule.

The second trial[9] evaluated alternative treatment schedules (Fig. 2.3.1). These schedules were designed to account for the specific physicochemical characteristics of itraconazole, its pharmacokinetic properties, and the formulation technology. They were aimed at decreasing the frequency of treatment with itraconazole, without increasing the total amount of product needed beyond the amounts required for 3 weeks of consecutive daily treatments. In this trial, the kinetic profile of itraconazole and its main metabolite, hydroxy-itraconazole, was monitored in plasma by

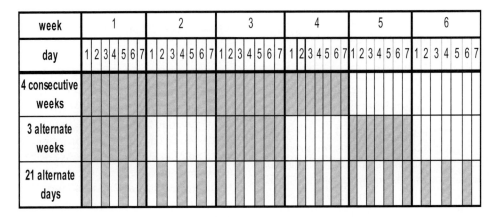

Fig. 2.3.1 Determination of treatment schedule; design of alternative schedules. ■, days with treatment; □, days without treatment.

HPLC.[10] The alternative schedules provided an even longer treatment duration than the 4-week consecutive treatment schedule. The alternative schedules resulted in higher mycological cure rates than the 4-week consecutive daily schedule. The final choice of the recommended treatment schedule was made taking into account the kinetic profile of each of these alternatives in cats.

Preliminary pharmacokinetic data

Based on the results of the dose-determination trial, a pilot pharmacokinetic trial was conducted in healthy short-haired cats with itraconazole at 5 and 10 mg/kg given orally once daily for 14 days.[6] Concentrations of itraconazole and hydroxyl-itraconazole were assayed in plasma by HPLC, and in hairs from different body regions by bioassay and HPLC. The plasma concentrations showed a clear dose-related effect. No concentrations were found in plasma 1 week after the end of treatment at either dose. Itraconazole was detected fairly rapidly in hairs of all body regions. In regions with fewer sebaceous glands or slower hair growth, lower concentrations were measured. The concentrations in hairs were also dose-related and measurable beyond the end of treatment, indicating a residual effect. The results of the HPLC analysis and the bioassay showed a comparable profile. As a consequence, the HPLC assay was validated and used for later development work. Quantification limits of this assay were: 5.0 ng/ml in plasma and 2.0 ng/sample in hairs for itraconazole, and 10 ng/ml in plasma and 5.0 ng/sample

in hairs for hydroxy-itraconazole. For itraconazole, the coefficient of variability (CV) on the percentage of accuracy ranged from 3.5% for concentrations of 600 ng/ml to 4.9% for concentrations of 15 ng/ml in plasma. The CV for concentrations in hairs ranged from 1.5% for concentrations of 750 ng per sample to 4.4% for concentrations of 15 ng per sample. In the case of hydroxy-itraconazole, CV ranged in plasma from 5.4% to 5.1% and in hairs from 4.2% to 3.4% for the same concentrations as evaluated for itraconazole.

The pharmacokinetic profile of Itrafungol™ is mainly determined by the specific physicochemical characteristics of itraconazole and the formulation. Due to its highly lipophilic character, itraconazole accumulates very well in adipose tissue and sebaceous glands.[1] As it is also keratinophilic, it readily incorporates into the stratum corneum and hairs.[1] Distribution to all these tissues is extensive and tissue concentrations are many times higher than plasma concentrations.[1] Itraconazole has a relatively long terminal half-life in plasma in cats. Following repeated administration, this half-life was 36 hours, substantially longer than after a single dose (12.1 hours).[11] Itraconazole is a very insoluble compound. However, by using hydroxypropyl-β-cyclodextrin as an excipient, it can be dissolved in water. Hence, oral absorption is enhanced compared with the pure compound and the capsule formulation that is available in human medicine.

All the above-mentioned factors, together with the fact that one of the authorised treatment schedules of these capsules in human medicine is 'pulse' therapy, supported the design of the two 'alternative' treatment schedules for evaluation: a 21-alternate-day schedule, and a schedule with three 1-week treatment periods, with each week of treatment followed by a week without treatment. After the end of treatment, no significant difference was seen in plasma concentrations of itraconazole and hydroxy-itraconazole in the alternative schedules. Seven days after the end of treatment, the plasma concentrations of hydroxy-itraconazole were below the quantification limit (10 ng/ml). Median concentrations of itraconazole in the alternate-week schedule were still 11.5 ng/ml 7 days after the end of treatment, whereas they were already below the quantification limit in the alternate-day schedule.[9]

The HPLC assay of plasma samples collected in this trial[10] demonstrated that in all treatment schedules the peak plasma levels of itraconazole were much higher than those of hydroxy-itraconazole. Plasma levels of both compounds at days 7, 21 and 35 were higher in the alternate-week schedule than in the alternate-day schedule. Taking into account that the target-tissue levels are correlated to the plasma levels, one could deduct that target-tissue levels were also higher in the alternate-week schedule than in the alternate-day schedule. Although the plasma levels decline during the week without treatment,[11] accumulation of itraconazole in the sebaceous glands and keratin-rich tissues[1] maintains the levels at the target sites and ensures sufficient drug concentrations to effectively treat the pathogen during that period. The plasma washout during the weeks without treatment may be of benefit from a safety point of view, compared to the alternate-day schedule, where plasma levels remained at a steady-state value over the complete treatment period. Hence, the alternate-week schedule was selected.

Pivotal pharmacokinetic trial

The results of the above-mentioned efficacy and pharmacokinetic studies suggested an optimal dose of 5 mg/kg orally once daily, administered according to a 3-alternate week schedule. Taking into account the fact that itraconazole accumulates in the skin structures according to a fixed-tissue versus plasma ratio[1] and that a positive correlation was observed between the bioassay and HPLC analyses, a GLP pharmacokinetic trial in cats was conducted at this dose and treatment schedule, to confirm the plasma and hair levels.[11] In total, 24 European short-haired cats were included, 8 females and 16 males. Blood and hair samples were

taken before, during and up to 2 weeks after the end of the treatment schedule. All samples were analysed for itraconazole and hydroxy-itraconazole by HPLC, with a quantification limit of 5 ng/ml plasma and 2 ng per hair sample for itraconazole, and 10 ng/ml plasma and 5 ng per hair sample for hydroxy-itraconazole. Both compounds were rapidly detectable.

Plasma concentrations of both compounds are given in Table 2.3.1. For days 1 and 7 of treatment, terminal half-life and area-under-the-curve (AUC) have been calculated (Table 2.3.2). Terminal half-life following repeated administration was 36 hours, substantially longer than the single dose estimate (12 hours). The AUC_{0-24h} was approximately threefold higher following repeated dosing than the single dose

Table 2.3.1 Pivotal pharmacokinetic trial: mean ± SD ($n = 12$ or 24) plasma concentrations of itraconazole (R051211) and of hydroxy-itraconazole (R063373) in cats following the proposed therapeutic treatment schedule of 5 mg/kg once daily for 3 alternate weeks of dosing

Treatment period	Day	Time (hours) post dose	R051211	R063373
1	1	0	ND*	ND†
		1	0.386 ± 0.249	ND†‡
		2	0.525 ± 0.336	0.016‡
		4	0.424 ± 0.211	0.025 ± 0.012
		8	0.219 ± 0.110	0.020‡
		12	0.157 ± 0.089	0.020‡
	2	24	0.085 ± 0.046	0.012‡
	7	1	1.05 ± 0.368	0.053 ± 0.020
		2	0.972 ± 0.391	0.051 ± 0.011
		4	0.947 ± 0.297	0.059 ± 0.017
		8	0.616 ± 0.223	0.046 ± 0.013
		12	0.580 ± 0.204	0.049 ± 0.015
	8	24	0.454 ± 0.167	0.045 ± 0.013
2	15	0	0.007‡	ND†‡
		2	0.553 ± 0.170	0.017‡
		4	0.473 ± 0.156	0.023 ± 0.007
	21	0	0.560 ± 0.245	0.051 ± 0.018
		2	1.21 ± 0.391	0.058 ± 0.016
		4	1.11 ± 0.370	0.061 ± 0.016
3	29	0	0.010‡	ND†‡
		2	0.731 ± 0.320	0.021 ± 0.007
		4	0.607 ± 0.224	0.028 ± 0.009
	35	0	0.599 ± 0.285	0.053 ± 0.021
		2	1.26 ± 0.503	0.060 ± 0.020
		4	1.16 ± 0.442	0.065 ± 0.020
	36	24	0.525 ± 0.291	0.044 ± 0.019
–	43		0.012‡	ND†
	49		ND*	ND†

ND, not detected. * ≤ 0.005 µg/ml. † ≤ 0.010 µg/ml. ‡Median.

Table 2.3.2 Pivotal pharmacokinetic trial: pharmacokinetic parameters of itraconazole (R051211) and of hydroxy-itraconazole (R063373) at day 1 and day 7 in cats following the proposed therapeutic treatment schedule of 5 mg/kg once daily for 3 alternate weeks of dosing

Parameter	R051211		R063373	
	Day 1	Day 7	Day 1	Day 7
$t_{1/2}$ [8–24 h] (hours)	12.10	35.8	20.200	97.70
AUC_{0-24h} (µg/h/ml)	5.09	15.4	0.416	1.17
$AUC_{0-\infty}$ (µg/h/ml)	6.57	–	0.766	–

value. Repeated administration for 1 week resulted in peak plasma levels of 1.05 µg/ml at 1 hour after the last dose of the week. Plasma concentrations dropped slowly during the week without treatment, mostly to below or marginally higher than the quantification limit, just before the start of the second and third treatment periods. This indicates almost complete plasma clearance. During the second and third treatment periods, there was a 20–30% increase in the 24-hour plasma concentrations towards the end of

these periods (Fig. 2.3.2). Plasma levels of hydroxy-itraconazole were considerably lower throughout the treatment period.

Median concentration of itraconazole in hair samples was 0.168 µg/g at 24 hours after the first dose (Fig. 2.3.3). After 1 week of treatment, the median concentration increased to 1.17 µg/g. The median concentration was 2.00 µg/g and 2.99 µg/g at the end of the second and third treatment periods, respectively. During the intermittent weeks without treatment, hair concentrations dropped 25–30%, to median values of 0.8–1.5 µg/g. Two weeks after the last dose of the full schedule, median hair concentrations were still 1.5 µg/g.

Although hair concentrations of hydroxy-itraconazole were below the quantification limit during the first and the second treatment periods, they were quantifiable in an increasing number of hairs after the last week of treatment, with concentrations between 0.058 and 0.186 µg/g. Concentrations of both compounds together, as well as itraconazole alone, were well above the MIC_{90} for *M. canis* strains from very shortly after

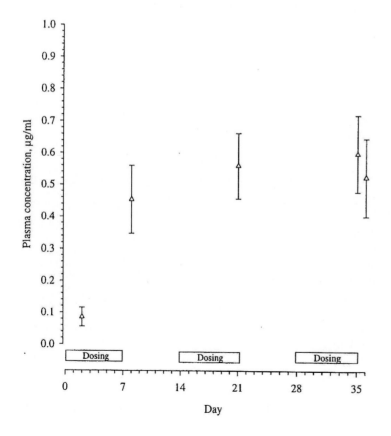

Fig. 2.3.2 Plasma concentrations of itraconazole. Mean trough plasma concentrations and 95% confidence intervals of itraconazole in the cat at 24 hours after dosing with 5 mg itraconazole/kg once daily following the proposed therapeutic treatment schedule of 3 alternate weeks of dosing; at the start of each treatment period, plasma levels were below or marginally higher than the quantification limit (0.005 µg/ml).

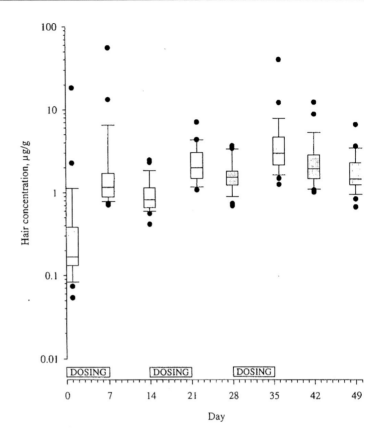

Fig. 2.3.3 Hair concentrations of itraconazole. Box plots of the hair concentrations of itraconazole in cats (*n* = 24) dosed at 5 mg/kg once daily according to the proposed therapeutic schedule of 3 alternate weeks. Boxes indicate the 25th and the 75th percentiles; the horizontal line in the boxes represents the median value; error bars indicate the 5th and the 95th percentiles. Individual values outside the 5th and 95th percentiles are represented by dots.

the first dose and up to at least 2 weeks after the last one.

Target animal safety data

A GLP Target Animal Safety Trial was conducted in adult cats.[12] Doses of 0, 5, 15 and 25 mg/kg once daily of itraconazole were administered orally for 6 consecutive weeks. The cats were evaluated up to 2 weeks after the end of treatment. The following parameters were assessed: mortality, clinical behaviour, body weight, food consumption, haematology, biochemistry, organ weight, gross pathology and histopathology. The target dose of 5 mg/kg appeared to be completely safe on all parameters monitored. A slight increase of bilirubin, an increase of alanine aminotransferase (ALT) and aspartate aminotransferase (AST) was observed at 15 mg/kg, together with a pale colour of the liver. At 25 mg/kg the increases in total bilirubin, ALT and AST were more pronounced. No increase in gamma-glutamyl transferase was observed. Clinical effects such as decreased

appetite, food consumption and body weight were also noted. However, all clinical and biochemical changes were reversible during the recovery period of 2 weeks.

Based on the outcome of this trial, the dose of 5 mg/kg was selected and a trial to evaluate the safety of this dose in kittens was conducted.[13] The kittens were 10 days old at the start of treatment. They were dosed for 4 consecutive weeks and no treatment-related side effects were observed.

Conclusion

This review has outlined the approach used to determine the dose and treatment schedule for itraconazole for *M. canis* infections in cats. Pharmacodynamic data (concentrations of itraconazole in hair) were generated concurrently with pharmacokinetic data.

The pivotal trial in cats was conducted at an itraconazole dose of 5 mg/kg body weight administered once daily for three 1-week periods, with each week of treatment followed by a week without treatment. Itraconazole levels in the hair were high enough to ensure adequate concentrations against *M. canis* for at least 7 weeks after the start of treatment. Consequently, the decision was made to confirm the selection of this dose and schedule in field circumstances. The validity of this approach was demonstrated in the European multinational, multicentre field trial, conducted according to Good Clinical Practice in a later phase of development, and in the recent marketing support trials conducted in the UK and Germany. Both the efficacy of Itrafungol™ against *M. canis* field strains and the safety profile of the product were confirmed.

References

1 Cauwenbergh, G. Skin kinetics of azole antifungal drugs. In: Borgers, M., Hay, R., Rinaldi, M.G., eds. *Current Topics in Medical Mycology*, Vol 4. Springer-Verlag, New York, 1992: 88–136.

2 Van Cutsem, J., Van Gerven, F., Janssen, P.A.J. The *in vitro* and *in vivo* antifungal activity of itraconazole. In: Fromtling, R.A., ed. *Recent Trends in Discovery, Development and Evaluation of Antifungal Agents*. J.R. Prous Science Publishers, Barcelona, 1987: 177–192.

3 Van Cutsem, J., Van Gerven, F., Janssen, P.A.J. Activity of orally, topically, and parenterally administered itraconazole in the treatment of superficial and deep mycoses: animal models. *Reviews of Infectious Diseases*, 1987; **9**: S15–S32.

4 Odds, F.C., Van Cutsem, J. Itraconazole: preclinical data *in vitro* and *in vivo* in cutaneous and other superficial mycoses. In: Rippon, J.W., Fromtling, R.A., eds. *Cutaneous Antifungal Agents*. Marcel Dekker, New York, 1993: 251–261.

5 Van Cutsem, J., Van Gerven, F. *Therapeutic oral treatment with itraconazole oral solution of experimental microsporosis in cats. Efficacy and hair antifungal levels. A dose-titration study*. Preclinical Research Report on R051 211, December 1991.

6 Jacobs, J., Odds, F., Woestenborghs, R., Engelen, M., Vlaminck, K. *Distribution and quantification of itraconazole in hairs after oral administration in cats: a pilot trial*. Preclinical Research Report on R051 211, June 1993.

7 Borgers, M., Van de Ven, M.A. Mode of action of itraconazole: morphological aspects. *Mycoses*, 1989; **32** (Suppl. 1): 53–59.

8 Engelen, M., Jacobs, J., Vlaminck, K. *Efficacy of oral itraconazole against* Microsporum canis *in naturally infected cats: preliminary evaluation of 3 treatment schedules*. Preclinical Research Report on R051 211/ R023979, March 1993.

9 Engelen, M., Jacobs, J., Odds, F., Van Gerven, F., Vlaminck, K. *Efficacy of oral itraconazole against* Microsporum canis *dermatophytosis in naturally infected cats: evaluation and comparison of 4 different treatment schedules under field conditions*. Preclinical Research Report on R051 211, September 1993.

10 Monbaliu, J., Heykants, J., Van Leemput, L., Woestenborghs, R. *Efficacy of oral itraconazole against* Microsporum canis *in naturally infected cats: comparison of 4 different treatment schedules. Addendum I: absorption and plasma levels of itraconazole (R51 211) and of hydroxyitraconazole (R 63 373)*. Preclinical Research Report on R051 211/ R063 373, October 1993.

11 Sterkens, P. *Pharmacokinetics of itraconazole and hydroxy-itraconazole in cats treated orally at 5 mg/kg/day following the proposed therapeutic treatment schedule*. Non-clinical Pharmacokinetics Report on R051211 FK-1855, November 1997.

12 Engelen, M., Vandenberghe, J., Lampo, A., Coussement, W., Van Cauteren, H. *Evaluation of the effects of exaggerated doses in cats (Repeated dosage for 6 weeks followed by a 2-week recovery)*. Non-clinical Laboratory Study, Experiment NO-2422, September 1993.

13 Engelen, M., Biermans, R. *Tolerance of oral itraconazole in kittens: pilot trial*. Preclinical Research Report on R051211, September 1993.

Evaluation of cephalexin intermittent therapy (weekend therapy) in the control of recurrent idiopathic pyoderma in dogs: a randomised, double-blinded, placebo-controlled study

D.N. Carlotti Doct-Vét[1], P. Jasmin Doct-Vét[2], L. Gardey Doct-Vét[2], A. Sanquer[2]

[1] Cabinet de dermatologie vétérinaire, Bordeaux-Mérignac, France (EU)
[2] Virbac SA, Carros, France (EU)

Summary

The purpose of this study was to evaluate the efficacy of cephalexin intermittent therapy 2 days a week (weekend therapy) in the prevention of relapses of recurrent idiopathic superficial or deep pyoderma in dogs. Idiopathic pyoderma was diagnosed in 28 dogs based on: (1) history, including at least two relapses cured in the previous 12 months; (2) clinical signs without underlying skin disease; and (3) appropriate diagnostic tests. In phase 1, dogs were treated with cephalexin (15 mg/kg twice daily) until 2 weeks after cure. In phase 2, the cured dogs were randomly and blindly allocated into two groups: group 1 received cephalexin (15 mg/kg twice daily) and group 2 received a placebo (given twice daily), on Saturdays and Sundays only, for 1 year. Dogs were examined every 3–4 weeks during phase 1 and every 2 months during phase 2, except in cases of relapse justifying an earlier examination. Clinical signs were scored at each examination (11 parameters scored 0–3). No topical antibacterial or anti-inflammatory treatments and no other systemic treatments were permitted. In phase 1, one case was lost to follow-up and four cases were excluded. In phase 2, there were 10 and 13 dogs allocated to group 1 and to group 2, respectively. The two groups were not statistically different according to age, weight, sex, number of previous relapses, clinical signs and duration of treatment in phase 1. The rate of relapse over time was significantly more rapid in group 2. Furthermore, two dogs in group 1 did not relapse. The average time until relapse in group 1 was significantly longer than in group 2. In this study, an increase in resistance to cephalexin was not demonstrated. We conclude that cephalexin weekend therapy can be beneficial in dogs with idiopathic recurrent pyoderma.

Introduction

Cutaneous flora in healthy dogs and dogs with pyoderma

Bacteria that are well adapted to the microenvironment of the superficial stratum corneum and the hair follicles colonise the skin surface of animals and humans. The normal flora contributes to skin immunity.[1]

Staphylococcus intermedius, a gram-positive coagulase-positive bacterium, is the most common infectious agent cultured in canine pyoderma. *Staphylococcus aureus* and *Staphylococcus hyicus* may also be isolated. Some healthy dogs carry these potential pathogens in low numbers on the skin surface, but it is likely that they have transient, rather than resident, status. In contrast, coagulase-positive staphylococci are frequently isolated from mucous membranes (anus, nose, genital tract, mouth, conjunctivae) and are probably residents at these sites. They might be seeded onto the skin and hair by grooming or licking.[2] Studies on isolates of *S. intermedius* from both normal dogs and dogs affected with pyoderma have failed to detect any evidence that different strains of this bacterium vary in pathogenicity.[3]

Predisposing factors for pyoderma in dogs

The stratum corneum is composed of squames (surface keratinocytes). Squames are compact plates of keratin embedded in an emulsion of sweat and lipids from the epidermis and sebum. This mixture forms a physical barrier limiting penetration of micro-organisms and their products.[4] In the dog, the stratum corneum is thinner and more compact than that of any other companion animal species, and there is a paucity of intercellular emulsion. Furthermore, the hair follicle infundibulum of the dog is open, lacking a sebum plug.[5,6]

Primary causes of pyoderma

Canine pyoderma is a common disease. It can be superficial (intertrigo, impetigo, folliculitis) or deep (furunculosis, cellulitis), based on the depth of extension of the infectious process in the hair follicles and skin. In most cases of pyoderma, an underlying cause can be identified and its control is beneficial to prevent relapses.[1,7–9]

Pathogenic staphylococci can easily colonise inflamed and excoriated, seborrhoeic skin. Self-trauma and excoriations due to pruritus further degrade the epidermal defences and allow inoculation of bacteria into the skin and leakage of serum, which is a source of nutrients for bacteria.[10] In addition, there is evidence from an experimental model of canine cutaneous type I hypersensitivity that intradermal injection of a mast cell degranulator, or histamine, renders the overlying epidermis more permeable to bacterial antigens.[11] Thus, allergic skin disease is probably one of the most common causes of secondary canine pyoderma.

Dogs affected with primary seborrhoea have markedly higher cutaneous bacterial counts than normal dogs, with a flora composed primarily of coagulase-positive staphylococci.[12] Any seborrhoeic skin disease, including allergic skin disease and endocrinopathies, is therefore a possible cause of secondary canine pyoderma. It seems likely that the majority of recurrent bacterial skin diseases in the dog result from surface abnormalities, which permit bacterial colonisation, and that immunological predisposing causes are relatively infrequent.[13]

However, deep pyoderma can be due to primary deficiency of specific cellular immunity. The best examples are juvenile-onset, generalised demodicosis and idiopathic deep pyoderma (cellulitis), particularly in German shepherd dogs. Also, acquired deficiency of specific immunity can lead to deep pyoderma. Examples in canine dermatology include endocrine diseases (hypothyroidism, hypercortisolism), leishmaniasis and adult-onset demodicosis.

Treatment for pyoderma in dogs

Cephalosporins are bactericidal antibiotics that act by destroying the bacterial cell wall. They have a broad spectrum of activity, including penicillinase-producing staphylococci. In addition, many cephalosporins can be given orally, particularly first-generation cephalosporins. Cephalexin is the most commonly used cephalosporin in canine dermatology based on its efficacy and safety.[7–9,14,15] Several studies have shown that a dose of 15 mg/kg twice daily[16–18] is effective, although higher doses have been used.[18,19] One study showed that a higher dose (30 mg/kg twice daily) did not give better results than the lower dose in deep pyoderma.[18] Cure, or clear improvement, is usually achieved in 2–8 weeks in superficial pyoderma, and 3–12 weeks in deep pyoderma.[16,17]

Recurrent pyoderma is usually due to an unresolved primary allergic skin disease. Idiopathic recurrent pyoderma (i.e. pyoderma without an underlying cause despite a thorough diagnostic work-up) also exists and is a real therapeutic challenge.[9,14] In such cases, non-specific (e.g. levamisole, cimetidine, interferon-alpha) or bacterial immunotherapy can be attempted.[9,14] Staphage Lysate (Delmont Laboratories, USA), which contains components of S. aureus, has been shown to be effective in the management of idiopathic recurrent pyoderma in a double-blinded, placebo-controlled study.[20] Immunoregulin (Immunovet, USA) contains Propionibacterium acnes and was successfully used along with antibiotics to treat chronic recurrent pyoderma in a randomised, double-blinded, placebo-controlled study.[21] Autogenous vaccines may also be considered, but adequate studies are lacking.[9] Only one study was placebo-controlled and showed efficacy in a limited number of dogs.[22]

Long-term antibacterial therapy may also be considered as an option in the management of recurrent canine pyoderma. Topical therapy is often insufficient on its own, and systemic antibiotics have to be administered for prolonged periods. Intermittent therapy using various empirical protocols has been reported.[9,14] Cephalexin at the dose of 15 mg/kg twice daily given 3 days per week has been shown to be helpful in recurrent pyoderma with underlying allergic dermatitis.[23] Results of a recent open study suggested that intermittent ('pulse') therapy with cephalexin at 25 mg/kg twice daily given on 2 consecutive days each week could be useful in the prevention of idiopathic recurrent deep pyoderma in German shepherd dogs.[24]

Study objective

The purpose of this study was to evaluate the efficacy of cephalexin intermittent therapy 2 days a week (weekend therapy [WET]) in the prevention of relapses of recurrent idiopathic superficial and deep pyoderma in dogs. Our hypothesis was that WET could decrease the frequency of, or prevent, relapses of recurrent idiopathic pyoderma.

Materials and methods

The trial was a prospective, randomised, double-blinded, placebo-controlled study.

Animal inclusion parameters

Informed consent of the owners was mandatory. Dogs of any breed, age or sex, with idiopathic recurrent pyoderma (at least two relapses in the last 12 months) were included. The two most recent relapses had to have been treated successfully by the investigator (D.N.C.).

Diagnosis of pyoderma was based on history, compatible clinical signs, and cytological examination (Diff Quik® stain) of exudate from an intact pustule, from beneath a crust, or from a fistula showing coccoid bacteria and phagocytosis.[8,9] Cultures were taken from lesions and isolation of Staphylococcus susceptible to cephalexin was required. Susceptibility to first-generation cephalosporins, including cephalexin, was evaluated with ATB VET (BioMérieux SA, Lyon, France), a susceptibility test for bacteria of animal origin using cephalothin at a concentration of 8 mg/L. However, two exceptions were permitted to this rule: (1) failure to culture Staphylococcus but with clear evidence of

cocci on cytology (two cases); and (2) isolation of a Staphylococcus resistant to cephalexin in a pyoderma responding rapidly and completely to cephalexin therapy (one case).

Animal exclusion parameters

Dogs allergic to penicillins or cephalosporins were excluded from the study. Dogs with secondary pyoderma were excluded, particularly dogs where underlying causes could be demonstrated by history, clinical signs and diagnostic tests, i.e. allergic skin disease (atopic dermatitis, flea allergy dermatitis, adverse food reactions, food allergy), scabies, demodicosis, Malassezia dermatitis, bacterial overgrowth,[25] dermatophytosis, endocrinopathies, leishmaniasis, ehrlichiosis and autoimmune dermatoses. Skin scrapings and surface (tape strip) cytological examination were performed systematically in all dogs and had to be negative. Routine blood tests (BUN, creatinine, glucose, cholesterol, alkaline phosphatase), serology for leishmaniasis and ehrlichiosis, and antinuclear antibody test were performed on all dogs with cellulitis, and were required to be within normal limits or negative.

Dogs requiring immunosuppressive, anti-inflammatory, or other antimicrobial treatments for any reason, and dogs previously treated with the following therapies, were excluded from the study: antibiotics within the previous 10 days; antibiotic intermittent therapy at any time; oral corticosteroids within the past 3 weeks or long-acting corticosteroids within the past 6 weeks; and other immune-modulating drugs within the previous 2 weeks.

Dogs which developed adverse reactions to the treatment, clinical signs of another disease other than pyoderma during treatment, or any deviation from the protocol were excluded. Dogs not responding to cephalexin after 2 months for superficial pyoderma or after 4 months for deep pyoderma were also excluded.

Protocol design and treatments

Study articles

The products used in this study were tablets containing 300 mg of cephalexin (Rilexine 300®, Virbac) and placebo tablets containing only Rilexine 300® excipients.

Dosage and administration

Phase 1 of the study: treatment of pyoderma

A case number and random allocation to the treatment or control group (for phase 2) were assigned for each dog at the time of inclusion in the study. Eleven clinical parameters associated with pyoderma were scored at each examination: erythema, papules, pustules, epidermal collarettes, furuncles, ulcers, crusts, fistulae, pruritus, pain, and extent of the body surface affected, utilising an arbitrary scale of 0–3 (0 = none, 1 = mild, 2 = moderate, 3 = severe for lesions, pruritus and pain; and 0 = < 10%, 1 = 10–25%, 2 = 25–50%, 3 = > 50% for extent of body surface affected).

All dogs were treated with cephalexin administered at 15 mg/kg twice daily until 2 weeks after cure, for a minimum of 4 weeks and a maximum of 2 and 4 months for superficial and deep pyoderma, respectively. The dose was rounded as closely as possible to the recommended dose of 15 mg/kg twice daily by dividing the tablets if necessary. The owners administered the tablets. The dogs were scored at the initiation of treatment, every 3–4 weeks during this treatment period, and at the end of treatment. A clinical cure was established when all the following specific lesions of pyoderma completely resolved (i.e. zero score): papules, pustules, furuncles, fistulae, epidermal collarettes and ulcers.

Phase 2 of the study: intermittent therapy (weekend therapy [WET])

When clinical cure of the pyoderma had been documented by the investigator, based on the clinical scoring forms at the end of treatment, the dogs were randomly assigned to one of two treatment groups for the next year of treatment: group 1 dogs received cephalexin (15 mg/kg twice daily on Saturdays and Sundays) and group 2 dogs received the placebo (twice daily on Saturdays and Sundays). The owners administered the tablets as in phase 1.

The dogs were kept under observation for up to 1 year after the start of treatment in phase 2. Re-examination was performed every 2 months during this period, except in cases of relapse justifying an earlier examination. At each consultation, a general and thorough dermatological examination of the animal was performed with clinical scoring as used in phase 1. In phase 2, a relapse of pyoderma was defined as the occurrence of any of the specific lesions of pyoderma regardless of the severity and extent. Relapse was con-

sidered a treatment failure and the dog was withdrawn from the study. A new swab for bacteriological culture and susceptibility testing was taken.

Associated treatments

Although not specifically mentioned in the inclusion or exclusion criteria for patient selection, the following treatments were authorised during both phases of the study: flea control, hair coat clipping and the use of a cleansing anti-seborrhoeic shampoo (Sebocalm®, Virbac, Carros, France).

Statistical analysis

The two groups were compared using Fisher's exact test for sex and clinical signs and the Wilcoxon rank-sum test for age, weight, number of relapses before inclusion and duration of treatment in phase 1. The number of dogs remaining free of relapse (rate of non-relapse over time) was compared between the two groups using a survival analysis with the log-rank test. The percentage of dogs that relapsed in the two groups was compared every month using Fisher's exact test. No adjustment for multiple comparisons was performed due to the high number of comparisons and the low number of groups. The average time before relapse was compared between the two groups using the Wilcoxon rank-sum test.

Results

Twenty-eight dogs were enrolled in phase 1 of the study. One case was lost to follow-up in phase 1. This dog would have been included in group 1 in phase 2. Four cases were excluded in phase 1: two because of treatment failure (one of these two cases had isolation of *Staphylococcus haemolyticus* with intermediate susceptibility to cephalexin); and two because of discontinuation of treatment after the return of unfavourable culture results (*Pseudomonas fluorescens* resistant to cephalexin and *S. aureus* with intermediate susceptibility to cephalexin) (Fig. 2.4.1). Three excluded cases would have entered group 1 and one would have entered group 2. The 23 remaining dogs were included in phase 2 of the study as they were affected with idiopathic recurrent pyoderma according to the inclusion criteria. No side effects were experienced by the dogs in either group.

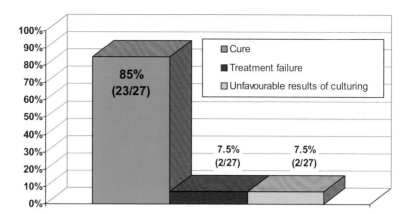

Fig. 2.4.1 Rate of cure in the 27 dogs with pyoderma included in phase 1 (treatment with cephalexin twice daily until 2 weeks after resolution).

The mean number of relapses in these 23 dogs had been 3.7 ± 1.3 in the previous year. Bacterial cultures showed various species of staphylococci at the time of inclusion, i.e. at the beginning of phase 1. Eight were considered non-pathogenic: *Staphylococcus xylosus* (*n* = 1), *S. simulans* (*n* = 2) and *S. hominis* (*n* = 5). Thirteen pathogens were isolated: *S. hyicus* (*n* = 2), *S. aureus* (*n* = 3), *S. intermedius* (*n* = 6) and *S. chromogenes* (*n* = 2).[1] *Staphylococcus* was not cultured in two cases for unknown reasons. Only one of the *S. aureus* isolates was resistant *in vitro* to cephalexin, but the dog was kept in the study because of a rapid (25 days) complete cure in phase 1. The rate of cure in phase 1 was 85% (23/27) (Fig. 2.4.1).

Among the 23 cases included in phase 2, 10 dogs were allocated to group 1 and 13 to group 2. There were 12 cases of folliculitis (52%), 6 of furunculosis (26%), 2 of furunculosis and folliculitis (9%), 1 of cellulitis (4%) and 2 of cellulitis, furunculosis and folliculitis (9%). There was no difference between the two groups according to the type of pyoderma (*p* = 0.7986) (Table 2.4.1) or sex (*p* = 0.5800) (Table 2.4.2). There were also no differences in age (*p* = 0.2491), weight (*p* = 0.1863),

number of relapses in the previous year (*p* = 0.2407) and duration of phase 1 (*p* = 0.3460) (Table 2.4.3).

Various breeds were represented: boxers (*n* = 3), German shepherd dogs (3), bull terriers (3), pointers (2), Yorkshire terriers (2), and 1 each of Catalan shepherd, golden retriever, Dogue de Bordeaux, Chinese Shar Pei, spitz, great Dane, Draahtar, bull mastiff, American cocker spaniel and West Highland white terrier.

There was a significant difference between the two groups in the rate of relapse during phase 2, which was more rapid in the dogs receiving placebo (*p* = 0.0102) (Fig. 2.4.2). The cumulative percentage of relapsing dogs was significantly higher in group 2 than group 1 from the fourth to the ninth month (*p* < 0.05) (Fig. 2.4.3).

The average time until relapse in group 1 (6.6 months) compared to group 2 (2.5 months) was significantly different (*p* = 0.0199) (Fig. 2.4.4). Two dogs in group 1 with three relapses of folliculitis in the previous year relapsed only at 10 and 11 months. Two other dogs in group 1, one with folliculitis and one with furunculosis, did not relapse during the year of follow-up, whereas they had relapsed three times and six times, respectively, during the previous year.

Table 2.4.1 Types of pyoderma in dogs in the study (group 1 vs group 2)

Type of pyoderma	Group 1 (cephalexin)	Group 2 (placebo)	Total
Folliculitis	6	6	12
Furunculosis	3 (2 with concurrent folliculitis)	5	8
Cellulitis	1	2 (both with concurrent folliculitis and furunculosis)	3
Total	10	13	23

Table 2.4.2 Sex of dogs in the study (group 1 vs group 2)

Sex	Group 1 (cephalexin)	Group 2 (placebo)	Total
Male	5	8	13
Female	5	5	10
Total	10	13	23

Parameter	Group 1 (cephalexin, $n = 10$)	Group 2 (placebo, $n = 13$)	Mean ± standard deviation ($n = 23$)
Average age (years)	6.1	4.6	5.3 ± 2.9
Average weight (kg)	32.9	25.0	28.6 ± 15.2
Average number of relapses in the previous year	4.1	3.4	3.7 ± 1.3
Average number of days in phase 1	65.0	40.8	51.3 ± 37.2

Table 2.4.3 Parameters of dogs in the study (group 1 vs group 2)

No statistical analysis was conducted to evaluate any possible correlation between the type and extent of lesion scoring and the efficacy of weekend treatment.

At the time of relapse, 10 staphylococci (*S. intermedius*, 3; *S. hyicus*, 1; *S. aureus*, 3; *S. simulans*, 2; *S. chromogenes*, 1), 1 beta-haemolytic *Streptococcus*, 1 *Citrobacter freundii* and 1 *Acinetobacter pseudomonas* were isolated in 13 dogs from the two groups (Table 2.4.4). Two cultures remained sterile. Six cultures were not obtained due to oversight, including three that were not performed because of continuation of WET in dogs with only a moderate relapse. Two cases did not relapse and thus were not sampled. Amongst the 13 cultured species, 5 were resistant to cephalexin, 3 from group 1 and 2 from group 2.

Discussion

Efficacy of weekend therapy

Cephalexin is widely used in veterinary dermatology to treat canine pyoderma.[1,7–9,14,15] The dose of 15 mg/kg twice daily has been demonstrated to be effective.[16–18] Among several options for treating idiopathic recurrent pyoderma, intermittent therapy has been recommended as a preventive method[9,14] and this form of therapy has been shown to be helpful in recurrent pyoderma with underlying allergic dermatitis at 15 mg/kg twice daily given on 3 days a week[23] and in the prevention of idiopathic recurrent deep pyoderma in German shepherd dogs at 25 mg/kg given on 2 days a week.[24] Thus, a controlled study of the efficacy of weekend treatment with cephalexin at the dose of 15 mg/kg twice daily given 2 days a week for the prevention of relapses of recurrent idiopathic canine pyoderma was justified.

Recruitment of dogs with idiopathic pyoderma is difficult. During this study, which lasted 3 years, we recruited only 28 dogs. In addition, one was lost to follow-up and four could not be included in phase 2 (Fig. 2.4.1). The rate of cure in phase 1 (85%) was comparable to previous data.[16–19]

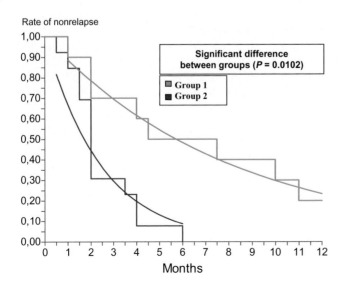

Fig. 2.4.2 Rate of non-relapse over time in the 23 dogs included in phase 2 (weekend treatment). Group 1, cephalexin; group 2, placebo.

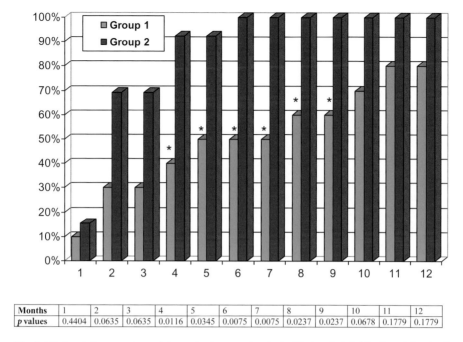

Months	1	2	3	4	5	6	7	8	9	10	11	12
p values	0.4404	0.0635	0.0635	0.0116	0.0345	0.0075	0.0075	0.0237	0.0237	0.0678	0.1779	0.1779

Fig. 2.4.3 Cumulative percentage of dogs relapsing over time in the 23 dogs included in phase 2 (weekend treatment). Group 1, cephalexin; group 2, placebo. *Significantly higher rate of relapse in group 2 compared to group 1.

At the time of inclusion in phase 2, there was no significant difference between the two groups (group 1 = cephalexin and group 2 = placebo) as regards age, weight, sex, type of pyoderma, average number of relapses in the previous year, and average number of days of treatment in phase 1. Consequently, the two groups were comparable and a statistical analysis on the efficacy of WET was valid.

As quickly as 2 months after the beginning of phase 2, 69% (9/13) of dogs relapsed in group 2 whereas only 30% (3/10) of dogs relapsed in group 1. At 4 months, 92% (12/13) of dogs had relapsed in group 2 whereas only 50% (5/10) relapsed in group 1 (Fig. 2.4.3). All dogs (13/13) relapsed before 6 months in group 2 whereas only 50% (5/10) of dogs had relapsed in group 1. The difference in rate of non-relapse over time between the two groups was

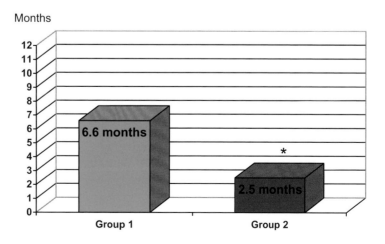

Fig. 2.4.4 Average time until relapse in the 23 dogs included in phase 2 (weekend treatment). Group 1, cephalexin; group 2, placebo. *Significantly more rapid time to relapse in group 2 compared to group 1.

Group	Case no.	Results at inclusion		Results at relapse	
		Isolate	Cephalexin susceptibility	Isolate	Cephalexin susceptibility
1	2	S. simulans	S	ND (maintenance of WET)	
	3	S. hominis	S	S. intermedius	S
	5	S. hominis	S	No relapse	
	7	Sterile culture		C. freundii	R
	9	S. hyicus	S	No relapse	
	11	S. aureus	R	ND (oversight)	
	16	Sterile culture		A. pseudomonas	S
	20	S. chromogenes	S	S. chromogenes	R
	22	S. simulans	S	S. aureus	R
	25	S. intermedius	S	S. simulans	S
2	1	S. xylosus	S	S. aureus	S
	4	S. hominis	S	S. intermedius	S
	6	S. hominis	S	Sterile culture	
	8	S. aureus	S	S. hyicus	S
	10	S. hominis	S	ND (oversight)	
	12	S. hyicus	S	β-haemolytic Streptococcus G	R
	13	S. aureus	S	S. intermedius	S
	15	S. intermedius	S	S. aureus	S
	18	S. intermedius	S	ND (maintenance of WET)	
	19	S. chromogenes	S	ND (maintenance of WET)	
	21	S. intermedius	S	Sterile culture	
	23	S. intermedius	S	ND (oversight)	
	26	S. intermedius	S	S. simulans	R

Table 2.4.4 Results of bacterial culture and susceptibility testing for cephalexin in dogs in the study at inclusion and at the end of phase 2

Group 1, cephalexin; group 2, placebo; S, susceptible to cephalexin; R, resistant to cephalexin; ND, not done; WET, weekend treatment.

statistically significant ($p = 0.0102$) (Fig. 2.4.2). Furthermore, two dogs did not relapse in group 1.

The percentage of relapsing dogs (Fig. 2.4.3) (significantly higher from the fourth to the ninth month, $p < 0.05$) would not have been significant if adjustment for multiple comparisons had been made. However, this was not done in this study because of the high number of comparisons and the existence of only two groups.

The average time until relapse was 2.5 months in group 2 and 6.6 months in group 1. Thus, the WET-treated dogs with idiopathic pyoderma remained free of relapse for a significantly longer period (2.5 times) than placebo-treated dogs.

The fact that all dogs in group 2 relapsed within 6 months following cure at the end of phase 1 confirms the recurrent nature of idiopathic pyoderma, with 70% and 90% of relapses at 2 and 4 months, respectively, and an average time until relapse of 2.5 months.

Bacteriological aspects

Among the 23 cases at time of inclusion, 2 had sterile cultures for unknown reasons. Twenty-one yielded a *Staphylococcus*, with 7 different species (3 considered as non-pathogenic and 4 as pathogenic[1]), whereas *S. intermedius* is the most common pathogen isolated from canine pyoderma.[1,26] The significance of this is unknown. It could be due to the selection of certain strains after multiple antibiotic treatments. In case of immunodeficiency leading to relapsing pyoderma, the pathogenicity of certain strains could be increased. Also, several strains of staphylococci can be isolated at the same time from a pyoderma lesion. Susceptibility can be tested on one strain only, possibly leading to misinterpretation. This might have happened at inclusion in one dog in group 1 where a *S. aureus* resistant to cephalexin was isolated, but the pyoderma resolved after 25 days of cephalexin treatment. This dog relapsed after 1 month of weekend treatment. Unfortunately sampling was not repeated at relapse due to an oversight.

Results of a previous study showed a discrepancy between *in vitro* susceptibility to cephalexin and *in vivo* clinical response to the antibiotic.[18] This could be due to the fact that serum, and not skin, concentrations are interpreted in relation to *in vitro* susceptibility of the organism. Also *in vitro* testing does not account for the immunological status of the patient or concurrent medical conditions.

Pulsed or intermittent antibiotic therapy could cause more resistance than continuous antibiotic administration, but this study could neither confirm nor exclude this phenomenon for cephalexin. The three dogs from group 1 from whom bacteria resistant to cephalexin were cultured at the time of relapse took only 1, 2 and 4 months to redevelop the pyoderma. More cases would be needed for a conclusion on this matter, with sampling done systematically at time of relapse, even if WET were to be continued.

Conclusions

This study confirmed that relapses are frequent in dogs with idiopathic pyoderma. It also showed that after resolution of clinical lesions with cephalexin (15 mg/kg twice daily), the rate of relapse of idiopathic pyoderma over time can be decreased, and time until relapse can be increased with WET with cephalexin (2 days a week at the same dosage), which was well tolerated. We conclude that WET with cephalexin can decrease the need for antibiotics in dogs with idiopathic recurrent pyoderma, which is beneficial both medically and economically.

Acknowledgement

The authors are grateful to Professor David Lloyd for his suggestions and corrections of the manuscript.

Funding

This study was funded by Virbac SA, France (EU).

References

1 Lloyd, D.H. Therapy for canine pyoderma. In: Kirk, R.W., Bonagura, J.D., eds. *Current Veterinary Therapy XI*. W.B. Saunders, Philadelphia, 1992: 539–544.

2 Saijonmaa-Koulumies, L.E., Lloyd, D.H. Colonization of the canine skin with bacteria. *Veterinary Dermatology*, 1996; **7**: 153–162.

3 Allaker, R.P., Lamport, A.I., Lloyd, D.H., Noble, W.C. Production of virulence factors by *Staphylococcus intermedius* isolated from cases of canine pyoderma and healthy carriers. *Microbial Ecology in Health and Disease*, 1991; **4**: 169–173.

4 Mason, I.S., Mason, K.V., Lloyd, D.H. A review of the biology of canine skin with respect to the commensals *Staphylococcus intermedius*, *Demodex canis* and *Malassezia pachydermatis*. *Veterinary Dermatology*, 1996; **7**: 119–132.

5 Lloyd, D.H., Garthwaite, G. Epidermal structure and surface topography of canine skin. *Research in Veterinary Science*, 1982; **33**: 99–104.

6 Mason, I.S., Lloyd, D.H. Scanning electron microscopical studies of the living epidermis and stratum corneum of dogs. In: Ihrke, P.J., Mason, I.S., White, S.D., eds. *Advances in Veterinary Dermatology*, Vol. 2. Pergamon Press, Oxford, 1993: 131–139.

7 Ihrke, P.J. Antibacterial therapy in dermatology. In: Kirk, R.W., ed. *Current Veterinary Therapy IX*. W.B. Saunders, Philadelphia, 1986: 566–571.

8 Fourrier, P., Carlotti, D.N., Magnol, J.-P. Les pyodermites du chien. *Pratique Médicale et Chirurgicale de l'Animal de Compagnie*, 1986; **23**: 462–535.

9 Scott, D.W., Miller, W.H., Griffin, C.E. *Muller and Kirk's Small Animal Dermatology*, 6th edn. W.B. Saunders, Philadelphia, 2001: 274–335.

10 Mason, I.S., Lloyd, D.H. The role of allergy in the development of canine pyoderma. *Journal of Small Animal Practice*, 1989; **30**: 216–218.

11 Mason, I.S., Lloyd, D.H. Factors influencing the penetration of bacterial antigens through canine skin. In: Von Tscharner, C., Halliwell, R.E.W., eds. *Advances in Veterinary Dermatology*, Vol. 1. Baillière Tindall, London, 1990: 370–374.

12 Ihrke, P.J., Schwartzman, R.M., McGinley, K.M., Horwitz, L.N., Marples, R.R. Microbiology of normal and seborrheic canine skin. *American Journal of Veterinary Research*, 1978; **39**: 1487–1489.

13 Halliwell, R.E.W., Gorman, N.T. *Veterinary Clinical Immunology*. W.B. Saunders, Philadelphia, 1989.

14 Kwochka, K.W. Recurrent pyoderma. In: Griffin, C.E., Kwochka, K.W., MacDonald, J.M., eds. *Current Veterinary Dermatology. The Science and Art of Therapy*. Mosby Year Book, St Louis, 1993: 3–21.

15 Carlotti, D.N. New trends in systemic antibiotic therapy of bacterial skin disease in dogs. *Supplement to the Compendium of Continuing Education for the Practicing Veterinarian*, 1996; **18**: 40–47.

16 Guaguère, E., Marc, J.-P. Utilisation de la céfalexine dans la traitement des pyodermites. *Pratique Médicale et Chirurgicale de l'Animal de Compagnie*, 1989; **24**: 124–129.

17 Guaguère, E., Picard, G. Essai clinique: Utilisation de la céfalexine et du lactate d'éthyle dans le traitement des pyodermites canines. *Pratique Médicale et Chirurgicale de l'Animal de Compagnie*, 1990; **25**: 547–551.

18 Guaguère, E., Salomon, C., Maynard, L. Utilisation de la céfalexine dans le traitement des pyodermites canines: comparaison de l'efficacité de différentes posologies. *Pratique Médicale et Chirurgicale de l'Animal de Compagnie*, 1998; **33**: 237–246.

19 Frank, L., Kunkle, G.A. Comparison of the efficacy of cefadroxil and proprietary cephalexin in the treatment of pyoderma in dogs. *Journal of the American Veterinary Medical Association*, 1993; **203**: 530–533.

20 DeBoer, D.J., Moriello, K.A., Thomas, C.B., Schultz, K.T. Evaluation of a commercial staphylococcal bacterin for management of idiopathic recurrent superficial pyoderma in dogs. *American Journal of Veterinary Research*, 1990; **51**: 636–639.

21 Becker, A.M., Janik, T.A., Smith, E.K., Sousa, C.A., Peters, B.A. *Propionibacterium acnes* immunotherapy in chronic recurrent canine pyoderma. An adjunct to antibiotic therapy. *Journal of Veterinary Internal Medicine*, 1989; **3**: 26–30.

22 Curtis, C.F., Lamport, A.I., Lloyd, D.H. Blinded, controlled study to investigate the efficacy of a staphylococcal autogenous bacterin for the control of canine idiopathic recurrent pyoderma (abstract). *Proceedings of the 16th Annual Meeting of the European*

Society of Veterinary Dermatology/European College of Veterinary Dermatology, Helsinki, Finland, 1999: 148.

23 Guaguère, E., Rème, C.A., Mondon, A., Salomon, C. Use of cephalexin intermittent therapy to prevent recurrent pyoderma in dogs with underlying allergic dermatitis: a double-blind placebo-controlled trial (abstract). In: *Proceedings of the 19th Annual Meeting of the European Society of Veterinary Dermatology/ European College of Veterinary Dermatology*, Tenerife, Spain, 2003: 144.

24 Bell, A. Prophylaxis of German shepherd recurrent furunculosis (German shepherd dog pyoderma) using cephalexin pulse therapy. *Australian Veterinary Practitioner*, 1995; **25**: 30–36.

25 Pin, D., Carlotti, D.N., Jasmin, P., DeBoer, D., Prélaud, P. A prospective study of the bacterial overgrowth syndrome (BOGs) in the dog. *Veterinary Record*, 2005 (in press).

26 Noble, W.C., Kent, L.E. Antibiotic resistance in *Staphylococcus intermedius* isolated from cases of pyoderma in the dog. *Veterinary Dermatology*, 1992; **3**: 71–74.

Comparison of bacterial organisms from otic exudate and ear tissue from the middle ear of untreated and enrofloxacin-treated dogs with end-stage otitis

L.K. Cole DVM, MS[1], K.W. Kwochka DVM[2], A. Hillier BVSc[1], J.J. Kowalski DVM, PhD[1], D.D. Smeak DVM[1], N.T. Kelbick PhD[3]

[1] Department of Veterinary Clinical Sciences, College of Veterinary Medicine, The Ohio State University, Columbus, Ohio, USA
[2] DVM Pharmaceuticals, Inc., Miami, Florida, USA
[3] Center for Biostatistics, The Ohio State University, Columbus, Ohio, USA

Summary

The objective of this study was to compare the organisms in the exudate and tissue from the middle ear of dogs with chronic end-stage otitis. In addition, the effect of concurrent antibiotic administration (enrofloxacin) on the organisms identified in the exudate and tissue was assessed. Samples for bacterial culture, one from tissue and one from exudate, were obtained from the middle ear of 23 dogs undergoing a unilateral total ear canal ablation and lateral bulla osteotomy. Nineteen dogs were randomised to the treatment group and received two intravenous (IV) doses of enrofloxacin prior to sampling (four received 5 mg/kg, five received 10 mg/kg, five received 15 mg/kg and five received 20 mg/ kg), while four (control group) did not receive any antibiotic. Bacterial organisms were identified biochemically and morphologically. The data were analysed using Fisher's exact test to compare differences in organisms identified among treatment groups. In all, 138 organisms were identified; 108 organisms (78%), 54 from tissue and 54 from exudate, matched biochemically and morphologically. Thirty organisms (22%) were unmatched, 17 from tissue and 13 from exudate. When treatment groups were combined, discrepancies between the organisms in the tissue and exudate were identified in 15 of 19 (79%) dogs that received enrofloxacin compared with only 1 of 4 dogs in the control group ($p = 0.067$), suggesting that it would be best to obtain cultures without concurrent antibiotic administration. In addition, samples for culture should be obtained from both tissue and exudate to identify all organisms. If only one sample is to be procured, a tissue sample would be preferred.

Introduction

The most common bacterial organisms isolated from the middle ear in dogs with otitis media are *Staphylococcus* spp. and *Pseudomonas* spp.[1–4] However, other bacterial organisms have also been identified including beta-haemolytic streptococcus, *Corynebacterium* spp., *Proteus* spp., *Enterococcus* spp. and *Escherichia coli*.[1,2] Therefore, in order to identify all the organisms isolated from the middle ear and choose an appropriate antibiotic for treatment, a bacterial culture and susceptibility test (C/S) should be performed.[5]

In the medical management of dogs with otitis media, culture samples of otic exudate are routinely obtained from the middle ear after flushing the exter-nal ear canal and evaluating the tympanic membrane. If the tympanic membrane is ruptured, samples for culture from the middle ear are obtained using a spinal needle or Tom cat catheter, saline flush and aspiration,[2] or a sterile swab.[1] If the tympanic membrane is intact, but abnormal, samples may be obtained as stated previously, after a myringotomy has been performed.[1,2] During a surgical procedure for the treatment of otitis media, such as a total ear canal ablation and lateral bulla osteotomy or ventral bulla osteotomy, samples for bacterial culture of otic exudate may be obtained via a swab sample[2] or the culture sample may be obtained from surgically excised tissue[4,6] from the middle ear. A surgical approach allows sample collection for culture from the exudates or tissue, or both, from the middle ear. To the authors' knowledge, there have been no studies performed to determine which technique (sampling the exudate or the tissue from the middle ear for bacterial culture) is the best method for identifying pathogenic organisms. If sampling is performed from the exudate or tissue only, all pathogenic organisms may not be identified, which could lead to treatment failure.

Prophylactic intravenous antibiotics are routinely administered prior to and during surgical procedures for otitis media.[7] In addition, dogs requiring medical management for otitis media may be on oral antibiotics when samples are obtained from the middle ear cavity for bacterial C/S. To the authors' knowledge, the effect of current antibiotic administration on the isolation of organisms from samples collected from the middle ear has not been reported.

The objective of this study was to compare the organisms in the exudate and tissue obtained from the middle ear of dogs with chronic end-stage otitis. Additionally, the effect of concurrent antibiotic (enrofloxacin) administration on the organisms identified from the exudate and tissue was assessed. It was hypothesised that the organisms identified from the exudate and tissue would match biochemically and morphologically regardless of antibiotic administration.

Materials and methods

Dogs

Thirty dogs with chronic end-stage otitis externa undergoing an elective unilateral total ear canal ablation and lateral bulla osteotomy (TECA-LBO) at The Ohio State University Veterinary Teaching Hospital were enrolled in a study measuring enrofloxacin concentrations in ear tissue. Chronic end-stage otitis externa was defined as ear disease that was non-responsive to medical management due to pathologic changes in the external ear canal (such as hyperplasia, stenosis, or calcification), or resistant bacterial infections. The hospital board at The Ohio State University reviewed and approved the study protocol. All clients signed a consent form prior to enrolment of their dog in the study. All the dogs had received topical and systemic medications before entering the study; however, none had any topical or systemic antimicrobial agent administered by the owner on the day of entry into the study. The

dogs were hospitalised overnight and the surgery was performed the following day.

The 30 dogs were randomised to one of four enrofloxacin-treatment groups (5 mg/kg, 10 mg/kg, 15 mg/kg or 20 mg/kg) or the control group. Each dog in the treatment group received two intravenous doses of enrofloxacin while the control group did not receive any antibiotic. For the dogs in the treatment group, the first dose of enrofloxacin was administered on day 1. No sooner than 20 hours later, the second dose of enrofloxacin was administered, and was timed to be administered 3 hours prior to surgical removal of the ear tissue, to coincide with the time of peak tissue concentration of enrofloxacin.[8] Twenty-three of the 30 dogs were selected for this study, since they all had bacterial cultures performed from both the middle ear tissue and middle ear exudate. Nineteen dogs were in the enrofloxacin-treatment group (four received 5 mg/kg, five received 10 mg/kg, five received 15 mg/kg and five received 20 mg/kg) and four dogs were in the control group.

Cultures of middle ear tissue and exudate

The TECA-LBO was performed as described previously.[7] After the ventral and lateral aspect of the tympanic bulla was removed with rongeurs, all epithelium and debris were curetted from the lumen.[7] The epithelium and debris were placed into a sterile bowl. One piece of the middle ear tissue epithelium was placed into a sterile vial for bacterial culture. A sterile swab was then inserted into the bulla for bacterial culture.

The sterile vial with the middle ear tissue and sterile swab were transported within 1 hour to the microbiology laboratory. The tissue was macerated and the tissue and swab samples were plated separately on blood agar and MacConkey agar and incubated at 35°C for 18–24 hours. Organisms were identified morphologically and by routine biochemical testing. For each bacterial organism, antimicrobial susceptibilities were performed using the antimicrobial disk diffusion test.[9] As different antibiotic panels were utilised for the organisms from the middle ear tissue and the organisms from the middle ear exudate, comparisons of antibiotic susceptibilities were not possible.

The organisms identified morphologically and by biochemical testing from the exudate and tissue from each middle ear were compared. If an organism from the middle ear exudate shared the same morphological and biochemical characteristics as an organism from the middle ear tissue, they were classified as similar organisms. For example, if two organisms were isolated from the same ear, one from the middle ear exudate and one from the middle ear tissue, and both were morphologically and biochemically classified as *Staphylococcus intermedius*, then these two organisms would be classified as similar organisms.

Statistical analysis

Differences in types of organisms detected between the middle ear exudate and middle ear tissue were evaluated by comparing the proportions of unmatched organisms between treatment and control groups using the Fisher's exact test. During the analysis, it was noted that a majority of the data were obtained from American cocker spaniels ($n = 12, 52\%$). The Wilcoxon rank sum test was used to compare differences in the age of onset of the otitis, age at presentation for surgery, and the length of time from the onset of the otitis until surgery between the American cocker spaniels and the other dogs. All comparisons were analysed using StatXact 6 Statistical Software (StatXact 6 for Windows, CYTEL Software Corp., 2003, Cambridge, MA, USA).

Results

Demographic data

Breeds represented included American cocker spaniel ($n = 12$), Labrador retriever (2), Basset hound (2) and one each of golden retriever, English mastiff, pug, American bulldog, English bulldog and English toy spaniel. There was one mixed-breed dog. There were 14 females (2 intact) and 9 males (4 intact). There was a significant difference between the age of onset of the otitis ($p = 0.0014$) and the age at presentation for surgery ($p = 0.0061$) between the American cocker spaniels (age of onset of 7 years old, age at presentation for surgery of 9.9 years old) and the other dogs (age of onset 3 years old, age at presentation for surgery 6.8 years). There was no significant difference between the length of time from the onset of the otitis until surgery between the two groups ($p = 0.3668$).

Administration of enrofloxacin

The dogs in the treatment group received their first dose of enrofloxacin on the day they entered the study (day 1). No sooner than 20 hours later, the second dose of enrofloxacin was administered, and was timed to be administered 3 hours prior to surgical removal of the ear tissue. The mean ($\pm$ standard deviation) of the timing of the second dose of enrofloxacin was 22 hours, 45 minutes ($\pm$ 1 hour, 53 minutes), while the range was 20 hours, 30 minutes to 26 hours, 25 minutes.

Culture results

In all, 138 organisms were identified, 71 (51.4%) from the middle ear tissue and 67 (48.6%) from the middle ear exudate. Of these, 108 organisms (78.3%), 54 from the middle ear tissue and 54 from the middle ear exudate, matched biochemically and morphologically. The 108 matched bacterial organisms isolated included *Staphylococcus intermedius* ($n = 30, 27.8\%$), *Enterococcus* spp. (22, 20.4%), *Pseudomonas aeruginosa* (14, 13%), *Corynebacterium* spp. (14, 13%), beta-haemolytic streptococcus (8, 7.4%), non-group D streptococcus (8, 7.4%), *Proteus* spp. (6, 5.6%), *Escherichia coli* (4, 3.7%) and coagulase-negative staphylococcus (2, 1.9%). Thirty organisms (21.7%) were unmatched; 17 (56.7%) from the middle ear tissue and 13 (43.3%) from the middle ear exudate. The 17 unmatched bacterial organisms from the middle ear tissue included *P. aeruginosa* (5, 29.4%), *S. intermedius* (3, 17.6%), beta-haemolytic streptococcus (3, 17.6%), *Corynebacterium* spp. (2, 11.8%), coagulase-negative staphylococcus (2, 11.8%), *Proteus* spp. (1, 5.9%) and *E. coli* (1, 5.9%). The 13 unmatched bacterial organisms from the middle ear exudate included *P. aeruginosa* ($n = 2, 15.4\%$), *S. intermedius* (2, 15.4%), beta-haemolytic streptococcus (2, 15.4%), *Corynebacterium* spp. (2, 15.4%), non-group D streptococcus (2, 15.4%), *E. coli* (2, 15.4%) and *Proteus* spp. (1, 7.7%).

There were no significant differences in the organisms identified morphologically and biochemically from the middle ear tissue compared to the organisms identified morphologically and biochemically from the middle ear exudate based on treatment group ($p = 0.230$). However, if differences in organisms isolated occurred between samples from the middle ear tissue and middle ear exudate, they were more likely to occur in those dogs treated with enrofloxacin. Fifteen of 19 (79%) of the enrofloxacin-treated dogs had discrepancies in the organisms isolated from the middle ear tissue and middle ear exudate (3 of 15 (20%) dogs had organisms isolated from the middle ear tissue only) compared with only 1 of 4 (25%) in the control group. This difference was not statistically significant ($p = 0.067$) at the 95% confidence level.

Discussion

In practice, cultures of otic exudate are the most common sample obtained from the middle ear of dogs with otitis media to identify infective organisms. However, in this study, slightly more organisms were isolated from cultures of the middle ear tissue (51.4%) than from the middle ear exudate (48.6%). When the number of unmatched organisms from the middle ear tissue and middle ear exudate from each ear were compared, 56.7% of the unmatched organisms were identified from the middle ear tissue and 43.3% from the middle ear exudate. These results are similar to a study comparing two culturing methods of 10 chronic wounds, in which 35 organisms (54.7%) were isolated from tissue cultures and 29 organisms (45.3%) were isolated from swab cultures, with 10 unmatched organisms (62.5%) from the tissue and 6 (37.5%) from the swab.[10] Therefore, based on the results from our study, samples from both the middle ear tissue and middle ear exudate should be obtained in order to identify all the organisms present in dogs with otitis media. Tissue samples from the middle ear of dogs with otitis media are easily obtained in dogs undergoing a TECA-LBO, as are swab samples of the exudate. However, samples from the middle ear tissue are virtually impossible to obtain in dogs being treated medically. In those cases, only a swab of the exudate for culture would be possible and a few organisms may be missed by not culturing the middle ear tissue.

Antibiotics are frequently administered during a TECA-LBO surgery as well as in the medical treatment of chronic otitis externa and otitis media prior to otic flushing. Administration of antibiotics prior to obtaining cultures may result in the recovery of fewer organisms.[11] In the study presented here, there were no differences in the organisms obtained from the middle ear tissue and middle ear exudate based on individual treatment groups. However, when enrofloxacin-treatment groups were combined and compared to the control group, 79% of dogs treated with enrofloxacin had discrepancies in the organisms isolated from the tissue versus the exudate, compared to one of four dogs in the control group. In addition, three dogs in the treatment

groups had organisms isolated from the middle ear tissue only. Although the difference was not statistically significant, probably a result of the small number of dogs in the control group, results suggest that it would be best to discontinue antibiotic administration prior to obtaining cultures from the middle ear.

In this study, 52% of the dogs were American cocker spaniels. This is consistent with other studies of chronic otitis externa and otitis media in which the American cocker spaniel breed is overrepresented.[1,2,12,13] Comparison of the age of onset of the otitis and age at the time of surgery between the American cocker spaniels and the other dogs revealed a significant difference between the two groups. The American cocker spaniels were significantly older when their otitis began (7 years old compared with 3 years old) and subsequently presented at an older age for surgery than the other dogs. This differs from a previous study in which there were no significant differences between the age at presentation for surgery between American cocker spaniels and other dogs, although the age of onset of the otitis was not reported.[14] In the current study, there were no significant differences between the two groups in the length of time from the onset of the otitis until surgery, suggesting that the progression of the chronic otitis externa to end-stage otitis externa requiring surgery is similar between the two groups.

Funding

This study was funded by Bayer Animal Health, The Ohio State University Canine Research Fund, the American College of Veterinary Dermatology and the Ohio Animal Health Foundation.

References

1 Cole, L.K., Kwochka, K.W., Podell, M., Hillier, A., Smeak, D.D. Evaluation of radiography, otoscopy, pneumotoscopy, impedance audiometry and endoscopy for the diagnosis of otitis media. In: Thoday, K.L., Foil, C.S., Bond, R., eds. *Advances in Veterinary Dermatology*, Vol. 4. Blackwell Science, Oxford, 2002: 49–55.

2 Colombini, S., Merchant, S. R., Hosgood, G. Microbial flora and antimicrobial susceptibility patterns from dogs with otitis media. *Veterinary Dermatology*, 2000; **11**: 235–239.

3 Beckman, S.L., Henry, W.B., Cechner, P. Total ear canal ablation combining bulla osteotomy and curettage in dogs with chronic otitis externa and media. *Journal of the American Veterinary Medical Association*, 1990; **196**: 84–90.

4 Sharp, N.J.H. Chronic otitis externa and otitis media treated by total ear canal ablation and ventral bulla osteotomy in thirteen dogs. *Veterinary Surgery*, 1990; **19**: 162–166.

5 Neer, T.M., Howard, P.E. Otitis media. *Compendium on Continu-*

ing Education, 1982; **4**: 410–417.

6 Vogel, P.L., Komtebedde, J., Hirsh, D.C., Kass, P.H. Wound contamination and antimicrobial susceptibility of bacteria cultured during total ear canal ablation and lateral bulla osteotomy in dogs. *Journal of the American Veterinary Medical Association*, 1999; **214**: 1641–1643.

7 Smeak, D.D. Total ear canal ablation and lateral bulla osteotomy. In: Bojrab, M.J., Ellison, G.W., Slocum, B., eds. *Current Techniques in Small Animal Surgery*, 4th edn. Williams & Wilkins, Baltimore, MD, 1998: 102–109.

8 DeManuelle, T.C., Ihrke, P.J., Brandt, C.M., Kass, P.H., Vulliet, P.R. Determination of skin concentrations of enrofloxacin in dogs with pyoderma. *American Journal of Veterinary Research*, 1998; **59**: 1599–1604.

9 Acar J.F., Goldstein, F.W. Disk susceptibility test. In: Lorian, V., ed. *Antibiotics in Laboratory Medicine*, 4th edn. Williams & Wilkins, Baltimore, MD, 1996: 1–51.

10 Neil, J.A., Munro, C.L. A comparison of two culturing methods for chronic wounds. *Ostomy/Wound Management*, 1997; **43**: 20–30.

11 Marangon, F.B., Miller, D., Alfonso, E.S. Impact of prior therapy on the recovery and frequency of corneal pathogens. *Cornea*, 2004; **23**: 158–164.

12 Smeak, D.D., Crocker, C.B., Birchard, S.J. Treatment of recurrent otitis media that developed after total ear canal ablation and lateral bulla osteotomy in dogs: nine cases (1986–1994). *Journal of the American Veterinary Medical Association*, 1996; **209**: 937–942.

13 Mason, L.K., Harvey, C.E., Orsher, R.J. Total ear canal ablation combined with lateral bulla osteotomy for end-stage otitis in dogs: results in thirty dogs. *Veterinary Surgery*, 1988; **17**: 263–268.

14 Angus, J.C., Lichtensteiger, C., Campbell, K.L., Schaeffer, D.J. Breed variations in histopathologic features of chronic severe otitis externa in dogs: 80 cases (1995–2001). *Journal of the American Veterinary Medical Association*, 2002; **221**: 1000–1006.

Absorption, bioavailability and activity of prednisone and prednisolone in cats

C.A. Graham-Mize DVM[1], E.J. Rosser Jr DVM[2], J. Hauptman DVM[2]

[1] Allergy and Dermatology Veterinary Referral Center, Milwaukie, Oregon, USA
[2] Department of Small Animal Clinical Sciences, College of Veterinary Medicine Michigan State University, East Lansing, Michigan, USA

Summary

The purpose of this study was to determine if a difference exists between the pharmacokinetics of oral prednisone and prednisolone in cats. A three-dose crossover trial was performed with a 14-day washout period, utilising six cats. The three treatment groups consisted of: treatment 1, oral prednisone tablets (a single dose of 10 mg); treatment 2, oral prednisolone tablets (a single dose of 10 mg); treatment 3, intravenous (IV) prednisolone (a single dose of 10 mg). Following oral treatments, blood samples of 1.5 ml were drawn at time 0 and post-treatment at 7, 18 and 30 minutes, and 1, 2, 4, 6, 12, 24 and 36 hours. Following IV treatment, blood samples of 1.5 ml were drawn at time 0 and post-

treatment at 1, 3, 6, 12, 18, 30 and 45 minutes, and 1, 1.5, 2, 2.5, 6, 12, 24 and 36 hours. Determination of glucocorticoid concentrations in serum was performed using high-pressure liquid chromatography-mass spectrometry (HPLC-MS). A paired t-test revealed that the maximum serum concentration (C_{max}) values of prednisolone were significantly greater for oral prednisolone than prednisone ($p = 0.001$), and that the reported area under the curve (AUC) values were significantly greater for oral prednisolone than prednisone ($p = 0.016$). These differences may be due to decreased gastrointestinal absorption of prednisone compared with prednisolone, or decreased hepatic conversion of prednisone to prednisolone in cats. These data indicate that oral prednisolone is the superior therapeutic choice for cats.

Introduction

Prednisone and prednisolone are commonly used glucocorticoids in clinical veterinary medicine. Prednisone is the inactive form of prednisolone and must be converted to prednisolone in the liver by the enzyme 11β-hydroxydehydrogenase. The reverse conversion of prednisolone to prednisone is carried out by 11-oxidation.[1] Equilibrium of this reaction greatly favours the formation of prednisolone. This is achieved on first pass metabolism through the liver.[1]

Prednisolone is often recommended in veterinary dermatology literature for use in cats rather than prednisone.[2–5] However, these recommendations are mostly based on clinical opinions, as the bioactivity and bioavailability of prednisone and prednisolone had not, until now, been determined in cats.

In humans, prednisone and prednisolone bioavailability for oral tablets does not appear significantly different.[1,6] In one of these studies, the data demon-

strated that prednisone and prednisolone tablets were bioequivalent, based on prednisone and prednisolone plasma concentrations.[6] It is apparent that the absorption of prednisone and conversion to the active metabolite, prednisolone, occurs in humans and also dogs.

In dogs both prednisone and prednisolone are rapidly absorbed and with high bioavailabilities. In addition, in the dog interconversion between prednisone and prednisolone occurs quite readily. Pharmacokinetics of prednisone and prednisolone have been studied in canine models. It was found, however, that the predominant drug in the serum is the drug that is administered, due to the fact that the form administered reaches the circulatory system more quickly than does the major metabolite.[7] In addition, the area under the serum concentration-time curve was larger for the drug administered than for the primary metabolite. Serum prednisone concentrations were significantly greater following prednisone administration than they were following prednisolone administration and serum prednisolone concentrations were significantly greater following administration of prednisolone than with prednisone. However, the combined prednisone and prednisolone areas under the serum concentration-time curves were similar for the two treatments. Peak serum concentrations were greater for prednisolone than for prednisone regardless of treatment. However, the difference in peak serum prednisolone concentrations was not significantly different with respect to treatment, and the combined prednisone-prednisolone peak serum concentrations were essentially equal. Also, there was no significant difference in the half-lives of the two treatments.[7] The conclusions were that the differences were not significant enough to predict any clinical difference of treatment with prednisone or prednisolone in the dog. In another study carried out in dogs, the investigators observed that hydrolysis of the phosphate ester to prednisolone in the body was rapid and complete after oral and intravenous dosing of prednisolone sodium phosphate.[8]

The pharmacokinetics of prednisone and prednisolone have been studied in other domestic species. In horses, oral prednisone is poorly absorbed and the active metabolite prednisolone is rarely produced when compared with oral administration of prednisolone.[9] This is in contrast to the findings in dogs and humans. In horses, clinical treatment for heaves has been based on human research studies of prednisone treatment for asthma. There has been a discrepancy in efficacy of this clinical treatment for horses. In research studies, the efficacy of oral prednisone has been questioned for treatment in respiratory diseases.[10–12] One study in horses showed that oral prednisone is poorly absorbed and the active metabolite prednisolone is rarely produced when compared with oral administration of prednisolone.[9] The resulting recommendations were in favour of prednisolone use over prednisone in horses.

The authors are not aware of any studies performed in cats that show a difference between prednisone and prednisolone pharmacokinetics. There is only limited information available regarding the efficacy of prednisone versus prednisolone in cats. For example, prednisolone was shown to suppress endogenous cortisol production for 14 days after oral administration.[13] There are no published studies which evaluate the efficacy of prednisone in cats. Therefore, the purpose of this study was to determine if there is a difference be-

tween the pharmacokinetics of prednisone and prednisolone when given orally to cats.

Materials and methods

Animals

Six adult cats were utilised for this study. A physical examination, complete blood count, serum chemistry panel and urinalysis were performed as baseline normal and to determine if the animals were healthy. Animals were housed in single cages in the same room. Animals were fed water *ad libitum* and a balanced adult dry cat food.

Study design

A three-dose crossover trial was performed with a 14-day washout period between each treatment. The three treatment groups consisted of: treatment 1, oral prednisone tablets (a single dose of 10 mg); treatment 2, oral prednisolone tablets (a single dose of 10 mg); treatment 3, intravenous (IV) prednisolone (a single dose of 10 mg). Anaesthesia was performed with isoflurane gas, and a single-lumen jugular intravenous catheter was placed. The animals were allowed to recover for 1 day after catheter placement, before starting the treatment protocol. Food was withheld for 12 hours before and for 6 hours after the treatment. Oral medication was placed on the base of the tongue and cats were observed for swallowing. Intravenous treatment was given via the cephalic vein.

On day 1, all animals received one of the three treatments. For intravenous treatment, blood samples of 1.5 ml were drawn immediately prior to drug administration and post-treatment at 1, 3, 6, 12, 18, 30 and 45 minutes, and 1, 1.5, 2, 2.5, 6, 12, 24 and 36 hours. As regards oral administration of treatments, blood samples of 1.5 ml were drawn immediately prior to drug administration and post-treatment at 7, 18 and 30 minutes, and 1, 2, 4, 6, 12, 24 and 36 hours. During sampling, residual fluid was withdrawn from the infusion set and set aside. After drawing the 1.5 ml blood sample the residual amount was reinfused and the catheter was then flushed with saline. Blood was collected into micro-serum collection tubes and allowed to clot at room temperature for 1 hour. Tubes were spun at 1000 *g* for 15 minutes to separate out the serum. The serum was collected and frozen for shipment (on dry ice) to the laboratory for analysis of serum concentration of prednisone, prednisolone and endogenous hydrocortisone. A 14-day washout period then occurred, followed by rotation of the treatment groups. This procedure was repeated until all cats had gone through the three treatment groups.

Samples

The serum was collected and frozen at –70°F for shipment to the K.L. Maddy Equine Analytical Chemistry Laboratory at the University of California-Davis for analysis. Determination of glucocorticoid concentrations in feline serum was performed using high-pressure liquid chromatography-mass spectrometry (HPLC-MS). Stock solutions (1 mg/ml) for prednisone, prednisolone, dexamethasone and hydrocortisone were prepared in acetonitrile. Feline serum samples were prepared for analysis by precipitating serum proteins with acidic acetonitrile and harvesting the supernatant. Serum calibration standards for prednisolone, prednisone and hydrocortisone were prepared by adding appropriate volumes of each stock solution to normal untreated cat serum to produce concentrations of 10, 20, 50, 100 and 500 ng/ml. For cortisol quantification, appropriate volumes of the dexamethasone stock solution, which was used as the internal standard, were added to extraction solvent, a 9:1 mixture of acetonitrile and 1 M acetic acid, to achieve a concentration of 417 ng/ml. Then 600 μl of the fortified extraction solvent was added to each test sample and each cortisol calibration standard in order to produce a final serum concentration of 500 ng/ml.[9]

Selected ion monitoring atmospheric pressure ionisation liquid chromatography-mass spectrometry (model 1100 LC/MSD, Agilent Technologies, Palo Alto, CA, USA) was used to detect the presence of analytes in protein-free supernatants. The concentrations of prednisone and prednisolone in the test samples were calculated from the slope and intercept of the calibration curve. The concentration of cortisol in test samples was determined by the internal standard method using the peak area ratio. The limits of quantification for the prednisolone, prednisone and hydrocortisone assays are 10 ng/ml, 20 ng/ml and 25 ng/ml, respectively. With HPLC-MS, cross-reactivity should not occur between prednisolone, prednisone and hydrocortisone.[9]

Statistics

The mean half-life for absorption ($T_{1/2\,Abs}$), mean half-life for excretion ($T_{1/2\,Exc}$), mean area under the curve (AUC), mean time to maximum serum concentration (T_{max}) and mean maximum serum concentration (C_{max}) were calculated and reported for each group above. The concentration data were fitted to a pharmacokinetic equation that assumes that prednisolone/prednisone is absorbed by first order kinetics and excreted by first order kinetics[14] as follows:

$$\text{concentration of prednisolone} = [k_1 \times F \times D \times (e^{-k_2 \times time} - e^{-k_1 \times time})]/[V \times (k_1 - k_2)]$$

In this equation, k_1 is the absorption rate constant, k_2 is the elimination rate constant, F is the fraction of the dose (D) absorbed after extravascular administration and V is an 'apparent' volume of distribution. F, D and V are all directly related, and are expressed as a constant.

The equation used for estimation of pharmacokinetic parameters is:

$$\text{concentration of prednisolone} = [k_1 \times constant \times (e^{-k_2 \times time} - e^{-k_1 \times time})]/(k_1 - k_2).$$

Results

Results revealed that when oral prednisolone was administered, serum prednisolone pharmacokinetics were: mean half-life for absorption ($T_{1/2\,Abs}$) = 0.47 h, mean half-life for excretion ($T_{1/2\,Exc}$) = 0.66 h, mean area under the curve (AUC) = 3230.55 ng/ml/h, mean time to maximum serum concentration (T_{max}) = 0.77 h, mean maximum serum concentration (C_{max}) = 1400.81 ng/ml (Table 2.6.1). Following the oral administration of prednisolone, the concentrations of prednisolone, prednisone and hydrocortisone are shown in Fig. 2.6.1.

When oral prednisone was administered, serum prednisolone pharmacokinetics were: $T_{1/2\,Abs}$ = 0.90 h, $T_{1/2\,Exc}$ = 2.46 h, mean AUC = 672.63 ng/ml/h, mean T_{max} = 1.44 h, mean C_{max} = 122.18 ng/m (Table 2.6.2). Following the oral administration of prednisone, the concentrations of prednisolone, prednisone and hydrocortisone are shown in Fig. 2.6.2.

A paired t-test was performed to compare the C_{max} and AUC of serum prednisolone, for prednisone versus prednisolone given orally. These calculations

Table 2.6.1 Absorption, bioavailability and activity of prednisolone after oral administration (single 10-mg dose) in cats.

Parameter	Prednisolone		Prednisone		Hydrocortisone	
	Mean	SEM	Mean	SEM	Mean	SEM
K_a	1.63	0.21	0.95	0.24	0.38	0.02
A	3260.38	424.82	183.80	18.79	466.78	124.93
K_e	1.19	0.19	0.58	0.09	0.38	0.02
R^2	0.88	0.03	0.87	0.01	0.79	0.07
$T_{1/2\,Abs}$ (hours)	0.47	0.07	0.91	0.16	1.83	0.10
$T_{1/2\,Exc}$ (hours)	0.66	0.11	1.37	0.25	1.83	0.10
AUC (ng/ml/h)	3230.55	698.37	362.71	66.27	1186.77	257.23
T_{max} (hours)	0.77	0.09	1.47	0.14	2.82	0.27
C_{max} (ng/ml)	1400.81	204.46	80.53	10.21	178.45	44.97

SEM, standard error of the mean; K_a, absorption; A, fraction of the dose absorbed after extravascular administration divided by the volume of distribution; K_e, excretion; R^2, correlation coefficient; $T_{1/2\,Abs}$, mean half-life for absorption; $T_{1/2\,Exc}$, mean half-life for excretion; AUC, mean area under the curve; T_{max}, mean time to maximum concentration; C_{max}, mean maximum serum concentration.

revealed that the C_{max} values of serum prednisolone (Tables 2.6.1 and 2.6.2) were significantly greater for oral prednisolone (C_{max} = 1400.81 ng/ml) than oral prednisone (C_{max} = 122.18 ng/ml) (p = 0.001). In addition, the AUC values of serum prednisolone were significantly greater for oral prednisolone (AUC = 3230.55 ng/ml/h) than oral prednisone (AUC = 672.63 ng/ml/h) (p = 0.016).

When intravenous prednisolone was administered, serum prednisolone pharmacokinetics were: mean half-life for distribution ($T_{1/2\,Distrib}$) = 0.027 h, $T_{1/2\,Exc}$ = 0.503 h (Table 2.6.3). The serum concentrations of prednisolone after intravenous administration are shown in Fig. 2.6.3. The estimation of the fraction of the dose absorbed (F = 1) after extravascular administration is shown in Fig. 2.6.4, which compares the intravenous administration of prednisolone to the oral administration of the drug.

Mean results for endogenous hydrocortisone with the three different treatment groups are shown in Fig. 2.6.5. The endogenous hydrocortisone concentrations were significantly greater for oral prednisone than both oral prednisolone and intravenous prednisolone (p < 0.0001). Oral prednisolone and intravenous prednisolone were not significantly different in their ability to suppress endogenous hydrocortisone.

Discussion

In this study, there was a significantly greater serum concentration (C_{max}) and mean area under the curve (AUC) for prednisolone after oral administration of prednisolone, in comparison with oral prednisone. As prednisone needs to be converted from this inactive form, to the metabolically active prednisolone, the results of this study support the proposition that

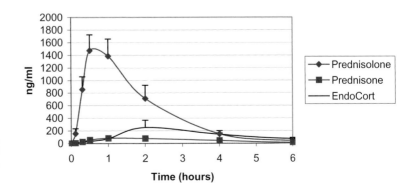

Fig. 2.6.1 Concentrations of prednisolone, prednisone and hydrocortisone following the oral administration of prednisolone (single 10-mg dose). EndoCort, hydrocortisone.

Parameter	Prednisolone Mean	Prednisolone SEM	Prednisone Mean	Prednisone SEM	Hydrocortisone Mean	Hydrocortisone SEM
K_a	2.39	1.62	2.53	1.59	0.77	0.21
A	303.28	147.78	578.77	163.88	1588.93	302.94
K_e	0.47	0.08	0.80	0.20	0.42	0.04
R^2	0.82	0.07	0.69	0.08	0.82	0.04
$T_{1/2\,Abs}$ (hours)	0.90	0.22	0.72	0.19	1.25	0.27
$T_{1/2\,Exc}$ (hours)	2.46	1.18	2.11	1.26	1.70	0.13
AUC (ng/ml/h)	672.63	259.16	842.02	235.22	3850.99	849.43
T_{max} (hours)	1.44	0.24	1.11	0.23	2.00	0.31
C_{max} (hours)	122.18	51.56	220.36	56.01	728.63	117.49

Table 2.6.2 Absorption, bioavailability and activity of prednisone after oral administration (single 10-mg dose) in cats.

See Table 2.6.1 for abbreviations.

prednisolone should be superior to prednisone in its clinical use as an anti-inflammatory or immunosuppressive drug in cats. Regarding the oral absorption of prednisolone, the estimation of the fraction of the dose absorbed after extravascular administration is equal to 1, and indicates nearly 100% absorption of the oral form of the drug (Fig. 2.6.4).

Superior suppression of endogenous hydrocortisone was observed for both IV prednisolone and oral prednisolone, when compared with oral prednisone, further supporting prednisolone's superior metabolic activity (Figs 2.6.1, 2.6.2 and 2.6.5). However, it is interesting to note that the baseline levels of endogenous hydrocortisone increased dramatically 2 hours after the sampling times for all cats in all three drug treatment groups. One possible explanation for this is that the cats are stressed during each blood sampling time period, and this stress response is reflected as an attempted increase in endogenous hydrocortisone over the next 2 hours. Even under these circumstances, both

IV prednisolone and oral prednisolone were superior in their ability to diminish this presumed endogenous hydrocortisone response, when compared with oral prednisone.

These reported differences in the pharmacokinetics of prednisone and prednisolone are most likely due to a decreased gastrointestinal absorption of prednisone, when compared with prednisolone. This is suggested in that the C_{max} for prednisolone after its oral administration is 1400.981 ng/ml of prednisolone, and the C_{max} for prednisone after its oral administration is 220.36

Table 2.6.3 Bioavailability of prednisolone after intravenous injection (single 10-mg dose)

Prednisolone	Mean	Standard error of mean
$T_{1/2}$ distribution (hours)	0.027	0.002
$T_{1/2}$ excretion (hours)	0.503	0.049

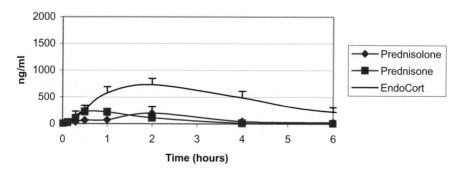

Fig. 2.6.2 Concentrations of prednisolone, prednisone and hydrocortisone following the oral administration of prednisone (single 10-mg dose). Endocort, hydrocortisone.

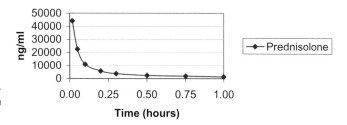

Fig. 2.6.3 Serum concentrations of prednisolone after intravenous administration (single 10-mg dose).

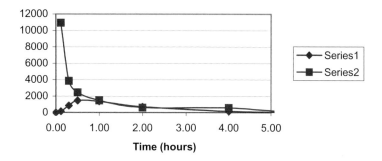

Fig. 2.6.4 Comparison of the intravenous administration of prednisolone to the oral administration of the drug. Series 1, oral prednisolone; Series 2, IV prednisolone.

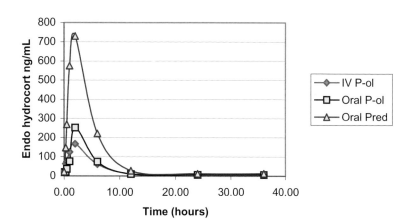

Fig. 2.6.5 Mean endogenous hydrocortisone concentrations for the three different treatment groups. IV P-ol, intravenous prednisolone; Oral P-ol, oral prednisolone; Oral Pred, oral prednisone.

ng/ml of prednisone (Tables 2.6.1 and 2.6.2). In addition there may be a reduced hepatic conversion of prednisone to prednisolone in cats when compared to other species; however, this was not one of the specific objectives of this study.

The results of this study support the proposition that prednisolone should be superior to prednisone in its clinical use as an anti-inflammatory or immunosuppressive drug in cats.

Acknowledgements

The authors would like to acknowledge Lara Maxwell and the K.L. Maddy Equine Analytical Chemistry Laboratory at the University of California-Davis for analysis of the samples.

Funding

Funding was supplied by the Companion Animal Fund, College of Veterinary Medicine, Michigan State University.

References

1 Begg, E.J., Atkinson, H.C., Gianarakis, N. The pharmacokinetics of corticosteroid agents. *Medical Journal of Australia*, 1987; **146**: 37–41.

2 Messinger, L.M. Therapy for feline dermatoses. *Veterinary Clinics of North America: Small Animal Practice,* 1995; **25**: 981–1005.

3 Power, H.T., Ihrke, P.J. Selected feline eosinophilic skin diseases. *Veterinary Clinics of North America: Small Animal Practice*, 1995; **25**: 833–850.

4 Power, H.T. Tips/Questions #6–8. Practice Tips. In: Roudebush, P., ed. *Derm Dialogue* 1993/1994; Winter: 7.

5 Rosser, E.J. Open Forum. In: Roudebush, P., ed. *Derm Dialogue* 1994; Summer: 11.

6 Ferry, J.J., Horvath, A.M., Bekersky, I., Heath, E.C., Ryan, C.F., Colburn, W.A. Relative and absolute bioavailability of prednisone and prednisolone after separate oral and intravenous doses. *Journal of Clinical Pharmacology*, 1988; **28**: 81–87.

7 Colburn, W.A., Sibley, C.R., Buller, R.H. Comparative serum prednisone and prednisolone concentrations following prednisone and prednisolone administration to Beagle dogs. *Journal of Pharmaceutical Sciences*, 1976; **65**: 997–1001.

8 Tse, F.L.S., Welling, P.G. Prednisolone bioavailability in the dog. *Journal of Pharmaceutical Sciences*, 1977; **66**: 1751–1754.

9 Peroni, D.L., Stanley, S., Kollias-Baker, C., Robinson, N.E. Oral prednisone is likely to have limited efficacy in horses. *Equine Veterinary Journal*, 2002; **34**: 283–287.

10 Traub-Dargatz, J.L., McKinnon, A.O., Thrall, M.A., *et al.* Evaluation of clinical signs of disease, bronchoalveolar and tracheal wash analysis, and arterial blood gas tensions in thirteen horses with chronic obstructive pulmonary disease treated with prednisone, methyl sulfonmethane, and clenbuterol hydrochloride. *American Journal of Veterinary Research*, 1992; **53**: 1908–1916.

11 Jackson, C.A., Berney, C., Jefcoat, A.M., Robinson, N.E. Environment and prednisone interactions in the treatment of recurrent airway obstruction (heaves). *Equine Veterinary Journal*, 2000; **32**: 432–438.

12 Robinson, N.E., Jackson, C., Jefcoat, A. Efficacy of three corticosteroids for the treatment of heaves. *Equine Veterinary Journal*, 2002; **34**: 17–22.

13 Middleton, D.J., Watson, D.J., Howe, C.J., Caterson, I.D. Suppression of cortisol responses to exogenous adrenocorticotrophic hormone, and the occurrence of side effects attributable to glucocorticoid excess, in cats during therapy with megestrol acetate and prednisolone. *Canadian Journal of Veterinary Research*, 1987; **51**: 60–65.

14 Gabrielson, J., Weiner, D. *Pharmacokinetic and Pharmacodynamic Data Analysis*. Swedish Pharmaceutical Press, Stockholm, 2000.

Diagnosis and treatment of pituitary pars intermedia dysfunction (classical Cushing's disease) and metabolic syndrome (peripheral Cushing's syndrome) in horses

H.C. Schott II DVM, PhD[1], E.A. Graves VMD, MS[1], K.R. Refsal DVM, PhD[2], R.J. Nachreiner DVM, PhD[2], S.W. Eberhart LVT[1], P.J. Johnson BVSc, MS[3], S.H. Slight PhD[4], N.T. Messer IV DVM[3], V.K. Ganjam DVM, PhD[3]

[1] Department of Large Animal Clinical Sciences, and [2] Diagnostic Center for Population and Animal Health, College of Veterinary Medicine, Michigan State University, East Lansing, Michigan, USA
[3] Departments of Veterinary Medicine and Surgery, and [4] Veterinary Biomedical Sciences, College of Veterinary Medicine, University of Missouri, Columbia, Missouri, USA

Summary

Study 1: Plasma adrenocorticotropin (ACTH) concentration, serum insulin concentration, and overnight low-dose dexamethasone suppression test (ODST) results and treatment responses (pergolide vs cyproheptadine vs no treatment) were compared in 56 horses with pituitary pars intermedia dysfunction (PPID, classical Cushing's disease). Both plasma ACTH and serum insulin concentrations were found to be unreliable single-sample diagnostic tests, in comparison to ODST results. In 24 horses (14 treated with pergolide, 6 treated with cyproheptadine and 4 that were not treated) that were re-examined after 6–12 months of therapy, clinical improvement and return to normal ODST results were greatest ($p < 0.05$) with pergolide treatment. These results provide further support that the ODST is the preferred diagnostic test for PPID and also provide strong evidence that

pergolide is a more effective treatment for PPID than cyproheptadine.

Study 2: Thyroid hormone responses to administration of thyrotropin-releasing hormone (TRH) stimulation test, and activity of 11-β-hydroxy-steroid dehydrogenase type 1 (11-β-HSD1) in subcutaneous adipose tissue were compared in nine horses afflicted with obesity-associated laminitis (equine metabolic syndrome, EMS) and seven control horses. No differences in TRH stimulation test results between EMS-affected horses and control horses were found. Although there was a tendency for greater 11-β-HSD1 activity in subcutaneous adipose tissue of EMS-affected horses, substantial variability in both groups precluded demonstration of a statistical difference. These results support the conclusions that hypothyroidism is not extant, but that altered cortisol metabolism in adipose tissue may be an important mechanism contributing to development of EMS.

Introduction

Pituitary pars intermedia dysfunction (PPID), or classical Cushing's disease, is the most commonly recognised endocrine disorder of horses. Although inappropriate hirsutism in older horses is considered pathognomonic, the two most important clinical complications of PPID are laminitis and type 2 diabetes.[1–4] Laminitis is also the most devastating complication associated with a syndrome of obesity in middle-aged horses. This latter syndrome has been recognised for many years, most commonly when equids, especially

ponies, are turned out to lush spring pasture. Despite the fact that insulin insensitivity was documented to be a consequence of obesity in horses nearly 20 years ago,[5] obesity-associated laminitis has commonly been attributed to hypothyroidism in horses.[6] In fact, horse owners spend more than one million dollars annually on thyroid hormone replacement therapy based on this diagnosis.[7]

With the increased recognition of obesity-associated disorders in human patients, grouped under the term human metabolic syndrome (HMS),[8] the term equine metabolic syndrome (EMS) has recently been advanced as a new descriptor for this apparently similar syndrome of obesity-associated laminitis in horses.[9] Patients afflicted with HMS typically have insulin insensitivity and obesity with central (omental) adiposity and suffer from complications including type 2 diabetes, dyslipidaemias, hypertension and cardiovascular disease.[8] In addition to insulin resistance (typically characterised by elevated fasting insulin concentrations and glucose intolerance), obesity in horses afflicted with EMS is also commonly accompanied by fat deposition in specific locations including the supraorbital fossa, crest of the neck, behind the shoulders and over the tail head. Accumulation of intra-abdominal fat has not been so well characterised in this species.[9] In both species, certain ethnic groups (humans) and breeds (horses) appear to be at higher risk of developing metabolic syndrome, indicating that genetic predisposition to the metabolic syndrome likely exists.[8,9] Further, recent data in people afflicted with HMS have implicated alterations in cortisol metabolism as one of several potential mechanisms involved in development of HMS.[10] Specifically, tissue variability in activity of the enzyme 11-β-hydroxysteroid dehydrogenase type 1 (11-β-HSD1), involved in regulation of cortisol at the tissue level, led to descriptors including 'Cushing's disease of the omentum' and 'peripheral Cushing's syndrome' as earlier terms advanced for the array of obesity-associated disorders now called HMS.[11]

Over the past few years, recognition and treatment of PPID has increased dramatically as horse owners have maintained their horses and ponies through the third and fourth decades of life. However, diagnosis and treatment of PPID remains controversial as opinions vary on what endocrine test is most diagnostic, and few data exist to document which treatments are most effective. Although the overnight low-dose dexamethasone suppression test (ODST) is the best documented endocrine test for evaluation of horses with PPID (when compared with necropsy findings),[12] measurement of plasma adrenocorticotropin (ACTH) and serum insulin concentrations have been advocated, in combination with clinical signs, as accurate single-sample endocrine tests.[3,13–15] The advantages of collecting a single blood sample, in comparison to performing an ODST, for ambulatory equine practitioners and their clients are clear. Further, although the phenomenon is poorly documented, concern is

widespread that administration of dexamethasone to a horse with PPID could either induce or exacerbate laminitis.

The two drugs most commonly used for treatment of PPID are cyproheptadine, a serotonin antagonist, and pergolide, a dopaminergic agonist.[1–4,16] Both are touted to decrease secretion of pro-opiomelanocortin (POMC) by the hyperplastic pars intermedia of the equine pituitary gland. Until recently, the cost of pergolide treatment was prohibitive for many clients ($300–500/month for 6 µg/kg once daily [equal to 3 mg/day] for a 500-kg horse), leading to selection of less costly cyproheptadine for treatment of many horses. However, in conjunction with the proliferation of compounding pharmacies that offer pergolide at a substantially lower cost, a clinical trial reported in 1995 found that a lower dose of pergolide (2 µg/kg once daily [equal to 1 mg/day] for a 500-kg horse) appeared to be effective for the control of clinical signs in equids with PPID.[17] However, a contemporary clinical report described improvement of clinical signs in 69% of horses and ponies treated with cyproheptadine.[15] Until recently, there have been no data comparing improvement in clinical signs and endocrine test results in equids treated with these two drugs.

As a consequence, the Michigan Cushing's Project (Study 1) was initiated in 1997 as a collaborative effort between Michigan veterinarians and Michigan State University (MSU) in an attempt to answer two questions: (1) How do plasma ACTH or serum insulin concentrations compare to ODST results in equids with PPID; and (2) Are there differences in clinical responses, laboratory data and endocrine test results in equids with PPID that are treated with cyproheptadine or pergolide or that are not treated (three comparison groups)?

During recruitment of horses for the Michigan Cushing's Project, equine veterinarians submitted samples from a number of non-hirsute, obese horses with laminitis as the primary clinical complaint (22 of 147 [15%] horses tested). The ODST results were normal in these horses; however, fasting hyperinsulinaemia was a common finding. Clearly, equine veterinarians were having difficulty discriminating between PPID and EMS as the underlying problem leading to laminitis. Further, despite the recent comparison of EMS to HMS, it should be emphasised that most of these laminitic horses were also being treated with exogenous thyroid hormone replacement therapy because hypothyroidism has long been propagated as the cause of obesity-associated laminitis.[6]

As a result of the apparent confusion between PPID and EMS as causes of insidious-onset laminitis in mature horses, and because thyroid hormone replacement therapy continues to be widespread in horses with obesity-associated laminitis, we compared the response of the pituitary-thyroid gland axis to administration of thyrotropin-releasing hormone (TRH) in horses with obesity-associated laminitis (EMS) with the response in control horses with other musculoskeletal disorders (Study 2). Additional aims of this study were to compare resting glucose and cortisol concentrations as well as 11-β-HSD1 activity in adipose tissue collected from the neck crest between the EMS-affected and control horses.

Materials and methods

Study 1

Animals, evaluation and treatments

Horses and ponies suspected to have PPID were identified by Michigan veterinarians. Initial evaluation included collection of historical and physical examination data (recorded on a standardised form) and blood samples for a complete blood count (CBC), serum biochemical profile and hormone analyses. Inclusion in the study required presence of clinical signs consistent with PPID and ODST results supportive of Cushing's disease (see below). In addition, plasma ACTH and serum insulin concentrations were measured in most equids for comparison to ODST results as single-sample diagnostic tests for equine Cushing's disease. Clinical examination, CBC and serum biochemistry, and endocrine testing were repeated after 6–12 months of treatment with pergolide (P) at a dose of 2 μg/kg administered orally once daily, or cyproheptadine (C) at a dose of 1.2 $mg/kg^{3/4}$ (e.g. 125 mg to a 500-kg horse – dose was based on estimated body surface area rather than body weight and participating veterinarians were provided with a table detailing doses over a range of body weights) administered orally once daily, or no treatment (NT). Clients made individual treatment decisions, in consultation with their veterinarians. No attempt was made to balance treatment group sizes with the exception that veterinarians were encouraged to enrol NT equids.

Endocrine testing

The ODST was performed as described previously;[12] however, to decrease participating veterinarians' concerns about induction or exacerbation of laminitis, dexamethasone was administered at a dose of ~20 μg/kg, rather than at the more commonly recommended dose of 40 μg/kg. Although there is no evidence that this lower dose of dexamethasone actually decreases the risk of laminitis, the lower dose was more acceptable to participating veterinarians. For the ODST, a blood sample was collected and 10 mg (or 5 mg for ponies) of dexamethasone was administered intramuscularly (IM) in the late afternoon. A subsequent blood sample was collected between 17 and 19 hours after dexamethasone administration (the following morning). Failure to suppress endogenous cortisol concentration below 30 pmol/L (~1 μg/dl) was interpreted as supportive of PPID. Although the lower dose of dexamethasone used could also increase the chance of 'false positive' diagnosis of PPID,[12] it should not have influenced assessment of response to treatment because the lower dose was used consistently across treatment groups. In addition to the ODST, ACTH concentration was measured in the pre-dexamethasone EDTA plasma sample, and a serum sample was collected at the same time for determination of fasting insulin concentration.

Participating veterinarians were instructed to process blood samples for hormone analyses as follows. (1) Cortisol and ACTH: blood samples were collected into vacutainer tubes containing EDTA and transferred within 15–30 seconds of collection to a plastic syringe or storage tube; samples were placed into a cooler or refrigerator and plasma harvested after centrifugation on the same day as collection (when the practitioner returned to the clinic), was then transferred to plastic storage tubes and samples were frozen. (2) Insulin: serum harvested from vacutainer tubes without anticoagulant was transferred to plastic storage tubes after centrifugation on the same day as collection and samples were refrigerated or frozen (veterinarians were encouraged to collect blood samples at least 4 hours after feeding of a grain meal but this criterion could not be strictly controlled). Participating veterinarians were further instructed to send all samples on ice packs directly to Michigan State University's Endocrinology Laboratory at MSU's Animal Health Diagnostic Laboratory by overnight or second-day express courier service. Upon receipt at the laboratory, samples were assayed in conjunction with other clinical samples received by the laboratory.

Sample analysis

Plasma cortisol concentration was determined using a commercially available solid-phase radioimmunoassay (Diagnostic Products Corp., Los Angeles, CA, USA) as described previously.[18] Assay of equine ACTH was performed using a commercially available immunoradiometric assay (Nichols Institute Diagnostics, San Clemente, CA, USA) for ACTH 1-39. The assay was performed with duplicate tubes for standards and samples as per the manufacturer's protocol with regards to sample volume and incubation times. Serum insulin concentration was measured using a commercially available radioimmunoassay (Diagnostic Products Corp.) that has also been used in previous equine studies.[19]

Data analysis

Categorical data including clinical parameters and ODST results (supportive or non-supportive of Cushing's disease) were subjected to chi-square analysis or Fisher's exact testing (when sample numbers were small). Laboratory data (glucose and hormone concentrations) were analysed using a paired t-test to compare values before and after 6–12 months of treatment, or by one-way analysis of variance, with Student-Newman-Keuls post hoc testing, for comparison of treatment groups. A p value < 0.05 was used to indicate significant differences, and all measures of variation were reported as standard error of the mean.

Study 2

Animals and clinical evaluation

Horses referred to Michigan State University's Veterinary Teaching Hospital for evaluation of laminitis were initially included in the study if they were obese (body condition score 6 or greater on a scale from 1 to 9),[20] or had abnormal fat deposition in the crest of the neck and over the tail head. Further inclusion criteria used to establish a diagnosis of EMS included an elevated fasting insulin concentration (> 300 pmol/L) and a normal ODST result (suppression of plasma cortisol concentration to < 30 pmol/L 17–19 hours after administration of 20 µg/kg dexamethasone IM). Control horses were matched on the basis of age, sex and presence of a musculoskeletal disorder resulting

in chronic lameness (usually osteoarthritis). Further inclusion criteria for control horses included a normal fasting insulin concentration (<300 pmol/L) along with a normal response to an ODST. Although used as an inclusion criterion for final case or control categorisation, the ODST was performed only once, after completion of the TRH stimulation test described below.

As certain medications can interfere with accurate measurement of thyroid hormone concentrations, all drugs were stopped for a minimum of 24 hours before blood samples were collected for a CBC, serum biochemistry profile and measurement of baseline serum concentrations of total thyroxine (TT4), free thyroxine (FT4), total triiodothyronine (TT3) and free triiodothyronine (FT3). For the TRH stimulation test, serum concentrations of TT4, FT4, TT3 and FT3 were repeated 2, 4 and 6 hours after administration of TRH (1 mg IV) (Sigma Chemical Co., St Louis, MO, USA).

At the time of initial blood sample collection, a disposable 6-mm skin biopsy instrument was used to make a circular incision through the skin of the mid-neck region (high under the mane, using local anaesthesia but not sedation). A bone ronguer was subsequently used to collect ~1 g of fat tissue from the subcutaneous (neck crest) area through the circular lesion created by the skin biopsy instrument. The fat sample was blotted free of excess blood and immediately frozen in liquid nitrogen and stored at −70°C until sent to the University of Missouri for assessment of 11-β-HSD1 activity. The incision was closed with one simple interrupted suture.

Sample analysis

The ODST was performed and plasma cortisol concentration was measured as described for Study 1. Thyroid hormone concentrations were measured using commercially available radioimmunoassays (Ciba Corning Diagnostics, East Walpole, MA, USA) as described previously.[21] The 11-β-HSD1 keto-reductase activity in subcutaneous neck crest fat samples was expressed as pmol per 100 mg of fat tissue per hour (based on conversion of added 11-dehydrocorticosterone to corticosterone), as described previously.[22]

Data analysis

Changes in thyroid hormone concentrations in EMS-affected and control horses were evaluated by a two-factor analysis of variance (main effects of group and time) and, when F ratios were significant ($p < 0.05$), a Student-Newman-Keuls post hoc test was performed to detect specific differences. Differences between single measurements (e.g. blood glucose concentration, plasma cortisol and serum insulin concentrations, and 11-β-HSD1 activity) between groups were compared by a non-paired t-test. All measures of variation are reported as standard error of the mean (SEM).

Results

Study 1

During the study period (1997–2000), samples collected from 147 equids were submitted to MSU for hormone analyses. Of these, 56 were initially included in the study on the basis of clinical signs characteristic of PPID and supportive ODST results. It should be emphasised that the diagnosis of PPID in these equids was presumptive because the nature of the field study precluded confirmation by necropsy examination. Of the remaining 91 animals that did not fulfil inclusion criteria, 35 with a variety of clinical signs had non-supportive ODST test results, 48 had characteristic clinical signs but an ODST was not performed, and 4 were excluded because they were already being treated with pergolide at the time of initial testing. Follow-up examination, CBC, serum biochemistry and endocrine testing were repeated after 6–12 months of treatment in 24 equids with P ($n = 14$), C ($n = 6$) or NT ($n = 4$). Of the 32 that did not complete at least 6 months of treatment, 5 died, 11 were euthanased and 16 were withdrawn from the study because the owners failed to continue treatment or follow-up testing was not performed. Chronic laminitis, a common complication of PPID, was reported to be the reason for euthanasia in 6 of 11 horses (55%).

The 56 equids initially enrolled in the study ranged in estimated age from 12 to 34 years (mean 22.8 years) and included a variety of breeds: Morgan ($n = 10$), quarter horse (6), Arabian (6), saddlebred (3), thoroughbred (2), Appaloosa (2), Tennessee walker (2), standardbred (1) and Paso Fino (1). Crossbreds (13) and ponies (10) were also affected. A sex predilection was not apparent as 27 (48%) were mares, 28 (50%) were geldings and 1 (2%) was a stallion. Hirsutism and delayed shedding of the winter hair coat was described in 46 of 56 (82%), and several equids had a history of abnormal shedding for 5 years or longer. The frequency of clinical signs and clinicopathologi-

Table 2.7.1 Frequency of clinical signs and abnormal laboratory values in 56 horses with presumptive Cushing's disease

Abnormality	Frequency reported
Clinical sign	
Hirsutism	82%
Chronic laminitis	52%
Muscle wasting	47%
Polyuria and polydipsia	34%
Hyperhidrosis	33%
Abnormal fat distribution	29%
Laboratory values	
GGT activity >25 IU/L	36%
Neutrophilia (>8000/µl)	33%
Hyperglycaemia (>120 mg/dl)	32%
Lymphopenia (<1500/µl)	29%
Hypercholesterolaemia (>120 mg/dl)	22%
Anaemia (PCV <30%)	17%
AST activity (>380 IU/L)	16%
AP activity (>300 IU/L)	4%

cal abnormalities consistent with PPID are detailed in Table 2.7.1.

Plasma ACTH concentration was elevated (>10 pmol/L [~45 pg/ml]) in 32/48 animals (67%) that had ODST results supportive of PPID (samples were not analysed in eight animals). Serum insulin concentration was elevated (> 300 pmol/L [~42 µU/ml]) in 39/55 (71%) that had ODST results supportive of PPID (sample was not analysed in one horse). Thus, of the 56 equids presumed to have PPID on the basis of clinical signs and supportive ODST results, a normal plasma ACTH concentration (< 10 pmol/L) was measured in 16/48 (33%) and serum insulin concentration was normal (< 300 pmol/L) in 16/55 (29%). Of further interest, of the 35 equids with non-supportive ODST results, 9/33 (27%) had a plasma ACTH concentration > 10 pmol/L and 22/34 (65%) had a serum insulin concentration > 300 pmol/L. The majority of the latter hyperinsulinaemic equids had laminitis as the major clinical problem and body condition recorded for 16 of these 22 animals was: fat (9), normal (6) or thin (1).

Follow-up evaluation after 6–12 months of treatment included overall assessment by the owner of whether the animal's condition had improved, was unchanged, or had deteriorated. Body condition, hair coat, hyperhidrosis and severity of laminitis were assessed and owners were again asked about excessive water consumption. Owners reported that improve-

Table 2.7.2 Clinical responses of horses with presumptive Cushing's disease after 6–12 months of treatment with pergolide (P), cyproheptadine (C) or no treatment (NT)

	No.	Overall assessment (I/U/D[a])	Hair coat Pre (N/A[b])	Hair coat Post (N/A[b])	PU/PD[c] (I/U/NR[a])	Laminitis[c] (I/U/NR[a])
P	14	12/2/0*	2/12	8/6*	4/1/1[†]	11/1/1[†]
C	6	2/3/1	0/6	1/5	0/1/0	0/1/0
NT	4	0/3/1	0/4	0/4	1/0/0	0/0/0

Pre, pre-treatment. Post, post-treatment.
[a]I, improved; U, unchanged; D, deteriorated; NR, not reported.
[b]N, normal; A, abnormal.
[c]Numbers are less than totals in each group because not all horses had polyuria and polydipsia (PU/PD) or laminitis.
*Chi-square test results indicated that distributions within a column were significantly different ($p < 0.05$).
[†]Low number of observations in C and NT groups precluded statistical analysis.

ment was most apparent with P (Table 2.7.2), although one horse was reported to have improved with C (improved attitude and energy level was described, rather than a substantial improvement in hair coat or other clinical signs). The NT mare that deteriorated developed a caudolateral abdominal wall hernia attributed to muscle wasting. Body condition and hair coat shedding improved significantly with P, but remained essentially unchanged with C and NT (Table 2.7.2). In addition, polyuria and polydipsia (PU/PD) and the severity of laminitis were also reported to improve in the majority of P-treated equids. When hyperhidrosis was reported at the initial evaluation, response to treatment was inconsistent and at least one animal in each treatment group was reported to have excessive sweating after 6–12 months when the

Table 2.7.3 Changes in overnight dexamethasone suppression test (ODST) results of 24 horses with presumptive Cushing's disease after 6–12 months of treatment with pergolide (P), cyproheptadine (C) or no treatment (NT)

	No.	ODST Pretreatment +/–	ODST Post treatment +/–	p value*
P	14	14/0	9/5	0.04
C	6	6/0	5/1	0.99
NT	4	4/0	3/1	0.99

+, supportive of Cushing's disease; –, not supportive of Cushing's disease.
*Fisher's exact test results.

problem had not been reported at the initial examination. This inconsistency may partly be explained by the fact that equids were initially enrolled and subsequently re-evaluated at different times of the year.

After 6–12 months of treatment, ODST results had returned to normal (non-supportive of Cushing's disease) for 5/14, 1/6 and 1/4 of P, C and NT equids, respectively (Table 2.7.3). Of interest, one horse had normal ODST results after 6–12 months of no treatment. Similarly, mean plasma ACTH concentration decreased significantly ($p < 0.05$) after 6–12 months of treatment with P in contrast to a lack of change with C or NT (Table 2.7.4). Although serum glucose concentration declined the most with P, significant differences in serum glucose and insulin concentrations before and after treatment were not detected.

Adverse treatment effects were not reported with C, but three P-treated horses were reported to have a decrease in appetite during the first week of treatment. Reduction of the dose for a few days appeared helpful in resolving the partial anorexia in these horses.

	No.	ACTH pre pmol/L	ACTH post pmol/L	Insulin pre pmol/L	Insulin post pmol/L	Glucose pre mg/dl	Glucose post mg/dl
P	14	27.4 ± 5.4 (3.8–65.8) n = 10	13.7 ± 2.2* (3.8–27.8) n = 10	675 ± 179 (127–2880) n = 12	497 ± 119 (110–1472) n = 12	131 ± 20 (75–288) n = 7	103 ± 6 (89–147) n = 7
C	6	20.4 ± 9.0 (3.7–58.3) n = 5	25.0 ± 8.1 (7.6–56.1) n = 5	1124 ± 406 (304–3152) n = 6	699 ± 119 (220–1068) n = 6	145 ± 34 (80–253) n = 5	176 ± 36 (83–316) n = 5
NT	4	19.9 ± 8.0 (5.7–45.8) n = 4	35.3 ± 15.0 (6.3–80.4) n = 4	727 ± 343 (138–1832) n = 4	449 ± 119 (44–628) n = 4	105 ± 8 (88–118) n = 3	104 ± 6 (90–112) n = 3

Table 2.7.4 Plasma hormone and glucose concentrations (mean ± SEM [range]) in 24 horses with presumptive Cushing's disease before (pre) and after (post) 6–12 months of treatment with pergolide (P), cyproheptadine (C) or no treatment (NT)

* Paired t-test results indicated a significant decrease after treatment ($p < 0.05$).

Study 2

During the study period, nine horses admitted for evaluation and treatment of obesity-associated laminitis had elevated serum insulin concentrations (909 ± 243 pmol/L) and were diagnosed with EMS. Affected horses ranged in age from 8 to 20 years (mean 14.5 years) and included a variety of breeds: Morgan (2), Paso Fino (2), saddlebred (2), Appaloosa (1), standardbred (1) and not indicated (1). A sex predilection was not apparent as four were mares and five were geldings. In addition, seven control horses with normal serum insulin concentrations (110 ± 22 pmol/L) were also studied. Control horses ranged in age from 8 to 19 years (mean 13.1 years) and also included a variety of breeds. Although serum glucose concentrations remained within the reference range for all horses, the mean value for EMS-affected horses (99.9 ± 3.3 mg/dl) was greater ($p < 0.05$) than that of control horses (85.0 ± 5.8 mg/dl).

In both EMS-affected and control horses, the TT4, FT4, TT3 and FT3 increased after administration of TRH (Table 2.7.5). In fact, the only significant differences between the groups were greater increases in TT3 at all times and in FT3 4 hours after TRH administration in EMS-affected horses. Although initial analysis did not reveal a significant difference ($p = 0.24$) in mean 11-β-HSD1 activity between EMS horses (mean 1.21 ± 0.24 pmol/100 mg tissue/h, range 0.24–2.33) and controls (mean 0.70 ± 0.33 pmol/100 mg tissue/h, range 0.15–2.63), four of nine EMS horses had an 11-β-HSD1 keto-reductase activity > 1.0 pmol/100 mg tissue/h, in comparison with only one of seven control horses (Fig. 2.7.1). Further, removing the outlying high value from the control group did result in a significant difference ($p < 0.03$) between 11-β-HSD1 keto-reductase activity in fat tissue collected from EMS-affected and control horses.

Discussion

Over the past decade, interest by both horse owners and equine practitioners in classical Cushing's disease (PPID) has increased dramatically. This phenomenon is a clear consequence of client demand for improved management and veterinary care of geriatric horses. An apparent offshoot of this phenomenon has been a similar increased interest in the syndrome of obesity-associated laminitis. Although recognised for decades, the latter syndrome has been confused with PPID and was often attributed to hypothyroidism. Recently, this condition was given the name 'peripheral Cushing's syndrome' (EMS) and subsequently 'equine metabolic syndrome' based on parallels to HMS.[9] Unfortunately, both PPID and EMS often have laminitis as the most serious complication. However, recent efforts in several laboratories around the world have led to better recognition that laminitis in these conditions develops as a consequence of underlying metabolic and endocrine disorders.[23] Although far from complete, the expanding knowledge base on PPID and EMS has led to improvements in understanding the development of PPID, as well as in the management and medical treatment of affected equine patients. For example, McFarlane and co-workers recently demonstrated that horses with PPID had greater evidence of oxidant-induced injury in hypothalamic dopaminergic neurons than in aged equids without PPID, or young horses.[24] This novel finding supports earlier suggestions that PPID is likely a consequence of loss of hypothalamic dopaminergic neurons, rather than a primary disease of the pars intermedia of the equine pituitary gland.[4,12]

Our research efforts described in this chapter focused on medical treatment of PPID and potential endocrine and metabolic derangements that accompany development of obesity in horses with EMS. The

Table 2.7.5 Serum concentrations of total thyroxine (TT4), free thyroxine (FT4), total triiodothyronine (TT3) and free triiodothyronine (FT3) in samples collected before (Pre) and 2, 4 and 6 hours after administration of 1 mg of thyrotropin-releasing hormone to nine EMS-affected horses and seven control horses

Hormone	Group	Pre	2 hours	4 hours	6 hours
TT4 (nmol/L)	EMS	22.8 ± 6.6	32.9 ± 5.8	$40.1 \pm 8.0^*$	$38.7 \pm 7.6^*$
	Control	25.7 ± 1.8	35.6 ± 2.1	$44.6 \pm 2.1^*$	$43.3 \pm 2.4^*$
FT4 (pmol/L)	EMS	13.2 ± 1.5	$17.1 \pm 1.3^*$	$20.6 \pm 1.3^*$	$19.3 \pm 2.1^*$
	Control	16.3 ± 1.1	$18.6 \pm 1.2^*$	$22.4 \pm 1.5^*$	$21.1 \pm 1.2^*$
TT3 (nmol/L)	EMS	0.8 ± 0.1	$2.6 \pm 0.2^{*\dagger}$	$1.9 \pm 0.3^{*\dagger}$	$1.4 \pm 0.2^{\dagger}$
	Control	0.6 ± 0.1	$1.8 \pm 0.3^*$	$1.3 \pm 0.1^*$	0.8 ± 0.1
FT3 (pmol/L)	EMS	3.7 ± 0.4	$7.7 \pm 0.9^*$	$5.8 \pm 0.6^{*\dagger}$	4.8 ± 0.5
	Control	2.7 ± 0.5	$5.4 \pm 0.7^*$	$3.9 \pm 0.4^*$	3.0 ± 0.4

*Significantly different from pre-value ($p < 0.05$).
†EMS-affected horses significantly greater than control horses ($p < 0.05$).

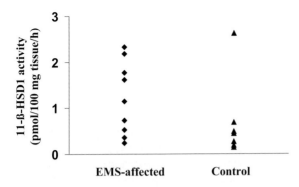

Fig. 2.7.1 11-β-hydroxysteroid dehydrogenase type 1 keto-reductase activity, expressed as conversion (in pmol/h) of added 11-dehydrocorticosterone to corticosterone per 100 mg of fat tissue, in subcutaneous fat collected from the neck crest of nine horses with obesity-associated laminitis and seven control horses.

results of our field study of animals with a presumptive diagnosis of PPID (Study 1) provide several important observations about the diagnosis, treatment and progression of this important problem of older equids. First, measurement of plasma ACTH and serum insulin concentrations was found to produce both false positive and false negative results, when compared to ODST results for diagnosis of PPID. Thus, the quest for a single-sample endocrine test for diagnosis and management of equids with PPID remains. Additionally, recent documentation of seasonal variation of plasma ACTH concentration (highest in the autumn) calls this diagnostic test into further question.[25] Second, treatment with pergolide clearly produced clinical and laboratory responses that were superior to treatment with cyproheptadine. Finally, identification of a group of obese equids with laminitis, but not hirsutism, that had elevated serum insulin concentrations and normal ODST results provided further support that EMS is an important endocrine disorder in horses. In addition to providing a stimulus for our group to pursue research of EMS, this latter observation is also important because equids with EMS would not be expected to improve with treatment aimed at counteracting excess production of POMC by the pars intermedia of the pituitary gland in horses with classical Cushing's disease.

At the time the Michigan Cushing's Project was completed, our findings corroborated the only other treatment comparison trial of equids with Cushing's disease that we could find.[26] In that report, limited to presentation as an abstract, horses and ponies treated with either 'high dose' (4–5 mg/day) or 'low dose' (1–2 mg/day) pergolide showed greater clinical improvement than cyproheptadine-treated animals. Subsequent to completion of the Michigan Cushing's Project, results of similar studies were reported by two other groups of investigators. Donaldson and co-workers found that 17/20 (85%) owners of horses and ponies treated with P (median dose of 1.5 mg/day) reported clinical improvement while only 2/7 owners of C-treated equids reported clinical improvement.[27] In this field study, plasma ACTH concentration, in conjunction with clinical signs, was used to diagnose PPID, and plasma ACTH concentration was significantly lower following treatment with P than after treatment with C.

In contrast, Perkins and co-workers found no difference in the percentage of horses and ponies that showed clinical improvement after treatment with C ($n = 32$) or P ($n = 10$).[28] In this study, > 80% of affected horses and ponies in both treatment groups had improvement in at least one clinical sign attributed to PPID, and 60–70% had a decrease in plasma ACTH concentration after treatment. Unfortunately, this study had several limitations in that not all cases included had convincing clinical signs of PPID (i.e. 20 horses were described as having 'possible equine Cushing's disease'), and clinical improvement was based on interviews with veterinarians who made the initial diagnosis and was likely affected by recall bias.

The discrepancy between these studies illustrates the importance of developing a more rigid case definition for PPID that can be used by various research groups in future studies. In our study, inclusion of a non-treated control group added strength to our findings, although ethical concerns must be considered when a no treatment or placebo group is studied. Finally, it also warrants emphasis that our study mandated specific doses of P and C. As a result, overall improvement with drug treatment could have been underestimated with both drugs. It has been our subsequent experience that horses that do not show substantial clinical improvement at these drug doses may subsequently improve if treated with higher doses, especially with P, that return ODST results to normal (non-supportive of PPID).

Taken together, the findings of our study and other recent studies provide reasonably strong support that pergolide is more effective than cyproheptadine as a treatment for PPID. However, it is also important to recognise that the number of horses reported by their owners to have improved was consistently higher than the number of horses that had endocrine test results return to normal (non-supportive of PPID). This discrepancy, observed with both P and C treatment, suggests that it is difficult to separate clinical improvement attributable to medication, from that attributable to improved management, particularly dentistry and nutrition. In our opinion, this observation also provides support for repeat endocrine testing (we recommend the ODST) in horses with PPID after 2–3 months of initiating P treatment. If the ODST remains abnormal, we increase the dose of P by 1 mg/day and repeat the ODST in 4–6 weeks to see if results have returned to normal (non-supportive of PPID). If the ODST remains supportive of PPID after the dose of P has been increased to 3 mg/day, we also recommend addition of C to the treatment regimen, as this drug combination has been effective in returning ODST results to normal in a few horses that we have treated in this manner. We should emphasise that these current recommendations are empiric at this time because they are based on clinical experience alone.

In Study 2 we elected to investigate thyroid gland function in horses with EMS due to the widespread empirical use of thyroid hormone replacement therapy in horses with obesity-associated laminitis. A potential limitation in assessment of thyroid gland function in this study was medication with phenylbutazone until 24 hours prior to measuring thyroid hormones. Administration of phenylbutazone has been demonstrated to affect measurement of FT4 and TT4 for as long as 2 and 10 days, respectively, after discontinuing treatment.[29] However, we thought that withholding this analgesic medication from acutely laminitic horses for more than 24 hours would be unethical. Although baseline serum concentrations of FT4 and TT4 tended to be lower in EMS-affected horses than in controls, these findings were not significant. Further, results of the TRH stimulation test clearly demonstrated that thyroid gland function in horses with EMS was no different from that in control horses with conditions accompanied by chronic pain. Although not detailed in this report, we also found that serum thyrotropin (thyroid stimulating hormone) concentrations in the two groups of horses in Study 2 were not different at rest or in response to TRH administration (unpublished data). Thus, the prior use of phenylbutazone in these patients does not appear to have confounded our overall assessment of thyroid gland function.

More importantly, our data support the notion that thyroid hormone replacement therapy does not appear to be warranted in EMS-afflicted horses as a treatment for decreased thyroid gland function. However, whether or not administration of additional thyroid hormone to EMS-afflicted horses will accelerate weight loss is unknown and remains a common, yet controversial, justification for supplementation. An additional reason that supplementation may continue to be common, despite our findings, is the frustration that other medications are currently unavailable for treatment of EMS-affected horses. As in people with HMS, diet and exercise are the mainstays of management of horses with EMS.[8,9] However, the pain of laminitis often precludes an increase in exercise. Thus, the most important role for equine practitioners is client education. The risks of obesity should be explained to owners of obese horses during annual health examinations and clients should be assisted with implementing dietary restriction and exercise programmes with a goal of preventing laminitis in at-risk horses.

In addition, Study 2 included a preliminary investigation into the possible role of 11-β-HSD1 activity in EMS because variation in activity of this enzyme has recently been implicated as a contributing mechanism in development of HMS.[10] This enzyme has both dehydrogenase (converting active cortisol to inactive cortisone) and keto-reductase (converting inactive cortisone to active cortisol) activities.[30] Although the presence of glucocorticoid receptors in various tissues has traditionally been considered the most essential requisite for glucocorticoid activity, this concept is currently being reassessed. Recently, 11-β-HSD1 activity has been advanced as a critical regulatory control point of glucocorticoid activity at the local tissue level.[30] Depending on the relative dehydrogenase and keto-reductase activities of 11-β-HSD1 in individual tissues, levels of cortisol available to bind to glucocorticoid receptors may vary considerably. Greater local cortisol activity at the cellular level, acting in a paracrine, an autocrine or an intracrine manner, would render affected tissues more resistant to insulin. This could also contribute to development of elevated circulating insulin concentrations, and eventually type 2 diabetes, in patients affected with both HMS and EMS.

In support of the hypothesis that pre-receptor modulation of circulating glucocorticoids by 11-β-HSD1 is an important contributor to development of HMS, Rask and co-workers found evidence that conversion of cortisone to cortisol by 11-β-HSD1 keto-reductase activity was increased in subcutaneous fat tissue collected from men.[10] This increased reactivation of cortisone to cortisol in fat tissue in obese men appeared to predispose them to enhanced fat deposition. Although an attractive concept, it warrants mention that altered cortisol metabolism is likely only one of several metabolic disturbances that lead to the overall condition of HMS.

In our horses in Study 2, two findings lend support for variation in peripheral cortisol metabolism in EMS-afflicted horses. First, plasma glucose concentration, although still within the reference range, was significantly higher in EMS-affected equids than controls. Second, 11-β-HSD1 keto-reductase activity in fat collected from the neck crest was higher in EMS-affected horses (when the value for the outlier control horse was excluded). However, further work is needed before tissue-specific variation in 11-β-HSD1 activity can be definitively implicated in the pathogenesis of EMS.

What does all of this have to do with development of laminitis in both PPID- and EMS-affected horses? Over the past decade, evidence for a 'metabolic theory' of equine laminitis, in addition to the more classical 'vascular theory', has been growing.[23] For example, explants of normal equine hoof wall have been demonstrated to have an absolute dependence on glucose to maintain integrity of the dermal–epidermal junction of the hoof capsule.[31] Thus, metabolic dysregulation (altered peripheral tissue cortisol activity and insulin insensitivity) could certainly impair glucose uptake by laminar basal epidermal cells and contribute to development of laminitis. Next, a recent report from one of the author's laboratories documented increased 11-β-HSD1 keto-reductase activity in both skin and lamellar tissue collected from horses with experimentally induced acute laminitis (carbohydrate overload model) and naturally occurring chronic laminitis.[22] Although these recent findings are only initial steps in furthering our understanding of the potential mechanisms involved in development of laminitis in both PPID- and EMS-affected horses, they are exciting observations because they further solidify the parallels between the metabolic and endocrine alterations observed in both HMS and EMS.

Further research is clearly needed but it appears that we may be on the right path to better understand the pathophysiology of the devastating complication of laminitis in horses with these endocrinopathies.

Hopefully, further understanding of the pathophysiology of laminitis will ultimately lead to development of interventional strategies (e.g. inhibitors of 11-β-HSD1) that may enhance our ability to both prevent development of laminitis and improve treatment of the disorder in affected equids.

Funding

These studies were supported by funds from the American Association of Equine Practitioners and the Michigan Veterinary Medical Association, as well as by endocrine testing by the Animal Health Diagnostic Laboratory at Michigan State University.

References

1 Love, S. Equine Cushing's disease. *British Veterinary Journal*, 1993; **149**: 139–153.
2 van der Kolk, J.H. Equine Cushing's disease. *Equine Veterinary Education*, 1997; **9**: 209–14.
3 van der Kolk, J.H. Diseases of the pituitary gland, including hyperadrenocorticism. In: Watson, T.D., ed. *Metabolic and Endocrine Problems of the Horse*. W.B. Saunders, London, 1998: 41–59.
4 Schott, H.C. Pituitary pars intermedia dysfunction: equine Cushing's disease. *Veterinary Clinics of North America: Equine Practice*, 2002; **18**: 237–270.
5 Jeffcott, L.B., Field, J.R., McLean, J.G., O'Dea, K. Glucose tolerance and insulin sensitivity in ponies and Standardbred horses. *Equine Veterinary Journal*, 1986; **18**: 97–101.
6 Sojka, J.E. Hypothyroidism in horses. *Compendium on Continuing Education*, 1995; **17**: 845–852.
7 Lori, D.N., MacLeay, J.M. Hypothyroidism in the horse. *Journal of Equine Veterinary Science*, 2001; **21**: 8–11.
8 Meigs, J.B. Epidemiology of the metabolic syndrome. *American Journal of Managed Care*, 2002; **8** (Suppl. 11): S83–S92.
9 Johnson, P.J. The equine metabolic syndrome: peripheral Cushing's syndrome. *Veterinary Clinics of North America: Equine Practice*, 2002; **18**: 271–293.
10 Rask, E., Olsson, T., Söderberg, S., *et al.* Tissue-specific dysregulation of cortisol metabolism in human obesity. *Journal of Clinical Endocrinology and Metabolism*, 2001; **86**: 1418–1421.
11 Bujalska, I.J., Kumar, S., Stewart, P.M. Does central obesity reflect 'Cushing's disease of the omentum'? *Lancet*, 1997; **349**: 1210–1213.
12 Dybdal, N.O., Hargreaves, K.M., Madigan, J.E., Gribble, D.H., Kennedy, P.C., Stabenfeldt, G.H. Diagnostic testing for pituitary pars intermedia dysfunction in horses. *Journal of the American Veterinary Medical Association*, 1994; **204**: 627–632.
13 van der Kolk, J.H., Kalsbeek, H.C., van Garderen, E., Wensing, T., Breukink, H.J. Equine pituitary neoplasia: a clinical report of 21 cases (1990–1992). *Veterinary Record*, 1993; **133**: 594–597.
14 van der Kolk, J.H., Wensing, T., Kalsbeek, H.C., Breukink, H.J. Laboratory diagnosis of equine pituitary pars intermedia adenoma. *Domestic Animal Endocrinology*, 1995; **12**: 35–39.
15 Couëtil, L., Paradis, M.R., Knoll, J. Plasma adrenocorticotropin concentration in healthy horses and in horses with clinical signs of hyperadrenocorticism. *Journal of Veterinary Internal Medicine*,

1996; **10**: 1–6.

16 Beech, J. Treatment of hypophyseal adenomas. *Compendium for Continuing Education*, 1994; **16**: 921–923.

17 Peters, D.F., Erfle, J.B., Slobojan, G.T. Low-dose pergolide mesylate treatment for equine hypophyseal adenomas (Cushing's syndrome). In: *Proceedings of the 41st Annual Convention of the American Association of Equine Practitioners*, 1995, Lexington, KY, 154–155.

18 van der Kolk, J.H., Nachreiner, R.F., Schott, H.C., Refsal, K.R., Zanella, A.J. Salivary and plasma concentration of cortisol in normal horses and horses with Cushing's disease. *Equine Veterinary Journal*, 2001; **33**: 211–213.

19 French, K., Pollitt, C.C., Pass, M.A. Pharmacokinetics and metabolic effects of triamcinolone acetonide and their possible relationships to glucocorticoid-induced laminitis in horses. *Journal of Veterinary Pharmacology and Therapeutics*, 2000; **23**: 287–292.

20 Henneke, D.R., Potter, G.D., Kreider, J.L., Yeates, B.F. Relationship between condition score, physical measurements and body fat percentage in mares. *Equine Veterinary Journal*, 1983; **15**: 371–372.

21 Messer, N.T., Johnson, P.J., Refsal, K.R., Nachreiner, R.F., Ganjam, V.K., Krause, G.F. Effect of food deprivation on baseline iodothyronine and cortisol concentrations in healthy, adult horses. *American Journal of Veterinary Research*, 1995; **56**: 116–121.

22 Johnson, P.J., Ganjam, V.K., Slight, S.H., Kreeger, J.M., Messer, N.T. Tissue-specific dysregulation of cortisol metabolism in equine laminitis. *Equine Veterinary Journal*, 2004; **36**: 41–45.

23 Moore, R.M., Eades, S.C., Stokes, A.M. Evidence for vascular and enzymatic events in the pathophysiology of acute laminitis: which pathway is responsible for initiation of this process in horses? *Equine Veterinary Journal*, 2004; **36**: 204–209.

24 McFarlane, D., Donaldson, M.T., Saleh, T.M., Cribb, A.E. The role of dopaminergic neurodegeneration in equine pituitary pars intermedia dysfunction (equine Cushing's disease). In: *Proceedings of the 49th Annual Convention of the American Association of Equine Practitioners*, 2003, New Orleans, LA, 233–237.

25 Donaldson, M.T., McDonnell, S.M., Schanbacher, B.J., Lamb, S.V., McFarlane, D., Beech, J. Variation in plasma ACTH concentration and dexamethasone suppression test results in association with season, age and sex in healthy ponies and horses (abstract). *Journal of Veterinary Internal Medicine*, 2004; **16**: 414.

26 Williams, P.D. Equine Cushing's syndrome – retrospective study of twenty four cases and response to medication (abstract). In: *Proceedings of the 34th British Equine Veterinary Association Congress*, 1995; 41.

27 Donaldson, M.T., LaMonte, B.H., Morresey, P., Smith, G., Beech, J. Treatment with pergolide or cyproheptadine of pituitary pars intermedia dysfunction (equine Cushing's disease). *Journal of Veterinary Internal Medicine*, 2002; **16**: 742–746.

28 Perkins, G.A., Lamb, S., Erb, H.N., Schanbacher, B., Nydam, D.V., Divers, T.J. Plasma adrenocorticotropin (ACTH) concentrations and clinical response in horses treated for equine Cushing's disease with cyproheptadine or pergolide. *Equine Veterinary Journal*, 2002; **34**: 679–685.

29 Ramirez, S., Wolfsheimer, K.J., Moore, R.M., Mora, F., Bueno, A.C., Mirza, T. Duration of effects of phenylbutazone on serum total thyroxine and free thyroxine concentrations in horses. *Journal of Veterinary Internal Medicine*, 1997; **11**: 371–374.

30 Stewart, P.M., Krozowski, Z.S. 11-β-hydroxysteroid dehydrogenase. *Vitamins and Hormones*, 1999; **57**: 249–324.

31 Pass, M.A., Pollitt, S., Pollitt, C.C. Decreased glucose metabolism causes separation of hoof lamellae in vitro: a trigger for laminitis? *Equine Veterinary Journal*, 1998; Suppl. 26: 133–138.

Part 3

Nutrition

A randomised, controlled, double-blinded, multicentre study on the efficacy of a diet rich in fish oil and borage oil in the control of canine atopic dermatitis

B. Baddaky-Taugbøl DVM[1], M.W. Vroom DVM[2], L. Nordberg DVM[3], M.H.G. Leistra DVM[4], J.D. Sinke DVM[4], R. Hovenier[5], A.C. Beynen MSc, PhD[5], F.J.H. Pastoor MSc, PhD[6]

[1] Dr. Baddakys Hudpraksis as, Skotterud, Norway
[2] Veterinaire Specialisten Oisterwijk, Oisterwijk, The Netherlands
[3] Trollesminde Dyreklinik, Hillerød, Denmark
[4] Dierenarts Specialisten Amsterdam, Amsterdam, The Netherlands
[5] Department of Nutrition, Faculty of Veterinary Medicine, Utrecht University, Utrecht, The Netherlands
[6] LEO Animal Health, Ballerup, Denmark

Summary

The efficacy of a diet with high levels of eicosapentaenoic acid (480 mg/MJ) and γ-linolenic acid (50 mg/MJ) in the control of clinical signs in strictly selected dogs with atopic dermatitis (AD) was evaluated. Dogs received the test diet plus a daily placebo capsule or a control treatment in the form of their habitual diet plus a daily placebo capsule, for 10 weeks. In a randomised, controlled design, 13 dogs received the control treatment and 15 dogs received the test diet. Subsequently, nine control dogs were also switched to the test diet. At weeks 0, 3, 6 and 10, the severity of clinical signs was scored. Scores were expressed as percentage of initial scores. At the end of the controlled study, intensity, the frequency and total score of pruritus (intensity $\times$ frequency) and score for erythema in dogs fed the test diet ($n = 15$) were significantly lower compared with control dogs, and significantly more dogs on the test diet had improved. The dogs' plasma and cutaneous fatty acid compositions changed significantly on the test diet. Of all 24 dogs that were fed the test diet (in both the controlled and crossover stages of the study), 54% improved. Non-responders more often had a positive reaction towards *Lepidoglyphus destructor* ($p < 0.05$) and had a higher pretrial incidence of secondary lesions on their limbs ($p < 0.01$). The cutaneous fatty acid concentrations were similar for responders and non-responders. This study demonstrates that the test diet rich in fish oil and borage oil significantly reduced the severity of pruritus and erythema in dogs with AD.

Introduction

Canine atopic dermatitis (AD) is a hereditary disorder with IgE-mediated hypersensitivity to environmental allergens as an important pathogenic factor. The disease has been estimated to affect up to 15% of the canine population.[1–3] The primary clinical sign of canine AD is pruritus, which is often associated with secondary infections.[1–4] Control of clinical signs in atopic dogs through avoidance of offending allergens is generally not possible, but allergen-specific immunotherapy (ASIT) is effective in about 70% of dogs with AD.[5] For dogs with AD that do not respond to ASIT, or when ASIT is not practical or desired, therapy is aimed at symptomatic relief of clinical signs. Systemic glucocorticoids and antihistamines form the basis of traditional management of canine pruritic skin disease.[3] However, due to side effects associated with long-term use of glucocorticoids, there is reluctance to use these drugs, and there is a need for alternative therapies.

During the last decade, there has been an increasing interest in fatty acid supplements as an alternative therapy for pruritic skin disease.[6] The potential beneficial effect of polyunsaturated fatty acids like γ-linolenic acid (GLA), α-linolenic acid (ALA), eicosapentaenoic acid (EPA) and docosahexaenoic acid (DHA) is attributed to a modification of the immune response. In theory, n-6 and n-3 fatty acids can compete for desaturation and elongation enzymes, incorporation into cell membranes, and for cyclooxygenase and lipoxygenase enzymes, leading to the production of several types of eicosanoids with different inflammatory effects.[6,7] Results of studies on the efficacy of fatty acid supplements in the treatment of allergic skin disease in dogs have been conflicting. This may be due to variations in the experimental design.[6,7] The first published studies[8–12] were all open uncontrolled studies using relatively low doses of supplemental fatty acids of 90 mg linoleic acid (LA), 3.4 mg GLA and 5 mg EPA (per MJ). The fatty acids were provided for a relatively short period of 1–2 weeks. Supplementation was reported as successful in 11–35% of patients,[8–12] but it cannot be excluded that the beneficial results were affected by a placebo effect or spontaneous fluctuations in the severity of the clinical symptoms. In two double-blinded crossover studies, supplementation with either 300 mg LA and 40 mg GLA, without or with 16 mg EPA (per MJ), did not result in a convincing difference compared to the control treatment.[13,14] Later studies with higher levels of GLA and EPA proved the efficacy of these fatty acids in the control of allergic dermatitis. In a double-blinded study involving 16 dogs with allergic dermatitis, a high dose of fish oil equivalent to 120 mg EPA and 80 mg DHA (per MJ), provided for 6 weeks, improved the skin and coat condition in 69% of the pruritic dogs.[15] In another double-blinded study, it was also shown that a high dose of 72 or 143 mg GLA (per MJ) improved clinical symptoms of atopic dogs after treatment for 8 weeks.[16] However, in a recently published study a diet supplemented with about 420 mg EPA (per MJ) did not affect the severity of clinical signs when compared to a diet without added EPA.[17]

The objective of the current study was to evaluate the efficacy of a commercial diet rich in fish oil and borage oil in the control of clinical signs in dogs with AD. When compared to test treatments used previously,[8–17] the diet is unique in that it combines a high concentration of EPA (480 mg/MJ) with an increased level of GLA (50 mg/MJ). The study was a randomised, controlled, double-blinded, multicentre trial with well-defined patients.

Materials and methods

The protocol of this study was approved by the animal experiments committee of the Veterinary Faculty of Utrecht University in the Netherlands and the required national authorities. Informed consent of the owner was obtained before any dog was enrolled in the study. Dog owners were allowed to withdraw from the study at any time for any reason.

Selection of dogs with AD

Dogs with perennial pruritic skin disease were chosen from patients from four referral practices of the investigators (BBT, MWV, LN, MHGL, JDS) in Norway, Denmark and the Netherlands. Selection occurred according to a strict protocol. Dogs were only selected if they met the diagnostic criteria for AD[18,19] and when AD was supported by a positive intradermal test (IDT) correlating with the history and clinical signs. The IDT was performed according to standard methods,[18] using the following allergens: pollens of grasses, trees, and weeds; epithelia from humans, cats and dogs; *Dermatophagoides farinae*; *Tyrophagus putrescentiae*; *Acarus siro*; *D. pteronyssinus*; *Lepidoglyphus destructor*; and flea antigen (Artuvetrin, Mycofarm, de Bilt, the Netherlands). Before selection, other possible causes of pruritus were ruled out by using a standardised 'preselection form'. This form systematically listed all required investigations, which are described below, so that for each case all investigations were performed and results were carefully documented. For at least 4 weeks, or 8 weeks in case of flea infestation, a strict flea-control regimen (monthly administration of lufenuron tablets and fipronil) was applied. Dogs with dermatophytosis or with ectoparasites diagnosed by skin scrapes, tape test, otoscopic examination and ear swabs, were excluded. Endoparasites were ruled out by anthelmintic treatment. Bacterial infections and secondary *Malassezia* were diagnosed by cytology and treated with antibiotics (cefadroxil, first generation cephalosporin, 10–30 mg/kg, two or three times daily) and/or topical lotion (chlorhexidine and enilconazole) before the start of the study. In all dogs, adverse reactions to food were ruled out by an elimination food trial with a home-made elimination diet or a commercial hypoallergenic diet for a period of at least 4–5 weeks; the average length of the elimination feeding trial was 53 ± 20 days (means ± SD). Dogs were only enrolled in the study if they were not currently being treated with ASIT. Any long-acting glucocorticoids and fatty acid supplementation was discontinued for at least 8 weeks, and any oral glucocorticoids, antihistamines or non-steroidal anti-inflammatory drugs (NSAIDs) were discontinued for at least 3 weeks prior to the study. Dogs with very severe clinical signs were excluded, because it was considered unacceptable that they may be withheld from any therapy during the study.

Study protocol

During the preselection period, a medical history of each dog was taken and characteristics of the dog were recorded. At week 0 (start of the study), the magnitude of the following clinical signs was scored by the investigators: pruritus (intensity and frequency), shedding, scaling, dryness of skin, erythema, alopecia, smell of coat and lustre of the coat. The magnitude of the clinical signs was scored on a continuous, anchored scale from 1 to 127. For instance, scores for the intensity of pruritus of 1, 26, 51, 76, 102 and 127 corresponded with none, minimal, mild, moderate, severe and extremely severe pruritus, respectively (Fig. 3.1.1). For pruritus a total score was calculated where total severity = intensity × frequency. Besides a score for the severity, the localisation of the clinical signs was recorded by using a ventral and dorsal sketch of the dog.[2]

Dog owners were requested to score their dog's skin and coat condition and to evaluate the incidence of gastrointestinal problems such as vomiting, diarrhoea and flatulence. Owners were also asked to complete a questionnaire regarding the dietary history of the dog and to deliver a sample of the dog's habitual diet for analysis of the fatty acid composition.

The dog owners were asked not to provide food to their dog for at least 12 hours prior to blood sampling. Blood samples were taken from the jugular or cephalic vein and whole blood activated coagulation time (ACT) was determined (Vacutainer ACT tube, Becton Dickinson, Rutherford, NJ, USA). For analysis of cutaneous and subcutaneous fatty acids, a 6-mm biopsy sample of skin with connecting subcutaneous fat tissue was taken from the dorsal area after local anaesthesia with 2% lidocaine hydrochloride and stored at –20°C.

The dogs were randomly assigned to one of two treatment groups. One group of dogs was fed with a commercial test food (SPECIFIC CΩD Eicosa, LEO Animal Health, Ballerup, Denmark) plus one placebo capsule per day. The other group of dogs remained on their habitual diet and also received one placebo capsule per day. The test diet had been developed for nutritional management of dermatological problems associated with hyperresponsive inflammatory reactions and was characterised by high levels of EPA and DHA (guaranteed analysis panel: 480 and 550 mg/MJ, respectively) derived from fish oil and a high level of GLA (50 mg/MJ) derived from borage oil. The test diet was composed of the following raw materials, listed in descending order of quantity: wheat, fish meal, rice, eggs, fish oil, animal fat, hydrolysed chicken protein, minerals, vitamin mix, powdered cellulose, borage oil, *Plantago psyllium* and sunflower oil. The placebo capsules were 250 μl non-transparent gelatin capsules filled with cellulose.

Randomisation occurred according to a computer-generated random number table. The assignment of the dogs was done with case record forms (CRFs) which were linked to a case number and a treatment. Dogs were assigned to a CRF according to the order of entry into the study. In order to blind the study for both the owners and the veterinarians, the case number of the dog was passed on to the study coordinator and the material for treatment (test diet and/or capsules) was sent directly to the owner's home address. Dog owners were instructed not to discuss the type of treatment with the veterinarian. Prior to the study, dog owners were informed that the test treatment could include a diet, capsules, or both, and that the diet, capsules or both could be a placebo. During the study, dogs were allowed to eat the test diet or their habitual diet (depending on their group assignment) only; no treats, snacks or other food was allowed.

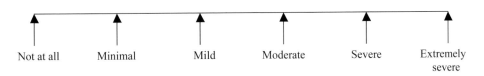

Fig. 3.1.1 Method for scoring of clinical signs. Example from questionnaire for scoring the the intensity of pruritus.

The treatment period lasted 10 weeks. After 3, 6 and 10 weeks of treatment, the severity of the clinical signs was scored without reference to the initial scores. As mentioned above, dog owners were requested to complete a questionnaire with respect to the dog's skin and coat condition, compliance to the treatment, the incidence of gastrointestinal problems, and the evaluation of changes in the dog's skin and coat condition since the start of the study (for example: 'How has the skin and coat condition of your dog changed, when compared to the start of the study? Is it much worse, worse, slightly worse, the same, slightly improved, improved, much improved?'). At week 10 (end of the study), blood samples were collected after the dog had been withheld from food for at least 12 hours and the ACT was determined. A skin biopsy, taken from the dorsal area close to the location of the first skin biopsy, was also obtained at this time.

Crossover design

The control group in the study would not have received a possibly effective treatment. All dogs (from both the control group and the treatment group) whose owners judged that the treatment during the study had not been effective, could participate in a double-blinded crossover period, during which the dog would then receive the other treatment for a period of 10 weeks. During the 10-week crossover period, the study remained double-blinded and the same measurements were performed as during the regular study.

Concomitant treatment during the study

During the entire study, snacks, supplements, glucocorticoids, NSAIDs and antihistamines were not allowed. During each visit, the use of these items was checked and documented in the questionnaire. For all dogs, the same strictly prescribed flea control regimen as applied during the pretrial selection period was continued during the course of the study. Secondary pyoderma was controlled with antibiotics (cefadroxil) and topical antibacterial lotion (chlorhexidine). Secondary Malassezia infection was controlled with topical application of a solution with enilconazole. The use of medication for control of secondary pyoderma and Malassezia infection was recorded as well as the frequency of bathing, swimming and shampooing.

Fatty acid analysis

Fat from plasma, food and skin biopsies was extracted by the method described by Folch et al.[20] Isolated fat and subcutaneous fat samples were saponified and methylated with boron trifluoride[21] and formed methyl esters were subjected to capillary gas chromatography, using a flame ionisation detector, a Chrompack column (Fused Silica, no. 7485, CP.FFAPCB 25 m × 0.32 mm, Chrompack, Middelburg, The Netherlands) and H_2 as carrier gas. Fatty acid methyl esters were expressed as fraction of the total amount.

For an adult dog with constant body weight and body composition, feed intake is determined by its energy requirement (on average 500 kJ/kg$^{0.75}$ daily) and the energy density of the food. As a consequence, nutrient intake depends on the nutrient:energy ratio in the food. The fatty acid composition of the dog's habitual diet and the test diet was therefore also expressed on an energy basis as mg per MJ (1000 kJ) of metabolisable energy. For this purpose, the dietary energy density was calculated on the basis of the analysed dietary crude fat content and the estimated sum of proteins and carbohydrates. It was assumed that all dry diets contained 6% ash, 2% crude fibre and 8% water. One dog in the study had a wet diet as its habitual diet; for this diet, the declared values for ash, crude fibre and water were used. The following conversion factors were used to calculate the metabolisable energy content of the diets: 1 g crude protein or carbohydrates = 16.7 kJ and 1 g crude fat = 37.6 kJ. It was assumed that 88% of the extracted fat was composed of fatty acids.

Statistical analysis

Data are expressed as means ± SEM. All statistical analyses were performed with the statistical program SPSS 10.1 for Windows (SPSS Inc., Chicago, IL, USA). The two-sided level of significance was pre-set at $p < 0.05$. Group means were compared by a Student's t-test or, when data were not linear or normally distributed, by the Mann–Whitney U test. Differences between groups regarding nominal data were evaluated by the chi-square test. Relationships between variables were evaluated by calculation of Pearson's or Spearman rank correlation coefficients. Time effects were evaluated by a paired Student's t-test.

Results

The study was performed between October 2000 and May 2003. Thirty dogs were selected for enrolment into the study. Two dogs dropped out during the first week of the study; one dog refused to eat the test diet, and the other dog was euthanised because of severe clinical signs. In total, 13 dogs receiving the control treatment and 15 dogs receiving the test diet completed the study. Of the 13 control dogs, 9 followed the initial controlled study with a subsequent crossover period on the test diet, so that the total number of dogs that had received the test diet was 24 by the end of the study. Treatment of dogs with the test diet during either the controlled study or the crossover period occurred partly simultaneously. Statistical analysis of the results of the controlled study alone gave similar results to the combined data from the controlled study and the crossover dogs. However, for the evaluation of the efficacy of the diet, only the results of the controlled study ($n = 13$ in the control group and $n = 15$ in the treatment group) were considered. Besides these data from the controlled study, the pooled data from all 24 dogs that received the test diet are shown as well.

Characteristics of dogs

There was no significant difference in age, age at onset of AD, body weight or gender between control dogs and dogs fed the test diet during the controlled study (Table 3.1.1). Eighteeen breeds were represented with the German shepherd dog ($n = 4$), golden retriever (4), Labrador retriever (2), boxer (2) and white elkhound (2) being the most common breeds. There was no difference in breed distribution between the two experimental groups.

The two groups did not differ regarding the first signs of AD, which included pruritus in 91% of dogs and erythema in 51%. Paws were first involved in 74% and ears first in 43%. The localisation of the first signs to the paws was significantly different between groups; 50% in the control group and 93% in the treatment group. In the majority of the dogs (70%), there was no seasonal fluctuation in the severity of clinical signs.

For all dogs in the controlled study, the average number of positive reactions on intradermal testing was 4.2 ± 0.3. There was no significant difference between the two groups for the total number of positive reactions or for reactions to individual allergens on the IDT. Positive reactions were most common with *D. farinae* (86%), *T. putrescentia* (75%), *A. siro* (68%), *L. destructor* (43%) and *D. pteronyssinus* (32%). When allergens were grouped in categories, all dogs had a positive reaction to at least one mite and 96% of dogs had a positive reaction to house dust mites (*D. farinae* and/or *D. pteronyssinus*).

The 24 dogs treated with the test diet (controlled and crossover study) did not differ from the control group (in the controlled study) regarding any of the characteristics mentioned above.

Fatty acid composition of the diet

The fatty acid composition of the habitual diet of the two groups prior to entry into the controlled study did not differ significantly, except for the level of EPA, which was higher in the habitual diet of the treatment group (Table 3.1.2). During the trial, the control dogs remained on their habitual diet and the dogs in the treatment group were switched over to the test diet. The change to the test diet for the treatment group resulted in significant

		Controlled, double-blinded study		Crossover study
Table 3.1.1 Characteristics of the dogs		Control group ($n = 13$)	Treatment group ($n = 15$)	All dogs treated with test diet ($n = 24$)
Features				
Age of dog (year)*		3.4 ± 0.7	4.5 ± 0.5	4.0 ± 0.5
Age at onset of AD (year)*		1.7 ± 0.4	2.0 ± 0.4	1.8 ± 0.3
Body weight (kg)*		24.3 ± 2.7	27.4 ± 4.3	26.8 ± 3.0
Sex	Female (%)	33.3	66.7	56.5
	Male (%)	66.7	33.3	43.5

*Values represent means $\pm$ SEM ($n = 12$–13 for the control group, $n = 15$ for treatment group, $n = 23$–24 for all dogs treated with the test diet).

Table 3.1.2 Analysed fatty acid composition of habitual diet and test diet of control and treatment groups

Fatty acids	Controlled study			Habitual diet of all dogs on test diet
	Habitual diet of control group	Habitual diet of treatment group	Test diet of treatment group	
Saturated FA				
C16:0	1497 ± 123 (21.5 ± 0.4)	1505 ± 102 (21.6 ± 0.3)	1964 (19.3) [c]	1471 ± 76 (21.4 ± 0.2)
C18:0	752 ± 110 (10.5 ± 0.9)	674 ± 65 (9.7 ± 0.9)	663 (6.5)	667 ± 50 (9.7 ± 0.6)
Monounsaturated FA				
C18:1n-9	2333 ± 194 (33.3 ± 0.8)	2346 ± 198 (33.1 ± 1.0)	2381 (23.4)	2309 ± 138 (33.3 ± 0.6)
Polyunsaturated FA				
Total n-6	1291 ± 121 (19.0 ± 1.6)	1325 ± 125 (19.1 ± 1.2)	1083 (10.7)	1303 ± 88 (19.2 ± 1.0)
LA	1236 ± 118 (18.2 ± 1.6)	1270 ± 120 (18.3 ± 1.1)	893 (8.8) [b]	1248 ± 85 (18.4 ± 0.1)
GLA	2 ± 1 (0 ± 0)	5 ± 2 (0 ± 0)	60 (0.6) [d]	4 ± 2 (0 ± 0)
DGLA	3 ± 2 (0 ± 0)	3 ± 1 (0 ± 0)	15 (0.2) [d]	4 ± 1 (0 ± 0)
AA	34 ± 5 (0.5 ± 0.1)	27 ± 3 (0.4 ± 0.1)	76 (0.8) [d]	28 ± 2 (0.4 ± 0.0)
Total n-3	205 ± 21 (3.1 ± 0.4)	230 ± 28 (3.6 ± 0.5)	1536 (15.1) [d]	225 ± 18 (3.6 ± 0.4)
ALA	144 ± 22 (2.3 ± 0.4)	104 ± 14 (1.5 ± 0.2)	97 (1.0)	121 ± 14 (1.9 ± 0.3)
EPA	12 ± 6 (0.2 ± 0.1)	46 ± 12 (0.7 ± 0.2) [a]	578 (5.7) [d]	35 ± 9 (0.5 ± 0.1)
DHA	26 ± 11 (0.4 ± 0.2)	55 ± 11 (1.0 ± 0.3)	690 (6.8) [d]	46 ± 9 (0.8 ± 0.2)

During the study, the dogs in the control group remained on their habitual diet. The dietary fatty acid levels are expressed in mg/MJ and values represent means ± SEM ($n =13$ for control group, $n = 14–15$ for treatment group, $n = 23–24$ for all dogs treated with the test diet). Data in parentheses indicate level of fatty acids expressed as percentage of total fatty acids (means ± SEM). AA, arachidonic acid (C20:4n-6); ALA, α-linolenic acid (C18:3n-3); DGLA, dihomo-γ-linolenic acid (C20:3n-6); DHA, docosahexaenoic acid (C22:6 n-3); EPA, eicosapentaenoic acid (C20:5n-3); FA, fatty acids; GLA, γ-linolenic acid (C18:3n-6); LA, linoleic acid (C18:2 n-6).
[a]Significant difference in fatty acid composition (expressed in mg/MJ) between habitual diet of control group and habitual diet of treatment group in the controlled study, $p < 0.05$.
[b]Significant difference in fatty acid composition (expressed in mg/MJ) between habitual diet of control group and test diet of treatment group in the controlled study, $p < 0.05$.
[c]Significant difference in fatty acid composition (expressed in mg/MJ) between habitual diet of control group and test diet of treatment group in the controlled study, $p < 0.01$.
[d]Significant difference in fatty acid composition (expressed in mg/MJ) between habitual diet of control group and test diet of treatment group in the controlled study, $p < 0.001$.

differences between groups regarding the dietary levels of most fatty acids. The relatively high content of fish oil in the test diet resulted in considerably increased levels of total n-3 fatty acids, EPA and DHA compared with the diet of the control group. The addition of borage oil to the test diet was associated with an increased level of GLA. The test diet contained less LA, and more DGLA and AA, than the habitual diet of the control dogs.

The body weight of the group of control dogs and the group of dogs fed the test diet did not change significantly during the study.

Clinical signs

The initial scores for clinical signs of the two groups in the controlled study are shown in Table 3.1.3, as well as the average initial scores for all 24 dogs receiving the test diet. At the start of the controlled study, the dogs of the treatment group had significantly higher scores (indicating more severe signs) for frequency of pruritus, total pruritus score, scaling, erythema and smell of coat. There were no significant differences in localisation of clinical signs. At the start of the study, the most common localisations for clinical signs were pruritus on the front legs including paws (93% of dogs), erythema on the front legs (85%), pruritus on the head (67%), pruritus on the hindquarters (63%) and erythema on the head (59%).

For each dog, the scores for clinical signs after 3, 6 and 10 weeks of treatment were expressed as a percentage of the initial score at week 0. The scores for intensity and frequency and total score for pruritus after 10 weeks of treatment were significantly reduced in dogs fed the test diet, when compared with control dogs in the controlled study (Fig. 3.1.2). After 10 weeks on the

Table 3.1.3 Initial scores for severity of clinical signs in dogs from the control and treatment group

Score for clinical sign[1]	Controlled, double-blinded study		All dogs treated with test diet
	Control group	Treatment group	
Pruritus, intensity	72 ± 6	85 ± 6	84 ± 4
Pruritus, frequency	64 ± 5	86 ± 6[b]	93 ± 5[d]
Pruritus, total[2]	4808 ± 631	7608 ± 862[a]	7202 ± 609[c]
Shedding	58 ± 6	58 ± 8	59 ± 6
Scaling	31 ± 5	51 ± 8[a]	50 ± 7
Dry skin and coat	53 ± 7	69 ± 6	63 ± 5
Erythema	51 ± 5	73 ± 5[b]	70 ± 5[c]
Smell of coat	21 ± 6	52 ± 9[a]	44 ± 6[c]
Alopecia	28 ± 5	30 ± 7	35 ± 6
General condition of skin and coat	81 ± 8	53 ± 9	59 ± 8
Lustre of fur	68 ± 7	56 ± 7	57 ± 6

Results are expressed as means ± SEM ($n = 11$–13 for control group, $n = $ 14–15 for treatment group, $n = $ 23–24 for all dogs treated with the test diet).

[1]Clinical signs were scored on a scale from 1 to 127. Higher scores for pruritus, shedding, scaling, dry skin, erythema, smell of coat and alopecia correspond to more severe clinical signs. Higher scores for general condition and lustre of coat correspond to a better skin and coat condition.

[2]Total score for pruritus was calculated as intensity × frequency.

[a]Significant difference between control and treatment group in controlled study, $p < 0.05$.

[b]Significant difference between control and treatment group in controlled study, $p < 0.01$.

[c] Significant difference between control group and all dogs treated with test diet, $p < 0.05$.

[d]Significant difference between control group and all dogs treated with test diet, $p < 0.01$.

test diet, the mean score for intensity, frequency and total pruritus score was reduced to 68, 63 and 52% of the initial score, respectively. Significant changes in pruritus were recorded after 6 weeks of treatment.

The score for erythema in dogs fed the test diet was significantly reduced to 62% of the initial score after 10 weeks of treatment. The difference in relative score for erythema between the two groups of the controlled study only reached significance after 10 weeks of treatment (Fig. 3.1.3).

At the end of the controlled study, there was no significant difference between the groups in the scores for shedding, scaling, dryness of skin, smell of coat, alopecia and lustre of the fur. However, the general condition of skin and coat of dogs fed the test diet had significantly improved compared with the control dogs (1367 ± 584 versus 94 ± 14%; $p < 0.05$).

After 10 weeks of treatment with the test diet, the 24 dogs on the test diet (dogs in the controlled study and crossover study together) had significantly different relative scores for pruritus (intensity, frequency and total score), erythema, general condition of skin and coat and lustre of the fur (67, 66, 53, 66, 1170 and 175% of the initial score, respectively), compared with the control group.

Owner's assessment of response

After 6 and 10 weeks of treatment, there was a significant difference between the two groups in the controlled study in owner's assessment of change in the dogs' skin

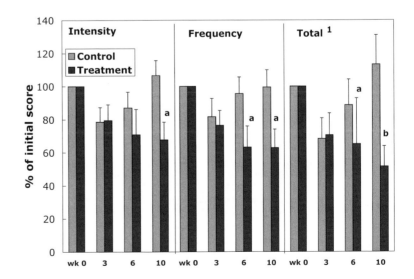

Fig. 3.1.2 Pruritus in dogs from the control and treatment group after 3, 6 and 10 weeks of treatment in the controlled study (week 0). The score for pruritus is expressed as percentage of the initial score at the start of the study (week 0). Values represent means ± SEM ($n = 13$ for control group, $n = 15$ for treatment group). 1, Total score for pruritus is calculated as intensity x frequency; a, Significant difference between groups (Mann–Whitney U test, $p < 0.05$); b, Significant difference between groups (Mann–Whitney U test, $p < 0.01$).

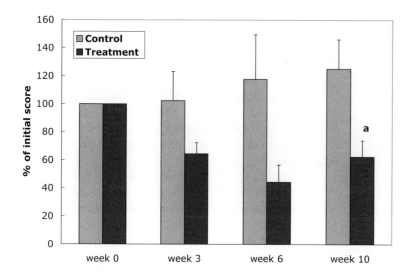

Fig. 3.1.3 Erythema in dogs from the control and treatment group after 3, 6 and 10 weeks of treatment in the controlled study. The score for erythema is expressed as percentage of the initial score at the start of the study (week 0). Values represent means ± SEM ($n = 13$ for control group, $n = 15$ for treatment group). a, Significant difference between groups (Mann–Whitney U test, $p < 0.05$).

and coat condition (Table 3.1.4). In the group of dogs that received the test diet, more owners indicated that the dog had improved, and the extent of improvement in these dogs was greater than in the control dogs. Further, when all 24 dogs fed with the test diet were considered together, the owners' assessments of the changes in skin and coat condition were significantly better than those of the owners of dogs fed the control diet.

Concomitant treatment and side effects

During the controlled study, approximately 20% of the dogs received antibiotics and 19% received local treatment for *Malassezia* dermatitis. There was no significant difference in use of medication between the two groups. The incidence of swimming, bathing or shampooing was similar for both groups. There was sporadic vomiting, diarrhoea and flatulence in the dogs, without any significant difference between groups. There were also no significant differences in the incidence of concomitant treatment or side effects between control dogs and all 24 dogs fed the test diet.

At the start of the study, the whole blood ACT was 118 ± 10 s in dogs from the treatment group and 116

Table 3.1.4 Owner's assessment of the dog's response to the treatment

	Controlled, double-blinded study								
	Control group			Treatment group			All dogs treated with test diet		
Assessment	wk 3	wk 6	wk 10	wk3	wk 6[a]	wk 10[a]	wk 3	wk 6[b]	wk 10[b]
Markedly worse	0	0	7.7	0	7.1	0	0	4.2	0
Worse	7.7	7.7	7.7	7.1	0	0	4.2	0	0
Somewhat worse	15.4	23.1	7.7	0	0	6.7	4.2	4.2	8.3
Unchanged	46.2	38.5	46.2	28.6	14.3	33.3	25	12.5	37.5
Somewhat improved	23.1	23.1	23.1	50	42.9	0	45.8	33.3	4.2
Improved	7.7	7.7	7.7	14.3	35.7	40	8.3	29.2	33.3
Markedly improved	0	0	0	0	0	20	12.5	16.7	16.7

Results are expressed as percentage of dogs.
[a]Significant difference between control and treatment group during controlled study in frequency distribution of owner's assessment of response at week 6 and week 10, $p < 0.05$.
[b]Significant difference between control group and all dogs fed the test diet in frequency distribution of owner's assessment of response after 6 and 10 weeks, $p < 0.05$.

± 8 s in the control dogs. After 10 weeks of treatment, the ACT in dogs fed with the test diet was 114 ± 9 s and 102 ± 4 s in the control dogs. There was no significant difference in ACT between groups, nor any time effect within groups. The whole blood ACT in the group of 24 dogs was 114 ± 7 s before and 107 ± 6 s after receiving the diet for 10 weeks.

Fatty acid composition of plasma, skin and subcutaneous fat

Plasma samples of seven dogs (four from the treatment group and three from the control group) were excluded from statistical analysis because of a temporary interruption of the electricity supply during storage of these samples. Analysis of the chromatogram of these samples showed increased levels of unidentified peaks, suggesting oxidation of the plasma fatty acids. The results for fatty acid composition of skin and subcutaneous fat in these dogs were not compromised. In contrast to fatty acids in an aqueous environment, polyunsaturated fatty acids in fat tissue are very stable[22] and the chromatograms of fatty acids in skin and fat tissue from these dogs did not show oxidation of fatty acids.

Initial fatty acid composition

The initial plasma fatty acid compositions of dogs are shown in Table 3.1.5. At the start of the controlled study, the plasma fatty acid composition of both groups was identical. Fatty acid composition in skin biopsies taken at the start of the study was similar for both groups, except for the level of palmitic acid (C16:0), which was significantly higher in the control group (Table 3.1.6). The fatty acid composition of subcutaneous fat tissue was almost identical to that of skin and did not differ between groups (data not shown).

There were significant correlations between the fatty acid levels in the habitual diet, plasma, skin and subcutaneous fat tissue at the start of the study (Table 3.1.7). The total dietary n-6 fatty acids correlated well with the total level of n-6 fatty acids in plasma, fat tissue and skin. A similar correlation was found for LA, the most abundant n-6 fatty acid. There was no correlation between the dietary level of AA and the AA level in plasma, fat tissue or skin.

Table 3.1.5 Plasma fatty acid composition in control and treatment group at week 0 and week 10

Fatty acids, % of total FA	Controlled, double-blinded study				All dogs treated with test diet	
	Control group		Treatment group			
	Week 0	Week 10	Week 0	Week 10	Week 0	Week 10
Saturated FA						
C16:0	14.7 ± 0.2	15.1 ± 0.1[a]	14.5 ± 0.4	13.2 ± 0.4[a,f]	14.7 ± 0.2	13.7 ± 0.3[b,j]
C18:0	21.7 ± 0.3	20.1 ± 0.4[b]	20.8 ± 0.4	20.6 ± 0.5	20.5 ± 0.3[h]	19.9 ± 0.4
Monounsaturated FA						
C18:1n-9	11.5 ± 0.4	12.2 ± 0.5	11.4 ± 0.5	10.2 ± 0.3[e]	11.6 ± 0.4	10.2 ± 0.2[b,j]
Polyunsaturated FA						
Total n-6	40.1 ± 1.1	40.2 ± 1.5	39.9 ± 1.1	28.6 ± 1.1[c,f]	40.1 ± 1.0	28.3 ± 0.8[b,j]
LA	21.8 ± 0.8	23.0 ± 1.1	23.7 ± 0.7	16.2 ± 0.9[c,f]	23.6 ± 0.6	16.5 ± 0.6[c,j]
GLA	0.1 ± 0.0	0.1 ± 0.0	0.1 ± 0.0	0.2 ± 0.0	0.1 ± 0.0	0.2 ± 0.0
DGLA	1.2 ± 0.1	1.1 ± 0.1	1.1 ± 0.1	0.8 ± 0.0[b,d]	1.1 ± 0.1	0.8 ± 0.0[c,i]
AA	16.3 ± 0.6	15.2 ± 0.9	14.4 ± 0.9	11.2 ± 0.5[b,e]	14.7 ± 0.6	10.7 ± 0.4[c,j]
Total n-3	5.2 ± 0.8	5.8 ± 1.2	7.2 ± 1.0	20.4 ± 1.2[c,f]	6.8 ± 0.9	20.5 ± 0.9[c,j]
ALA	0.2 ± 0.1	0.3 ± 0.1	0.1 ± 0.1	0.1 ± 0.0	0.2 ± 0.1	0.2 ± 0.0
EPA	1.0 ± 0.2	1.3 ± 0.4	2.3 ± 0.5	9.8 ± 0.8[c,f]	1.9 ± 0.4	10.4 ± 0.7[c,j]
DHA	2.0 ± 0.5	2.3 ± 0.7	2.8 ± 0.4	8.4 ± 0.5[c,f]	2.7 ± 0.4	8.0 ± 0.4[c,j]

Values are expressed as means ± SEM. See Table 3.1.2 for explanation of fatty acid abbreviations.
Significant difference within group between week 0 and week 10: [a] $p < 0.05$; [b] $p < 0.01$; [c] $p < 0.001$.
Significant difference at same date between control group and treatment group in the controlled study: [d] $p < 0.05$; [e] $p < 0.01$; [f] $p < 0.001$.
Significant difference at same date between control group and all dogs treated with the test diet: [h] $p < 0.05$; [i] $p < 0.01$; [j] $p < 0.001$.

Fatty acids, % of total FA	Controlled, double-blinded study				All dogs treated with test diet	
	Control group		Treatment group			
	Week 0	Week 10	Week 0	Week 10	Week 0	Week 10
Saturated FA						
C16:0	15.7 ± 0.3	15.5 ± 0.2	14.4 ± 0.5^d	14.3 ± 0.5	14.9 ± 0.3	14.9 ± 0.4
C18:0	5.4 ± 0.3	5.2 ± 0.3	5.1 ± 0.3	4.9 ± 0.3	5.2 ± 0.3	4.9 ± 0.2
Monounsaturated FA						
C18:1n-9	45.6 ± 0.7	46.6 ± 0.9^a	45.7 ± 0.9	45.7 ± 1.0	45.8 ± 0.7	44.7 ± 0.8^a
Polyunsaturated FA						
Total n-6	13.2 ± 0.9	12.7 ± 0.9	14.1 ± 0.9	13.1 ± 0.6^a	13.8 ± 0.7	12.7 ± 0.5^b
LA	12.8 ± 0.8	12.4 ± 0.8	13.7 ± 0.8	12.7 ± 0.6^a	13.4 ± 0.6	12.3 ± 0.5^b
GLA	0.0 ± 0.0	0.0 ± 0.0	0.0 ± 0.0	0.0 ± 0.0	0.0 ± 0.0	0.0 ± 0.0
DGLA	0.1 ± 0.1	0.0 ± 0.0	0.0 ± 0.0	0.0 ± 0.0	0.0 ± 0.0	0.0 ± 0.0
AA	0.3 ± 0.0	0.2 ± 0.1^a	0.2 ± 0.0	0.2 ± 0.1	0.2 ± 0.0	0.3 ± 0.0
Total n-3	1.3 ± 0.1	1.2 ± 0.1	1.3 ± 0.1	1.6 ± 0.2	1.3 ± 0.1	1.9 ± 0.2^{c,e}
ALA	0.8 ± 0.1	0.8 ± 0.1	0.7 ± 0.1	0.7 ± 0.0	0.8 ± 0.1	0.7 ± 0.0
EPA	0.0 ± 0.0	0.0 ± 0.0	0.0 ± 0.0	0.2 ± 0.1^{b,f}	0.0 ± 0.0	0.3 ± 0.0^{c,f}
DHA	0.0 ± 0.0	0.0 ± 0.0	0.0 ± 0.0	0.3 ± 0.1^{c,e}	0.0 ± 0.0	0.4 ± 0.1^{c,f}

Table 3.1.6 Fatty acid composition in skin in dogs from control and treatment group at week 0 and week 10

Values are expressed as means ± SEM. See Table 3.1.2 for explanation of fatty acid abbreviations. Significant difference within group between week 0 and week 10: $^a p < 0.05$; $^b p < 0.01$; $^c p < 0.001$. Significant difference at same date between control group and treatment group in the controlled study: $^d p < 0.05$.
Significant difference at same date between control group and all dogs treated with the test diet: $^e p < 0.01$; $^f p < 0.001$.

Table 3.1.7 Pearson's correlation coefficients between fatty acid levels in diet, plasma, skin and subcutaneous fat tissue at the start of the study

Fatty acid	Significant Pearson's correlation coefficients between				
	diet and plasma (n = 27)	diet and fat tissue (n = 35)	diet and skin (n = 35)	plasma and skin (n = 27)	fat tissue and skin (n = 36)
Saturated FA					
C16:0	–	–	–	0.40^b	0.84^c
C18:0	–	0.38^b	–	–	0.84^c
Monosaturated FA					
C18:1n-9	–	–	–	–	0.84^c
Polyunsaturated FA					
Total n-6	0.60^a	0.50^a	0.58^c	–	0.92^c
LA	0.40^b	0.49^a	0.57^c	–	0.93^c
GLA	–	–	–	*	*
DGLA	–	0.36^b	–	–	–
AA	–	–	–	0.44^b	0.49^a
Total n-3	0.62^c	0.64^c	0.73^c	–	0.83^c
ALA	0.81^c	0.57^c	0.77^c	0.60^a	0.96^c
EPA	0.80^c	0.34^b	0.60^c	0.59^a	0.64^c
DHA	0.90^c	0.48^a	0.40^b	–	0.86^c

See Table 3.1.2 for explanation of fatty acid abbreviations.
*Correlation could not be calculated, because all values were below the detection limit.
$^a p < 0.05$; $^b p < 0.01$; $^c p < 0.001$.

There was a significant correlation between the dietary total n-3 fatty acids, as well as ALA, EPA and DHA and the levels in plasma, fat tissue and skin. However, it should be noted that for almost all habitual diets, the levels of EPA and DHA in fat tissue and skin were 0 (i.e. below the detection limit). The significant correlation was therefore based only on a few cases with higher levels of EPA and DHA in skin and fat tissue. Except for AA, no correlation was found between the level of n-6 fatty acids in plasma and skin. For the n-3 fatty acids, only ALA and EPA had significant correlation between plasma and skin levels. The fatty acid levels of GLA and DGLA in fat tissue and skin were too low to detect any correlation. However, for all other fatty acids, there was a high correlation between the fatty acid composition of skin and subcutaneous fat tissue.

Post-trial fatty acid composition

During the controlled trial, the control dogs remained on their habitual diet. As expected, the fatty acid composition of plasma (Table 3.1.5) and skin (Table 3.1.6) from control dogs changed very little during the study. In the dogs fed the test diet, the plasma fatty acid composition changed considerably (Table

3.1.5). The level of palmitic acid (C16:0) decreased compared with initial values and the level of palmitic acid (C16:0) and oleic acid (C18:1n-9) was significantly different from the control group. These differences reflect the levels of palmitic and oleic acid in the test diet, expressed as percentage of total fatty acids rather than as mg/MJ. The plasma levels of total n-6 fatty acids and LA in dogs fed the test diet were significantly reduced compared with initial values and post-trial levels in the control dogs. Although the test diet had a much higher level of GLA than the habitual diet, the plasma level of GLA in dogs fed the test diet did not increase significantly. Even though the levels of DGLA and AA in the test diet were increased compared with the dogs' habitual diet, the plasma levels of these fatty acids decreased after eating the test diet. The increased levels of EPA, DHA and total n-3 fatty acids in the test diet were associated with a significant increase in the plasma levels of EPA, DHA and total n-3 fatty acids.

The most abundant type of fatty acid in skin was oleic acid. The post-trial cutaneous level of oleic acid in the control group was increased compared with initial values, but there was no difference between groups (Table 3.1.6). The level of total n-6 fatty acids and LA in skin from dogs fed the test diet was slightly reduced compared with baseline. The switch to the test diet was associated with a significant, although small, increase in the cutaneous content of EPA and DHA. The response in fatty acid composition in subcutaneous fat was almost identical to that in skin (data not shown).

The response in fatty acid composition of plasma, skin and subcutaneous fat in the group of all 24 dogs that were fed the test diet was similar to the response of the treatment group during the controlled study. The increase in the cutaneous level of n-3 fatty acids, which failed to reach statistical significance in the treatment group of the controlled study, was significant for the group of all 24 dogs receiving the test diet.

Comparison of responders and non-responders of dogs fed the test diet

The relative score for clinical signs and the owners' assessments of the dogs' response to the test diet did not differ significantly between the subgroup of dogs that received the test diet during the crossover period ($n = 9$) and the subgroup of dogs that received the test diet during the controlled study ($n = 15$).

Of all 24 dogs fed the test diet, 46% of the owners indicated that the dog did not improve (non-responders, owner's assessment: 'markedly worse', 'worse', 'somewhat worse' or 'unchanged'), whereas 54% of the owners indicated that the dog improved on the diet (responders, owner's assessment: 'somewhat improved', 'improved', or 'markedly improved') (Table 3.1.4). Responders and non-responders differed significantly regarding the relative score for intensity, frequency and total score for pruritus, erythema and alopecia (Table 3.1.8).

There were no significant differences between responders and non-responders as to age, age at onset of AD, body weight, breed, gender, type and localisation of the first signs of AD or seasonal fluctuation of clinical signs. There was no significant difference between study centres in frequency distribution of responders and non-responders.

The responders and non-responders did not differ regarding the total number of offending allergens, but significantly more non-responders than responders had a positive reaction towards *L. destructor*; 63.6% of the non-responders had a positive intradermal test towards *L. destructor*, compared with 15.4% of the responders.

The initial score for severity of clinical signs of the responders and non-responders did not differ, except for the score for the frequency of pruritus. There was no significant correlation between the initial severity of the clinical signs and the extent of response to the test diet.

There was a significant difference between responders and non-responders concerning the incidence of secondary lesions on the limbs at the start of the study. In the group of non-responders, 63.6% of the dogs had secondary lesions such as crusts, hyperpigmentation, hyperkeratosis and hypertrophy on their limbs, compared with 7.7% of the dogs in the group of responders. The responders and non-responders did not differ in use of medication and incidence of bathing, swimming and shampooing.

The fatty acid composition of the habitual diet of responders and non-responders was similar as well, as were the initial fatty acid composition of plasma, skin and subcutaneous fat tissue. However, there was a trend that the responders had higher initial levels of total n-6 fatty acids and LA in their subcutaneous fat tissue; the level of total n-6 fatty acids was $13.1 \pm 0.9\%$ in non-responders and $16.0 \pm 1.1\%$ in responders (Student's t-test, $p = 0.059$); the level of LA was $12.8 \pm$

Table 3.1.8 Comparison between responders and non-responders fed the test diet for selected variables

Variable	Responders ($n = 13$)	Non-responders ($n = 115$)
Relative score at week 10 for		
Pruritus, intensity	48 ± 10	90 ± 9[a]
Pruritus, frequency	50 ± 10	86 ± 12[a]
Pruritus, total	34 ± 10	79 ± 16[a]
Erythema	43 ± 10	93 ± 19[a]
Alopecia	54 ± 12	526 ± 294[a]
Number of offending allergens	3.9 ± 0.4	4.4 ± 0.5
Positive reaction towards Glycophagus, Lepidoglypus destructor, %	15.4	63.6[a]
Initial score for		
Pruritus, intensity	84 ± 6	83 ± 8
Pruritus, frequency	86 ± 8	79 ± 3[a]
Pruritus, total	7699 ± 1044	6615 ± 499
Erythema	77 ± 6	62 ± 6
Incidence of secondary lesion on limbs, %	7.7	63.6[b]
Fatty acids in plasma at week 10, % of total FA		
Total n-6	27.9 ± 1.1	28.7 ± 1.3
LA	15.6 ± 0.7	17.4 ± 1.0
GLA	0.2 ± 0.0	0.2 ± 0.0
DGLA	0.8 ± 0.0	0.7 ± 0.1
AA	11.2 ± 0.7	10.2 ± 0.5
Total n-3	21.9 ± 1.1	19.0 ± 1.5
ALA	0.1 ± 0.0	0.3 ± 0.0[a]
EPA	10.9 ± 0.9	9.8 ± 1.0
DHA	8.7 ± 0.5	7.2 ± 0.4[a]
Fatty acids in skin at week 10, % of total FA		
Total n-6	13.4 ± 0.8	11.9 ± 0.6
LA	12.9 ± 0.7	11.5 ± 0.6
AA	0.3 ± 0.1	0.3 ± 0.1
Total n-3	1.9 ± 0.2	2.0 ± 0.3
ALA	0.7 ± 0.0	0.7 ± 0.1
EPA	0.3 ± 0.1	0.3 ± 0.1
DHA	0.4 ± 0.1	0.5 ± 0.1

Values represent means ± SEM, unless indicated otherwise. See Table 3.1.2 for explanation of fatty acid abbreviations and Table 3.1.3 for explanation of clinical scores.
Significant difference between responders and non-responders: [a] $p < 0.05$; [b] $p < 0.01$.

0.8% in non-responders and 15.7 ± 1.1% in responders (Student's t-test, $p = 0.057$). At the end of the study, responders had a somewhat lower level of ALA and a higher level of DHA in their plasma (Table 3.1.8).

At the start of the study, all dogs had cutaneous levels of EPA below the detection limit. In the group of dogs eating the test diet, the average cutaneous level of EPA increased significantly during the study, with a considerable variation between dogs. However, there was no significant difference between the responders and non-responders with respect to the cutaneous level of EPA at the end of the study. In the group of responders, there were five dogs which still had cutaneous levels of EPA below the detection limit at the end of the study. The post-trial levels of other fatty acids in the skin and subcutaneous fat were also similar for responders and non-responders. The change during the study in the level of total n-3 fatty acids, ALA, EPA or DHA in the skin, expressed as either percentage of total fatty acids or as percentage of initial values, did not differ between responders and non-responders. For all 24 dogs fed the test diet, there was no correlation between the change in total n-3 fatty acids, ALA, EPA or DHA or the final level of total n-3 fatty acids, ALA, EPA or DHA in the skin on the one hand, and the relative scores for clinical signs at week 10 on the other hand.

Discussion

In this controlled, double-blinded, multicentre trial with atopic dogs, a switch from the dogs' habitual diet to a diet rich in fish oil and borage oil resulted in a significant reduction of the scores for pruritus and erythema, when compared with the group of control dogs. Pruritus and erythema had been identified in the study as the first and most prevalent clinical signs of AD. The reduction in the severity of pruritus and erythema became significant after 6–10 weeks of treatment. In other double-blinded studies a similar period was required before any significant effect of fatty acid supplementation could be detected.[15,16] In some open trials[8–12] and a single-blinded study,[23] effects were already reported after 1–3 weeks of supplementation. It cannot be excluded that the results of these latter studies were affected by a placebo effect, spontaneous fluctuations of clinical symptoms,[8–12] or interference by adverse food reactions (food allergy),[23] especially as the time required to alter the fatty acid composition of skin is more than 6 weeks.[7]

After 6 and 10 weeks of treatment, significantly more owners of dogs eating the test diet indicated that the dog had improved, compared with owners of dogs in the control group. In the controlled study, 40% of the dogs did not respond to the test diet, whereas 60% of the dogs improved. In other studies on the efficacy of fatty acid supplementation in the control of AD, it was also found that only a fraction of the dogs responded.[8–12,15,16,23] In the group of responders in this study, the average post-trial score for intensity, frequency and total score for pruritus, erythema and alopecia was reduced to 48, 50, 34, 43 and 54% of the initial score, respectively. Thus, although the diet was effective in reducing the severity of clinical signs, the clinical signs may not completely disappear. The test diet should therefore not be regarded as a single treatment for complete control of AD.

The finding that almost all dogs were allergic to house dust mite indicates that it is almost impossible to avoid contact with the offending allergen. In about 70% of the atopic dogs, ASIT can be effective.[5] During ASIT, and in all other cases where ASIT is not possible or desired, the clinical signs of AD should be controlled by several measures such as flea control, control of secondary pyoderma or *Malassezia* infection, bathing, optimal nutrition, medications, etc. By a combination of measures, it may be possible to reduce the degree of pruritus below the pruritic threshold. The finding that some control dogs improved during the study could also be explained by the combination of measures taken and thorough clinical management during the study. The use of a diet rich in fish oil and borage oil can make an important contribution to the reduction of the degree of pruritus, possibly to a level below the pruritic threshold.

It has been suggested that high doses of fish oil can be associated with side effects such as prolonged bleeding time, vomiting, diarrhoea, flatulence and *in vivo* lipid oxidation. Studies on the incidence of these side effects are not consistent.[6] In this study, the use of a test diet with high levels of fish oil and borage oil was not associated with an increased incidence of vomiting, diarrhoea, flatulence or whole blood ACT. During this study, we did not measure the dogs' antioxidant status. However, in another study with healthy dogs, we found that the dogs' antioxidant status improved on the test diet (after 60 days on the diet, the plasma total antioxidant status significantly increased from 0.91 ± 0.06 to 1.00 ± 0.06 mmol/L, unpublished results). This finding is probably related to the use of a mix of antioxidants (butylhydroxytoluene, ascorbyl palmitate, propyl gallate and citric acid monoglyceride ester) and a high level of vitamin E (30 mg/MJ) in the test diet.

Historical features and clinical signs of responders and non-responders were almost identical. However, significantly more non-responders had a positive intradermal test towards *L. destructor*. It is not clear if and how a positive reaction towards *L. destructor* can affect the response to the test diet. In a study on the response to ASIT, it was noted that there was a lower response in case of positive reactions towards certain allergens, but not in relation to a positive reaction towards *L. destructor*.[5] The fact that 15% of the responders had a positive IDT to *L. destructor* indicates that hypersensitivity to *L. destructor* does not necessarily indicate that a dog will not respond to the diet. At the start of the study, non-responders also had a significantly higher incidence of secondary lesions on their limbs. It remains unknown if this affected the response to the diet.

During the study, the dogs in the treatment group received the test diet and a daily placebo capsule, whereas the control dogs remained on their habitual diet and also received a daily placebo capsule. The only difference between the treatment group and the control group was thus a switch from the dogs' habitual diet to the test diet. Although it is hypothesised that the observed effect of the test diet can be ascribed to its fatty acid content, we cannot exclude that other nutrients in the test diet also contributed to the diet's efficacy. In order to support an optimal skin and coat condition, the test diet contained increased levels of total fat, vitamin A, vitamin E, protein, zinc and selenium (declared values: 11 g, 1200 IU, 30 mg, 14.5 g, 20 mg and 0.040 mg/MJ, respectively). These values are increased within the range of 1.2–2-fold for fat, vitamin A, protein, zinc and selenium and within the range of 1–5-fold for vitamin E, when compared with values in usual diets. As the major difference between the test diet and the habitual diet was a 30-fold increase in the dietary level of GLA and a 48-fold increase in the dietary level of EPA, it seems reasonable to conclude that the test diet's efficacy was related to its fatty acid composition. The observed effect of the test diet on the reduction of clinical signs of AD is comparable to results of studies on supplementation with high levels of EPA[15] and GLA.[16] The hypothesised mechanism of its efficacy through modification of the immune response by altered eicosanoid production is supported by the observation that the test diet reduced the chemotaxis of neutrophils towards interleukin-8 in healthy dogs (unpublished results). In other studies, increased dietary levels of n-3 fatty acids were associated with a reduction of plasma levels of PGE_2[17] and LTB_4 and an increase of the plasma level of LTB_5,[24] indicating the production of less inflammatory mediators.

A major drawback of several studies on the efficacy of fatty acid supplementation is the lack of information on the dog's habitual diet.[7,16] In this study, owners were asked to complete a questionnaire concerning the dog's dietary history and habitual diet. The change in plasma fatty acid composition in dogs that were switched to the test diet and also the almost stable plasma fatty acid composition in the control dogs confirmed the owners' excellent compliance with use of the diet. Minor changes in the fatty acid composition in the control dogs may be explained by the fact that snacks or table scraps were no longer allowed during the trial. For most fatty acids, the relative levels in the diet, plasma, skin and subcutaneous fat tissue were significantly correlated (Table 3.1.7). This implies that, in situations where information on the dogs' habitual diet is lacking, the fatty acid composition of plasma, skin or subcutaneous fat tissue can be used as biomarker for the dietary fatty acid intake in the past. The plasma fatty acid composition gives an indication of the dietary fatty acid intake over the last weeks,[25] whereas the fatty acid composition of skin or subcutaneous fat tissue can be used as index of habitual dietary fatty acid intake over a few months.[22]

Even though the test diet had a much higher level of GLA than the dogs' habitual diet, dogs eating the test diet did not show an increase in their plasma level of GLA. This finding may be explained by the fact that blood samples were taken after the dogs had been fasted for at least 12 hours; plasma levels of GLA are only increased for 2 hours after feeding.[26] Apparently GLA is rapidly cleared and/or converted into other fatty acids. The increase in the level of EPA in the test diet was associated with a significant rise in the plasma level of EPA in all dogs fed the test diet. However, not all dogs eating the test diet had an increased level of EPA in their skin. There was no significant difference between responders and non-responders regarding the cutaneous level of EPA; some of the responders had cutaneous EPA levels below the detection limit. This suggests that an increase in the cutaneous level of EPA is not a prerequisite for responding to the diet. However, it cannot be excluded that EPA in the skin of some responders had already been metabolised into other active components. There was no correlation between the post-trial cutaneous level (or change in the cutaneous level) of total n-3 fatty acids, ALA, EPA or DHA and the relative scores for clinical signs. Differences in response to the diet may therefore be related to other factors involved in the production of inflammatory mediators and modulation of the immune response. Responsiveness to the diet may

also be related to the individual dog's degree of pruritus in relation to its pruritic threshold.

At the end of the study, the group of responders had somewhat lower plasma levels of ALA and higher levels of DHA. It is not clear if this could have affected the response to the diet. Responders and non-responders did not differ in cutaneous fatty acid composition. The finding that responders and non-responders had almost identical initial and post-trial plasma and cutaneous fatty acid composition is in contrast with results of the study by Scott et al.[23] They suggested that subsets of atopic dogs with different fatty acid metabolism responded differently to fatty acid supplementation. In their study, responders had higher post-trial levels of ALA, whereas in our study, responders had somewhat lower post-trial levels of ALA than non-responders. Furthermore, in their study, there were excellent correlations between plasma GLA to DGLA, and AA to C22:4n-6 in both responders and non-responders, and a correlation between plasma LA and GLA in responders only. In our study, these correlations were not detected. This may be related to the fact that in our study blood was collected in fasted dogs and plasma levels of GLA were therefore very low.

It has been suggested that several clinical dermatological conditions are associated with an aberrant cutaneous fatty acid composition.[6] In atopic dogs, plasma levels of DGLA were lower than in dogs without skin problems.[27,28] As we only analysed the cutaneous fatty acid composition in dogs with AD, it cannot be evaluated if the cutaneous fatty acid composition of these dogs with AD was significantly different from healthy dogs.

In summary, in this randomised, controlled, double-blinded clinical trial, a switch from the dogs' habitual diet to a diet rich in fish oil and borage oil significantly reduced the severity of pruritus and erythema in dogs with AD. The diet may therefore contribute to a reduction in the degree of pruritus, possibly to below the individual pruritic threshold, in dogs with AD.

Acknowledgements

The authors would like to thank the owners of the dogs involved in this study for their participation.

Funding

The study was funded by LEO Animal Health, Ballerup, Denmark.

References

1 Chamberlain, K.W. Atopic (allergic) dermatitis. *Veterinary Clinics of North America*, 1974; **4**: 29–39.

2 Scott, D.W., Miller, W.H., Griffin, C.E. In: *Muller and Kirk's Small Animal Dermatology*, 5th edn. W.B. Saunders, Philadelphia, 1995: 500–518.

3 Reedy, L.M., Miller, W.H., Willemse, T. In: *Allergic Skin Diseases of Dogs and Cats*, 2nd edn. W.B. Saunders, Philadelphia, 1997: 32–149.

4 Zur, G., Ihrke, P.J., White, S.D., Kass, P.H. Canine atopic dermatitis: a retrospective study of 266 cases examined at the University of California, Davis, 1992–1998. Part I. Clinical features and allergy testing results. *Veterinary Dermatology*, 2002; **13**: 89–102.

5 Zur, G., White, S.D., Ihrke, P.J., Kass, P.H., Toebe, N. Canine atopic dermatitis: a retrospective study of 266 cases examined at the University of California, Davis, 1992–1998. Part II. Response to hyposensitization. *Veterinary Dermatology*, 2002; **13**: 103–111.

6 Campell, K.L. Clinical use of fatty acid supplements in dogs. *Veterinary Dermatology*, 1993; **4**: 167–173.

7 Remillard, R.L. Omega 3 fatty acids in canine and feline diets: a clinical success or failure? *Veterinary Clinical Nutrition*, 1998; **5**: 6–11.

8 Lloyd, D.H., Thomsett, L.R. Essential fatty acid supplementation in the treatment of canine atopy. A preliminary study. *Veterinary Dermatology*, 1989; **1**: 41–44.

9 Miller, W.H., Griffin, C.E., Scott, D.W., Angarano, D.K., Norton, A.L. Clinical trial of DVM Caps in the treatment of allergic disease in dogs: a nonblinded study. *Journal of the American Animal Hospital Association*, 1989; **25**: 163–168.

10 Paradis, M., Lemay, S., Scott, D.W. The efficacy of clemastine (Tavist), a fatty acid-containing product (Derm Caps), and the combination of both products in the management of canine pruritus. *Veterinary Dermatology*, 1991; **2**: 17–20.

11 Scott, D.W., Buerger, R.G. Nonsteroidal antiinflammatory agents in the management of canine pruritus. *Journal of the American Animal Hospital Association*, 1988; **24**: 425–428.

12 Scott, D.W., Miller, W.H. Nonsteroidal management of canine pruritus: chlorpheniramine and a fatty acid supplement (DVM Derm Caps) in combination, and the fatty acid supplement at twice the manufacturer's recommended dosage. *Cornell Veterinarian*, 1990; **80**: 381–387.

13 Scarff, D.H., Lloyd, D.H. Double blind, placebo-controlled, crossover study of evening primrose oil in the treatment of canine atopy. *Veterinary Record*, 1992; **131**: 97–99.

14 Sture, G.H., Lloyd, D.H. Canine atopic disease: therapeutic use of an evening primrose oil and fish oil combination. *Veterinary Record*, 1995; **137**: 169–170.

15 Logas, D., Kunkle, G.A. Double-blinded cross-over study with marine oil supplementation containing high-dose eicosapentaenoic acid for the treatment of canine prurutic skin disease. *Veterinary Dermatology*, 1994; **5**: 99–104.

16 Harvey, R.G. A blinded, placebo-controlled study of the efficacy of borage seed oil and fish oil in the management of canine atopy. *Veterinary Record*, 1999; **144**: 405–407.

17 Nesbitt, G.H., Freeman, L.S., Hannah, S.S. Effect of n-3 fatty acid ratio and dose on clinical manifestations, plasma fatty acids and inflammatory mediators in dogs with pruritus. *Veterinary Dermatology*, 2003; **14**: 67–74.

18 Willemse, T. Atopic skin disease: a review and a reconsideration of diagnostic criteria. *Journal of Small Animal Practice*, 1986; **27**: 771–778.

19 Prélaud, P., Guagaère, E., Alhaidari, Z., Faivre, N., Héripret, D., Gayerie, A. Re-evaluation of diagnostic criteria in atopic dermatitis. *Révue de Médecine Vétérinaire*, 1998; **149**: 1047–1064.

20 Folch, J., Lees, M., Sloane Stanley, G.H. A simple method for the isolation and purification of total lipids from animal tissues. *Journal of Biological Chemistry*, 1957; **226**: 497–509.

21 Metcalfe, L.D., Schmitz, A.A., Pelka, J.R. Rapid preparation of fatty acid esters from lipids for gas chromatographic analysis. *Analytical Chemistry*, 1966; **318**: 514–517.

22 Deslypere, J.P., Van de Bovenkamp, P., Harryvan, J.H., Katan, M.B. Stability of n-3 fatty acids in human fat tissue aspirates during storage. *American Journal of Clinical Nutrition*, 1993; **57**: 884–888.

23 Scott, D.W., Miller, W.H., Reinhart, G.A., Mohammed, H.O., Bagladi, M.S. Effect of an omega-3/omega-6 fatty acid containing commercial lamb and rice diet on pruritus in atopic dogs: results of a single-blinded study. *Canadian Journal of Veterinary Research*, 1997; **61**: 145–153.

24 Vaughn, D.M., Reinhart, G.A., Swaim, S.F., *et al*. Evaluation of effects of dietary n-6 to n-3 fatty acid ratios on leukotriene B synthesis in dog skin and neutrophils. *Veterinary Dermatology*, 1994; **5**: 163–173.

25 Hansen, R.A., Ogilvie, G.K, Davenport, D.J., *et al*. Duration of effects of dietary fish oil supplementation on serum eicosapentaenoic acid and docosahexaenoic acid concentrations in dogs. *American Journal of Veterinary Research*, 1998; **59**: 864–868.

26 Taugbøl, O., Baddaky-Taugbøl, B., Saarem, K. The postprandial plasma concentration of fatty acids in dogs. In: von Tscharner, C., Kwochka, K.W., Willemse, TW., eds. *Advances in Veterinary Dermatology*, Vol. 3. Butterworth Heinemann, Oxford, 1998: 251–257.

27 Taugbøl, O., Baddaky-Taugbøl, B., Saarem, K. The fatty acid profile of subcutaneous fat and blood plasma in pruritic dogs and dogs without skin problems. *Canadian Journal of Veterinary Research*, 1998; **62**: 275–278.

28 Saevik, B.K., Thoresen, S.I., Taugbøl, O. Fatty acid composition of serum lipids in atopic and healthy dogs. *Research in Veterinary Science*, 2002; **73**: 153–158.

Part 4

Skin biology

Reduction of scarring following injury and surgery

M.W.J. Ferguson BSc, BDS, PhD, DMedSci

Faculty of Life Sciences, University of Manchester, Manchester, UK

Summary

Scarring following injury or surgery is a major medical and veterinary problem. We discovered that wounds made on early embryos heal perfectly with no scar. Investigation of the cellular and molecular differences between scar-free embryonic wound healing and scar-forming adult wound healing resulted in the discovery of mechanistic variables which could be experimentally or pharmacologically manipulated to prevent or reduce scarring in adults. This chapter briefly reviews our research in this field which, although primarily directed at the development of potential new human pharmaceuticals, could find application in the veterinary field.

Scarring

Scarring occurs after trauma, injury or surgery to any tissue or organ in the body. Scars are a consequence of a repair mechanism that replaces the missing normal tissue with an extracellular matrix consisting predominantly of abnormally aligned fibronectin and collagen types I and III; as such, scarring represents a failure of tissue regeneration.

It is not surprising that the skin represents the most frequently injured tissue, and dermal scarring after injury, trauma or surgery results in adverse medical and veterinary consequences, including adverse aesthetics, loss of function, restriction of tissue movement and or growth, and adverse psychological effects. Further adverse consequences of scarring in other organ systems include: (1) in the eye, scarring can cause hazy vision or blindness; (2) in the peripheral and central nervous systems, glial scarring prevents neuronal reconnections and hence restoration of neuronal function; (3) in the internal gastrointestinal and reproductive organs, scarring causes strictures and adhesions which can give rise to serious or life-threatening conditions, such as infertility or failure of bowel function; and (4) in tendons and ligaments, scarring restricts movement, decreases strength and prevents normal function.

A scar in the skin may be defined as 'a macroscopic disturbance of the normal structure and function of the skin architecture, resulting from the end product of a healed wound'.[1] The severity of skin scarring in man and laboratory animals can be measured clinically (macroscopically) by using a variety of criteria such as scar volume, colour, pliability, contour, etc., and both clinically and histologically (microscopically) by using a visual analogue scale, whereby 0 represents normal skin and 10 a very poor scar.[2] There are currently no registered mechanistic-based therapies, i.e. pharmaceutical drugs, to prevent or improve scarring. Current therapies such as pressure garments, silicone dressings and hydrocortisone injections are empirical, unpredictable and largely ineffective.[3]

In man, it is known that the severity of scarring varies by:

- Tissue site – e.g. the shoulders and upper chest scar badly, whereas gums hardly scar at all.
- Sex – males generally have worse scars than females, and fertile females have worse scars than post-menopausal females.
- Race – coloured-skinned races such as negroids and mongoloids have worse scars than white-skinned races such as Caucasians.

- Age – young people, particular teenagers and those in their early twenties, have worse scars than older people.
- Magnitude of injury – larger wounds produce worse scars.
- Wound contamination – the more contaminated the wound, the worse the scar.

Scar-free embryonic wound healing

In the early 1990s, we discovered that skin wounds on early mouse embryos healed perfectly with no signs of scarring and complete restitution of the normal skin architecture.[4] We conducted systematic experiments making defined skin wounds on mouse and sheep embryos at different stages of development.[4–6] These *in vivo* surgical experiments demonstrated that skin wounds made during the first one-third to one-half of gestation healed perfectly with no scars, whereas wounds made later in gestation and during adult life heal with a scar.[1,7,8] In mice, the latest time a small incisional skin wound heals with no discernible scar is embryonic day 16 (the time of birth is normally embryonic day 20 or day 21). The transition from scar-free embryonic wound healing to scar-forming adult wound healing is gradual, and is characterised by the progressively abnormal organisation of the newly formed dermis. The abnormal deposition of small parallel bundles of extracellular matrix consisting predominantly of collagen types I and III and fibronectin leading to scar formation, as opposed to the deposition of large bundles of extracellular matrix in a normal basket-weave orientation in the normal skin and in the newly formed dermis of an embryonic (pre-day 16) wound. Scarring is, therefore, not only a biochemical problem, but predominantly a morphogenetic problem, i.e. a failure of the regeneration of the normal skin structure.

We then investigated and compared the cellular and molecular differences between embryonic wounds (pre-embryonic day 16 in the mouse) that heal without a scar and adult or late-fetal wounds, which heal with a scar. There are a large number of differences, but many of these are epiphenomena (i.e. not causative of the scar-free healing phenotype), because embryos are still developing and changing rapidly at that time.

From a mechanistic and therapeutic perspective, the key point is to determine which of these numerous differences are involved in embryonic scar-free healing and adult scar-forming healing. In addition to mere presence or absence of scarring in embryonic and adult wounds, several criteria must be fulfilled to demonstrate causality.[1] First, manipulation of the cellular or molecular variable should induce an improvement or absence of scarring in the adult (which normally heals with a scar) and a manipulation in the reverse direction should induce scarring in the early embryonic wound (which normally heals without a scar). When such stringent criteria are employed, only a few of the myriad of cellular and molecular differences between embryonic and adult healing remain as potential mechanisms, and therapeutic targets, involved in skin scarring.[1,7,8]

Firstly, embryonic wounds elicit a very different inflammatory response compared to adult wounds.[9] The immune system in the embryo is in a developmental stage and the response to injury of the primitive immune cells is different from that in the adult. As a consequence, embryonic wounds have far fewer inflammatory cells, the inflammatory cells present are less differentiated, and the length of time that the inflammatory cells are present is markedly reduced compared with adult wounds. Therefore, highly selected strategies to manipulate the inflammatory response of adult wounds were investigated with a view to the prevention or reduction of scarring in the adult.

Second, the embryo is developing and growing rapidly, with a considerable expansion of skin volume on a daily basis. Consequently, normal embryonic skin and embryonic wounds contain high levels of morphogenetic factors involved in skin growth, remodelling and morphogenesis. Therefore, studies involving the manipulation of the levels of skin morphogenetic factors, such as transforming growth factor (TGF)-β_3, were conducted to prevent or reduce scarring during adult healing.[8]

Largely as a consequence of these two principal variables (altered inflammatory response and skin morphogenesis), the growth factor profile at a healing embryonic wound is very different qualitatively (i.e. the types of growth factor present), quantitatively (i.e. the amounts of such growth factors present) and temporally (i.e. the length of time the growth factors are present), compared with an adult wound.[5,7,8,10] Thus, for example, there are major differences in the TGF-β isoforms present in embryonic and adult wounds. Embryonic wounds express very high levels of TGF-β_3, a skin morphogenetic factor predominantly synthesised by keratinocytes and fibroblasts, and very low levels of

TGF-β_1 and TGF-β_2.[5] By contrast, adult wounds contain predominantly TGF-β_1 (and TGF-β_2), which is derived initially from degranulating platelets and subsequently from inflammatory cells such as monocytes and macrophages. Likewise, adult wounds contain large quantities of platelet-derived growth factor (PDGF), which is virtually absent in embryonic wounds owing to the lack of platelet degranulation.[5]

Experimental manipulation of adult wound healing

Using information on the cellular and molecular differences between scar-free embryonic wound healing and scar-forming adult wound healing, we experimentally manipulated the healing wounds of adult mice, rats and pigs.[7,8,11–14] These manipulations have been conducted with potential pharmacological and genetic approaches in transgenic mice. For example, application of exogenous TGF-β_3, or neutralising agents against TGF-β_1 and TGF-β_2, or neutralising agents against PDGF, result in healing with markedly improved or absent scarring of experimental wounds on adult animals.

We have investigated when potential pharmaceutical agents should be applied to elicit their scar-improving effects during healing.[11–13] We have shown that early application at the time of wounding, or shortly thereafter (within 48 hours), produces the best results, despite the fact that scars are the final end point of a healed wound. In rodents, scars are not normally stable and mature until some 70–80 days post-wounding. Likewise in man, scars are not normally mature and stable until at least 6 months post-injury. Despite this long time-frame for normal scar maturation, we have shown that acute administration of scar-preventing pharmaceuticals at the time of wounding, or shortly after, is sufficient to realise the full beneficial effects; there are negligible additional benefits from more prolonged application. This may be explained by the fact that the initial wound healing response is triggered by a small number of effector molecules which rapidly induce overlapping and redundant signalling and cellular cascades. Consequently, early intervention at the time of wounding, or shortly thereafter, results in major long-term effects due to the establishment of altered auto-inductive regulatory cascades. As normal wound healing rapidly progresses, additional cytokine, growth factor

and cellular cascades are induced, resulting in a multiply-redundant and robust response, which is fairly resistant to meaningful pharmaceutical manipulation at later time points.

In clinical practice, this timing is advantageous, and not problematic. During surgical operations, the timing of wounding can be anticipated accurately and is precisely known. In the case of major traumatic injury, e.g. road traffic accidents, sporting injuries, domestic accidents, burns, violence, etc., patients are transported rapidly to the hospital, where any scar-improving drug could be appropriately administered within the critical 48-hour therapeutic period. Indeed, the discovery that experimental or therapeutic agents appear necessary only in acute doses in the early phases of healing is a major clinical advantage, obviating the necessity of developing long-term dosing strategies, ensuring patient compliance, and facilitating the administration of a scar-improving human pharmaceutical via intradermal injection into the margins of the wound or wound sites.

Despite its morphological appearance, a skin scar is actually weaker than the normal surrounding skin. With our scar-improving and scar-preventing experimental and therapeutic regimens, we observed: no decrease in the tensile strength of the wounds (often they were stronger than normal scars as the extracellular matrix was more normally aligned), no decrease in the rate of wound healing (often the wounds healed faster compared with controls), and no increase in the incidence of wound complications, e.g. dehiscence or wound infection.[11–13]

Central role of TGF-β_3

Various experiments in mice and rats strongly suggest that TGF-β_3 is involved in the mechanistic pathway for scar prevention.

- TGF-β_3 is present at high levels in developing embryonic skin and in embryonic wounds that heal with no scar. In contrast, it is present at low levels in adult wounds that scar. TGF-β_3 is known to play a role in embryonic skin morphogenesis. Exogenous addition of TGF-β_3 by intradermal injection to experimental wounds, either before wounding or to the wound margins, results in markedly reduced or absent scarring. Dose-response experiments indicate that in rats the optimum dose is 50 ng TGF-β_3

per 100 µl per l cm of wound, administered at the time of wounding and 24 hours later.[13]

- Whereas neutralisation of TGF-β_1 and TGF-β_2 at the wound site prevents or reduces scarring, pan-neutralisation of all three TGF-β isoforms (TGF-β_1, TGF-β_2 and TGF-β_3) does not improve scarring, suggesting that neutralisation of TGF-β_3 may be detrimental.[12,13]

- Genetic deletion of TGF-β_3 in mice using transgenic technology results in scarring following embryonic wounding, whereas the wild-type litter mates, with two normal copies of the TGF-β_3 gene, heal with no scar. The abnormal, slowly healing, scar-forming embryonic wounds in the TGF-β_3-null mice indicate a defect in cell migration. Fibroblasts recovered from TGF-β_3-null skin migrate significantly more slowly in a collagen filter-migration assay, compared with fibroblasts from normal TGF-β_3-positive skin. This deficit in TGF-β_3-null fibroblast cell migration can be rescued by exogenous addition of TGF-β_3 to the culture medium, but not by addition of exogenous TGF-β_1 or TGF-β_2. This indicates a TGF-β_3 isoform-specific effect on cell migration. By contrast, the effects of TGF-β_1, TGF-β_2 and TGF-β_3 on fibroblast cell proliferation are similar. These data clearly indicate that among the three TGF-β isoforms, there are both promiscuous (cell proliferation) and isoform-specific (cell migration) effects. Stimulation of fibroblast cell migration into a healing wound results in a more normal basket-weave organisation of the fibroblasts and the extracellular matrix molecules which they deposit, thus restituting the normal dermal architecture and producing a marked improvement in, or absence of, scarring. Enhancement of keratinocyte migration by exogenous addition of TGF-β_3 also results in more rapid wound re-epithelialisation (closing).

Physiologically, this active TGF-β_3 molecule binds at the TGF-β receptor. The TGF-β receptor is a heterotetromer, consisting of two R1 and two R2 subunits. Ligand binding brings the receptor subunits into close proximity and allows phosphorylation of their cytoplasmic tails. It appears that TGF-β_1, TGF-β_2 and TGF-β_3 all bind at the same receptor. The documented isoform-specific effects of TGF-β_3 are likely the result of the TGF-β_3 ligand engaging the TGF-β receptor subunits in a slightly different conformation (compared to TGF-β_1 or TGF-β_2 engagement with the receptor), resulting in the exposure or masking of different phosphorylation sites, which in turn result in an altered second-messenger signal and isoform-specific effects, e.g. on cell migration. Equally, the promiscuous effects of TGF-β_1, TGF-β_2 and TGF-β_3 are caused by phosphorylation of common cytoplasmic domains that are available, irrespective of which ligand binds the receptor.

We have developed TGF-β_3 as a potential human pharmaceutical agent for the prevention and reduction of scarring and demonstrated clinical and statistical evidence of efficacy in early human clinical trials.

Scarring and evolution

Scarring is often thought to be an inevitable consequence of injury or surgery and, by inference, to be an evolutionarily optimised end point. We have challenged that view and argued that most wounds in primitive animals (for example from bites, blows, contusions, degloving injuries, fight wounds, etc.) would involve widespread tissue damage, haematoma formation and bruising, and would frequently be contaminated with dirt, wood splinters, bacteria, etc.[8] We hypothesise that the evolutionary forces shaping healing in these wounds have been directed to the prevention of infection, the walling off of foreign bodies and the rapid restitution of missing tissue, i.e. scarring.[8] However, these are not the types of wounds commonly encountered today. Sharp injuries such as those inflicted by surgical instruments, mechanical equipment, glass and weapons are a very modern invention of the last 500 years; indeed, sharp clean injuries with close approximation of the wound margins such as those that occur after surgery or surgical repair are very new and completely unoptimised by the forces shaping natural wound healing mechanisms. In brief, we hypothesise that surgical wounds, the most common wound in contemporary man or animals, heal by inappropriate and suboptimal cellular and molecular mechanisms that have been selected over a long period of time for the healing of a different type of wound (bite, blow, contusion, etc.) with different degrees of tissue damage, wound infection, foreign body involvement and different wound morphology (no approximation of the wound margins).[8] We hypothesise that the normal response to a wound made with a sharp object under clean conditions and with approximation of its margins is inappropriate, indeed pathological, and that therapeutic manipulation of these normal, but inappropriate, healing mechanisms can result in the improved healing response of reduced scarring and/or tissue regeneration and it is to these ends that our novel pharmaceuticals are directed.

Potential veterinary applications

Although our efforts in the prevention and reduction of scarring are primarily directed towards potential human applications, all of our preclinical studies have been effectively conducted in a variety of animals: mice, rats, sheep, pigs and marsupials.[7,8,11–15] Potential veterinary applications include the prevention or reduction of skin scarring in horses or domestic animals following injury or surgery, the prevention of abdominal adhesions in horses, and the acceleration of repair and prevention of scarring in equine tendon injury.

Acknowledgements/Funding

Worked reviewed in this chapter has been funded by a variety of sources over the past 20 years: most recently by the MRC/BBSRC/EPSRC as part of a large grant for the UK Centre for Tissue Engineering. Many scientists, clinicians and students have contributed to the original research. All of the therapeutic developments of scar improving drugs have been conducted by staff within a biotechnology company, Renovo Ltd, of which Professor Ferguson is the Co-Founder and Chief Executive Officer.

References

1 Ferguson, M.W.J., Whitby, D.J., Shah, M., Armstrong, J., Siebert, J.W., Longaker, M.T. Scar formation: the spectral nature of fetal and adult wound repair. *Plastic and Reconstructive Surgery*, 1996; **97**: 854–860.

2 Beausang, E., Floyd, H., Dunn, K.W., Orton, C.I., Ferguson, M.W.J. A new quantitative scale for clinical scar assessment. *Plastic and Reconstructive Surgery*, 1998; **102**: 1954–1961.

3 Bayat, A., McGrouther, D.A., Ferguson, M.W.J. Skin scarring. *British Medical Journal*, 2003; **326**: 88–92.

4 Whitby, D.J., Ferguson, M.W.J. The extracellular matrix of lip wounds in fetal, neonatal and adult mice. *Development*, 1991; **112**: 651–668.

5 Whitby, D.J., Ferguson, M.W.J. Immunohistochemical localisation of growth factors in fetal wound healing. *Developmental Biology*, 1991; **147**: 207–215.

6 Whitby, D.J., Longaker, M.T., Adzick, N.S., Harrison, M.R., Ferguson, M.W.J. Rapid epithelialisation of fetal wounds is associated with the early deposition of tenascin. *Journal of Cell Science*, 1991; **99**: 583–586.

7 McCallion, R.L., Ferguson, M.W.J. Fetal wound healing and the development of anti-scarring therapies for adult wound healing. In: Clarke, R.A.F., ed. *The Molecular and Cellular Biology of Wound Repair*, 2nd edn. Plenum Press, New York, 1996: 561–600.

8 Ferguson, M.W.J., O'Kane, S. Scar-free healing: from embryonic mechanisms to adult therapeutic intervention. *Philosophical Transactions of the Royal Society of London. Series B: Biological Sciences*, 2004; **359**: 839–850.

9 Cowin, A.J., Brosnan, M.P., Holmes, T.M., Ferguson, M.W.J. Endogenous inflammatory response to dermal wound healing in the fetal and adult mouse. *Development Dynamics*, 1998; **212**: 385–393.

10 O'Kane, S., Ferguson, M.W.J. Transforming growth factor betas and wound healing. *International Journal of Biochemistry and Cell Biology*, 1997; **29**: 63–78.

11 Shah, M., Foreman, D.M., Ferguson, M.W.J. Control of scarring in adult wounds by neutralising antibodies to transforming growth factor beta (TGFβ). *Lancet*, 1992; **339**: 213–214.

12 Shah, M., Foreman, D.M., Ferguson, M.W.J. Neutralising antibody to TGFβ1,2, reduces scarring in adult rodents. *Journal of Cell Science*, 1994; **107**: 1137–1157.

13 Shah, M., Foreman D.M., Ferguson, M.W.J. Neutralisation of TGFβ1 and TGFβ2 or exogenous addition of TGFβ3 to cutaneous rat wounds reduces scarring. *Journal of Cell Science*, 1995; **108**: 985–1002.

14 Shah M., Rorison P., Ferguson M.W.J. The role of transforming growth factors beta in cutaneous scarring. In: Garg, H.G., Longaker, M.T., eds. *Scarless Wound Healing*. Marcel Dekker, New York, 2000: 213–226.

15 Armstrong J.R., Ferguson, M.W.J. Ontogeny of the skin and the transition from scar free to scarring phenotype during wound healing in the pouch young of a marsupial *Monodelphis domestica*. *Developmental Biology*, 1995; **169**: 242–260.

Optical biopsy: non-invasive tissue evaluation utilising optical coherence tomography

R.S. Walton DVM, MS[1], E.J. Dick DVM[1], G. Woong PhD[2], J. Zhang PhD[2], Z. Chen PhD[2], G.M. Peavy DVM[2], J.S. Nelson MD, PhD[2]

[1] U.S. Army Institute of Surgical Research, San Antonio, Texas, USA
[2] Beckman Laser Institute, School of Medicine, University of California, Irvine, California, USA

Summary

The accurate non-invasive assessment of traumatic wound depth and serial evaluation of wound healing is an active and ongoing research goal of our laboratories. A large number of non-invasive modalities have been evaluated. Due to various limiting factors, non-invasive technologies have not improved the clinician's ability to assess tissue viability beyond simple observation. Histological assessment is invasive and has a slow turn-around time, even when frozen section techniques are utilised.

Polarisation-sensitive optical coherence tomography (PS-OCT) and optical coherence tomography/Doppler tomography (OCT/ODT) devices have recently been developed that have the potential to assess tissue viability non-invasively in a real-time mode. The technology is analogous to ultrasound except that the images are created with echoes of infrared light rather than sound. Using a thermal injury model and inhalation injury models in several species, we have qualitatively compared the results of this instrument to standard histopathology. Four different histology staining techniques (haematoxylin and eosin, Masson's trichrome, Movat's pentachrome and nitro blue tetrazolium – a vital stain) were compared to the PS-OCT and OCT/ODT device results. The OCT measurement contained less variability site-to-site when compared with standard histology techniques. We also found that the PS-OCT technique provided an accurate assessment of wound depth when compared with histology specimens. We evaluated 366 biopsy pairs which appear to have excellent gross morphologic correlation.

Further studies are planned with OCT/ODT technology in skin and other tissues. Preliminary work with this device in the airway, gastrointestinal tract and muscle appears promising. Utilisation of these combined non-invasive imaging technologies has the potential to improve assessment of traumatically and thermally injured patients in real time, thereby improving overall wound care.

Introduction

No affliction of mankind challenges the patient and health care professional as much as that of traumatic and burn injuries.[1] Traumatic injury is one of the leading causes of death in humans under the age of 40 years worldwide, and is also one of the most common reasons pet owners seek emergency care. The accurate non-invasive assessment of traumatic wound depth, tissue viability and serial evaluation of wound healing is an active and ongoing research goal of our laboratories. A large number of non-invasive modalities have been evaluated. These include the use of vital dyes, indocyanine green dye fluorescence, fluorescein fluorometry, laser Doppler flowmetry (LDF), thermography, ultrasound, nuclear magnetic resonance imaging and spectral analysis of light reflectance.[2–12] Due to various limiting factors, these non-invasive technologies have not improved the clinician's ability to assess tissue viability beyond simple observation. The four 'C's' (colour, consistency, contractility and circulation) have remained the surgeons' gold standard of tissue viability for the last 100 years.

Debridement of traumatised tissue back to 'bleeding' tissue is still the standard in most practices. Many instances exist where excessive debridement is neither indicated, nor desirable, from a cosmetic or functional standpoint. Histological assessment to determine tissue viability is invasive and has a slow turn-around time even when frozen section techniques are utilised. The distinction between viable and non-viable tissue is often not immediately evident by visual inspection, but an accurate early assessment is a critical factor to provide appropriate therapeutic intervention.

Treatment plans vary considerably depending on the severity of the injury.[5,10] Thermally and traumatically injured skin sustains extensive damage to dermal arterioles, capillaries and venules, which results in decreased blood flow to the skin. This can be detected with laser Doppler flowmetry. Recent research has focused on the use of LDF, but LDF is limited because it cannot resolve depth in tissue or specific blood flow; LDF only measures perfusion over an entire volume of section of tissue. Problems with accuracy have limited the clinical usefulness of LDF.[11,12]

The Beckman Laser Institute (Irvine, CA, USA) has recently developed new polarisation-sensitive optical coherence tomography (PS-OCT) and optical coherence tomography/Doppler tomography (OCT/ODT) devices that could potentially assess thermal and traumatically injured tissue non-invasively in a 'real-time' mode. OCT is an imaging modality where the location and relative strength of embedded structures can be deduced. In OCT, light is emitted from a low coherence source and coupled into a Michelson interferometer where the light is split into two paths. The light used is a low coherence source which differs from a coherent light source (laser) in that the light is emitted over a range of wavelengths. After being split, the beam is directed toward the sample material and the reference mirror equally. Light backscattered by the sample is recombined with the reflected light from the reference mirror to produce an inference pattern that corresponds to the specific depth with a test material and results in high spatial and axial resolution. The polarisation state of this beam can be evaluated, allowing assessment of change in collagen that uses coherence gating to image tissue birefringence with high spatial resolution due to its inherent changes with tissue damage.

Pilot research with these prototype instruments has produced excellent correlation to histology in a rodent thermal injury model,[13,14] rodent skin and mesentery model,[15–18] as well as endoscopic application.[19–23] The devices have also successfully imaged blood flow and structure in normal human skin.[24,25]

Utilisation of these combined non-invasive imaging technologies has the potential to accurately assess the patient in real time, giving the surgeon the ability to make rapid accurate assessment of injury and tissue viability, thereby improving patient care. The purpose of this study was to compare tissue injury and viability using PS-OCT and OCT/ODT to standard histopathology using a thermal injury model and inhalation injury models in several species.

Methods

Instrumentation

The PS-OCT/OCT/ODT instrument was designed and constructed by the Beckman Laser Institute Research Laboratories, School of Medicine, University of California at Irvine. The instrument was designed to image tissue structure and blood flow simultaneously. The systems use a fibreoptic Michelson interferometer with a broadband light source (1300 nm). A schematic diagram of the instrument is shown in Fig. 4.2.1. Light from this broadband partially coherent light source is coupled into a fibre interferometer by a 2×2 fibre coupler and then split equally into reference and target arms of the interferometer. Light backscattered from the turbid sample is coupled back into the fibre and forms interference fringes with the light reflected from the reference arms. High axial spatial resolution is possible because interference fringes are observed only when the path length differences between the light from the sample arm and reference arm are within the coherence length of the source.

ODT combines Doppler principles with OCT structural imaging into extremely high-resolution tomographic images. The principle of the ODT portion is based on the Doppler effect where the backscattered light undergoes a frequency shift that is dependent on the velocity of the moving structures (red blood cells) in the sample. This frequency information is the Doppler spectrum and provides information on the velocity distribution and concentration of the local microcirculation. Therefore, ODT can obtain tomographic images of blood flow as well as tissue structure simultaneously from a single scan, giving it a distinct advantage over existing technologies.

PS-OCT is an imaging technology that uses coherence gating to image tissue birefringence with high spatial resolution. Skin contains collagen, a weakly birefringent material. When collagen is exposed to temperatures of 56–65°C, it denatures and loses its birefringence. Through an analysis process of the polarisation state of

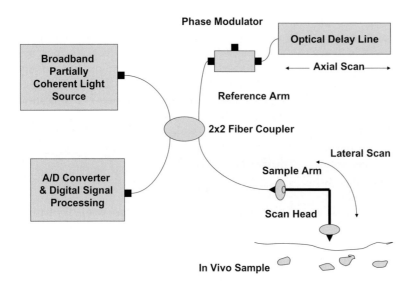

Fig. 4.2.1 Schematic of the prototype OCT/ODT instrument.

light reflected from various depths in a sample, PS-OCT is able to provide information on the amount and condition of collagen in an *in vivo* sample.

The OCT/ODT system has also been adapted to fibreoptic acquisition that allows accurate sampling over a large luminal surface area. Longitudinal probe systems allow maintenance of focal distance limits in large lumen systems without the need for optical coupling sites. By extrapolating these data, ODT essentially combines the LDF with OCT to produce high-resolution tomographic images of static and moving constituents in biologic tissues.

Subjects

The subjects were evaluated first with the non-invasive scanners. This scanner is set up with a fixed micromanipulator stage, portable handpiece or endoscopic fibre. The tissues evaluated were: normal rodent skin; partial and full thickness rodent thermally injured skin; and rodent, lagomorph, porcine, caprine and ovine normal and inhalation injured airway. A biopsy sample corresponding exactly to the optical scan was taken and placed in formalin. The image generated by the non-invasive 'optical biopsy' was evaluated in a blind fashion. A standard histopathology sample from the same location was evaluated separately and pairs were coded so that the investigators did not know their relationship. The images were digitally recorded and stored. A calibrated grid was overlaid on the standard histology images. Optical images generated were compared to histopathology specimens for depth and structural similarities. Polarisation images assigned an arbitrary colour value to changes in collagen birefringence and allowed the digital creation of phase maps indicating damaged tissue areas. Doppler images were assigned standard coloration of red and blue based on flow toward and away from the probe, respectively.

Data analysis

The same pathologist and investigator evaluated each case. The optical biopsy and histopathology images were graded using a numerical scoring system. The pathologist and investigator were blinded to treatment group. A qualitative assessment of positive or negative correlation was performed on the basis of haematoxylin and eosin-stained biopsy being the 'gold standard'. As with many new and evolving technologies, direct comparison to a 'gold standard' is difficult. The entire data analysis was qualitative only; available statistical testing methods and image comparison data did not provide a reasonable or valid system for a more accurate analysis. Currently we are working on a digital overlay system to accurately and mathematically compare structural similarities of the data sets.

Results

Tissue samples submitted for histopathology were converted to digital images with a depth-indexing grid attached (Fig. 4.2.2). A phase map was created using

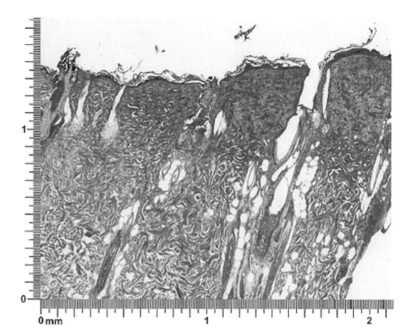

Fig. 4.2.2 Example of a standard full-thickness biopsy specimen of a third-degree thermal injury in a rodent model across the transition zone of intermediate zone of stasis (left) to coagulative necrosis (right). Digital overlay of a calibrated grid allows the pathologist to measure precise regions of injury depth.

an arbitrary colour selected by the investigator to define a regional difference between tissues (Fig. 4.2.3).

Our primary area of interest was the transition from normal to abnormal tissue. Good structural similarity

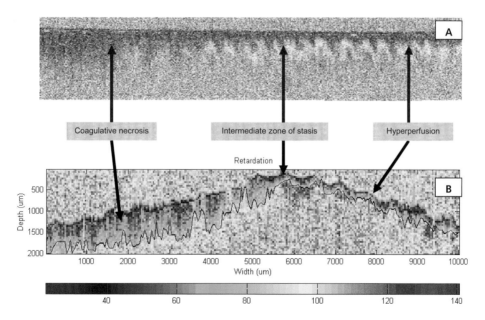

Fig. 4.2.3 (A) Standard monochromatic PS-OCT image of third-degree thermal injury represented in Fig. 4.2.2. Injury zones are labelled coagulative necrosis (third degree), intermediate zone of stasis (second degree) and zone of hyperperfusion (first degree). (B) Colorised phase map of collagen birefringence with thermal injury biopsy specimen pictured in Fig. 4.2.2. Blue coloration assigned to reflect change in birefringence properties of collagen. Collagen markedly changes its birefringence properties when thermally injured, and assigning a numerical index to the change in collagen birefringence allows precise calculation of burn depth.

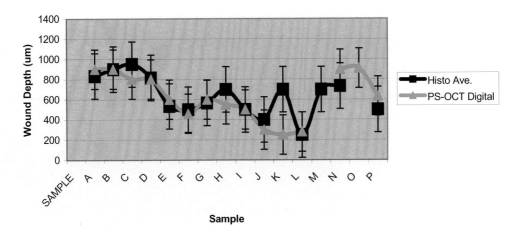

Fig. 4.2.4 Wound depth measures with polarisation-sensitive optical coherence tomography (PS-OCT). Samples A–P represent locations arranged clockwise on the dorsum of subjects ($n = 20$). The optical depth is measured in micrometres. Histology measures are numerical average of haematoxylin and eosin, Masson's trichrome and Movat's pentachrome of 312 sample pairs of rodent thermally injured skin.

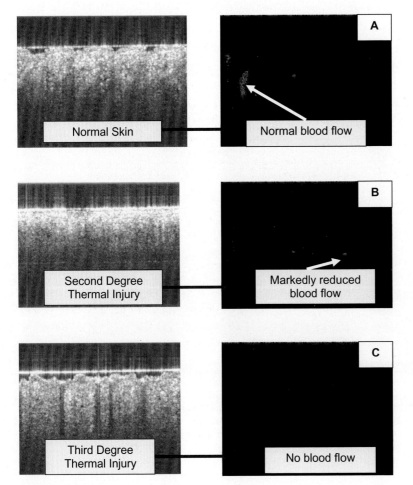

Fig. 4.2.5 Panels (A–C) The monochromatic polarisation-sensitive OCT (PS-OCT) image is on the left side of each panel. A colorised image of the optical Doppler tomography (ODT) is on the right side. (A) Normal skin PS-OCT scan colorised ODT image on the right indicating normal blood flow. (B) Second-degree thermal injury monochromatic PS-OCT image and ODT image indicating decreased blood flow. (C) Third-degree thermal injury with ODT indicating absent blood flow.

was noted between the images, especially the relationship to thermal injury depth. Figure 4.2.4 shows the correlation of burn depth measures, PS-OCT instrument reading and standard histopathology techniques in 20 thermally injured rodent subjects with over 312 biopsy pairs evaluated to date. The ODT images have been good (Fig. 4.2.5), but were inconsistent due to movement artifacts causing image degradation. Probe stabilisation was a critical issue *in vivo*. Structural comparisons to date have been qualitative with the overall impression being good. Early evaluation of airway tissue with bronchoscopically delivered probes has also produced very good images in several species (Figs 4.2.6 and 4.2.7).

Discussion

The results of this study have demonstrated our ability to rapidly acquire and consistently produce images with the OCT and PS-OCT probe. The qualitative results of this study are similar to those reported by other investigators with respect to cutaneous and endoscopic imaging.[13,14,19–25] The technical issues of

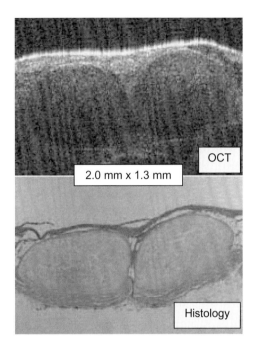

Fig. 4.2.6 Endoscopic image of a normal rabbit trachea with fibre-based monochromatic OCT image probe (top). The histology specimen biopsy (haematoxylin and eosin) corresponding to the optical image for comparison (bottom).

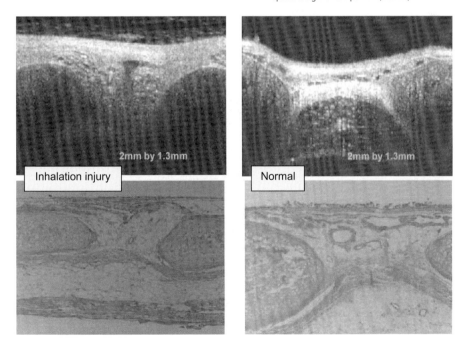

Fig. 4.2.7 Comparison of monochromatic OCT images ('optical biopsy images') of normal and inhalation injury model rabbit trachea to corresponding standard haematoxylin and eosin-stained biopsy segments. Note marked mucosal thickening in the inhalation injury tissue.

digital image layering and differences in structure between preserved histological specimens and *in vivo* digital images have made quantitative comparison of the images difficult. Qualitatively the images have marked similarity in structure and gross morphology. We are currently working on a digital image layering comparison technique to allow rapid and statistically valid comparisons of the data sets.

In conclusion, OCT is a novel non-invasive, non-contact imaging system that uses coherence gating to obtain high-resolution cross-sectional images of tissue microstructure. This system can simultaneously obtain *in situ* images of tissue structure, blood flow velocity and birefringence properties. Good correlation of tissue structure measured by standard means has great potential for basic biomedical application and clinical medicine. Miniaturisation and image stabilisation are the challenges facing future designs.

Acknowledgement

The authors would like to thank the dedicated technical staff of the US Army Institute of Surgical Research, San Antonio, Texas and the Beckman Laser Institute, University of California at Irvine for making this project possible.

Funding

This is a self-supported study through the United States Department of Defense.

References

1 Dressler, D.P., Hozid, J.L., Nathan, P. *Thermal Injury*. Mosby, St Louis, 1998: 1–7.
2 Greenfield, E., Defazio, D.M. Burn management. *Nursing Clinics of North America*, 1997; **32**: 237–273.
3 Carrougher, G.J. *Burn Care and Therapy*. Mosby, St Louis, 1998: 1–33.
4 American Burn Association. Hospital and pre-hospital resources for optimal care of patients with burn injury: guidelines for operation and development of burn centers. *Journal of Burn Care and Rehabilitation*, 1990; **11**: 98–104.
5 Shirani, K.Z., Vaughan, G.M., Mason, A.D., et al. Update on current therapeutic approaches in burns. *Shock*, 1996; **5**: 4–16.
6 Brigham, P., McLoughlin, E. Burn incidence and medical care use in the United States: estimates, trends and data sources. *Journal of Burn Care and Rehabilitation*, 1996; **17**: 95–107.
7 Sheridan, R.L., Schomaker, K.T., Lucchina, L.C., et al. Burn depth

8 Smahel, J. Viability of skin subjected to deep partial thickness thermal damage: experimental studies. *Burns*, 1991; **17**: 17–24.
9 Kaufman, T., Lusthaus, S.N., Sagher, U., Wexler, M.R. Deep partial skin thickness burns: a reproducible animal model to study burn wound healing. *Burns*, 1990; **16**: 13–16.
10 Heimbach, D., Engrav, L., Grube, B., Marvin, J. Burn depth: a review. *World Journal of Surgery*, 1992; **16**: 10–15.
11 Park, D.H., Hwang, J.W., Lang, K.S., et al. Use of laser Doppler flowmetry for estimation of depth of burns. *Plastic and Reconstructive Surgery*, 1998; **101**: 1516–1523.
12 Yeong, E.K., Mann, R., Goldberg, M., Heimbach, D. Improved accuracy of burn wound assessment using laser Doppler. *Journal of Trauma*, 1996; **40**: 956–962.
13 de Boer, J.F., Srinivas, S.M., Malekafzali, A., Chen, Z., Nelson, J.S. Imaging thermally damaged tissue by polarization sensitive optical coherence tomography. *Optics Express*, 1998; **3**: 212–218.
14 Park, B.H., Saxer, C., Srinivas, S.M., et al. In vivo burn depth determination by high-speed fiber-based polarization sensitive optical coherence tomography. *Journal of Biomedical Optics*, 2001; **6**: 474–479.
15 Chen, Z., Milner, T.E., Srinivas, S., et al. Noninvasive imaging of in vivo blood flow velocity using optical Doppler tomography. *Optics Letters*, 1997; **22**: 1119–1121.
16 Lindmo, T., Smithies, D.J., Chen, Z., Nelson, J.S., Milner, T.E. Monte Carlo simulation studies of optical coherence tomography (OCT) and optical Doppler tomography (ODT). *SPIE*, 1998; **3251**: 114–125.
17 Chen, Z., Milner, T.E., Srinivas, S., Nelson, J.S. Optical Doppler tomography: imaging in vivo blood flow dynamics following pharmacological intervention and photodynamic therapy. *Photochemistry and Photobiology*, 1998; **67**: 56–60.
18 Major, A., Kimel, S., Mee, S., et al. Microvascular photodynamic effects determined in vivo using optical Doppler tomography. *IEEE Journal of Selected Topics in Quantum Electronics*, 1999; **5**: 1168–1175.
19 Tearney, G.J., Brezinski, S.F., Bouma, B.E., et al. In vivo endoscopic optical biopsy with optical coherence tomography. *Science*, 1997; **276**: 2037–2039.
20 Tearney, G.J., Brezinski, J.F., Southern, B.E., et al. Optical biopsy in human gastrointestinal tissue using optical coherence tomography. *American Journal of Gastroenterology*, 1997; **92**: 1800–1804.
21 Herz, P.R., Chen, Y., Aaron, D., et al. Ultrahigh resolution optical biopsy with endoscopic optical coherence tomography. *Optic Express*, 2004; **12**: 3532–3542.
22 Poneros, J.M., Brand, S., Bouma, B. Diagnosis of specialized intestinal metaplasia by optical coherence tomography. *Gastroenterology*, 2001; **120**: 7–12.
23 Brand, S., Poneros, J.M., Bouma, B.E., Tearney, G.J. Optical coherence tomography in the gastrointestinal tract. *Endoscopy*, 2000; **32**: 796–803.
24 Pierce, M.C., Strasswimmer, J., Park, B.H., et al. Advances in optical coherence tomography imaging for dermatology. *Journal of Investigative Dermatology*, 2004; **123**: 458–463.
25 Pircher, M., Goetzinger, E., Leitgeb, R., Hitzenberger, C.K. Three dimensional polarization sensitive OCT of human skin in vivo. *Optics Express*, 2004; **12**: 3236–3244.

estimation by use of indocyanine green fluorescence: initial human trial. *Journal of Burn Care and Rehabilitation*, 1995; **16**: 602–604.

4.3

Influence of purinergic substances on proliferation of murine keratinocytes and full-thickness skin healing

M. Braun Dr med vet, K. Lelieur, M. Kietzmann Dr med vet

Department of Pharmacology, Toxicology and Pharmacy, University of Veterinary Medicine, Hannover Foundation, Hannover, Germany

Summary

Purinoceptors are membrane-bound receptors for adenosine, purines and pyrimidines that are expressed in nearly all cell types throughout the organism. Previous studies have demonstrated that they are involved in the regulation of proliferation and differentiation of most target cells. As it is well-known that several purinoceptors are expressed in skin keratinocytes, we were interested in examining their involvement in wound healing.

The expression of the receptors A_{2B}, $P2Y_1$, $P2Y_2$ and $P2Y_6$ was previously demonstrated in the murine keratinocyte cell line MSC-P5.[1] Therefore, we performed proliferation assays with various purinoceptor agonists and antagonists in these cells. The proliferation was determined by incorporation of 5-bromo-2-deoxyuridine (BrdU).

The purinoceptor agonists adenosine triphosphate (ATP), uridine triphosphate (UTP) and 5'-(N-ethyl)-carboxamidoadenosine (NECA) enhanced the cell growth of MSC-P5 cells *in vitro*. The mitogenic effect of ATP and UTP was inhibited by the non-selective P2Y-receptor antagonist suramin, while the effect of NECA was inhibited by the selective A_{2B}-receptor antagonist enprofylline.

For *in vivo* studies, female NMRI mice were used. To impair the wound healing process, animals were treated once daily with dexamethasone. After a week of treatment, full-thickness wounds were set with biopsy punches in depilated back skin and the purinoceptor agonists and antagonists were administered once daily topically on the wound area. The wound healing process was measured by determination of the wound area. Topical treatments with both NECA and UTP induced better wound healing in dexamethasone-treated mice, which was comparable to the control group without dexamethasone treatment.

These studies confirm that pharmacological actions via purinoceptors offer an intriguing possibility in the treatment of impaired wound healing. Nevertheless, further investigations are needed to fully elucidate the role of purinergic mechanisms involved in wound healing.

Introduction

Wound healing is a complex process that takes place to restore the anatomical and functional integrity of damaged tissue. As the undisturbed healing process cannot be accelerated,[2,3] important research efforts have been made to maintain an optimal environment for 'normal' healing and to counteract retarded wound healing, such as that induced by immunosuppression or metabolic disorders like diabetes mellitus.[2–4]

Purinoceptors are membrane-bound receptors for adenosine, purines and pyrimidines.[5] Their discovery led to intensive research, especially concerning their role in neurotransmission and regulation of the cardiovascular system.[6] It was also demonstrated that purines and pyrimidines are involved in the proliferation and differentiation of various cell types, including keratinocytes. These findings led to the assumption that the purinergic system may be a promising target in the pharmacological manipulation of wound healing.

Purinoceptors are expressed in nearly all types of cells throughout the mammalian organism. Depending on their physiological agonist, the purinoceptors are divided into P1 adenosine receptors (natural ligand adenosine) and P2 receptors (natural ligands adenosine triphosphate [ATP] and adenosine diphosphate).[6] The G protein-coupled adenosine receptors are further classified into the A_1, A_{2A}, A_{2B} and A_3 subtypes based on different molecular, biochemical and pharmacological properties.[6] The P2 receptors on the other hand are divided into the ion channel-coupled P2X and the G protein-coupled P2Y receptor family, which are subdivided into subtypes $P2X_{1-7}$ and $P2Y_{1,2,4,6,11-14}$, respectively.[6]

Since the expression of various purinoceptors (namely A_{2B}, $P2Y_1$, $P2Y_2$, $P2Y_4$, $P2Y_6$ and $P2X_7$) was demonstrated in primary cultured murine keratinocytes and also in a murine keratinocyte cell line,[1] the present studies were performed to elucidate the influence of purinergic substances on the proliferation and differentiation of these cells *in vitro*. Table 4.3.1 summarises the test substances and their effects on the respective purinoceptors. It was furthermore tested whether those substances are promising candidates for pharmacological treatment of wounds by using a well-established animal model of impaired wound healing.[7,8]

Materials and methods

Test substances

All test substances were purchased from Sigma-Aldrich (Steinheim, Germany). For cell culture experiments, ATP was used at concentrations of 0.01, 0.1, 1, 10 and 100 µmol/L. Uridine triphosphate (UTP) and 5'-(N-ethyl)-carboxamidoadenosine (NECA) were applied at concentrations of 0.1, 1, 10 and 100 µmol/L. For uridine diphosphate (UDP) and 2-methylthio-ATP (2-Me-S-ATP) the concentrations 1, 10 and 100 nmol/L as well as 1, 10 and 100 µmol/L were used. As antagonists, suramin and enprofylline were used at

Table 4.3.1 Test substances and their purinergic properties

Substance	Purinoceptor specifity	Effect on receptor
ATP	$P2Y_1$, **$P2Y_2$, $P2Y_4$**, $P2Y_{11}$, $P2Y_{13}$	Agonist
UTP	**$P2Y_2$, $P2Y_4$**, $P2Y_6$	Agonist
UDP	**$P2Y_6$**	Agonist
2-Me-S-ATP	**$P2Y_1$**, $P2Y_6$, $P2Y_{11}$, $P2Y_{13}$	Agonist
Suramin	$P2Y_1$, $P2Y_2$, $P2Y_6$, $P2Y_{11}$	Antagonist
NECA	A_1, A_{2A}, A_{2B}, A_3	Agonist
Enprofylline	A_{2B}	Antagonist

Bold font indicates receptor preferences of the substances.

concentrations of 10 µmol/L and 100 µmol/L, respectively.

For *in vivo* experiments, UTP and NECA were used topically in gel formulations of 1 mmol/L and 100 µmol/L, respectively. Topical treatment with suramin and enprofylline was performed with solutions of 1 mmol/L and 100 µmol/L, respectively.

Cell culture of the permanent murine keratinocyte cell line MSC-P5

MSC-P5 cells (CLS, Heidelberg, Germany) were cultured in RPMI 1640 medium (Biochrom, Berlin, Germany) supplemented with 10% fetal calf serum (FCS; Biochrom) in a humidified atmosphere at 37°C and 5% CO_2, as described in detail by Hoppmann.[9]

Influence of test substances on the proliferation of murine keratinocytes

For the *in vitro* experiments, MSC-P5 cells were seeded in 96-well microtitre plates (Greiner Bio-One, Frickenhausen, Germany) at a density of 10 000 cells/cm². After incubation for 24 hours, the supernatant was removed and the cells were treated with the substances diluted in pure RPMI 1640 medium. Cells treated with RPMI 1640 medium without FCS supplementation served as the control group. Determination of cell proliferation was performed after 96 hours of treatment by the measurement of 5-bromo-2'-deoxyuridine (BrdU) incorporation, using the Cell Proliferation Biotrak ELISA System, version 2 (Amersham Biosciences, Freiburg, Germany), according to the manufacturer's protocol.

In vivo *experiments on impaired wound healing*

The animal experiment had been registered by the Bezirksregierung (district administration) Hannover, Germany (ref. no. 509.6-42502-03/706). All procedures were carried out in agreement with the German Act on the Protection of Animals.

Thirty-six female NMRI mice (Charles River, Sulzfeld, Germany), weighing 25 g each were used. Six animals per treatment group were housed per cage at 22°C with a 12-hour light/dark cycle. They were fed a standard diet (Altromin, Lage/Lippe, Germany) and received fresh water *ad libitum*.

For the induction of retarded wound healing, the animals were treated once daily for 18 days with dexamethasone at 1 mg/kg body weight subcutaneously (Dexa 8 Inject, Jenapharm, Jena, Germany). After 7 days of dexamethasone treatment and under ether anaesthesia, the back skin was depilated and a full-thickness wound was cut using a 6-mm diameter punch (Stiefel Laboratorium GmbH, Offenbach, Germany). Immediately after wounding and once daily thereafter, the wounds were treated topically with the test substances or vehicle (Dermatest Basis-Gel, P&M Cosmetics GmbH & Co. KG, Puchenau, Austria). The amount applied was approximately 100 mg gel and 100 µl solution. In the experiments where sequential treatments with agonist and antagonist were performed, the antagonist solution was administered first and allowed to dry for 1 hour before treatment with the gel formulation of the agonist. After every treatment, the animals were separated and monitored for 1 hour to prevent them from licking. The wounds were left uncovered.

The wound area was measured by planimetry directly after wounding and after 1, 3, 6, 8 and 10 days. To acquire a normal, undelayed wound healing rate, wound areas were measured in six mice without dexamethasone treatment. These animals were treated topically with vehicle once daily.

Statistical analysis

To enable better comparison of the single experiments, cell culture results were expressed as percentages, adjusted to the respective control group (= 100%). In the *in vivo* experiments, the wound area measured on day 0 was set to 100% and the subsequent measurements were adjusted accordingly.

For statistical calculation of differences ($p < 0.05$) in the proliferation of MSC-P5 cells or differences in the wound healing process, depending on the treatment with purinergic substances, Mann–Whitney's rank sum test for unpaired matches (U-test) was performed after Kruskal-Wallis ANOVA on ranks revealed significant differences.

Results

Influence of purinergic substances on the proliferation of murine keratinocytes

Determination of BrdU incorporation after 4 days of

treatment showed that the purinoceptor agonists ATP and UTP significantly ($p < 0.05$) enhanced the proliferation of MSC-P5 cells, with a most effective concentration at 1 µmol/L (Figs 4.3.1 and 4.3.2). These effects were totally inhibited ($p < 0.01$) by simultaneous treatment with the non-selective P2Y-receptor antagonist suramin at a concentration of 10 µmol/L (Fig. 4.3.3).

The P2Y$_1$-selective agonist 2-Me-S-ATP and the P2Y$_6$-selective agonist UDP had no influence on the cell proliferation (data not shown).

The non-selective adenosine receptor agonist NECA significantly ($p < 0.01$) enhanced the proliferation of MSC-P5 cells at concentrations of 10 and 100 µmol/L (Fig. 4.3.4). This effect was totally inhibited ($p < 0.05$) by simultaneous treatment with the selective-A$_{2B}$ antagonist enprofylline (Fig. 4.3.5).

In vivo *influence of purinergic substances on impaired wound healing*

Once-daily treatment of mice with dexamethasone (1 mg/kg body weight) resulted in significantly ($p <$

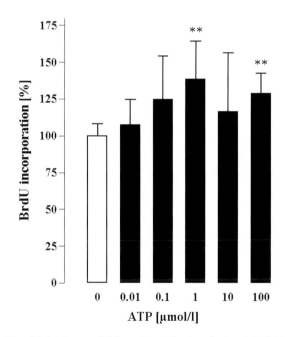

Fig. 4.3.1 Influence of ATP on the proliferation of cultured MSC-P5 cells. Measurement of BrdU incorporation after 4 days of treatment with various ATP concentrations in RPMI medium without FCS. Data are given as percentage of control without ATP supplementation (= 100%). Significant enhancement of cell proliferation by ATP at 1 and 100 µmol/L (**$p = 0.00433$, U-test).

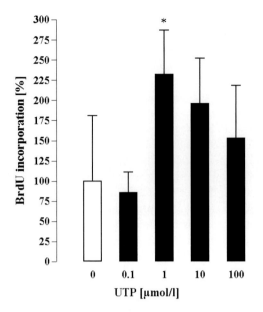

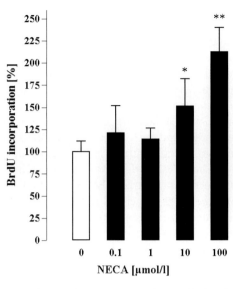

Fig. 4.3.2 Influence of UTP on the proliferation of cultured MSC-P5 cells. Measurement of BrdU incorporation after 4 days of treatment with various UTP concentrations in RPMI medium without FCS. Data are given as percentage of control without UTP supplementation (= 100%). Significant enhancement of cell proliferation by UTP at 1 µmol/L ($*p = 0.0411$, U-test).

Fig. 4.3.4 Influence of NECA on the proliferation of cultured MSC-P5 cells. Measurement of BrdU incorporation after 4 days of treatment with various NECA concentrations in RPMI medium without FCS. Data are given as percentage of control without NECA supplementation (= 100%). Significant enhancement of cell proliferation by NECA at 10 and 100 µmol/L ($*p = 0.00433$, $**p = 0.00216$, U-test).

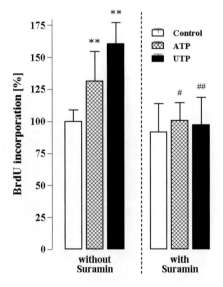

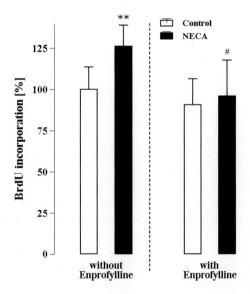

Fig. 4.3.3 Inhibition of the proliferation enhancing effects of ATP and UTP (1 µmol/L) on MSC-P5 cells by simultaneous treatment with suramin (10 µmol/L). Measurement of BrdU incorporation after 4 days of treatment with the respective substances in RPMI medium without FCS. Data are given as percentage of control without supplementation (= 100%). Significant enhancement of cell proliferation by ATP and UTP at 1 µmol/L ($**p = 0.00216$, U-test). Significant inhibition of the enhanced proliferation by suramin at 10 µmol/L ($\#p = 0.0152$, $\#\#p = 0.00216$, U-test).

Fig. 4.3.5 Inhibition of the proliferation enhancing effects of NECA (100 µmol/L) on MSC-P5 cells by simultaneous treatment with enprofylline (100 µmol/L). Measurement of BrdU incorporation after 4 days of treatment with the respective substances in RPMI medium without FCS. Data are given as percentage of control without supplementation (= 100%). Significant enhancement of cell proliferation by NECA at 100 µmol/L. ($**p = 0.00216$, U-test). Significant inhibition of cell proliferation by enprofylline at 100 µmol/L ($\#p = 0.0260$, U-test).

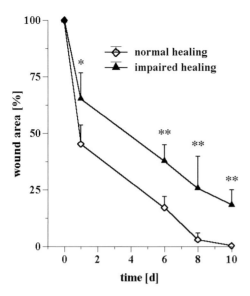

Fig. 4.3.6 Impaired wound healing in mice induced by once-daily subcutaneous treatment with dexamethasone (1 mg/kg body weight). Mean and standard deviation of wound areas (% of wound area on day 0) of six mice. Significant retardation of wound healing compared to wound healing without dexamethasone treatment (*$p = 0.00866$, **$p = 0.00216$, U-test) at days 1, 6, 8 and 10.

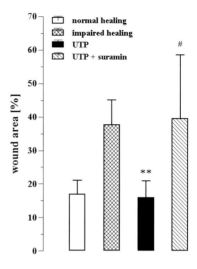

Fig. 4.3.7 Influence of daily topical treatment with a gel formulation of UTP (1 mmol/L) on impaired wounds (dexamethasone treated) in mice and antagonistic effects of suramin (1 mmol/L). Mean and standard deviation of wound areas (% of wound area on day 0), 6 days after wounding ($n = 6$). Topical treatment with UTP significantly (**$p = 0.00216$, U-test) improves impaired wound healing and is significantly antagonised by sequential topical treatment with suramin (#$p = 0.0152$, U-test).

0.05) impaired wound healing, apparent from day 1 after wounding (Fig. 4.3.6). Topical treatment with both NECA at 100 µmol/L and UTP at 1 mmol/L induced significantly ($p < 0.01$) better wound healing from day 6 in dexamethasone-treated mice (Figs 4.3.7 and 4.3.8). The time course of wound healing in NECA- and UTP-treated mice was comparable to the control without dexamethasone treatment (data not shown).

After 6 days of simultaneous topical treatment, suramin (1 mmol/L) resulted in a significant ($p < 0.05$) antagonism of the effect of UTP (Fig. 4.3.7). Simultaneous topical treatment with enprofylline (100 µmol/L) significantly ($p < 0.05$) antagonised the effect of NECA after 6 days (Fig. 4.3.8).

Discussion

The involvement of purinoceptors in the regulation of a variety of cell functions such as differentiation and proliferation is well-known.[10–15] For human skin keratinocytes, it was demonstrated that several P2Y and adenosine receptors are expressed and that their stimulation leads to enhanced cell proliferation, predominantly mediated by elevation of intracellular Ca^{2+} and increased

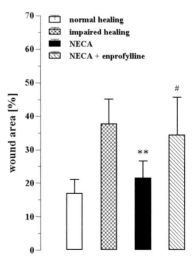

Fig. 4.3.8 Influence of daily topical treatment with a gel formulation of NECA (100 µmol/L) on impaired wounds (dexamethasone treated) in mice and antagonistic effects of enprofylline (100 µmol/L). Mean and standard deviation of wound areas (% of wound area on day 0) 6 days after wounding ($n = 6$). Topical treatment with NECA significantly (**$p = 0.00216$, U-test) improves impaired wound healing and is significantly antagonised by sequential treatment with enprofylline (#$p = 0.0411$, U-test).

cAMP production due to enhanced adenylate cyclase activity.[16-18] Previous studies in our laboratory showed that the purinoceptor expression profile in murine keratinocytes is comparable to that described for human keratinocytes.[1,19] Therefore, we examined whether several purinergic substances that are known to stimulate the proliferation of cultured human keratinocytes have the same effects on murine cells.

As shown by determination of the BrdU incorporation, both ATP and UTP significantly enhance the proliferation of MSC-P5 cells, which is inhibited by simultaneous treatment with the non-selective P2Y antagonist suramin. Since treatment with the $P2Y_1$-selective agonist 2-Me-S-ATP and the $P2Y_6$-selective agonist UDP does not result in comparably enhanced proliferation, it is very likely that the growth stimulation in the MSC-P5 cells is mediated via the $P2Y_2$ receptor subtype, especially as the cell line does not express the $P2Y_4$ subtype, which is also preferentially stimulated by ATP and UTP. These observations are consistent with data previously reported for canine keratinocytes[20] and primary human keratinocytes.[18,19] However, a study performed on primary cultured human keratinocytes describes a positive proliferative effect of other compounds, like the selective $P2Y_1$ agonist 2-Me-S-ADP.[21] The differences can be explained by species-specific responses on purinoceptor binding and by a possible idiosyncrasy in the MSC-P5 cells due to their immortalisation.

Concerning the role of adenosine receptors, the results after treatment with the non-selective agonist NECA give evidence of involvement of these purinoceptor-types in the induction of cell proliferation.[15] As the simultaneous treatment with enprofylline inhibits the effect of NECA, it can be postulated that the proliferative stimulus is mediated via the A_{2B} receptor.

Based on the results from the *in vitro* tests, the efficacy of UTP and NECA was further tested in a well-characterised *in vivo* model of impaired wound healing in mice, achieved by daily systemic treatment with a high dose of dexamethasone.[7,8] In this study, dexamethasone treatment started 7 days prior to wounding and was continued for a total of 18 days. Six days after wounding, a significant delay in wound healing, compared with normal wounds in untreated mice, was determined by measurement of the wound area. Daily topical treatment of the impaired wounds with a gel formulation of UTP improved their healing rate to that of normal, undisturbed wounds. To our knowledge this is the first *in vivo* investigation of the positive effects of topical UTP on skin wounds, although there are several reports of its efficacy *in vitro* using cultured keratinocytes and skin explants.[16,17,21,22] Furthermore, an improved effect of UTP on the healing rate in the n-heptanol wounded rabbit cornea was recently reported.[23] To demonstrate the specificity of the UTP action, i.e. stimulation of the respective purinoceptor(s), simultaneous topical treatment with the non-selective P2Y antagonist suramin was performed. As suramin fully antagonised the effect of UTP on the impaired wounds, the specificity of the improvement seems likely. These data lead to the assumption that the stimulating effect of UTP in impaired wound healing is mediated via the $P2Y_2$ receptor, which is in accordance with the observation of an alteration in the expression pattern of several P2 receptors during wound healing.[24]

Similar to UTP, topical treatment with a gel formulation of NECA improves the impaired wound healing to the rate of normal wounds. Comparable results were reported for the A_{2A} selective agonist 4-([N-ethyl-5'-carbamoyladenos-2-yl]-aminoethyl)-phenylproprionic acid (CGS-21680) in wounded healthy mice and rats, as well as in artificially rendered diabetic rats.[25,26] The positive effect of CGS-21680 is antagonised by the A_{2A}-selective antagonist 3,7-dimethyl-1-propargyl-xanthine (DMPX).[26] In our studies, the positive effect was antagonised by simultaneous topical treatment with the selective A_{2B} antagonist enprofylline, suggesting a dominant role of this adenosine receptor in wound healing. Whether these differences are due to the different mouse strains (Montesinos *et al.* used BALB/c mice,[25,26] whereas our experiments were performed in NMRI mice) or species variations between mice and rats remains to be investigated.

In conclusion, the present study demonstrates the suitability of purinoceptor agonists in the stimulation of keratinocyte growth *in vitro* as well as the improvement of impaired wound healing *in vivo*. Although further investigations are needed to fully elucidate the role of purinergic mechanisms involved in wound healing, research on purinergic substances offers intriguing possibilities for development of new drug targets in pharmacological wound care.

References

1 Lelieur, K., Leeb, T., Kietzmann, M. Purinoceptors in murine and human keratinocytes: detection by RT-PCR and influence on proliferation. *Naunyn-Schmiedeberg's Archives of Pharmacology*, 2003; **367** (Suppl. 1): R35.

2 Niedner, R., Schopf, E. Inhibition of wound healing by anti-septics. *British Journal of Dermatology*, 1986; **115** (Suppl. 31): 41–44.

3 Sedlarik, K. M. *Wundheilung*, 2nd edn. Gustav Fischer, Stuttgart, 1993.

4 Swaim, S.F., Lee, A.H. Topical wound medications: a review. *Journal of the American Veterinary Medical Association*, 1987; **190**: 1588–1593.

5 Sattin, A., Rall, T.W. Effect of adenosine and adenine nucleotides on cyclic adenosine 3',5'-phosphate content of guinea pig cerebral cortex slices. *Molecular Pharmacology*, 1970; **6**: 13–23.

6 Ralevic, V., Burnstock, G. Receptors for purines and pyrimidines. *Pharmacological Reviews*, 1998; **50**: 413–492.

7 Kietzmann, M., Lubach, D., Swoboda, M., Geisler, A. Effects of pale ichthyol in a model of impaired wound healing. In: Altmeyer, P., Hoffmann, K., el Gammal, S., Hutchinson, J., eds. *Wound Healing and Skin Physiology*, 1st edn. Springer, Berlin, 1995: 609–615.

8 Kietzmann, M. Improvement and retardation of wound healing: effects of pharmacological agents in laboratory animal studies. *Veterinary Dermatology*, 1999; **10**: 83–88.

9 Hoppmann, J. *Beitrag zur Rolle von Keratinozyten für die Aktivierung und Regulierung von immunologisch bedingten Abwehrreaktionen der Haut.* Thesis, Universitaet Giessen, 2002.

10 Huang, N.N., Wang, D.J., Heppel, L.A. Extracellular ATP is a mitogen for 3T3-cell, 3T6-cell, and A431-cell and acts synergistically with other growth-factors. *Proceedings of the National Academy of Sciences of the United States of America*, 1989; **86**: 7904–7908.

11 Rathbone, M.P., Middlemiss, P.J., Gysbers, J.W., Deforge, S., Costello, P., Delmaestro, R.F. Purine nucleosides and nucleotides stimulate proliferation of a wide range of cell-types. *In Vitro Cellular and Developmental Biology*, 1992; **28A**: 529–536.

12 Rathbone, M.P., Deforge, S., Deluca, B., *et al.* Purinergic stimulation of cell-division and differentiation – mechanisms and pharmacological implications. *Medical Hypotheses*, 1992; **37**: 213–219.

13 Rathbone, M.P., Christjanson, L., Deforge, S., *et al.* Extracellular purine nucleosides stimulate cell-division and morphogenesis – pathological and physiological implications. *Medical Hypotheses*, 1992; **37**: 232–240.

14 Thellung, S., Florio, T., Maragliano, A., Cattarini, G., Schettini, G. Polydeoxyribonucleotides enhance the proliferation of human skin fibroblasts: involvement of A(2) purinergic receptor subtypes. *Life Sciences*, 1999; **64**: 1661–1674.

15 Yuh, I.S., Sheffield, L.G. Adenosine stimulation of DNA synthesis in mammary epithelial cells. *Proceedings of the Society for Experimental Biology and Medicine*, 1998; **218**: 341–348.

16 Dixon, C.J., Bowler, W.B., Littlewood-Evans, A., *et al.* Regulation of epidermal homeostasis through P2Y(2) receptors. *British Journal of Pharmacology*, 1999; **127**: 1680–1686.

17 Lee, W.K., Choi, S.W., Lee, H.R., Lee, E.J., Lee, K.H., Kim, H.O. Purinoceptor-mediated calcium mobilization and proliferation in HaCaT keratinocytes. *Journal of Dermatological Science*, 2001; **25**: 97–105.

18 Pillai, S., Bikle, D.D. Adenosine-triphosphate stimulates phosphoinositide metabolism, mobilizes intracellular calcium, and inhibits terminal differentiation of human epidermal-keratinocytes. *Journal of Clinical Investigation*, 1992; **90**: 42–51.

19 Burrell, H.E., Bowler, W.B., Gallagher, J.A., Sharpe, G.R. Human keratinocytes express multiple P2Y-receptors: evidence for functional P2Y(1), P2Y(2), and P2Y(4) receptors. *Journal of Investigative Dermatology*, 2003; **120**: 440–447.

20 Suter, M.M., Crameri, F.M., Slattery, J.P., Millard, P.J., Gonzalez, F.A. Extracellular ATP and some of its analogs induce transient rises in cytosolic free calcium in individual canine keratinocytes. *Journal of Investigative Dermatology*, 1991; **97**: 223–229.

21 Greig, A.V.H., Linge, C., Terenghi, G., McGrouther, D.A., Burnstock, G. Purinergic receptors are part of a functional signaling system for proliferation and differentiation of human epidermal keratinocytes. *Journal of Investigative Dermatology*, 2003; **120**: 1007–1015.

22 Greig, A.V.H., Linge, C., Healy, V., *et al.* Expression of purinergic receptors in non-melanoma skin cancers and their functional roles in A431 cells. *Journal of Investigative Dermatology*, 2003; **121**: 315–327.

23 Pintor, J., Bautista, A., Carracedo, G., Peral, A. UTP and diadenosine tetraphosphate accelerate wound healing in the rabbit cornea. *Ophthalmic and Physiological Optics*, 2004; **24**: 186–193.

24 Greig, A.V.H., James, S.E., McGrouther, D.A., Terenghi, G., Burnstock, G. Purinergic receptor expression in the regeneration epidermis in a rat model of normal and delayed wound healing. *Experimental Dermatology*, 2003; **12**: 860–871.

25 Montesinos, M.C., Desai, A., Chen, J.F., *et al.* Adenosine promotes wound healing and mediates angiogenesis in response to tissue injury via occupancy of A(2A) receptors. *American Journal of Pathology*, 2002; **160**: 2009–2018.

26 Montesinos, M.C., Gadangi, P., Longaker, M., *et al.* Wound healing is accelerated by agonists of adenosine A(2) (G(alpha s)-linked) receptors. *Journal of Experimental Medicine*, 1997; **186**: 1615–1620.

Factors associated with *Malassezia* colonisation in the ear canals of dogs without clinical signs of otitis externa

C.A. Rème DVM

Medical Department, Virbac SA, Carros, France

Summary

This study analysed the relationships between animal characteristics and clinical signs, and *Malassezia* populations in the ear canals of dogs without clinical signs of otitis externa, but with cerumen readily visible at the opening of the ear canal. Forty-two dogs were studied. The dogs had not received any treatment in the previous week. Quantity of cerumen in ears, malodour and erythema were graded on a five-point severity scale. *Malassezia* populations were recorded by cytology from ear swabs. No yeast was detected in 12 (28.6%) of the dogs. Mean yeast numbers in the range of 0.1–1.3 and 1.5–3.5 organisms/oil immersion field (OIF, ×1000) were demonstrated in 21 (50%) and 7 dogs (16.7%) respectively.

Only two dogs (4.7%) yielded mean yeast counts in the range of 4–5 organisms/OIF. Breeds documented to be at higher risk for ear disease did not harbour higher *Malassezia* counts as compared to other breeds represented. Dogs with pendulous ears were not more prone to yield higher yeast counts as compared to dogs with erect ears. Dogs' age and sex, cerumen consistency and quantity, and aural malodour were not found to be associated with *Malassezia* numbers in smears. However, dogs' weight, cerumen colour and intensity of aural erythema correlated positively with yeast counts (p ≤ 0.05). This study confirms the high prevalence of Malassezia in the ear canals of dogs without clinical signs of otitis externa. Good clinical prognostic variables to predict the importance of yeast colonisation in the ear canals could not be identified.

Introduction

The lipophilic yeast *Malassezia pachydermatis* is frequently isolated from the external ear canal of healthy dogs. The fungus is part of the normal cutaneous microflora, but may proliferate under favourable environmental conditions (e.g. moisture, epidermal barrier dysfunction) and play an important role in the development of otitis externa.[1] The key factors associated with colonisation of the aural epithelium and resident yeast carriage in the external ear canal remain to be identified. Breed, ear conformation, density of hair in the canal, and living conditions are usually thought to be important predisposing factors.[2,3]

Investigators have reported isolation of yeast from 15–50% of normal canine ear canals.[4–7] Only one semi-quantitative cytological study has addressed the impor-

tance of commensal *Malassezia* populations residing in healthy ears.[8] Recommendations as to the number of yeast per high power microscopic field that should be considered normal differ among authors.[8–10]

The purpose of this study was to evaluate *Malassezia* populations in ear swab smears from dogs without clinical signs of otitis externa, but with cerumen visible at the opening of the ear canal, and to analyse the relationships between animal characteristics and clinical signs, and the yeast counts.

Materials and methods

Animal selection

Forty-two dogs without clinical signs of otitis externa,

of any breed, sex or age, were selected from five veterinary clinics in France. The presence of cerumen (greasy malodorous debris) readily visible at the opening of the ear canal was the inclusion criterion. Exclusion criteria were signs of otitis externa (marked ear canal irritation, exudate, pruritus, pain), any other ear disease, treatment in the previous week with systemic or otic antimicrobial or anti-inflammatory agents, and treatment in the previous 3 weeks with long-acting injectable corticosteroids. Animal characteristics (breed, age, sex, weight) and recent history, as well as any relevant background information (e.g. allergic condition), were recorded on standard case report forms.

Evaluation criteria

Clinical scores
Veterinarians performed visual examination of the pinnae, olfactory evaluation of the ear canal openings, and otoscopic inspection of the ear canals, together with cerumen sampling for cytological examination. Quantity of cerumen in ears, malodour and associated erythema were graded on a five-point severity scale. Cerumen consistency (soft or dry) and colour (yellowish or brown) were also recorded.

Cytological examination
Both ears of each dog were sampled with cotton-tipped swabs. The swabs were inserted into the vertical canal and rotated through 180°. The samples were rolled onto clean slides (three bands) and allowed to dry. The slides were scanned for mites. Diff-Quik® staining procedure was performed and the samples were allowed to dry completely. The slides were scanned at low magnification (4–10× objective) to determine if all areas of the smears were stained adequately and to select representative areas. Then, *Malassezia* counts were performed on 10 contiguous oil immersion fields (OIF, ×1000 with oil immersion objective).

Statistics

Spearman rank correlation coefficients (r) were calculated to examine the relationships among *Malassezia* counts, animal characteristics and clinical signs. Differences in the numbers of *Malassezia* among subgroups of dogs were tested by the Kruskal-Wallis analysis of variance. Data analyses were performed with commercial statistical software (NCSS 2000, NCSS, Kaysville,

UT, USA) and differences were considered to be significant at $p \leq 0.05$.

Results

Animal characteristics

Dogs included in the study represented a large variety of breeds, sizes and ages (Table 4.4.1). Breeds most represented were Bassets, Labrador retrievers, poodles, spaniels and setters (59.5% of dogs). Dogs with pendulous ears were more common (76.2%) than those with erect pinnae. Young (4–8 months) as well as old (12–15 years) dogs were included in the study,

Table 4.4.1 Demographic data and clinical scores of dogs included in the study

Characteristic	All dogs included in the study ($n = 42$)
Sex	
Female	18
Male	24
Breed	
Basset Artésien Normand	9
Beauce shepherd	3
Brittany spaniel	3
English setter	2
Labrador retriever	6
Lhasa apso	2
Samoyed	2
Poodle	4
Other*	11
Age (years)	
Median	6
Range	0.25–15
Weight (kg)	
Median	17
Range	4.1–40
Cerumen quantity in ears (0–4 severity score)	
Median	2
Range	1–4
Aural malodour intensity (0–4 severity score)	
Median	2
Range	0–4
Aural erythema intensity (0–4 severity score)	
Median	1
Range	0–2

*Other breeds represented by a single individual included bichon frise, fox terrier, German shepherd dog, Griffon Vendéen, Siberian husky, Jagd terrier, Labrit, pinscher, rottweiler, Shih Tzu and cocker spaniel.

but overall middle-aged (2–7 years) dogs represented the majority of cases (52.4%). The sex ratio was approximately equal.

Correlation of clinical parameters and yeast counts between left and right ears

Good correlation was found for the quantity of cerumen and intensity of odour and erythema between left and right ears ($0.75 \leq r \leq 0.83$, $p < 0.0001$). Strong correlation was detected for *Malassezia* counts in ear samples from both ears ($r = 0.93$, $p < 0.0001$). Consequently, only the average scores and counts of both ears were considered for each individual, in order to obtain independent data for statistical tests.

Clinical scores

Cerumen accumulation was rated as moderate to marked for 73.8% of dogs by the investigators. Cerumen consistency was soft in the vast majority of cases (85.7%) and brown was the predominant colour (64.3%). Moderate to strong unpleasant odour was detected at close examination for 59.5% of dogs. There was no erythema of the pinna or ear canal in 33.3% of cases, only slight redness of the epithelial lining in 45.2%, and moderate redness in 21.5% of cases.

Malassezia counts by cytology

Malassezia organisms could be detected in the majority of dogs (71.4%). Mean yeast counts very rarely exceeded four organisms/OIF (Fig. 4.4.1). Variation was significant among investigators because no *Malassezia* organisms could be detected in smears at one clinic (Table 4.4.2). This site included five dogs in the study: one Beauce shepherd, one Griffon Vendéen, two Lhasa apsos and a pinscher.

Variations in yeast counts were observed among breeds at all clinics (Table 4.4.2). The English setter ($n = 2$) was the only breed in which no *Malassezia* could be found. Yeast counts were not significantly different among other breed groups (Fig. 4.4.2). Ear conformation, breed predisposition for ear disease, available historical information and cerumen consistency were qualitative factors not associated with the number of *Malassezia* organisms in smears. Brown cerumen colour was more frequently associated with increased yeast counts (Table 4.4.2).

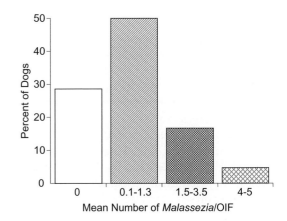

Fig. 4.4.1 *Malassezia* counts determined by microscopic examination of 10 representative contiguous fields (OIF, ×1000 magnification) in smears obtained from the ear canals of healthy dogs.

As for animal characteristics and clinical signs, only the animal body weight and intensity of erythema of the pinna or ear canal correlated significantly with yeast counts in smears, although the degree of linear relationship was moderate (Table 4.4.3). The mean yeast count was twice as high for the heavier dogs (>15 kg) presenting with aural erythema (1.3 *Malassezia*/OIF), as compared to the lighter dogs without erythema (0.6 *Malassezia*/OIF). Quantity of cerumen in ears and aural malodour did not correlate with *Malassezia* numbers (Table 4.4.3).

Discussion

This study confirms the high prevalence of *Malassezia* yeast in the ear canals of dogs without clinical signs of otitis externa. Frequency of yeast detection in this study (71.4%) was higher than previously reported (15–50%),[4–7] possibly because dogs with visible accumulation of cerumen were selected for the study. The presence of yeast alone cannot be equated with true ear infection. Indeed, studies suggest that the incidence of *Malassezia* is similar for both normal and diseased ears.[4,9]

The number of yeast organisms in stained smears is thought to be more indicative of infection.[9] There is some debate, however, as to the number of *Malassezia* organisms per microscopic field that should be considered normal. Our results suggest that in a majority of cases, < 3.5 yeast/oil immersion field (×1000)

Table 4.4.2 Association between qualitative variables and the number of *Malassezia* organisms per oil immersion field (×1000 magnification) counted from microscopic examination of ear samples

Variable	Category	Number of dogs	Median *Malassezia* counts/OIF (min–max)	Kruskal-Wallis test *p* value
Investigating site	1	5	0 (0–0)	0.005*
	2	9	1.3 (0.4–4.8)	
	3	2	2.3 (0.5–4.2)	
	4	20	0.8 (0–3.4)	
	5	6	0.3 (0–1.2)	
Sex	Female	18	0.7 (0–2.8)	0.9
	Male	24	0.6 (0–4.8)	
Breed	Labrador	6	0.7 (0–4.2)	0.04*
	Basset	9	1.3 (0.4–4.8)	
	Poodle	4	0.3 (0.1–1.0)	
	Setter	2	0 (0–0)	
	Spaniel	4	1.0 (0–2.2)	
	Other breed	17	0.3 (0–2.3)	
Risk for ear disease	High[a]	30	0.8 (0–4.8)	0.2
	Low	12	0.3 (0–2.3)	
Ear conformation	Pendulous	32	0.7 (0–4.8)	0.3
	Erect	10	0.3 (0–2.3)	
Past episodes of otitis	Yes	5	1.0 (0.6–4.2)	0.06
	No	37	0.6 (0–4.8)	
Episodes of pruritus/head shaking	Yes	12	0.4 (0–3.4)	0.5
	No	30	0.6 (0–4.8)	
Rancid odour/seborrhoea	Yes	14	0.5 (0–3.4)	0.5
	No	28	0.8 (0–4.8)	
Cerumen consistency	Soft	36	0.8 (0–4.8)	0.4
	Dry	6	0.3 (0–4.2)	
Cerumen colour	Brown	27	0.8 (0–4.8)	0.02*
	Yellowish	15	0 (0–3.4)	

[a] The following breeds were considered to be at high risk for ear disease: Basset Artésien Normand, bichon frise, poodle, cocker and other spaniels, Labrador retriever, Labrit, Lhasa apso, English setter and German shepherd dog.
*Significant at $p \leq 0.05$.

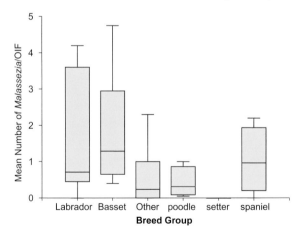

Fig. 4.4.2 Box and whisker plot of *Malassezia* counts by breed group. The top and bottom of the shaded boxes are the 25th and 75th percentiles. The length of the boxes is the interquartile range (IQR) and represents the middle 50% of the data. The lines crossing the shaded boxes represent medians. The whiskers extend to the most extreme observation that is less than 1.5 × IQR from the upper and lower limits of the IQR.

can be found on average in ears without clinical signs of infection. This finding agrees with an earlier report indicating that < 10 yeasts per high-power dry field (×400) should be considered normal, a figure approximately equivalent to ≤ 4 yeasts per oil immersion field (×1000).[11] However, in another report the authors concluded that mean counts > 5 yeasts per high-power dry field are abnormal.[8] The proposed upper limit of normality for *Malassezia* yeast cells per field found in the present study on healthy dogs is in agreement with recent clinical studies of antimicrobial preparations for the treatment of canine otitis that use a minimum average of 3–4 yeast/OIF for the cytological diagnosis of yeast overgrowth.[12,13]

Few factors were found to be significantly associated with the number of yeast organisms in smears. Variation in yeast counts among investigators mainly reflected the absence of findings at one clinic. Values

Table 4.4.3 Correlation between quantitative variables and the number of *Malassezia* organisms per oil immersion field (×1000 magnification) counted from microscopic examination of ear samples

Variable	Sample size	Spearman rank correlation coefficient, r	Significance level, p value
Age	42	0.22	0.2
Weight	41	0.36	0.02*
Cerumen quantity	42	0.24	0.1
Malodour intensity	42	0.25	0.1
Erythema intensity	42	0.30	0.05*

recorded at every other site were consistent and may have reflected stricter compliance with the specified standard sampling procedure and counting method. Given that the numbers of *Malassezia* organisms vary greatly from field to field by microscopic examination,[14] the most critical parameter to decrease variability among sites is the proper selection criteria of 'representative fields' for counting.

No variation in *Malassezia* carriage was demonstrated among breed groups in our study, with the exception of the two setters which were free of aural yeast. The findings contrast with earlier reports suggesting breed predisposition in the levels of resident yeast carriage on canine skin. In one study, both the number of organisms and frequency of isolation in ears were significantly greater for 20 kennelled beagles as compared to a random sample of 20 healthy pet dogs.[3] However, the two groups differed in their environmental parameters in addition to breed category. Higher basal yeast carriage has been described in Basset hounds,[2] but this particular breed was not represented in the present study.

No influence of ear type (pendulous or erect) was found on yeast counts, although this factor is commonly mentioned as playing a role in *Malassezia* colonisation.[2,15] *Malassezia* is primarily affected by alterations in the microclimate of the ear canal. Recent evidence supports the fact that the ear type does not affect the retention of heat and moisture in the ear canal as much as previously thought.[6] By contrast, the external ear canal temperature (EECT) was more readily influenced by body weight, a factor significantly correlated with yeast counts in our study. Smaller animals indeed have decreased EECT,

possibly as a result of a more rapid rate of heat loss via aural skin.[16]

Dog breeds documented to be at higher risk for ear disease did not harbour higher *Malassezia* counts than non-predisposed breeds. Thus, development of otitis may be more readily related to a multiplicity of internal and external factors that allow a basal opportunistic *Malassezia* population to proliferate and become pathogenic (e.g. alteration of host defence mechanisms, underlying disease, exposure to water, climatic changes, traumatic or irritating ear cleaning).

Slightly increased skin redness was the only quantitative clinical parameter correlated with *Malassezia* counts. This may correspond to slight reaction of the epithelial lining to developing yeast populations, or the subclinical expression of an underlying allergic condition. It is noteworthy that the absolute quantity of cerumen in ears is poorly predictive for yeast numbers, despite the fact that cerumen is a favourable substrate for yeast development.[2] However, all dogs in this study had some kind of cerumen accumulation, which could have sustained *Malassezia* colonisation. The brown colour of cerumen material was more indicative of higher basal yeast counts.

The study found that *Malassezia* is a frequent commensal in the ear canal of dogs without clinical signs of otitis externa, but with visible cerumen accumulation. The fact that these dogs had cerumen but no signs of otitis externa does not imply that in the general population the ear canals will always be totally normal. A large quantity of wax and slight erythema could still be found and may correspond to subclinical, early stage, developing disease. Ears with greasy debris without obvious signs of otitis may provide a favourable medium for the establishment of permanent yeast populations, prompting the need for regular ear cleansing. Many of the factors that govern yeast ecology remain obscure and good prognostic variables to predict the importance of yeast colonisation in the ear canals could not be identified in this study.

Acknowledgements

The author would like to thank Drs Jean-François Marty, Olivier Ramette, Bernard Coubray, Marc Boulet and Yvan Cochin for their active participation in the trial.

Funding

This study was funded by Virbac SA.

References

1 Bond, R. Pathogenesis of *Malassezia* dermatitis. In: Thoday, K.L., Foil, C.S., Bond R., eds. *Advances in Veterinary Dermatology*, 4th edn. Blackwell Science, Oxford, 2002: 69–75.

2 Guillot, J., Guého, E., Mialot, M., Chermette, R. Importance des levures du genre *Malassezia* en dermatologie vétérinaire. *Le Point Vétérinaire*, 1998; **29**: 691–701.

3 Bond, R., Saijonmaa-Koulumies, L.E., Lloyd, D.H. Population sizes and frequency of *Malassezia pachydermatis* at skin and mucosal sites on healthy dogs. *Journal of Small Animal Practice*, 1995; **36**: 147–150.

4 McKeever, P.J., Torres, S.M.F. Ear disease and its management. *Veterinary Clinics of North America: Small Animal Practice*, 1997; **27**: 1523–1536.

5 Kumar, A., Singh, K., Sharma, A. Prevalence of *Malassezia pachydermatis* and other organisms in healthy and infected dog ears. *Israel Journal of Veterinary Medicine*, 2002; **57**: 145–148.

6 Yoshida, N., Naito, F., Fukata, T. Studies of certain factors affecting the microenvironment and microflora of the external ear of the dog in health and disease. *Journal of Veterinary Medical Science*, 2002; **64**: 1145–1147.

7 Crespo, M.J., Abarca, M.L., Cabanes, F.J. Occurrence of *Malassezia* spp. in the external ear canals of dogs and cats with and without otitis externa. *Medical Mycology*, 2002; **40**: 115–121.

8 Ginel, P.J., Lucena, R., Rodriguez, J.C., Ortega, J. A semiquantitative cytological evaluation of normal and pathological samples from the external ear canal of dogs and cats. *Veterinary Dermatology*, 2002; **13**: 151–156.

9 Kowalski, J.J. The microbial environment of the ear canal in health and disease. *Veterinary Clinics of North America: Small Animal Practice*, 1988; **18**: 743–754.

Part 5

Infectious and parasitic diseases

Part 5

Infectious and parasitic diseases

Mycobacterial diseases of cats and dogs

R. Malik BVSc, DipVetAn, MVetClinStud, PhD

Post Graduate Foundation in Veterinary Science, The University of Sydney, New South Wales, Australia

Summary

Mycobacterial diseases are an uncommon but fascinating cause of cutaneous lesions in cats and dogs. In some cases disease is restricted to the skin, whilst in others skin involvement is merely a reflection of a disseminated disease process. The author's experience in treating these cases has been limited to Australia, a continent virtually free of tuberculosis. Accordingly, this presentation is biased towards non-tuberculous mycobacterial disease conditions of companion animals.

It is useful to consider infectious diseases in light of a widely applicable conceptual framework which takes into account the mammalian host, the bacterial parasite and the environment. Accordingly, as well as considering patho-anatomic syndromes, we will consider mycobacterial diseases of cats and dogs under the following categories:

- Diseases caused by obligate mycobacterial parasites.
- Localised disease caused by saprophytic mycobacteria in immunocompetent hosts:
  - where the infection is self-limiting, i.e. the immune response eventually eliminates the causal organisms, or
  - where the infection remains localised, but requires veterinary intervention to effect a cure.
- Disseminated diseases caused by mycobacteria in immunodeficient hosts.

Diseases caused by members of the *Mycobacterium tuberculosis* complex (including *M. microti*) generally represent infection by obligate mycobacterial parasites, i.e. primary pathogens that are sufficiently host-adapted that they require a suitable mammalian host for survival. Some feline infections caused by the rat leprosy bacillus *M. lepraemurium* also fit into this category. Canine leproid granulomas are caused by a fastidious, presumably slow-growing, mycobacterium, and generally give rise to limited infections of the skin that are eventually terminated by a successful immune response. Rapidly growing mycobacteria such as *M. fortuitum* and *M. smegmatis* give rise to localised invasive and often refractory disease in immunocompetent hosts, but can be permanently cured using appropriate antimicrobial agents, and sometimes surgery. In contrast, disseminated disease occurs in immuno-incompetent hosts due to infection with a range of saprophytic mycobacteria including *M. avium* complex, novel fastidious mycobacterial species that produce feline leprosy in elderly cats, and *M. genavense* infections in cats and ferrets.

Towards a conceptual framework

Mycobacteria are gram-positive rods which have a cell wall rich in high molecular weight fatty acids and waxes as their distinguishing feature. The name *Mycobacterium* (fungus-bacterium) is a consequence of the hydrophobic nature of the lipid-rich cell wall which gives them the tendency to grow as mould-like pellicles on the surface of liquid medium. The major lipid in the cell wall is mycolic acid, which imparts two characteristic features to the genus: (1) a capacity for survival and replication within phagocytes; and (2) the ability to retain carbol fuchsin stain after heating and exposure to acid and/or alcohol.

Historically, mycobacteria have been divided into three groups: (1) obligate pathogens such as *M. tuberculosis*, *M. bovis* and *M. microti*, which do not normally multiply outside vertebrate hosts; (2) facultative pathogens which normally exist as saprophytes in the environment and only sporadically cause disease; and (3) those environmental saprophytes which almost never cause disease. However, the situation has recently been made more complex. *M. avium* subsp. *paratuberculosis*, for example, may or may not be an obligate pathogen of ruminants, while a number of formerly non-pathogenic species have been reported to cause significant disease in HIV/AIDS patients.

Mycobacteria of clinical importance to man and animals include the well-known pathogenic species *M. tuberculosis*, *M. leprae* and *M. avium* subsp. *paratuberculosis* that give rise to tuberculosis, leprosy and Johne's disease, respectively. Tuberculosis in cats can be caused by *M. tuberculosis*, *M. bovis* and *M. microti*. As these diseases have been reviewed recently,[1–3] they will not be covered in any detail here. Classical tuberculosis in cats is caused by *M. bovis* and occasionally *M. tuberculosis*.[3] 'Feline tuberculosis syndrome' is caused by a mycobacterium with characteristics intermediate between *M. bovis* and *M. tuberculosis* and it seems most likely to result from infection with *M. microti* strains[3] inoculated during altercations with voles.[1,2]

As well as these well-known agents of disease, there are many different saprophytic mycobacterial species that, under certain circumstances, are capable of producing opportunistic infections in both immunocompetent and immunoparetic patients. It is this latter group of organisms, and the diseases they produce in cats and dogs, that are the subject of this review.

Although by no means a common cause of disease in small animal practice, mycobacteria are important 'unusual' agents of infectious disease. Recent developments in antimicrobial chemotherapy and reconstructive surgery have enabled most mycobacterial infections encountered in cats and dogs to be potentially curable, given committed owners and patients with an agreeable disposition.

When mycobacteria give rise to stereotypical clinical syndromes, diagnosis is usually straightforward, providing the opportunity for a successful outcome. However, when mycobacteria give rise to 'atypical' disease, such as granulomatous pneumonia or disseminated disease with peripheral lymph node and/or internal organ involvement, the clinical picture can be suggestive of neoplasia (such as lymphosarcoma); hence, animals can sometimes be euthanased on the basis of having an untreatable terminal disease unless appropriate specimens are collected for laboratory examination.

We have adopted a collaborative approach to the diagnosis and management of small animals with myco-bacteriosis. Our group consists of a team of interested small animal practitioners, veterinary cytopathologists and microbiologists with a special interest in diseases caused by unusual pathogens, a specialist surgeon interested in novel reconstructive approaches to extensive cutaneous disease, and similarly interested medical colleagues and mycobacteriologists at research institutes, reference laboratories and human hospitals.

Non-tuberculous mycobacteria give rise to a number of different patho-anatomic syndromes in small animal practice, although sometimes the distinction between these syndromes can become blurred. In the main part of this chapter, the clinical features of mycobacterial disease in cats and dogs will be discussed according to a simple classification scheme (Box 5.1.1), although only dermal syndromes will be covered in detail.

Although clinicians are comfortable working with such a 'syndromic' classification, a deeper insight can be provided by a scheme which classifies disease on the basis of the interaction between the mammalian host, the bacterial agent of disease, and the environment in which the host and pathogen interact. Such a conceptual framework would divide the mycobacterial diseases of cats and dogs into the categories defined in Box 5.1.2.

Obviously these schemata are arbitrary, and one of the purposes of this review is to reconcile the different ways of classifying mycobacterial disease with respect to the infections seen in cats and dogs (Table 5.1.1). Thus, diseases caused by members of the *M. tuberculosis* complex (including *M. microti*) generally represent infection by an obligate mycobacterial parasite, i.e. a primary pathogen that is sufficiently host-adapted that it must have a suitable mammalian host in order to survive. In contrast, canine leproid granulomas are caused by a fastidious, presumably slow-growing mycobacterium, that generally gives rise to limited infections of the skin that are eventually terminated by a successful immune response. Rapid-growing mycobacteria such as *M. fortuitum* and *M. smegmatis* give rise to localised, invasive, and often refractory, disease in immunocompetent hosts. Such infections

---

Box 5.1.1 Historical and patho-anatomic classification of non-tuberculous mycobacterial syndromes encountered in companion animal practice

A. Mycobacterial panniculitis due to rapidly growing myco-bacteria (RGM)
B. Localised or disseminated cutaneous/subcutaneous disease due to fastidious mycobacterial species
C. Disseminated mycobacterial infection, with lymph node and/or internal organ involvement and sometimes lesions of the skin and subcutis
D. Miscellaneous localised mycobacterial infections, e.g. mycobacterial pneumonia, keratitis, etc.

Box 5.1.2 Classification scheme for mycobacterial disease based on inherent virulence of the organism and the immunological response of the host, taking into account host/pathogen/environment interrelationships

1. Diseases caused by obligate mycobacterial parasites
2. Localised disease caused by saprophytic mycobacteria in immunocompetent hosts:
   (a) where the infection is self-limiting, i.e. the immune response eventually eliminates the causal organisms, or
   (b) where the infection remains localised but requires veterinary intervention to effect a cure
3. Disseminated diseases caused by mycobacteria in immunodeficient hosts

require a combination of factors to develop, such as an especially large inoculum of organisms, sufficiently traumatised host tissue, a microenvironment rich in fat with a limited blood supply, and perhaps an anatomic region relatively inaccessible to self-cleaning. Even though the resulting lesions can become extensive, it is vital to appreciate that the cell-mediated immune

response of the host is typically competent, and thus debridement and adjunctive antibacterial therapy can permanently clear the infection. A very different situation exists when disseminated disease occurs in immune incompetent hosts. This may involve infection with one of a number of saprophytic mycobacteria including: (1) members of the *M. avium* complex (MAC) (in Abyssinian and Somali cats with a familial immune deficiency); (2) novel mycobacterial species that produce feline leprosy lesions in elderly cats with concurrent renal disease and/or long-standing FIV infection; or (3) *M. genavense* infections in cats and ferrets. Importantly, some organisms behave in a different fashion according to the immune competence of the mammalian host. For example, *M. lepraemurium* may produce either localised disease in young cats that resolves spontaneously (rarely) or following simple surgical excision. Alternately, this infection may result in widely disseminated disease in older cats with immune compromise.

A feature of mycobacterial disease is the associated inflammatory response, which is generally granulomatous or pyogranulomatous, as might be expected for an infection in which cell-mediated

Table 5.1.1 Composite categorisation of mycobacterial infections in cats and dogs taking into account the patho-anatomic distribution of lesions, growth characteristics of the organism, and the immunological relationship between the patient and the agent of disease

Patho-anatomic and immunological characteristics	Disease syndrome and causative organisms
Obligate mycobacterial parasites, typically in immune competent hosts. Such infections may remain localised if effectively constrained by the immune response, or become generalised following dissemination from the primary site of infection	Tuberculosis (caused by members of the *M. tuberculosis* complex including *M. tuberculosis*, *M. bovis* and *M. microti*). Feline leprosy caused by *M. lepraemurium* in young adult cats
Localised disease caused by saprophytic mycobacteria, generally in immune competent hosts. Infections are generally self-limiting	Canine leproid granuloma syndrome caused by an unnamed fastidious novel mycobacterial species
Localised disease caused by saprophytic mycobacteria in immune competent hosts, but where the infection remains 'localised' to the subcutis and skin. Infections generally require veterinary intervention to effect a cure	'Panniculitis syndrome' caused by rapidly growing mycobacterial species (e.g. *M. smegmatis*, *M. fortuitum*, *M. chelonae*). Lobar pneumonia caused by rapidly growing mycobacteria. Localised infections of the skin/subcutis caused by *M. avium* complex (MAC). Localised keratitis due to MAC
Disseminated diseases caused by mycobacterial species in immunodeficient hosts. Mycobacterial species that give rise to these infections frequently involve species of such limited pathogenicity that they rarely (if ever) give rise to disease in immune competent hosts	A. MAC infections in young adult Abyssinian cats. B. *M. genavense* infections in ferrets and old cats with long-standing FIV infection. C. Feline leprosy caused by *M. visibilis* and unnamed fastidious novel mycobacterial species in old cats. Some cases of feline leprosy are caused by *M. lepraemurium* in cats that due to age, genetic make-up, or concurrent disease, have increased susceptibility to mycobacteria

immunity (CMI) is required to activate mononuclear phagocytes to combat bacteria capable of intracellular survival. Pyogranulomatous inflammation most usually accompanies disease associated with saprophytic mycobacteria, whether slow-growing (MAC, *M. marinum*, *M. xenopi* or *M. scrofulaceum*) or rapid-growing species (*M. fortuitum, M. smegmatis, M. chelonae* or *M. thermoresistible*). Similar pathology may be seen with diseases associated with other bacteria with high lipid content in their cell walls (such as members of the genera *Corynebacterium*, *Nocardia* and *Rhodococcus*) and with some fungal infections. The pathology, however, is clearly distinguishable from that associated with parasitic (tuberculous) mycobacteria (*M. tuberculosis, M. bovis, M. africanum* and *M. microti*) where granulomatous inflammation dominates the cellular response in immunocompetent hosts.[4,5]

Although many other disease processes and agents give rise to (pyo)granulomatous inflammation, for example feline infectious peritonitis virus and the other microorganisms mentioned earlier, mycobacteria should be considered in the differential diagnosis when cytopathology demonstrates mixtures of lymphoid cells and mononuclear phagocytes. Under these circumstances, the diagnostic laboratory should be requested to perform special stains to demonstrate mycobacteria, including both modified acid-fast stains to directly demonstrate the acid-fast bacilli (AFB) and Romanowsky-type stains (such as DiffQuik® which 'negatively' stain the bacilli). Furthermore, material should be collected for mycobacterial culture which involves using a variety of special media, incubation conditions and preparatory techniques to maximise the likelihood of isolating causal organisms. It is prudent also to freeze representative tissue from these suspect cases, as molecular studies such as those using hybridisation probes and 16S ribosomal RNA (16S rRNA) polymerase chain reaction (PCR) may be contemplated at a later date. These molecular techniques have had an enormous impact on the management of mycobacterial infections in human patients, as they have the potential to provide an aetiological diagnosis more rapidly than culture. Further, they are highly sensitive even when low numbers of organism may be present, whereas routine mycobacterial culture may be negative because of the fastidious nature of disease-producing strains.

Before discussing specific entities seen clinically in cats and dogs, it is worth emphasising again that non-tuberculous mycobacterial disease should be considered in distinct conceptual categories. Firstly, there are those immunocompetent patients in whom some breach in normal defence mechanisms allows mycobacteria to enter the host tissues and give rise to (relatively) localised disease. In this type of scenario, organisms are inoculated into an otherwise sterile site, e.g. following disruption of the skin by a penetrating injury, or aspiration of abnormal material into the respiratory tract. Secondly, there are cases where the host has some immunological defect, typically affecting CMI, which allows saprophytic mycobacteria to produce disseminated disease, often without an obvious breach in epithelial integrity to account for the site of primary infection. In these cases, it is suspected that organisms colonise some region, such as the gastrointestinal or respiratory tract, and spread haematogenously to skin, peripheral and internal lymph nodes, lungs, liver, spleen and bone marrow, tissues which favour multiplication of mycobacteria for some reason.

Some mycobacterial species, such as the rapid-growing *M. fortuitum* and *M. smegmatis*, are strongly linked with localised infections in immunocompetent hosts. Other species, such as *M. avium* complex, can produce either localised disease in an immunocompetent host, or disseminated infections in immunodeficient hosts. This distinction is clinically important, as cats in the latter category may have identifiable causes of immune compromise, such as inherited immune deficiency (e.g. in certain lines of Abyssinian and Somali cats), retroviral infections, or a history of immunosuppressive therapy, and may be at risk of developing other diseases associated with immune dysfunction at some point in the future, presupposing that the mycobacterial infection can be treated successfully.

Infections caused by rapidly growing mycobacteria

Aetiology

Rapidly growing mycobacteria (RGM) are a heterogeneous group of organisms that produce colonies on synthetic media within 7 days when cultured at 24–45°C. They are distributed ubiquitously in nature and can be isolated from soil, dirt and bodies of water (including tap water).[6] Members of the RGM group include the *M. fortuitum* group (including *M. fortuitum*, *M. peregrinum* and the third biovariant complex), the *M. chelonae/abscessus* group (including *M. chelonae* and *M. abscessus*), the *M. smegmatis* group (including *M. smegmatis* sensu stricto, *M. goodii* and *M. wolinskyi*) and a variety of other species including *M. phlei* and *M. thermoresistibile*. The taxonomy of this group has been revised recently and because of this, the word 'group' is used when referring to isolates recorded in early publications.[6]

In both humans and animals, RGM are strongly linked with localised infections of immunocompetent hosts.[3, 6–9] This is because they are well adapted to a saprophytic existence and have low inherent virulence for mammals. Thus, they do not produce disease unless a breakdown in normal defence barriers provides them with a portal of entry to a favourable tissue environment. Once introduced, RGM are generally constrained by a vigorous immunological response that may or may not eradicate them from the tissues, but is effective enough to prevent haematogenous or lymphatic spread. The RGM can produce widely disseminated disease, but only in severely immunocompromised individuals; they are, however, much less common pathogens in this cohort of patients than other mycobacterial species, such as the *M. avium* complex.[6] The RGM produce three different syndromes in cats and dogs: (1) mycobacterial panniculitis; (2) pyogranulomatous pneumonia; and (3) disseminated systemic disease.[10] In certain dairy herds, RGM are a significant cause of mastitis.[11]

Mycobacterial panniculitis refers to a syndrome characterised by chronic infection of the subcutis and skin with RGM.[3] This condition is quite common in cats, especially in Australia, and series of up to 49 cases have been reported.[8,9,12] The condition is less common in dogs.[8,13,14] The organisms replicate in mammalian tissues when introduced through a breach in the skin. This typically follows penetrating injury, especially when the wound is contaminated by dirt or soil. Preference of RGM for fat is a key factor in the pathogenesis of these infections, and results in a tendency for disease to occur in obese individuals and in tissues rich in lipid, such as the subcutaneous panniculus and especially the inguinal fat pad of cats. Experimental infections cannot be induced in cats that do not have appreciable subcutaneous fat depots.[15] Likewise, experimental infections of the ovine mammary gland requires instillation of oil in

addition to organisms, to induce mastitis. The same phenomenon accounts for situations where RGM gives rise to human infections, e.g. athletes who inject anabolic steroids in oily vehicles from contaminated multi-use vials, as a complication of lipoid pneumonia, and following augmentation mammoplasty, liposuction and median sternotomy.[6] Adipose tissue offers a favourable environment for survival and proliferation of RGM by providing triglycerides for growth of organisms or protecting them from the phagocytic or immune responses of the host.

Initial reports suggested that mycobacterial panniculitis was more common in warm humid climates;[8] however, cats and dogs from temperate regions, including parts of Australia, Canada, Finland and Germany, have subsequently been reported to develop these infections, and RGM can be cultivated from soil samples from Japan and throughout the USA.[6] In Australia, the *M. smegmatis* group accounts for the majority of feline cases, but it is a much less common cause of equivalent infections in human patients, where the *M. fortuitum* group are the predominant pathogens.[9] Interestingly, the swimming pool/fish tank bacillus, *M. marinum*, a common cause of subcutaneous mycobacterial disease in people, has not been isolated from feline or canine patients.

Mycobacterial pneumonia has been reported in several dogs[14,16–18] and a few cats.[3,19] Insufficient cases have been recorded to identify predisposing factors, apart from a cat examined by Wilkinson where the infection was thought to be secondary to aspiration of liquid paraffin administered as a fur-ball treatment.

Clinical signs

In cats, infections tend to start in the inguinal region, usually following environmental contamination of cat-fight injuries, e.g. raking wounds inflicted with the hind claws. The infection may spread to contiguous subcutaneous tissues of the ventral and lateral abdominal wall and perineum. Penetrating injury by sticks, metallic objects, and vehicular trauma may also give rise to these infections, as can cat and dog bite injuries contaminated with soil or dirt. Sometimes infections start in the axillae, flanks or dorsum and spread into adjacent tissues.[3]

Early in the clinical course, infections can resemble cat-fight abscesses, but without the characteristic foetid odour and turbid pus. Instead, a circumscribed

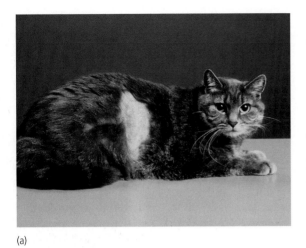

(a)

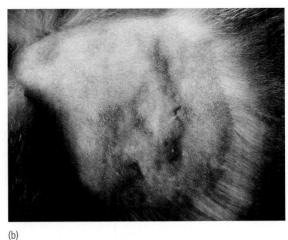

(b)

Fig. 5.1.1 (a) Panniculitis due to *M. smegmatis* on the lateral trunk of a cat. The area of localised panniculitis has been shaved for better visualisation of the skin lesions. (b) Closer view of the affected area. Note the punctate ulcer and purple-coloured depressions. (Courtesy of Dr Andrew Hillier, The Ohio State University, Columbus, OH, USA.)

plaque or nodule is apparent at the site of injury. Later, there is progressive thickening of the nearby subcutis to which overlying skin becomes adherent. Affected areas become denuded of hair and numerous punctate fistulae appear, discharging a watery exudate. Fistulae are intermingled with focal purple depressions, which correspond to thinning of the epidermis over accumulations of pus (Figs 5.1.1 and 5.1.2). The lesion gradually increases in area and depth, and may eventually involve the entire ventral abdomen, adjacent flanks or limbs. If cats are presented promptly

for veterinary attention and the lesion is confused with an anaerobic cat bite abscess, surgical drainage and administration of synthetic penicillin is typically followed by wound breakdown and development of non-healing suppurating tracts surrounded by indurated granulation tissue. Some affected cats with severe infections develop constitutional signs; they become depressed, pyrexic, inappetent, lose weight and are reluctant to move. Occasionally, cats develop hypercalcaemia of granulomatous disease, although this is rarely, if ever, symptomatic. Surprisingly, other

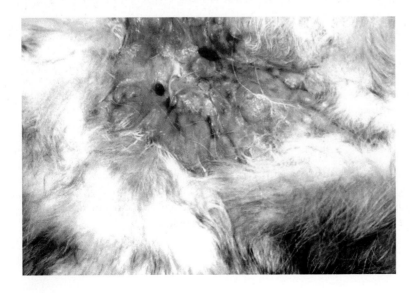

Fig. 5.1.2 Inguinal panniculitis due to *M. smegmatis* in a cat prior to therapy. Note the punctate ulcers and fistulae and the presence of purulent exudate on the skin.

cats remain comparatively well despite extensive disease. Usually the problem remains localised to the skin and subcutis. Although adjacent structures such as the abdominal wall may eventually be affected, spread to internal organs or lymph nodes is very unusual.[3]

In dogs, RGM infections should be suspected by veterinarians when confronted with patients with chronic non-healing wounds that are unresponsive to drainage and conventional antimicrobial therapy. Lesions typically consist of firm to fluctuant subcutaneous swellings (Fig. 5.1.3) or nodules which ulcerate, drain, and spread centrifugally (with the development of new lesions at the edges of older lesions). Some infections behave differently and instead spread widely to produce multifocal lesions through the entire panniculus. Lesions tend to be neither painful nor pruritic, and are generally located in regions subjected to bite wounds or injections, such as the neck, shoulders, flank or dorsum. There is usually a prior history of penetrating injury, e.g. a bite wound or veterinary intervention (injections, previous surgery). A minority of animals may demonstrate pyrexia, pain or lameness.[8,13,14,20]

Dogs and cats with pyogranulomatous pneumonia present for coughing, dyspnoea, fever, malaise and often have lost weight due to poor appetite. Young dogs appear to be over-represented. One patient developed hypertrophic osteopathy secondary to the pulmonary pathology.[18]

Diagnosis

Sample collection, cytology and histology

A tentative diagnosis of mycobacteriosis can be confirmed by collection of pus or deep tissue specimens. This material is used to confirm the diagnosis using appropriately stained cytology preparations, histopathology and mycobacterial culture. A histological diagnosis is unnecessary if appropriate samples for cytology and culture have been procured.[9,12] It is vital to give the laboratory warning that a mycobacterial aetiology is suspected so that special procedures for processing the specimens can be adopted.

In our experience, samples of pus obtained from needle aspirates of affected tissues through intact skin provide the best laboratory specimens in cases of panniculitis. This material can be obtained from a palpably abnormal portion of the subcutis. The overlying skin should be carefully disinfected with 70% ethanol prior to obtaining the specimen to preclude the isolation of saprophytic mycobacteria residing on the skin surface. It may be necessary to carefully move the needle in the subcutaneous space, whilst applying constant negative pressure, until a pocket of purulent material is encountered (Fig. 5.1.4). High resolution ultrasound can be useful in canine patients to identify anechoic foci suitable for aspiration. Aspirated purulent fluid should be submitted to the laboratory for cytology and mycobacterial culture, or inoculated immediately into a commercially prepared mycobacteria

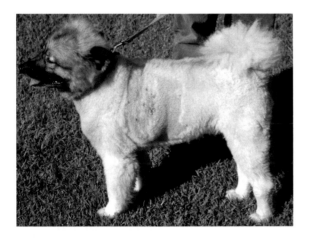

Fig. 5.1.3 Panniculitis due to *M fortuitum* on the lateral thorax of a keeshond. There was palpable subcutaneous oedema; pockets of fluid were visualised using a high resolution ultrasonography, facilitating aspiration of material for cytology and culture.

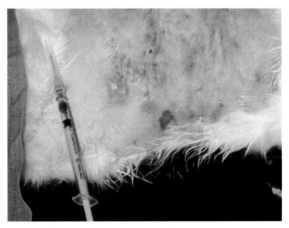

Fig. 5.1.4 Panniculitis of the lateral chest of a cat due to *M. smegmatis*. Needle aspiration through disinfected, intact skin produced approximately 0.1 ml of haemopurulent material. This provided an excellent specimen for cytological examination and culture.

culture bottle which is subsequently submitted to the laboratory. It is only necessary to suck a small amount of liquid material into the hub of the syringe. It is easiest to submit the entire syringe to the laboratory after replacing the needle with a sterile cover. Exudate from draining sinus tracts is heavily contaminated with secondary invaders and represents an inferior sample. If deep biopsies are obtained, they should be triturated in brain heart infusion broth using a sterile mortar and pestle to produce a tissue homogenate suitable for cytology and culture. In cases suspected of having mycobacterial pneumonia, deep bronchial washings, bronchoalveolar lavage specimens, or ultrasound-guided transthoracic fine needle aspirates provide optimal specimens.

Smears prepared from aspirates of purulent exudate, bronchial washings, or tissue homogenates should be stained using DiffQuik®, Burke's modification of the Gram stain, and a modified acid-fast procedure (decolorising with 5% sulphuric acid for only 3–5 minutes, as RGM are not as acid-fast as other mycobacteria). Cytology invariably demonstrates pyogranulomatous inflammation and it is generally possible to visualise gram-positive and/or acid-fast bacilli (AFB) in smears, although an exhaustive search of several smears is sometimes required.[9,12] Organisms often demonstrate beading. Speckled structures or non-staining 'ghosts', corresponding to poorly staining or non-staining bacilli, may be observed in smears stained with Romanowsky-type stains,[14] but are much harder to appreciate than in *M. avium* infections, feline leprosy or canine leproid granuloma cases.

Histologically, there is pyogranulomatous inflammation of subcutaneous adipose tissue, overlying dermis and underlying abdominal fascia and musculature. It may be difficult, or impossible, to find AFB in Ziehl-Neelsen (ZN)-stained tissue sections. The bacteria are often located in lipid vacuoles.

Bacteriology and antimicrobial susceptibility testing

Tissue homogenates and pus should be streaked onto duplicate 5% sheep blood agar plates and a mycobacterial medium such as Lowenstein-Jensen medium or 1% Ogawa egg yolk medium, and incubated aerobically at 37°C and 25°C. If available, the BACTEC system can also be utilised. Moderate to heavy growth of pin-point, non-haemolytic colonies is usually detected after 2–3 days (occasionally longer) on sheep blood

agar at 37°C. Where only contaminated specimens are available, tissue homogenates can be treated with 4% sodium hydroxide followed by neutralisation with dilute hydrochloric acid prior to inoculation onto media. Another method which can be used to selectively differentiate RGM from contaminant flora is by primary isolation around antibiotic sensitivity discs (first generation cephalosporins or isoxazolyl penicillins) applied to the plate after inoculation. We prefer this method to alkali pretreatment when dealing with specimens contaminated with staphylococci.

There is great value in determining species identification and susceptibility data in every case, as this has a significant impact on antimicrobial drug strategies. Species identification can be carried out in a well-equipped veterinary bacteriology laboratory, although it is often more convenient to send the strain to a mycobacteria reference laboratory, following primary isolation. Identification takes into account the following phenotypic features: organism morphology in ZN-stained smears of growth taken from Lowenstein-Jensen medium; colonial morphology (rough or smooth); pigmentation in the dark and light; degree of acid-fastness; rate of growth at room temperature and 37°C; ability to grow at 42°C and 52°C; arylsulphatase activity at 3 days; iron uptake; p-amino salicylic acid (PAS) degradation; nitrate reduction; β-galactosidase activity; acid production from carbohydrates (glucose, inositol, mannitol); utilisation of compounds (glucose, fructose, inositol, mannitol, citrate) as the sole carbon source; tolerance to 5% sodium chloride in Lowenstein-Jensen medium; and susceptibility to polymyxin B, trimethoprim and tobramycin. In specialised laboratories, a variety of molecular techniques are also utilised.[6,9]

Minimum inhibitory concentrations (MICs) for ciprofloxacin, gentamicin, trimethoprim, clarithromycin and doxycycline can be determined easily using the Etest (AB Biodisk, Solna, Sweden) method.[21] This methodology is less demanding than the 'gold standard' of broth microdilution. Antimicrobial susceptibility of clinical isolates can also be determined using disc diffusion methodology. Typically, isolates are tested against discs containing representative antimicrobials including doxycycline (30 μg), gentamicin (10 μg), ciprofloxacin (5 μg), trimethoprim (5 μg), tobramycin (10 μg), polymyxin B (300 μg), enrofloxacin (5 μg) and clarithromycin (30 μg). Some antibiotics are included to determine a suitable agent for long-term oral therapy, while others (trimethoprim, polymyxin B, tobramycin) are used to provide phenotypic information concerning strains. Suspensions of each organism in saline or nutrient broth are grown on sensitivity agar and incubated at 37°C. Results are recorded after incubation for 48 and 72 hours.[9]

Therapy

The management of mycobacterial panniculitis continues to evolve over time according to ongoing clinical experience, availability of new antimicrobial agents, and development of new surgical techniques.[9,12] There is great variation in the severity and extent of lesions from patient to patient. Difficulty in making a prompt diagnosis is partly responsible for the chronicity, severity and refractory nature of these infections.[14] Briefly, treatment should commence with oral antimicrobial(s) (doxycycline, a fluoroquinolone and/or clarithromycin), initially chosen empirically, but subsequently on the basis of *in vitro* susceptibility data. Sometimes, long-term administration of such an agent (or agents) is sufficient to effect a cure. However, in more severe cases it is eventually necessary to surgically resect recalcitrant tissues so that oral antimicrobial therapy will be able to cure the infection permanently. Given the extent and severity of the pathology in many of these cases, it is understandable that adequate levels of antimicrobials may not be achieved throughout all affected tissues; in these cases the best chance for a successful outcome is to remove as much infected tissue as possible following preliminary antimicrobial therapy.[22] Residual foci of infection can then be targeted by the high concentrations of antibiotics achieved during and after surgery. Peri- and postoperative antimicrobial therapy is vital to ensure primary intention healing of the surgical incision.

Once a tentative diagnosis of mycobacterial panniculitis is made, it is desirable to start treatment immediately. As positive primary culture takes 3–4 days, with a similar additional period required for susceptibility testing, the initial choice of antimicrobial(s) must be guided by retrospectively acquired microbiology data. These data vary from region to region. In Australia, *M. smegmatis* and *M. fortuitum* infections are encountered with similar frequency in companion animals, whereas in the southern USA, *M. fortuitum* and *M. chelonae* infections predominate.[8,13,14] *M. smegmatis*

strains are susceptible to a wide range of antimicrobial agents suitable for treating chronic infections, except for clarithromycin to which a majority of strains show inherent resistance. In contrast, *M. fortuitum* strains generally demonstrate resistance to one or more agents and often have higher MICs for agents to which strains are susceptible, while *M. chelonae* strains tend to be resistant to all common agents available for oral dosing apart from clarithromycin, gatifloxacin and linezolid.[6] In Australia, doxycycline or a fluoroquinolone are thus sensible choices for first-line therapy, whereas in the USA clarithromycin is the drug of choice for empiric therapy. Current recommendations from human infectious disease experts emphasise the possibility of RGM developing resistance to fluoroquinolones during a course of therapy.[6] Thus, it may be prudent to use fluoroquinolones strategically after surgical debulking, or to use them initially in concert with another effective antimicrobial to reduce the likelihood of resistance developing. Such considerations are not thought to be applicable to doxycycline or clarithromycin.[6] For this reason, many veterinary dermatologists in Australia routinely use combination therapy with doxycycline and a fluoroquinolone from the outset. It should be emphasised that, although some RGM strains show *in vitro* susceptibility to amoxycillin clavulanate, this drug combination has no efficacy *in vivo*.

Once susceptibility data become available, the optimal drug(s) is selected. The response *in vivo* to a drug (or drugs) known to be effective *in vitro* can then be assessed. It general, it is necessary to use the highest possible doses because affected subcutaneous tissues are not well perfused, and considerable diffusion barriers prevent blood levels of antibiotics reaching organisms in fat. Treatment should commence using standard dose rates. Subsequently, the dose is increased slowly (over several weeks) until adverse side effects (inappetence, vomiting) suggest the need for slight dose reduction, or until a convincing clinical improvement is observed.

Some cases treated in a preliminary fashion using orally administered agents respond progressively to such an extent that surgery becomes unnecessary. These cases can be cured using medical therapy alone, although treatment with oral antimicrobials for 3–12 months may be required. Generally, cases that resolve without the need for surgical intervention tend not to involve deep tissue as much as those cases that require surgery. Some cases are so severe, however, that only a limited improvement can be achieved with antimicrobial therapy alone, and surgical intervention is required to effect a cure. As it is impossible to predict which cases will require operative debridement, our current recommendation is to start empiric antimicrobial therapy, determine the *in vitro* susceptibility pattern, then re-assess the patient every 3–4 weeks to determine whether continued improvement is occurring, or whether therapy has plateaued and surgery is required. Preliminary medical therapy is of great benefit because firstly, it reduces the amount of tissue requiring resection, and secondly, it minimises the possibility of wound dehiscence.

If surgery is required, a drug with known efficacy against the causal strain that can be administered by injection, e.g. gentamicin, should be administered intra-operatively (2 mg/kg three times daily or 6 mg/kg once daily either intravenously or subcutaneously) and in the early postoperative period (ideally for several days if finances permit). Gentamicin is a good choice because it is bactericidal, available in a parenteral form, inexpensive and displays good *in vitro* activity against all RGM. Amikacin is superior to gentamicin, although it is substantially more expensive in Australia. The critical surgical consideration is to remove as much abnormal subcutaneous tissue as possible, which in some cases may necessitate the removal of very large portions of infected tissue. Severe cases benefit from the radical excision technique developed by Hunt *et al.* where infected tissues are resected *en bloc*, followed by re-arrangement of nearby skin to fill the often substantial tissue deficits created.[7,23] In some cases, however, there is such extensive panniculitis that this is not feasible. Advanced cases, with extensive lesions, optimally require the skill of an experienced soft tissue surgeon to reconstruct the resulting wound without undue tension, particularly in feline cases. The large amount of dead space created by the debridement requires judicious use of latex or closed-suction drains for several days postoperatively.

Following surgery, drugs thought to be of greatest theoretical efficacy against the causal organism are used to ensure that primary intention healing occurs. Residual bacteria at the wound margins are thus targeted by high levels of effective agent(s). Generally, because of cost considerations and other practicalities, the choice comes down to one (or a combination) of a fluoroquinolone, doxycycline, or clarithromycin, based on *in vitro* susceptibility.

Of the agents suitable for postoperative therapy, the fluoroquinolones (ciprofloxacin [10–20 mg/kg twice daily], enrofloxacin [5–15 mg/kg once daily], marbofloxacin, orbifloxacin, gatifloxacin) and doxycycline (5–10 mg/kg twice daily) are generally the agents of choice for treating RGM infections in Australia where *M. smegmatis* and *M. fortuitum* strains predominate. In the USA, clarithromycin (10–15 mg/kg orally twice daily) and/or fluoroquinolones represent the cornerstones of therapy for RGM, although doxycycline still has a place in the treatment of susceptible strains.

Fluoroquinolones are bactericidal, have good tissue penetration (including fat), and are concentrated in polymorphonuclear cells and macrophages. Current concerns for the retinotoxic potential of enrofloxacin when given to cats in daily doses exceeding 5 mg/kg probably preclude its use in this species, where ciprofloxacin, gatifloxacin or other veterinary fluoroquinolones are safer choices at the high dosages likely to be required for these infections. To the best of our knowledge, retinal toxicity in cats has not been reported for fluoroquinolones other than enrofloxacin. The author has no experience using marbofloxacin or orbifloxacin in the treatment of mycobacterial infections and unfortunately no published data on their use are available. Doxycycline has a cost advantage over the fluoroquinolones, and based on our experience, has similar efficacy, and is equally suited to long-term oral therapy. Doxycycline monohydrate is the tetracycline of choice for use in small animal patients, being well tolerated, present in a readily available form (Vibravet tablets; Pfizer, Australia) and having good lipid solubility. The monohydrate form of doxycycline is not freely available in the USA or Europe, which is problematic as other doxycycline salts are more irritant, causing vomiting, or worse, oesophageal ulceration.[24] For this reason, doxycycline should be either given immediately before meals, or be followed by a small amount of liquid. Clarithromycin, a macrolide with an extended spectrum of activity and prolonged pharmacokinetics, has proved extremely useful in treating RGM infections in human and veterinary patients. Its major disadvantage is its present high cost, which becomes an issue in large dogs. There is insufficient information to currently recommend routine combination therapy in these cases, but the possibility of resistance emerging during therapy should be considered in cases where a favourable response (especially to fluoroquinolones) is not sustained during a course of therapy, or if relapse occurs.

In human infections due to RGM, single-drug therapy is recommended for localised or minor disease. In contrast, severe or disseminated disease and pulmonary infections usually require multiple antimicrobials, including both intravenous (e.g. amikacin) and oral medications (e.g. clarithromycin or ciprofloxacin), at least for the first 2 weeks of therapy.

The total duration of therapy should be in the order of 3–12 months. Agents should be administered for at least 1–2 months after affected tissues look and feel completely normal. In occasional refractory cases, clofazimine,[25] cefoxitin or amikacin may be used for monotherapy, or in conjunction with other agents shown to be effective *in vitro*. Cefoxitin and amikacin can only be given by injection. Several new oral agents for treating refractory RGM infections have recently become available, including gatifloxacin and linezolid.[6] Although these agents hold great promise for some previously untreatable mycobacterial infections, high cost currently precludes their routine use. We have had limited experience with gatifloxacin in feline patients, where it has proven to be well tolerated and helpful in two refractory cases. This drug has greater activity against *M. fortuitum* and *M. chelonae* strains than older fluoroquinolones such as ciprofloxacin.[26]

In summary, mycobacterial panniculitis is an eminently treatable disease. Diagnosis is straightforward, especially for practitioners familiar with the syndrome. The prognosis is excellent, even in cases with severe, extensive and long-standing disease. Treatment involves long courses of antimicrobials chosen on the basis of laboratory testing, sometimes combined with extensive surgical debridement and wound reconstruction. Finally, the routine prophylactic use of doxycycline following treatment of penetrating injuries in obese dogs and cats may prevent the development of these deep-seated infections.

Similar considerations apply to the treatment of pyogranulomatous pneumonia due to RGM. Empiric treatment should be started immediately after obtaining diagnostic specimens for cytology and culture. Therapy may need to be altered in the light of susceptibility data. Treatment should initially consist of high levels of two agents known to be effective *in vitro*, including intravenous gentamicin or amikacin. Nebulisation using gentamicin or amikacin is likely to be a useful adjunct to systemic therapy. Pulmonary lesions that respond incompletely to appropriate medical therapy may need to be surgically resected in order to effect a cure.[14,16–19]

Canine leproid granuloma syndrome ('canine leprosy')

Aetiology, epidemiology and clinical findings

Canine leproid granuloma syndrome (CLGS), or canine leprosy, is the most common mycobacterial disease of dogs in Australia. Although the causal organism has a worldwide distribution, its prevalence in other countries has not been documented. Patients with this infection present with one or more nodules of the subcutis or skin, but are otherwise healthy.[27–33] The condition was first described in a boxer and a bull mastiff from Zimbabwe in 1973, with similar reports from Australia appearing soon afterwards.

Primary skin lesions consist of single or multiple, well-circumscribed nodule(s). These lesions can appear anywhere on the dog, although they are usually located on the head and typically on the dorsal fold of the ears (Fig. 5.1.5). The nodules are firm, painless, and vary in size from 2 mm up to 5 cm in diameter. Small nodules are detected as firm subcutaneous lumps, while larger nodules may show superficial hair loss. Very large lesions may ulcerate (Fig. 5.1.6). Leproid granulomas are confined to the subcutis and skin and do not involve regional lymph nodes, nerves or internal organs. Consequently, affected dogs suffer no apparent systemic effects. This suggests that the causal organism has low pathogenicity or special prerequisites, such as a requirement for low temperature, which permits them to survive and multiply in superficial tissues only. Lesions can be disfiguring and cause irritation, especially when lesions are multiple and secondarily infected with *Staphylococcus intermedius*.

CLGS has a wide geographic distribution, with cases recorded from coastal and inland regions of all states of Australia. The causal organism is likely to have a worldwide distribution, as the condition has also been reported in New Zealand, Zimbabwe, Brazil, California and Florida. The authors are also aware of unreported cases of affected boxers in New York and foxhounds in Georgia in the USA. The condition would seem to be especially common in Australia and Brazil.

Interestingly, there is a strong propensity for short-coated breeds to be affected, with boxer and boxer-

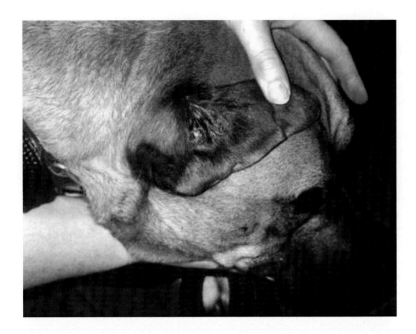

Fig. 5.1.5 Canine leproid granuloma syndrome; solitary lesion on the dorsal fold of the ear pinna of a bull mastiff.

cross dogs accounting for nearly half of the cases reported. Despite the fact that CLGS was first reported nearly 30 years ago, its aetiopathogenesis has not been fully elucidated. The initial report of the disease by Richard Smith stated that 'lesions appear suddenly, and are usually seen on dogs pestered by biting flies'. This might suggest that flies, or some other biting arthropod (such as midges or mosquitoes), inoculate mycobacteria from an environmental niche into susceptible tissues. The predilection for lesions to develop in regions favoured by biting insect vectors, such as the head and particularly the ears, is consistent with this hypothesis, as is the overrepresentation of short-coated, large-breed dogs (which are generally housed outdoors).

Diagnosis

The diagnosis is usually straightforward, as the distribution of lesions (especially the propensity for the dorsal ear fold to be affected), coupled with the tendency for lesions to be multiple, particularly in at-risk breeds, is strongly suggestive of CLGS. Diagnosis can

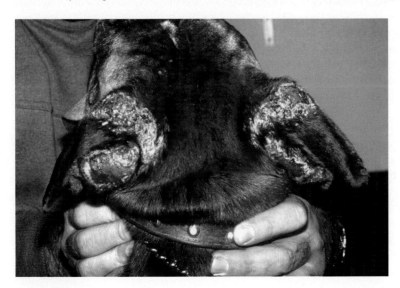

Fig. 5.1.6 Canine leproid granuloma syndrome; multiple, ulcerated lesions on both ear folds of a boxer dog.

be confirmed by obtaining specimens of representative lesions for cytologic or histologic examination.[28] DiffQuik®-stained smears from needle aspirates typically demonstrate numerous macrophages with variable numbers of lymphocytes and plasma cells and lower numbers of neutrophils. Usually few-to-moderate numbers of negatively stained, medium-length bacilli can be detected within macrophages or extracellularly. Histologically, lesions within the subcutis and dermis consist of pyogranulomas composed chiefly of epithelioid macrophages, Langerhans-type giant cells and scattered neutrophils, plasma cells and small lymphocytes. The number and morphology of AFB in ZN-stained sections is highly variable from case to case. Currently, it is impossible to confirm the diagnosis by culture, as the *in vitro* growth requirements for this fastidious organism have not been determined. A negative culture, however, can exclude other mycobacterial aetiologies. It is vital to thoroughly disinfect the skin surface prior to obtaining specimens for culture, as saprophytic mycobacteria can be cultured erroneously from dirt present on canine skin (P. Martin and R. Malik, unpublished observations).

Recently, PCR methodologies using 'universal primers' designed to amplify regions of the bacterial 16S rRNA gene have been performed on leproid granuloma specimens from dogs. Using sequence capture PCR for paraffin-embedded specimens and nested PCR on DNA from fresh-tissue specimens, a novel PCR product has been identified with identical sequence over a 350-bp region. Analysis of the partial 16S rRNA sequence supports the notion that the novel species is a fastidious, slow-growing mycobacterium. In total, molecular methodologies identified this proposed novel mycobacterial sequence in material from in excess of 16 Australian cases of CLGS, indicating that the species represented by this sequence is probably the principal causative agent of CLGS.[29] Our continuing experience, and that of colleagues in California[29] and Brazil, support this contention. Interestingly, the species represented by this sequence has never been recorded from mycobacterial granulomas affecting the skin or subcutis of cats, horses, people, or other non-canine mammalian species. Hence, there is thought to be no public health risk to the owners of affected dogs.

Treatment

Very little has been written concerning the treatment of CLGS. Many cases are self-limiting, with the nodular skin lesions regressing spontaneously with time, typically within 1–3 months of appearing. The stated time-frame is based on our experiences consulting with veterinarians regarding cases diagnosed histologically; by the time the sections have been submitted, processed and reported, and we have established a dialogue with the clinician, lesions are often already starting to regress, either spontaneously, or in response to antimicrobials (useful for secondary *Staphylococcus intermedius*, but with unlikely efficacy for mycobacteria). This 'self-cure' occurs presumably as a result of an effective CMI response mounted by the patient.

In cases with a limited number of lesions, surgical excision can be curative and provides material with which to confirm the diagnosis histologically and using PCR. In other cases, however, the infection progresses to produce chronic, disfiguring lesions that may persist indefinitely. Limited information suggests that treatment with conventional antimicrobial regimens using β-lactam drugs or doxycycline (as monotherapy) fails to have a significant impact on the course of infection,[27] although these drugs may be of some benefit by effectively treating secondary pyogenic infections. One report concerning two dogs from Brazil suggested that topical antibacterial treatment and orally administered rifampicin may be effective. Our experience treating 'canine leprosy' suggests that this infection responds to therapy with combinations of antimicrobial agents known to be effective against non-tuberculous mycobacteria, including rifampicin, clarithromycin, clofazimine and doxycycline. Based on our evolving experience, a combination of rifampicin (10–15 mg/kg administered orally once daily) and clarithromycin (15–25 mg/kg total daily dose; divided and given orally two to three times daily) is currently recommended for treating severe or refractory CLGS cases.[32] Unfortunately, the clarithromycin component of therapy is, at present, extremely expensive in large dogs. A more affordable combination consists of rifampicin (at the same dose) and doxycycline (5 mg/kg [or higher] twice daily); further studies may prove this to have similar efficacy to the former regimen. Treatment should be continued until lesions are substantially reduced in size (typically for 4–8 weeks) and ideally until lesions have resolved completely. It is prudent to monitor hepatic function periodically during treatment, as rifampicin may cause hepatotoxicosis in some patients. A topical formulation containing clofazimine in petroleum jelly may be used as an adjunct to systemic drug therapy. This can be prepared by crushing (with a hammer) forty 50 mg clofazimine 'capsules' within a plastic bag; the extracted liquid dye is mixed into an ointment with 100 g of petroleum jelly.[32] Further work is required to determine the most cost-effective treatment regimen for this condition; to this end a topical treatment using multiple chemotherapeutic agents in a permeant vehicle is currently under development in Australia.

Feline leprosy syndromes

Aetiology, epidemiology and clinical signs

The term feline leprosy is used to refer to a mycobacterial disease in which single or multiple granulomas form in the skin or subcutis in association with large numbers of AFB which are non-culturable using standard methods. The condition was first recorded in the literature by Australian and New Zealand researchers in the early 1960s. Since then, the disease has been reported in western Canada, the Netherlands, France, the UK and the USA.[3,34]

Feline leprosy is more common in certain geographical locations such as the North Island of New Zealand, the Netherlands and British Columbia. Furthermore, it appears to be more prevalent in temperate coastal areas and port cities, as opposed to inland or tropical habitats. Historically, the causative agent of feline leprosy was purported to be *M. lepraemurium*. This bacterium causes murine leprosy, a systemic mycobacterial infection of rats. Cats are thought to contract *M. lepraemurium* following bite injuries from infected rodents.[3,34]

M. lepraemurium is a fastidious, slow-growing mycobacterial species which, with difficulty, can be cultured from large inoculae on Ogawa's egg yolk medium under strictly controlled conditions, or in enriched liquid medium at a critical pH. Although a few investigators have successfully grown *M. lepraemurium* from infected cats, the basis of ascribing this bacterium as the aetiological agent of feline leprosy was dependent on transmission studies and the results of delayed hypersensitivity reactions to intradermally injected tissue extracts. Several groups were able to show that material obtained from feline lesions can be used to transmit disease to rats, and subsequently back to cats. In such studies, the incubation period varied from 2 months to 1 year or more. Interestingly, some cats appeared much more susceptible to infection than others.

According to the literature, cats with feline leprosy are typically young adults (<5 years old), perhaps with a preponderance of males. Presumably these patient characteristics reflect the need for the cat to interact with a rat to become infected. The initial lesion is a focal granuloma of the subcutis. Owners become aware of solitary, or multiple (more commonly), painless, raised, fleshy, tumour-like lesions, from a few millimetres up to 4 cm in diameter. These granulomas are freely movable over underlying tissues. Lesions can develop rapidly and may ulcerate when large. Infection spreads to adjacent areas and may invade underlying tissues and drain to regional lymph nodes. Lesions can occur anywhere on the body, but tend to be concentrated on the head and limbs. Small lesions are occasionally found on the tongue, lips and nasal planum. Lesions, even if multiple, tend to be initially concentrated in one region and have the propensity to recur following excision. In some cases widespread cutaneous lesions develop.

Pathologically, feline leprosy was subdivided into lepromatous or tuberculoid forms on the basis of the number of AFB present (multibacillary versus paucibacillary) and the host immunological response (lepromatous versus tuberculoid). As the causal mycobacteria are slow-growing organisms capable of intracellular survival, the histologic picture depends on the host's immune response. When this response is poor, lepromatous (multibacillary) disease develops with infiltration of the dermis with large sheets of 'incompetent' foamy macrophages containing enormous numbers of organisms. The AFB are usually arranged in the cytoplasm of macrophages as dense parallel accumulations which displace the nucleus to an eccentric position. Lymphoid cells and plasma cells are virtually absent from the lesions. If the host's immune response is more effective, histiocytic cells are accompanied by moderate numbers of lymphoid cells and plasma cells and multiplication of the organism is limited; the so-called tuberculoid response. The tuberculoid form accounts for perhaps two-thirds of the cases in western Canada, a large proportion of cases in New Zealand and the Netherlands, but only a minority of the cases encountered in Australia. Invasion of local nerves, a prominent feature of human leprosy, is rarely observed in patients with feline leprosy, although a recent report described a cat without skin lesions which presented for mycobacterial infiltration of one sciatic nerve.

AFB in smears and tissue sections appear as long slender rods. In smears stained with Romanowsky stains, such as DiffQuik® or Giemsa, organisms appear as negative-staining bacilli. In smears or sections stained with modified acid-fast stains such as Ziehl-Neelsen (ZN) or Fite's stain, organisms take up the carbol fuschin and are acid/alcohol-fast.

Molecular insights

Molecular methodologies have recently been used to investigate presumptive feline leprosy. Of eight cases of invasive or disseminated cutaneous mycobacterial disease investigated by Hughes and colleagues using material collected largely from New Zealand cats, four were shown to have *M. lepraemurium* infections. Of the remaining cases, one cat had a disseminated *M. avium* infection, one was of undetermined aetiology and in two cases infection was attributable to a novel mycobacterial species.[35] This information encouraged a reappraisal of Australian feline leprosy cases. Interestingly, cats could be divided into two groups on the basis of the patient's age, lesion histology, clinical course and sequence of 16S rRNA PCR amplicons obtained from lesions.[36]

One group consisted of young cats (typically <4 years) which initially developed localised nodular disease affecting the limbs. Lesions progressed rapidly and sometimes ulcerated. Sparse to moderate numbers of AFB were identified using cytology or histology, typically in areas of caseous necrosis and surrounded by pyogranulomatous tuberculoid inflammation. Organisms did not stain with haematoxylin and ranged from 2 to 6 μm (usually 2–4 μm). *M. lepraemurium* was diagnosed based on the sequence of a 446-bp fragment encompassing the V2 and V3 hypervariable regions amplified from lesions using PCR and universal primers. Based on gene sequence data, *M. lepraemurium* showed greatest nucleotide identity with *M. avium* subsp. *paratuberculosis* and *M. avium*. The clinical course of *M. lepraemurium* infections was aggressive, with a tendency towards local spread, ulceration, recurrence following surgery and development of widespread lesions over several weeks. Cats resided in suburban or rural areas.

A second group consisted of old cats (>9 years old) with generalised nodular skin lesions (Fig. 5.1.7) associated with multibacillary lepromatous histology. Some cats initially had localised disease which subsequently became widespread, while others had generalised disease from the outset. Disease progression

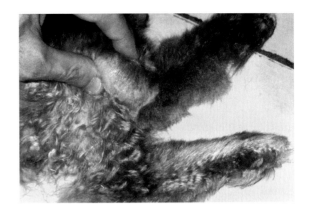

Fig. 5.1.7 Nodule on the hock of an 11-year-old, FIV-negative Persian cat infected with the novel *Mycobacterium* sp. Although this was the largest lesion evident, numerous similar lesions were present elsewhere over the integument.

was protracted, typically taking months to years, and skin nodules did not ulcerate. Microscopically, lesions consisted of sheets of epithelioid macrophages containing large to enormous numbers of AFB of 2–8 μm (mostly 4–6 μm) which also stained with haematoxylin. A single unique sequence spanning a 557-bp fragment of the 16S rRNA gene was identified in lesions from these patients. The sequence was characterised by a long helix 18 in the V3 region, suggesting that the new species was likely to be a fastidious, slow grower. The 16S rRNA sequence had greatest nucleotide identity with *M. leprae*, *M. haemophilum* and *M. malmoense*, and contained an additional 'A' nucleotide at position 105 (the only other mycobacterial database sequence with the same extra nucleotide being *M. leprae*). A very slow, pure growth of a mycobacterium species was observed on Lowenstein-Jensen medium (supplemented with iron) and semi-solid agar in one of three cases in which culture was attempted at a reference laboratory. The environmental niche of this new mycobacterial species has yet to be determined, although the preponderance of cases from rural or semi-rural areas suggests it is a saprophyte found more commonly in these locations than in metropolitan environments. The organism may normally reside in soil or stagnant watery environments that favour the proliferation of saprophytic mycobacteria and subsequently become inoculated into the subcutis through contamination of traumatic injuries (from cats or possums), or via a biting arthropod.

The establishment or spread of infection with the novel mycobacterial species suggests a requirement for decreased immunological surveillance to permit the development of disease with an organism of limited virulence. Furthermore, the aetiopathogenesis needs to account for the absence of young cats among this cohort of patients. The presence of a foamy histiocytic infiltrate of the dermis and subcutis in human patients with mycobacteriosis is observed almost exclusively in association with profound immunodeficiency, such as that seen with terminal HIV infection. Feline leprosy caused by the novel mycobacterial species may likewise represent a manifestation of deteriorating immune competence in elderly cats with long-standing FIV infection, and indeed half of the cats so far tested in Australia have been FIV-positive. Decreased cellular immunity associated with renal disease may also predispose cats to infection, as renal disease is common amongst infected cats. Alternately, renal disease may occur as a consequence of the mycobacterial infection, as it does in rats with disseminated *M. lepraemurium* infection, presumably as a result of immune complex deposition in glomeruli. Thankfully, these infections seem quite sensitive to antimycobacterial therapy.[35]

These findings suggest that feline leprosy comprises two clinical syndromes, one tending to occur in young cats caused by *M. lepraemurium* and another in immunosuppressed elderly cats caused by a single novel mycobacterium species. To make matters even more complex, recent work by Appleyard and Clark[37,38] and Foley and colleagues (see Chapter 5.2) has demonstrated a third mycobacterial syndrome in cats from western Canada, and several states within the USA, called 'feline multisystemic granulomatous mycobacteriosis'. This disease is caused by a slow-growing species provisionally called *M. visibilis* that gives rise to diffuse (rather than nodular) cutaneous disease and widespread dissemination to multiple internal organs. Sequence analyses demonstrate a number of nucleotide differences between *M. visibilis* and both *M. lepraemurium* and the novel species reported by Hughes and colleagues.

The existence of multiple diseases, rather than one, clearly has important implications for prevention, diagnosis and therapy. For example, most authors recommend wide surgical excision as the treatment of choice for localised feline leprosy cases.[3] This is a practical option in *M. lepraemurium* infections, at least when cats are presented for treatment in a timely manner

when lesions are localised. On the other hand, although surgery may have a place in reducing particularly large lesions in infections caused by the novel mycobacterial species, combination drug therapy generally represents a better first line of treatment.

Diagnosis

Diagnosis of the 'feline leprosy' syndromes is usually straightforward, provided that the clinician has a high index of suspicion for the condition. Needle aspirates, crush preparations of biopsy material and histological sections stained with ZN or similar methods contain easily demonstrable AFB surrounded by variable granulomatous to pyogranulomatous inflammation (Fig. 5.1.8). In DiffQuik®-stained smears, mycobacteria can be recognised by their characteristic negative-staining appearance and location within macrophages and giant cells (Fig. 5.1.9).

Material should also be submitted for culture, because occasionally slowly growing species such as *M. avium* complex (MAC) and *M. genavense*[39] and the tubercle bacillus (*M. bovis* or *M. microti*[2]) can produce an identical clinical presentation; in such cases optimal antimycobacterial therapy can be selected more readily on the basis of *in vitro* susceptibility results and information available in the literature. In the majority of cases, however, conventional mycobacterial culture is negative due to the fastidious nature of the causal organisms and a mycobacterial aetiology can only be proven using molecular techniques such as PCR amplification and nucleotide sequence determination of gene fragments. PCR has the additional advantage of providing a rapid diagnosis. Fresh (frozen) tissue delivered to a mycobacterium laboratory with PCR facilities provides the optimal sample, although freeze-dried specimens may be more conveniently sent where tissues need to travel long distances. Sometimes PCR can be performed successfully on formalin-fixed paraffin-embedded material, although fixation conditions invariably cause some DNA degradation which may limit the success of the procedure. Recently, Hughes and colleagues have developed specific PCR assays to diagnose infections due to *M. lepraemurium* and the novel species;[40] furthermore, use of a simple restriction enzyme digest allows these assays to distinguish *M. visibilis* strains as well.

M. lepraemurium infections have a number of distinguishing features that suggest this aetiology even

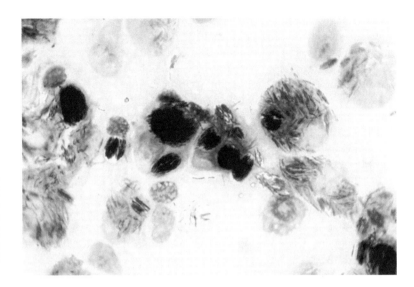

Fig. 5.1.8 Smear made from biopsy material from a cat infected with the novel *Mycobacterium* sp. Macrophages laden with abundant intracellular acid-fast bacteria (AFB) appear pink as a result of taking up the carbol fuchsin stain, which is acid/alcohol-fast. The AFB are often grouped in ovoid bundles. (Original magnification ×330.)

where molecular testing is not practicable (see above). Although a young age at presentation supports the diagnosis of *M. lepraemurium* infection, age alone is not a reliable criterion, as we have recently diagnosed *M. lepraemurium* in cats as old as 9 years of age.

Therapy

Too few cases with a documented aetiology have been reported to provide definitive treatment guidelines. Although *M. lepraemurium* and the novel species can be cultured *in vitro*, it is currently not routine or reliable to isolate these organisms due to their slow growth and fastidious requirements. Determination of *in vitro* susceptibility data for individual isolates is therefore not possible.

Only limited experimental studies have been undertaken to determine effective drug therapy for *M. lepraemurium in vitro* or *in vivo*, and as yet we have limited data only for the novel mycobacterial species. Portaels and colleagues[41] found the minimum inhibitory concentration for rifampicin of two strains of *M. lepraemurium* to be 4 and 8 μg/ml, levels that should be just obtainable *in vivo* based on extrapolation from

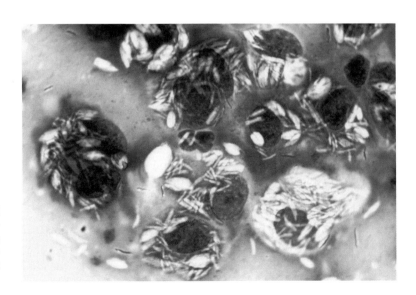

Fig. 5.1.9 Smear made from biopsy material from a cat infected with the novel *Mycobacterium* sp. Negatively-stained bacilli are evident individually, and in bundles, predominantly within macrophages. (DiffQuick stain, original magnification ×330.)

pharmacokinetic studies in humans and dogs. Other drugs shown to have activity against *M. lepraemurium in vitro* include ansamycin compounds (rifabutin) and sulpha drugs. There is a good deal of evidence that clofazimine has efficacy *in vivo*, while it is likely that clarithromycin would be also be effective based on its wide spectrum of activity against slow-growing mycobacterial species.[42]

The literature suggests that when *M. lepraemurium* infection is diagnosed early, while disease is localised, wide surgical excision of infected tissues provides the best chance to simply and rapidly effect a cure.[3] Aggressive resection techniques should be adopted, with *en bloc* resection of all lesions, and reconstruction of resulting tissue deficits using appropriate surgical techniques. Such an approach should be combined with adjunct antimicrobial therapy beginning a few days prior to surgery, so that effective levels of drugs are present in blood and tissues intra- and postoperatively to ensure primary intention healing.

Clofazimine (at a dose of up to 10 mg/kg once daily orally; typically 25–50 mg every 1–2 days) has the best reported success rate, although it is likely that combination therapy using two or more drugs will eventually prove superior. Drugs that could be combined with clofazimine include rifampicin and clarithromycin, although sulpha drugs, doxycycline, new fluoroquinolones such as gatifloxacin, or amikacin may in time also prove to be useful.

In feline leprosy cases caused by the novel mycobacterium species, we believe combination therapy using two or three of clofazimine (25–50 mg per cat orally once daily to once every 2 days), clarithromycin (62.5 mg twice daily) or rifampicin (10–15 mg/kg once daily) represents optimal therapy. However, we are currently unsure as to which will prove to be the best combination, and side effects in individual cats may affect which two drugs are used in a given patient. Currently, we recommend a combination of rifampicin and clarithromycin as initial therapy.

Clofazimine 'capsules' (which contain 50 mg of the dye) can be cut into halves using a scalpel blade while wearing disposable gloves, and the two portions placed into gelatin capsules to facilitate dosing. Rifampicin is made up by dividing the contents of a 150-mg capsule and reformulating the dose in a gelatin capsule. Alternatively, a compounding pharmacist can be used to produce optimal dosage formulations. As clofazimine and rifampicin can both produce reversible hepatotoxicity, biochemical monitoring of cats regularly during therapy is mandatory, while vomiting and/or inappetence suggests the need for dosage reduction or temporary discontinuation of therapy. We have encountered photosensitivity and pitting corneal lesions in some cats during clofazimine therapy. Of these different agents, clarithromycin is the least likely to cause worrisome side effects; however, monotherapy with this agent is not recommended because of the possibility of resistance developing during treatment.

Guidelines for duration of therapy are hard to define, although mycobacterial infections should generally be treated for several months and continued for at least 2 months (the life of a macrophage in the tissues) after disappearance of lesions.

Treatment has only been attempted in one cat with *M. visibilis* infection, which was cured using clofazimine and clindamycin.[1]

Acknowledgements

The material presented here was performed in collaboration with a large number of veterinary clinicians and laboratory scientists. Most of the cytopathology was performed by Patricia Martin. Denise Wigney assisted in collating the information, and did the initial bacteriological investigations in some patients. Siobhan Hughes and Greg James, and their respective teams, did the molecular studies. Sharon Chen and David Mitchell assisted in formulating treatment regimens for companion animals. Vanessa Barrs, Sue Foster and Carolyn O'Brien treated many of the cases included here. Finally, Daria Love provided the inspiration to do this work.

Funding

Abbots Australia provided generous supplies of clarithromycin in support of these studies, and this permitted many animals to be treated that otherwise would not have been included in these investigations.

References

1　Gunn-Moore, D.A., Jenkins, P.A., Lucke V.M. Feline tuberculosis: a literature review and discussion of 19 cases caused by an unusual mycobacterial variant. *Veterinary Record*, 1996; **138**: 53–58.
2　Cavanagh, R., Bego, M., Bennett, M., *et al. Mycobacterium microti* infection (vole tuberculosis) in wild rodent populations. *Journal of Clinical Microbiology*, 2002; **40**: 3281–3285.
3　Wilkinson, G.T., Mason, K.V. Clinical aspects of mycobacterial infections of the skin. In: August, JR, ed. *Consultations in Feline*

Internal Medicine. W.B. Saunders, Philadelphia, 1991: 129–136.

4 Grange, J.M. The biology of the genus *Mycobacterium. Journal of Applied Bacteriology Symposium Supplement*, 1996; **81**: 1S–9S.

5 Wolinsky, E. Mycobacteria. In: Davis, B.D., Dulbecco, R., Eisen, H.N., Ginsberg, H.S., Wood, W.B., eds. *Microbiology.* Harper and Row, Hagerstown, 1973: 884.

6 Brown-Elliot, B.A., Wallace, R.J. Jr. Clinical and taxonomic status of pathogenic nonpigmented or late-pigmenting rapidly growing mycobacteria. *Clinical Microbiology Reviews*, 2002; **15**: 716–746.

7 Hunt, G.B. Skin-fold advancement flaps for closing large sternal and inguinal wounds in cats and dogs. *Veterinary Surgery*, 1995; **24**: 172–175.

8 Kunkle, G.A., Gulbas, N.K., Fakok, V., Halliwell, R.E.W., Connelly, M. Rapidly growing mycobacteria as a cause of cutaneous granulomas: report of five cases. *Journal of the American Animal Hospital Association*, 1983; **19**: 513–521.

9 Malik, R., Wigney, D.I., Dawson, D., Martin, P., Hunt, G.B., Love, D.N. Infection of the subcutis and skin of cats with rapidly growing mycobacteria: a review of microbiological and clinical findings. *Journal of Feline Medicine and Surgery,* 2000; **2**: 35–48.

10 Grooters, A.M., Couto, C.G., Andrews, J.M., Johnson, S.E., Kowalski, J.J., Esplin, R.B. Systemic *Mycobacterium smegmatis* infection in a dog. *Journal of the American Veterinary Medical Association,* 1995; **206**: 200–202.

11 Thomson, J.R., Mollison, N., Matthews, K.P. An investigation of mastitis due to *S. agalactiae, S. uberis* and *M. smegmatis* in a dairy herd. *Veterinary Record*, 1988; **122**: 271–274.

12 Malik, R., Hunt, G.B., Goldsmid, S.E., Martin, P., Wigney, D.I., Love, D.N. Diagnosis and treatment of pyogranulomatous panniculitis due to *Mycobacterium smegmatis* in cats. *Journal of Small Animal Practice*, 1994; **35**: 524–530.

13 Gross, T.L., Connely, M.R. Nontuberculous mycobacterial skin infections in dogs. *Veterinary Pathology*, 1983; **20**: 117–119.

14 Jang, S.S., Hirsh, D.C. Rapidly growing members of the genus *Mycobacterium* affecting dogs and cats. *Journal of the American Animal Hospital Association*, 2002; **38**: 217–220.

15 Lewis, D.T., Hodgin, E.C., Foil, C.S., Cox, H.U., Roy, A.F., Lewis, D.D. Experimental reproduction of feline *Mycobacterium fortuitum* panniculitis. *Veterinary Dermatology*, 1994; **5**:189–195.

16 Irwin, P.J., Whithear, K., Lavelle, R.B., Parry, B.W. Acute bronchopneumonia associated with *Mycobacterium fortuitum* in a dog. *Australian Veterinary Journal*, 2000; **78**: 254–257.

17 Turnwald, G.H., Pechman, R.D., Turk, J.R., *et al.* Survival of a dog with pneumonia caused by *Mycobacterium fortuitum. Journal of the American Veterinary Medical Association*, 1988; **192**: 64–66.

18 Wylie, K.B., Lewis, D.D., Pechman, R.D., Cho, D.Y., Roy, A. Hypertrophic osteopathy associated with *Mycobacterium fortuitum* pneumonia in a dog. *Journal of the American Veterinary Medical Association*, 1993; **202**: 1986–1988.

19 Foster, S.F., Martin, P., Davis, W., Allan, G.S., Malik, R. Chronic pneumonia caused by *Mycobacterium thermoresistibile* in a cat. *Journal of Small Animal Practice*, 1999; **40**: 433–438.

20 Malik, R., Shaw, S.E., Griffin, C., *et al.* Infections of the subcutis and skin of dogs caused by rapidly growing mycobacteria. *Journal of Small Animal Practice*, 2004; **45**: 485–494.

21 Hoffner, S., Klintz, L., Olsson-Liljequist, B., Bolstrom, A. Evaluation of Etest for rapid susceptibility testing of *Mycobacterium chelonae* and *M. fortuitum. Journal of Clinical Microbiology*, 1994; **32**: 1846–1849.

22 Plaus, W.J., Hermann, G. The surgical management of superficial infections caused by atypical mycobacteria. *Surgery*, 1991; **110**: 99–103.

23 Hunt, G.B., Tisdall, P.L.C., Liptak, J.M., Beck, J.A., Swinney, G.R., Malik, R. Skin-fold advancement flaps for closing large proximal limb and trunk defects in dogs and cats. *Veterinary Surgery*, 2001;

30: 440–448.

24 Melendez, L.D., Twedt, D.C., Wright, M. Suspected doxycycline-induced esophagitis with esophageal stricture formation in three cats. *Feline Practice*, 2000; **28**: 10–12.

25 Michaud, A.J. The use of clofazimine as treatment for *Mycobacterium fortuitum* in a cat. *Feline Practice,* 1994; **22**: 7–9.

26 Brown-Elliot, B.A., Wallace, R.J. Jr, Crist, C.J., Mann, C.J., Wilson, R.W. Comparison of in vitro activities of gatifloxacin and ciprofloxacin against four taxa of rapidly growing mycobacteria. *Antimicrobial Agents and Chemotherapy*, 2002; **46**: 3283–3285.

27 Malik, R., Love, D.N., Wigney, D.I., Martin, P. Mycobacterial nodular granulomas affecting the subcutis and skin of dogs (canine leproid granuloma syndrome). *Australian Veterinary Journal*, 1998; **76**: 403–407.

28 Charles, J., Martin, P., Wigney, D.I., Malik, R., Love, D.N. Pathology of canine leproid granuloma syndrome. *Australian Veterinary Journal*, 1999; **77**: 799–803.

29 Hughes, M.S., James, G., Ball, N., *et al.* Identification by 16S rRNA gene analysis of a potential novel mycobacterial species as an aetiological agent of canine leproid granuloma syndrome. *Journal of Clinical Microbiology*, 2000; **38**: 953–959.

30 Foley, J.E., Borjesson, D., Gross, T.L., Rand, C., Needham, M., Poland, A. Clinical, microscopic and molecular aspects of canine leproid granuloma in the United States. *Veterinary Pathology*, 2002; **9**: 234–239.

31 Malik, R., Martin, P., Wigney, D.I., *et al.* Treatment of canine leproid granuloma syndrome: preliminary findings in seven dogs. *Australian Veterinary Journal*, 2001; **79**: 30–36.

32 Mason, K.V., Wilkinson, G.T., Blacklock, Z. Some aspects of mycobacterial diseases of the dog and cat (abstract). In: *Proceedings of the Annual Meeting of the American Academy of Veterinary Dermatology/American College of Veterinary Dermatology,* Davis, California, 1989: 36.

33 Ralph, H. Mycobacterial granuloma in dogs. In: *Proceedings of the Post Graduate Foundation of Veterinary Science of the University of Sydney,* 1979; **37**: 157–164.

34 Rojas-Espinosa, O., Lovic, M. *Mycobacterium leprae* and *Mycobacterium lepraemurium* infections in domestic and wild animals. *Revue Scientifique et Technique Office International des Epizooties*, 2001; **20**: 219–251.

35 Hughes, M.S., Ball, N.W., Beck, L-A., de Skuce, R.A., Neill, S.D. Determination of the etiology of presumptive feline leprosy by 16S rRNA gene analysis. *Journal of Clinical Microbiology*, 1997; **35**: 2464–2471.

36 Malik, R., Hughes, M.S., James, G., *et al.* Feline leprosy: two different clinical syndromes. *Journal of Feline Medicine and Surgery*, 2002; **4**: 43–59.

37 Appleyard, G.D., Clark, E.G. Histologic and genotypic characterization of a novel *Mycobacterium* species found in three cats. *Journal of Clinical Microbiology*, 2002; **40**: 2425–2430.

38 Matthews, J.A., Liggitt, H.D. Disseminated mycobacteriosis in a cat. *Journal of the American Veterinary Medical Association*, 1983; **183**: 701–702.

39 Hughes, M.S., Ball, N.W., Love, D.N., *et al.* Disseminated *Mycobacterium genavense* infection in an FIV-positive cat. *Journal of Feline Medicine and Surgery*, 1999; **1**: 23–30.

40 Hughes, M.S., James, G., Taylor, M.J., *et al.* PCR studies of feline leprosy cases. *Journal of Feline Medicine and Surgery*, 2004; **6**: 235–243.

41 Portaels, F., Pattyn, S.R., Francken, A. In vitro sensitivity of *Mycobacterium lepraemurium* for antimycobacterial drugs. *Arzneimittel-Forschung*, 1982; **32**: 1123–1124.

42 Peters, D.H., Clissold, S.P. Clarithromycin. A review of its antimicrobial activity, pharmacokinetic properties and therapeutic potential. *Drugs*, 1992; **44**: 117–164.

Clinical, pathological and molecular characterisation of feline leprosy syndrome in the western USA

J.E. Foley DVM, PhD[1,2], T.L. Gross DVM[3], N. Drazenovich MS[2], F. Ramiro-Ibanez DVM, PhD[3], E. Anacleto[2]

[1] School of Veterinary Medicine, Department of Medicine and Epidemiology, University of California, Davis, California, USA
[2] School of Veterinary Medicine, Center for Vectorborne Diseases, University of California, Davis, California, USA
[3] IDEXX Veterinary Services, West Sacramento, California, USA

Summary

Eleven cats with skin lesions characteristic of feline leprosy syndrome were included in this retrospective clinical, histopathological and molecular study of feline leprosy syndrome (FLS). Nine of 11 cats were from coastal cities of Hawaii, Washington or California, while two cats were from the coastal mountain range in California, approximately 30 miles inland. Potential environmental risk factors included place of domicile, access to the outdoors (nine cats) and hunting (four cats). Skin lesions ranged from mildly alopecic and swollen to nodular and ulcerated. Lesions were evaluated histopathologically for necrosis, number and distribution of acid-fast bacteria (AFB), and visibility of organisms in haematoxylin and eosin (H&E)-stained sections. Polymerase chain reaction (PCR) and DNA sequencing of a fragment of the 16S rRNA gene was performed in all cases. Lesions from four cats yielded *Mycobacterium visibilis* (three cats) or the *Mycobacterium* species IWGMT 90242 species (one cat), similar to findings previously reported in North American, but not Australian, cases. In these cases, large numbers of AFB were seen diffusely within non-necrotic lesions, and the organisms stained with haematoxylin. This group was designated as group 1. Lesions from five cats were associated with

M. lepraemurium: three had necrosis with few (three cases) to moderate (one case) numbers of AFB that were not visible upon H&E examination. Organisms tended to cluster in necrotic foci. This group was designated as group 2. One cat with *M. lepraemurium* did not conform well to this morphology but was intermediate between the two groups. The lesions from the two remaining cats were associated with *Rhodococcus erythropolis* and *M. kansasii/gastri*, respectively; both of these had *M. lepraemurium*-type histomorphology (group 2). Clinically, group 1 cats with *M. visibilis*/IWGMT infection tended to be older and have larger numbers of lesions with recurrence, unexplained mortality, or concurrent disease (one cat co-infected with *Toxoplasma gondii*). Cats of group 2 with *M. lepraemurium*, or histomorphologically similar *R. erythropolis* and *M. kansasii/gastri* infections, were younger and tended to have few lesions. These cases responded completely to excision and treatment with miscellaneous broad-spectrum antibiotics. Based on this study and previous literature, it appears that, in western North America, FLS is caused by multiple species of mycobacteria, including most commonly *M. lepraemurium* and *M. visibilis*. This case series documents that FLS can occur as a result of infection with multiple mycobacterial pathogens, with important clinical and prognostic distinctions among the subtypes.

Introduction

Feline leprosy syndrome (FLS) is an uncommon, primarily cutaneous or cutaneolymphatic disease of cats.[1-3] The condition varies in severity from mild often self-limiting nodular dermatopathy, to chronic or recurring ulcerative lesions of skin and occasional draining lymph nodes. Currently, at least two histomorphological forms of feline leprosy have

been recognised, 'lepromatous' and 'tuberculoid' leprosy.

Evaluation of appropriate therapeutic modalities and predicting outcome and prognosis are problematic due to clinical heterogeneity. The aetiological organisms typically are difficult or impossible to culture, forcing veterinarians to rely on histopathology or molecular methods of diagnosis in most cases. Progress in studying and treating feline leprosy has been slow, in part because of a lack of tools for identifying and manipulating the causative bacteria.

Based on molecular analysis and fulfilment of Koch's postulates, the aetiological agent of FLS was originally reported to be *Mycobacterium lepraemurium*, an agent associated with systemic mycobacteriosis in rats.[1,4] However, recent studies have documented the presence of DNA of other *Mycobacteria* spp. in lesions of feline leprosy and suggest that FLS may be a complex of related host responses to a variety of related bacteria. Diverse mycobacteria and actinomycetes implicated in FLS have included *M. lepraemurium, M. visibilis, M. avium, Rhodococcus* spp. and others.[5–8] With several distinct aetiological agents likely involved in FLS, it is important to ascribe specific clinical and diagnostic characteristics to the appropriate agent and to evaluate the ecology, prognosis and appropriate treatment for each agent separately.

In this study, a case series of 11 cats with FLS was evaluated retrospectively to define the aetiological agents using molecular techniques, and to correlate these with clinical findings, host and environment risk factors, response to therapy and prognosis, and histomorphological features of skin biopsy. Further, the roles of tuberculoid and lepromatous histological subtypes were investigated as potential predictors of specific aetiological agents and clinical syndromes.

Materials and methods

Animals

Cats from the western continental USA and Hawaii were included in the case series on the basis of clinical signs and histopathological findings consistent with FLS. Criteria for inclusion in the study were nodular to ulcerative skin lesions characterised by pyogranulomatous to granulomatous dermatitis and panniculitis with acid-fast bacteria (AFB). For each case, a questionnaire was sent to the clinic of the referring veterinarian to evaluate host and environmental factors for the disease, and outcome of the case. Information obtained included age and home location of the cat. To evaluate environmental risk, clinics were asked: whether cats lived indoors, outdoors or both; whether the cat was known to hunt prey or have a history of fighting prior to the onset of the disease; and whether the cat lived near a sea port. To evaluate the history of the illness,

clinicians were asked to describe any wounds observed prior to the diagnosis of feline leprosy, to give the locations of the wounds on the cat and numbers of lesions, and to describe the clinical progression of the disease. Lesions were classified by referring veterinarians as nodular, alopecic or ulcerative (or any combination), with or without pruritus or apparent pain. Systemic or concurrent illness was reported, as was any attempted therapy and the outcome of the case.

Histopathology

Lesions were characterised independently by two pathologists (FRI, TLG) after paraffin-embedded, formalin-fixed tissue samples were stained with haematoxylin and eosin (H&E) and Fites acid-fast stain. Without prior knowledge of clinical features or PCR results, lesions were evaluated for necrosis, density and distribution of organisms with Fites staining, and visibility of organisms with H&E; these features were selected based on previous familiarity with tuberculoid and lepromatous forms of FLS.

DNA extraction, PCR and sequencing

For DNA extraction, a 50-μm thick section was obtained from each paraffin block of tissue using a new, disposable microtome blade. Sections were deparaffinised with xylene, the xylene was removed with three washes in absolute ethanol, and the ethanol was allowed to evaporate. Samples were then agitated with 0.1 mm zirconia silicon beads for 5 minutes (Biospec Products, Bartlesville, OK, USA). The DNA was extracted with the Qiagen Dneasy Tissue Kit (Qiagen, Valencia, CA, USA) according to the manufacturer's instructions. DNA was resuspended after extraction in 50 μl of water.

Nested PCR was performed with conserved bacterial primers 246 and 247 for round 1, and M1 and R7 for round 2, modified from previously described protocols.[9] Each 25-μl reaction contained 1× buffer, 1.5 mM $MgCl_2$, 400 nmol of each primer, 100 μM dNTPs and 0.5 U *Taq* DNA polymerase (Sigma, St Louis, MO, USA) and 2.5 μl DNA extract. Amplifying conditions were denaturation at 95°C for 5 min, 40 cycles of 96°C for 10 s, annealing at 68°C for 2 min and extension at 74°C for 3 min, followed by a 10-min final extension at 74°C. For the second round, 2 μl of first-round product was added to the same composition PCR mix and amplifying conditions were as before except only 25 rounds were performed. The approximately 469-bp amplicon spanned the V2 and V3 hypervariable regions of the 16S rDNA gene. The PCR testing was performed under conditions designed to minimise potential contamination, including running DNA extraction, PCR and electrophoresis in separate rooms, using plugged pipette tips and including negative controls in each PCR and electrophoresis run.

Amplicons were resolved in 1% (w/v) agarose gels stained with ethidium bromide (0.5 μg/μl) and visualised with an Alpha Innotech Imager (Alpha Innotech Corp., San Leandro, CA, USA). The PCR products were purified with Microcon columns (Millipore Corp., Bedford, MA, USA) and both strands of each amplicon were sequenced using PCR primers M1 and R7 using the Big Dye Terminator cycle sequencing kit (Applied Biosystems, Foster City, CA, USA). The sequences were analysed with the software program Chromas (Technelysium, Queensland, Australia) and compared to sequences maintained in Genbank using the BLAST algorithm from the National Center for Biotechnology

Information. A dendrogram was generated by the program SeqWeb (GCG, Madison, WI, USA) by sequence comparison using the Cantor-Jukes correction, followed by distance calculations using the UPGMA algorithm.

Statistical analysis

Data were maintained in Excel 2002 (Microsoft, Redmond, WA, USA) and analysed in 'R' (The R-Development Core Team, http://www.r-project.org). Differences in mean age, duration of lesion and number of lesions were compared among cats with M. visibilis and M. lepraemurium infection by t-test, with a cut-off for inferring statistical significance of $p = 0.05$.

Results

Clinical features and correlation with PCR (Tables 5.2.1 and 5.2.2)

The mean age of cats affected with FLS in this study was 7.2 ± 1.4 years (median = 7, range 1–14 years)

Table 5.2.1 Clinical and molecular findings in 11 cats with feline leprosy syndrome

Cat no.	Age (years)	Duration of lesion (months)	Lesion	No. of lesions	Lesion location	Treatment	Outcome	Sequence	Percentage homology to reported sequence
2	9	0.25	Swollen/nodular	1	Forelimb	Enrofloxacin/doxycycline	Recovered	M. kansasii/gastri	100
8	7	2	Nodular	1	Hindlimb (proximal)	Amoxicillin-clavulanate	Recovered	R. erythropolis	99
3	NA	0.5	Nodular	5	Head	Excised	Recovered	M. lepraemurium	99
4	NA	NA	NA	Too numerous to count	NA	NA	NA	M. lepraemurium	100
5	1	0.1	Alopecic/nodular	2	Hindlimb, abdomen	Doxycycline/amoxicillin-clavulanate	Recovered	M. lepraemurium	99
6	5	2	Nodule progressing to fistulous, ulcerated	1	Foreleg	Amoxicillin	Recovered	M. lepraemurium	99
7	2	1	Nodular	3	Hindlimb, tail	NA	Recovered	M. lepraemurium	99
1	9	0.5	Nodular/ulcerated	2	Head	Excision/clofazimine	Recurred	IWGMT 90242	100
9	14	4	Nodular/ulcerated	6	Abdomen, forelimbs, tail	Enrofloxacin	Found dead	M. visibilis	99
10	6	2	Nodular/pruritic	4	Head, neck, hindlimbs	Clindamycin/clofazimine	Recovered	M. visibilis	99
11	12	NA	NA	4	Neck, trunk	NA	NA	M. visibilis	99

NA, data were not available.

Table 5.2.2 Summary of clinical and microscopic findings of two feline leprosy syndrome groups

	Leprosy syndrome	
	Group 1	Group 2
Mean age of onset	10.3 years	2.7 years
Mean no. of lesions	4	2.75
Outcome of infection	Recurring or chronic	Complete recovery
PCR results	*M. visibilis*/IWGMT	*M. lepraemurium**
H&E	Diffuse inflammation with pale or vacuolated macrophages, few or no neutrophils, pale grey visible bacteria	Pyogranulomatous inflammation, often with necrosis, no visible organisms
Pathology	Lepromatous	Generally tuberculoid; rarely lepromatous (case no. 4)
Acid-fast stain	Massive diffuse acid-fast bacteria	Low to moderate acid-fast bacteria often in necrotic foci

*This group also included one cat with *M. kansasii/gastri* and one cat with *Rhodococcus erythropolis*.

and the mean reported duration of the lesion prior to biopsy was 1.4 ± 0.42 months (median = 1, range 3 days to 4 months). Of the 11 cats, two were from Hawaii, one from Washington state, and six from cities or towns in California adjacent to the Pacific Ocean; two additional Californian cats were from the coast range mountains approximately 30 miles inland from the Pacific Ocean. Possible environmental risk factors could be detected in nine of the cats, including nine that were allowed to roam outside the house, four of which were observed hunting, and one which fought. However, none of the lesions appeared to be associated directly with prior trauma.

Skin lesions in all cats in the series were present within the subcutaneous and dermal tissue and ranged from foci of mild alopecia and swelling to nodules with variable ulceration. The mean number of lesions among all cats with feline leprosy was 2.9 ± 1.8 (median = 2.5, range 1 to 'too numerous to count'), where the report with 'too numerous to count' was arbitrarily set at 6 (the maximum quantified lesion number in other cats) in the calculation of the mean (Table 5.2.2). Anatomical sites of lesions were head (*n* = 3), neck (2), proximal hindleg (5), distal hindleg (1), abdomen (3) and tail (2) (Table 5.2.1). Pruritus was reported in three cats and apparent pain in two.

DNA sequencing of PCR products supported the division of these FLS cases into two groups: one due to *M. visibilis* and the other primarily (although not exclusively) due to *M. lepraemurium* (Tables 5.2.1 and 5.2.3). Three cases of feline leprosy were associated with an organism with amplicon homology of

99–100% to *M. visibilis* and one with 100% homology with an isolate designated previously as IWGMT-90242. One cat (no. 10) in this group was systemically ill, a cat with concurrent *M. visibilis* and *Toxoplasma gondii* infection, based on lymphadenopathy, anaemia, anorexia and positive *T. gondii* IgM titre. This cat had generalised lymphadenopathy, with nodular cutaneous lesions due to *M. visibilis*. Acid-fast stain of the lymph nodes confirmed the presence of mycobacteria associated with moderate granulomatous lymphadenitis. Following treatment with clindamycin and clofazamine, the cat's FLS lesions resolved completely. An additional cat in this group was found dead but a necropsy was not performed.

Table 5.2.3 Histopathological findings in 11 cats with feline leprosy syndrome

Case no.	Necrosis	Visible on H&E	Visible on acid-fast	Sequence
2	Y	Low to moderate	Low numbers	*M. kansasii/gastri*
8	Y	N	Low numbers	*R. erythropolis*
3	Y	N	Low numbers	*M. lepraemurium*
4	N	Faintly	High numbers	*M. lepraemurium*
5	Y	N	Low numbers	*M. lepraemurium*
6	N	N	Low numbers	*M. lepraemurium*
7	Y	N	Moderate numbers	*M. lepraemurium*
1	N	Y	High numbers	IWGMT 90242
9	N	Y	High numbers	*M. visibilis*
10	N	Y	High numbers	*M. visibilis*
11	N	Y	High numbers	*M. visibilis*

Y, yes; N, no.

Cats with *M. visibilis* or IWGMT-90242 infection were significantly older (mean age 10.3 years, $p = 0.008$), and had more lesions (mean = 4) compared to cats with *M. lepraemurium* (mean = 2), although the latter difference was not statistically significant. Treatments included enrofloxacin, clindamycin plus clofazamine (in the cat co-infected with *T. gondii)*, enrofloxacin plus amoxicillin-clavulanate, and clofazamine alone; nevertheless, recurrence or chronicity was reported in two of four cats with *M. visibilis* infection.

In five cats, PCR and partial 16S rRNA gene sequences with 99–100% nucleotide identity over 450 bp to *M. lepraemurium* 16S rRNA gene sequences were detected. All cats from Hawaii ($n = 2$) and Washington state (1) had *M. lepraemurium* DNA amplified from their lesions. These cats were significantly younger (mean age 2.7 years) and tended to have fewer lesions than the *M. visibilis* group. Complete recovery after excision and treatment with doxycycline, amoxicillin, or amoxicillin-clavulanate was reported in all five cats with *M. lepraemurium* infection. There was no evidence of recurrence in any of these cats.

In two additional cats, apparent *R. erythropolis* and *M. kansasii/gastri* were detected by PCR and DNA sequencing. The cat with DNA with 99% sequence homology to *Rhodococcus erythropolis* was 7 years old and had a 2-month duration of a single lesion on the proximal hindlimb. He was successfully treated with

amoxicillin-clavulanate and the lesion did not recur. The cat with DNA with 100% sequence homology to *M. kansasii* and *M. gastri* (indistinguishable on 16S sequencing) was 9 years old and had only a 1-month duration of a single lesion on the right carpus. This lesion resolved completely after treatment with enrofloxacin and doxycycline.

Histopathological features and correlation with PCR (Tables 5.2.2 and 5.2.3)

Lesions were principally one of two types based on microscopic features. In group 1 (four cats), there was diffuse inflammation composed of macrophages that appeared pale or vacuolated; neutrophils were typically not prominent (Figs 5.2.1 and 5.2.2). Necrosis was not evident. Large numbers of organisms were visible in H&E-stained sections, and were pale grey and filamentous, often stacked up within the cytoplasm of macrophages. Fites staining revealed massive numbers of AFB throughout the lesions. This group was designated as 'lepromatous'. PCR testing of this group revealed *M. visibilis* in three cats and IWGMT-90242 in one cat.

In group 2 (six cats), inflammation was more pyogranulomatous in nature and included more neutrophils than in the *M. visibilis* group (Fig. 5.2.3). Necrosis was present within lesions of five of the six

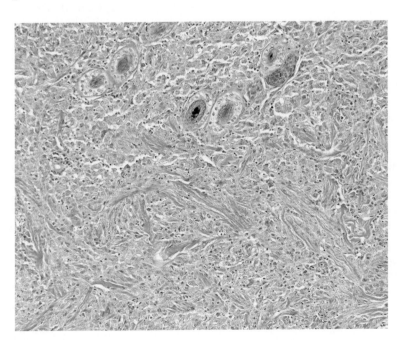

Fig. 5.2.1 Lepromatous leprosy. Diffuse granulomatous inflammation comprises predominantly pale or vacuolated macrophages. PCR testing and DNA sequencing of this sample revealed DNA with 99% sequence homology in the 16S rRNA gene to *Mycobacterium visibilis* (H&E).

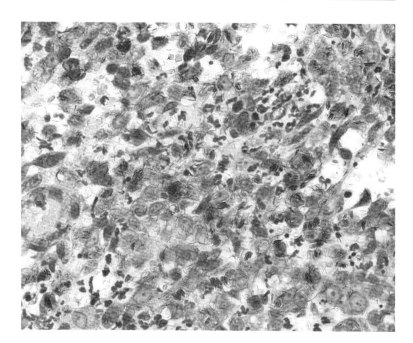

Fig. 5.2.2 Fites stain of section described in Fig. 5.2.1, revealing massive numbers of acid-fast bacteria throughout the lesions. Notice the 'stacked' pattern of bacteria within macrophages.

cats. Organisms were not visible on H&E examination. Fites staining revealed low to moderate numbers of organisms, always of lower density than in the *M. visibilis* group. Organisms were confined predominantly to necrotic foci in five cats; one additional cat without necrosis had low numbers of organisms distributed sporadically. This group was designated as 'tuberculoid'. Of the six cats, PCR and sequence analysis revealed *M. lepraemurium* sequences in four, *M. kansasii/gastri* in one and *R. erythropolis* in one. Both the *M. kansasii/gastri* and *R. erythropolis* cats had necrotic lesions.

Fig. 5.2.3 Tuberculoid leprosy. Granulomatous inflammation surrounds prominent central necrosis. Bacterial organisms were not visible on H&E examination. PCR testing and DNA sequencing of this sample revealed DNA with 99% sequence homology in the 16S rRNA gene to *M. lepraemurium* (H&E).

One cat (no. 4) did not fit well into either group. In this cat, there was diffuse granulomatous inflammation composed of pale macrophages; neutrophils were sparse. Organisms were faintly visible on H&E evaluation, but were shorter, creating a granular appearance to the cytoplasm, in contrast to the clearly delineated organisms in the *M. visibilis* group. Necrosis was not present. Organisms were abundant with Fites staining but were not as intensely present as in the *M. visibilis* group. The PCR testing recovered *M. lepraemurium* sequence from this cat's lesions.

Discussion

Data presented in this paper support important clinical and pathological distinctions between at least two groups of FLS: a more severe, older age-onset syndrome attributable to *M. visibilis*/IWGMT (group 1); and a milder disease with a generally better prognosis in young cats, usually attributable to *M. lepraemurium* (group 2). Unfortunately, comprehensive health information on the cats in the present study, including FeLV or FIV infection status, neoplasia or renal disease, was not consistently available, but may be relevant in some cases of FLS.

Histopathological features of group 1, designated as lepromatous, were easily visible organisms on H&E examination, intense numbers of organisms visible with Fites staining, and predominantly granulomatous inflammation with no necrosis. This group revealed *M. visibilis*/IWGMT-94202 with PCR and DNA sequencing. In group 2, organisms were not stained by H&E and were low to moderate in density with Fites staining; inflammation was pyogranulomatous, usually with foci of necrosis. Group 2 comprised multiple species based on PCR analysis and DNA sequencing; *M. lepraemurium*, *M. kansasii/gastri* and *R. erythropolis*. Microscopic features correlated with, and were thus predictive of, the clinical groups in all but one cat (cat no. 4 with *M. lepraemurium*, which could not be assigned to either group). This occurred despite variability in PCR-determined aetiologies, particularly in group 2.

Other researchers have also found a diversity of mycobacteria associated with cutaneous lesions of cats clinically and histologically consistent with feline leprosy. Retrospective evaluation of published FLS cases is difficult because many of those cases previously believed to be associated with *M. lepraemurium* may have been due to other mycobacteria instead. Classical FLS

has been described as a disease of relatively young cats (<5 years old), with focal cutaneous and subcutaneous granulomas which may ulcerate and invade muscles, fascia and lymph nodes.[3,4,10] Disease was reported in association with weight loss and systemic dissemination of the mycobacteria, often with local, or less commonly, disseminated caseous necrosis and lymphadenopathy possibly progressing to unencapsulated granulomas invading tissue. The variability in clinical leprosy was hypothesised to be due to differences in host susceptibility.[11]

More recent literature (including the present study) has identified the mycobacterial agents with DNA sequencing. Retrospective evaluation of 30 FLS cases from the USA, UK, New Zealand and Australia documented DNA sequences characterised as *M. lepraemurium*, *M. intracellulare*, *M. szulgai*, *M. visibilis*-like and *M. tilburgii*-like, although that study did not correlate pathogen identification with clinical syndromes.[5] Interestingly, the *M. tilburgii*-like organism is genetically very closely related or identical to the organism described in canine leproid granuloma syndrome.[12]

DNA sequence data from this and the majority of previous studies indicate that cases due to *M. lepraemurium* generally have relatively mild clinical signs, with relatively few but often necrotic lesions, in younger cats; these may contain low numbers of bacteria. In our study, one cat with *M. lepraemurium* (no. 4) deviated from typical group 2 (tuberculoid) microscopic features, and had unusually high numbers of organisms and few neutrophils. These lesions had an intact epidermis and contained no necrosis. The authors propose that early lesions of *M. lepraemurium* infection are more likely to contain higher numbers of organisms which may then be dissipated by a progressive necrotising inflammatory host response in older lesions.

A lepromatous form of leprosy in older cats, associated with a reportedly novel bacterium with close DNA sequence homology to *M. malmoense* and *M. haemophilum*, was reported to generalise slowly to systemic disease.[6] In cats in the present study, bacteria that were closely related to *M. malmoense* or the strain described previously were not detected. In contrast, *M. visibilis* has not so far been reported from FLS cases from Australia and New Zealand. In cases from Idaho, Oregon and western Canada, a mycobacterium named *M. visibilis* was associated with fasciitis, granulomatous dermatitis with foamy vacuolation in macrophages and visible organisms on H&E evaluation that were dense with acid-fast staining. *M. visibilis* infection produced relatively severe clinical disease in that study, characterised by open sores, swelling, severe alopecia, pruritus and extensive internal organ involvement.[7] Similar to that study, cases due to *M. visibilis* in the present series were more severe than cases due to *M. lepraemurium*.

The mycobacteria associated with FLS do not appear to constitute a monophyletic clade (Fig. 5.2.1). *M. visibilis* is related to a species designated IWGMT 90242 and disease associated with both was clinically and histopathologically very similar. Thus, cases in this study were analysed together. *M. lepraemurium* is somewhat distantly related to *M. visibilis,* while *M. malmoense*, the novel mycobacterial species in FLS cases in Australia and *M. kansasii* are genetically clustered together. All of these pathogens are more distantly related to *M. leprae*, the agent of human leprosy. The finding of a diversity of mycobacteria in FLS, particularly in the stereotypic histopathological group 2 described in this study, is of great interest and may suggest that some feline hosts have a limited repertoire of host responses to a multitude of opportunistic organisms.

Two cases in the present series, otherwise fitting group 2 (tuberculoid) criteria, were not attributable to either *M. visibilis* or *M. lepraemurium*, including one case from which the DNA sequence identified *R. erythropolis*. The clinical significance of the amplification of *R. erythropolis* DNA is not clear. Genetically, the *Rhodococcus* spp. are within the same subfamily Mycobacterinae, possibly accounting for the amplification of *Rhodococcus* spp. with a *Mycobacterium*-generic PCR protocol, although previous assessment of the specificity of these primers indicates that the assay should not amplify bacteria in this genus.[13] *Rhodococcus equi* is a facultatively intracellular pathogen associated with suppurative bronchopneumonia and enteritis in foals and a variety of opportunistic diseases in immunocompromised humans.[14] In cats, *R. equi* has been reported in pyogranulomatous lesions, abscesses and cellulitis, particularly on the legs and neck, including a case in which macrophages in cutaneous pyogranulomatous lesions contained large numbers of visible rhodococci.[15–17] *R. erythropolis* infection was reported in a 24-year-old human patient with AIDS and multiple subcutaneous nodules at various sites on the extremities, each with granulomatous inflamma-

tion containing acid-fast rods,[18] and in a South African cat with FLS.[19]

In the case in the present study, AFB were visualised within lesions, which would suggest that the recovery of *R. erythropolis* was not consistent with environmental contamination, as suggested recently based on amplification of rhodococcal DNA in miscellaneous inflammatory and non-inflammatory skin lesions as well as internal viscera of dogs and cats.[20] In the future, if *R. erythropolis* or *R. equi* isolates were cultured, it might be diagnostically valuable to assay for virulence plasmids, which often are missing from soil strains but common in strains invading mammalian hosts.[21] However, evaluation of feline *R. equi* isolates from Texas, Ontario (Canada), New Zealand and Brazil revealed that many feline isolates lacked virulence plasmids.[22]

This appears to be the first published report of *M. kansasii* or *M. gastri* dermatitis in a cat; this cat had clinical morphologic features of group 2 (tuberculoid) leprosy. Based on 16S rRNA gene sequencing, the two organisms cannot be distinguished. *M. kansasii* is a serious opportunistic pathogen in humans, often associated with pulmonary disease similar to tuberculosis as well as dermatitis and associated lymphadenitis.[23] We found only one previous report of its isolation in a dog which presented with chronic severe lung lobe torsion and pleural effusion.[24] The diagnosis in that case was made on the basis of culture, PCR analysis and DNA sequencing. In contrast, *M. gastri* is very rarely found in association with disease and thus is generally not considered a pathogen.[23]

Understanding of FLS is emerging as a result of evaluating cases using combined molecular, clinical and histopathological lines of evidence. The results of this study show two distinct groups of FLS that are predictable in most cases by histopathological and molecular findings. This type of correlative analysis may allow further progress in the ecology, medical management and prognostication of FLS. In the future, it will be necessary to accurately identify the aetiological agent in each case of FLS so as to untangle the roles of the bacterial genotype and host immunity in the ultimate manifestation of FLS.

Acknowledgements

We thank referring veterinarians and clinics for their assistance with the clinical outcome questionnaire. Jen Olsen provided valuable laboratory assistance.

References

1   Lawrence, W., Wickham, N. Cat leprosy: infection by a bacillus resembling *Mycobacterium lepraemurium*. *Australian Veterinary Journal*, 1963; **39**: 390–393.

2   McIntosh, D. Feline leprosy: a review of forty-four cases from western Canada. *Canadian Veterinary Journal*, 1982; **23**: 291–295.

3   Pedersen, N. *Feline Infectious Diseases*. American Veterinary Publisher, Goleta, CA, 1988.

4   Lewis, D., Kunkle, G. Feline leprosy. In: Greene, C., ed. *Infectious Diseases of the Dog and Cat*. W.B. Saunders, Philadelphia, 1998: 321–324.

5   Davies, J., Sibley, J., Clark, E., Appleyard, G.D. Feline leprosy syndrome is associated with several mycobacterium species: a histologic and genotypic retrospective study on formalin-fixed and paraffin-embedded tissues. *Veterinary Pathology*, 2003; **40**: 613.

6   Malik, R., Hughes, M., James, G., *et al.* Feline leprosy: two different clinical syndromes. *Journal of Feline Medicine and Surgery*, 2002; **4**: 43–59.

7   Appleyard, G.D., Clark, E.G. Histologic and genotypic characterization of a novel *Mycobacterium* species found in three cats. *Journal of Clinical Microbiology*, 2002; **40**: 2425–2430.

8   Hughes, M.S., Ball, N.W., Beck, L.A., de Lisle, G.W., Skuce, R.A., Neill, S.D. Determination of the etiology of presumptive feline leprosy by 16S rRNA gene analysis. *Journal of Clinical Microbiology*, 1997; **35**: 2464–2471.

9   Hughes, M.S., James, G., Ball, N., *et al.* Identification by 16S rRNA gene analyses of a potential novel mycobacterial species as an etiological agent of canine leproid granuloma syndrome. *Journal of Clinical Microbiology*, 2000; **38**: 953–959.

10 Wilkinson, G., Mason, K. Clinical aspects of mycobacterial infections of the skin. In: August, J., ed. *Consultations in Feline Internal Medicine*. W.B. Saunders, Philadelphia, 1991: 129–136.

11 Grange, J., Yates, M. Infections caused by opportunistic mycobacteria. *Journal of the Royal Society of Medicine*, 1986; **79**: 226–229.

12 Foley, J., Borjesson, D., Gross, T., Rand, C., Needham, M., Poland, A. Clinical, microscopic, and molecular characterization of canine leproid granuloma in North America. *Veterinary Pathology*, 2002; **39**: 234–239.

13 Böddinghaus, B., Rogall, T., Flohr, T., Blöcker, H., Böttger, E.C. Detection and identification of mycobacteria by amplification of rRNA. *Journal of Clinical Microbiology*, 1990; **28**: 1751–1759.

14 Prescott, J.F. *Rhodococcus equi*: an animal and human pathogen. *Clinical Microbiology Reviews,* 1991; **4**: 20–34.

15 Elliott, G., Lawson, G.H., Mackenzie, C.P. *Rhodococcus equi* infection in cats. *Veterinary Record,* 1986; **118**: 693–694.

16 Fairley, R., Fairley, N. *Rhodococcus equi* infections of cats. *Veterinary Dermatology,* 1999; **10**: 43–46.

17 Patel, A. Pyogranulomatous skin disease and cellulitis in a cat caused by *Rhodococcus equi*. *Journal of Small Animal Practice*, 2002; **43**: 129–132.

18 Vernazza, P., Bodmer, T., Galeazzi, R. *Rhodococcus erythropolis* infection in HIV-associated immunodeficiency. *Schweizerische Medizinische Wochenschrift*, 1991; **121**: 1095–1098.

19 Last, R.D., Appleyard, G.D. Canine leproid granuloma: a South African perspective (abstract). *Proceedings of the 18th Annual Congress of the European Society of Veterinary Dermatology/European College of Veterinary Dermatology*, Nice, France, 2002: 242.

20 Ramiro-Ibanez, F., Foley, J.A., Gross, T.L. *Rhodococcus* spp. as ubiquitous contaminants of paraffin-embedded tissues in PCR analysis for *Mycobacterium* spp. skin infections. In: Hillier, A., Foster, A.P., Kwochka, K.W., eds. *Advances in Veterinary Dermatology*, Vol. 5. Blackwell Publishing, Oxford, 2005, 247–254.

21 Takai, S. Epidemiology of *Rhodococcus equi* infections: a review. *Veterinary Microbiology*, 1997; **56**: 167–176.

22 Takai, S., Martens, R.J., Julian, A., *et al.* Virulence of *Rhodococcus equi* isolated from cats and dogs. *Journal of Clinical Microbiology*, 2003; **41**: 4468–4470.

23 Wayne, L.G., Sramek, H.A. Agents of newly recognized or infrequently encountered mycobacterial diseases. *Clinical Microbiology Reviews,* 1992; **5**: 1–25.

24 Pressler, B.M., Hardie, E.M., Pitulle, C., Hopwood, R.M., Sontakke, S., Breitschwerdt, E.B. Isolation and identification of *Mycobacterium kansasii* from pleural fluid of a dog with persistent pleural effusion. *Journal of the American Veterinary Medical Association*, 2002; **220**: 1336–1340.

Rhodococcus spp. as ubiquitous contaminants of paraffin-embedded tissues in PCR analysis for *Mycobacterium* spp. skin infections

F. Ramiro-Ibanez DVM, PhD[1], J.E. Foley PhD[2], T.L. Gross DVM[3]

[1] IDEXX Veterinary Services, West Sacramento, California, USA
[2] Center for Vectorborne Diseases, School of Veterinary Medicine, UC Davis, California, USA
[3] IDEXX Veterinary Services and California Dermatopathology Service, West Sacramento, California, USA

Summary

As part of a study to characterise the aetiology of feline leprosy, biopsies from nodular pyogranulomatous lesions lacking visible acid-fast organisms were analysed by nested PCR and DNA sequencing. The DNA of nodular skin lesions from 12 cats was extracted and amplified with generic mycobacterial primers targeting the 16S rRNA gene. Amplified fragments were sequenced in an automated sequencer, analysed and compared by computer analysis with known sequences of related organisms. Controls consisting of inflamed and normal, cutaneous and visceral, feline and canine tissues (14 samples) were also analysed. The results revealed DNA sequences homologous to the comparable gene in *Rhodococcus erythropolis* in 9/12 of the acid-fast bacteria-negative nodules. Additionally, 9/14 control tissues showed similar amplification of a bacterium with high homology to *R. erythropolis* and occasionally other actinomycetes. Based on these results, two main scenarios may be in play. First, in lesions with histologically undetectable acid-fast organisms, the amount of mycobacterial DNA may be very low and other dominant contaminant organisms such as *Rhodococcus* spp. may be preferentially amplified. Second, a negative acid-fast result obtained histologically may accurately predict an absence of infection with *Mycobacterium* spp., and only contaminant DNA is amplified by PCR. In summary, the significance of *Rhodococcus* spp. as aetiological agents in nodular dermal lesions with no recognisable acid-fast organisms should be questioned (when results are obtained exclusively by PCR analysis), and further investigation using other complementary diagnostic procedures is indicated.

Introduction

The genus *Mycobacterium* of the order actinomycetales consists of a diverse group of acid-fast bacilli that may act as primary or opportunistic pathogens.[1] These organisms and other actinomycetales are often involved in opportunistic infections in humans and animals.[2-5] Other important actinomycete genera described in opportunistic infections include *Streptomyces* spp.,[6] *Rhodococcus* spp.[5,7-10] and *Corynebacterium* spp.[11] For some infectious agents, such as *Mycobacterium* spp., identification to species level is relevant for establishing appropriate therapy and for epidemiological studies.[12-14]

Molecular diagnosis has significantly broadened the capabilities of diagnostic laboratories and research facilities, particularly in circumstances in which aetiological agents are difficult to culture.[15] Amplification of DNA by polymerase chain reaction (PCR) is the most widespread molecular technique used for diagnosis.[15]

PCR techniques used in the characterisation of *Mycobacterium* spp. and other organisms are frequently based on the amplification and sequencing of the ribosomal RNA genes (rRNA), which is highly conserved among species. Of these genes, 16S rRNA is one of the most extensively used for identification purposes and phylogenetic studies of bacterial organisms.[3,12,16-18]

Ordinarily, a diagnostic approach for unknown aetiological microorganisms is based on the use of universal or generic primers for highly conserved regions of the 16S rDNA that span the variable regions, followed by either hybridisation with specific oligoprobes,[19] sequencing of the amplified gene and comparison with published bacterial databases,[3] or identification by restriction endonuclease analysis.[4,17]

Despite the wide applicability and efficacy of the PCR technique, there are some drawbacks derived from the potential presence of contaminant organisms or DNA.[20,21] In this retrospective study, we report the presence of contaminant DNA of actinomycetales, predominantly *Rhodococcus erythropolis*, in DNA extracted from paraffin-embedded tissue samples. These contaminants may be considered true opportunistic aetiological agents of skin diseases in cats and potentially other species as well.

Materials and methods

Specimens

A retrospective search for cases of nodular pyogranulomatous or granulomatous dermatitis and/or panniculitis was performed. Paraffin-embedded, formalin-fixed tissue samples received between the years 2000 and 2003 were selected from the tissue collection of the laboratory. The selection was based on examination by two pathologists (FRI, TLG) of 5-µm sections stained with haematoxylin and eosin (H&E). Twelve skin lesions from 12 different cats were selected based on histological similarity to lesions containing acid-fast organisms, as seen in feline leprosy syndrome.[4] All selected cases were additionally examined with Fites modified acid-fast (referred to hereafter as acid-fast technique) and Grocott's methenamine silver (GMS) stains for the presence of acid-fast bacteria and fungi,[22] respectively. Five selected samples positive by PCR were also sent to a reference laboratory (UC Davis Immunohistochemistry Laboratory) for anti-BCG immunohistochemistry, a more sensitive technique used for the detection of actinomycetes and fungi.[23] Paraffin-embedded, formalin-fixed tissue samples of inflammatory and non-inflammatory skin lesions from dogs ($n = 5$) and cats (3) were further included as controls: canine inflammatory lesions (2) were diagnosed as mild allergic dermatitis; feline lesions (3) lacked inflammation, and were

clinically consistent with psychogenic alopecia; and canine dermal neoplasms (3). Non-cutaneous paraffin-embedded samples, including normal spleen, liver and lung from both cats and dogs ($n = 6$), were similarly processed and analysed for the presence of amplifiable DNA. Additional controls included PCR solutions and reagents with no added DNA.

DNA extraction

DNA was extracted from each tissue sample following standard laboratory protocols. Briefly, a 50-µm thick section was obtained from each paraffin block using a new disposable microtome blade and transferred to a sterile tube. All the specimens were handled with latex gloves. Sections obtained were deparaffinised with xylene and then agitated with 0.1-mm zirconia-silicon beads for 5 minutes (Biospec Products, Bartlesville, OK, USA). The DNA was extracted with the Qiagen DNA Kit (Qiagen, Valencia, CA, USA) according to the manufacturer's instructions.

PCR amplification

Nested 16S rRNA gene PCR was performed with 16S rDNA generic mycobacterial primers 246 (16SF) and 247 (16SR) for round 1 and MycoM1 and MycoR7 for round 2, as described previously.[24] All reactions, including controls, were repeated twice in separate experiments. Each 25-µl reaction consisted of 1× buffer, 1.5 µM $MgCl_2$, 3.2 pmol of each primer, 100 nM dNTPs, 0.02 units of *Taq* DNA polymerase (Sigma Chemical Co.), and 2.5 µl DNA (round 1) or 0.5 µl DNA (round 2). Thermocycling conditions consisted of an incubation at 95°C for 5 min, then 40 cycles of 96°C for 10 s, 68°C for 2 min, 74°C for 3 min, followed by 74°C for 10 min (round 1) and 25 cycles of 94°C for 30 s, 68°C for 1 min, 74°C for 15 s, followed by 74°C for 5 min (round 2). The 469-bp region amplified spanned the V2 and V3 hypervariable regions of the gene. The position and sequences of the primers for the first (16SF and 16SR) and second (MycoM1 and MycoR7) rounds have been published.[24] The PCR testing was performed under conditions designed to minimise potential contamination, as previously specified,[12] including running DNA extraction, PCR and electrophoresis in separate rooms, using plugged pipette tips and running negative and positive controls in each PCR and electrophoresis.

PCR product analysis

Amplicons (10 μl) were resolved in 1% (w/v) agarose gels stained with ethidium bromide (0.5 μg/μl) and visualised with an Alpha Innotech Imager (Alpha Innotech Corp., San Leandro, CA, USA). The PCR products were purified with Microcon columns (Millipore Corp., Bedford, MA, USA) and DNA was sequenced with the MycoR7 primer by Davis Sequencing using the Big Dye Terminator cycle sequencing kit (Applied Biosystems, Foster City, CA, USA). The sequences were analysed with the software program Chromas (Technylysium, Queensland, Australia). DNA sequences were compared to sequences maintained in Genebank using the BLAST algorithm from the National Center for Biotechnology Information.

Results

Nodular skin lesions (Table 5.3.1)

Clinically, all the lesions were nodular, solitary ($n = 10$) or multiple (2), and affected the face, trunk and extremities. All samples were characterised histologically as nodular pyogranulomatous to granulomatous dermatitis and/or panniculitis (Fig. 5.3.1). The infiltrates were predominantly formed by epithelioid macrophages, intermingled with variable numbers of neutrophils, peripheral lymphocytes and plasma cells, and rare eosinophils. Areas of central necrosis were seen in a few cases (Fig. 5.3.2). Samples were negative for acid-fast organisms by routine acid-fast stain ($n = 12$), for fungi by GMS stain (12) and negative with anti-BCG immunohistochemistry (5) (Fig. 5.3.3).

Table 5.3.1 Clinical, molecular and histopathological data of feline nodular skin lesions included in the study

Case	Breed	Age (years)/sex	Lesion	Sequence	Homology
Fel 1	Oriental- SH	3/m	Nodular granulomatous dermatitis	*R. erythropolis*	100%
Fel 2	DSH	12/m	Coalescing pyogranulomatous dermatitis	*R. erythropolis*	99%
Fel 3	DSH	2/m	Nodular to diffuse pyogranulomatous dermatitis and panniculitis	*R. erythropolis*	99%
Fel 4	DLH	8/m	Diffuse pyogranulomatous panniculitis with necrosis	*R. erythropolis*	100%
Fel 5	DSH	10/m	Coalescing granulomatous to pyogranulomatous dermatitis	Negative	
Fel 6	DSH	11/f	Granulomatous dermatitis	*R. erythropolis*	99%
Fel 7	DSH	2/m	Nodular pyogranulomatous panniculitis	*R. erythropolis*	99%
Fel 8	DLH	4/f	Nodular to coalescing pyogranulomatous dermatitis	*R. erythropolis*	99%
Fel 9	DSH	4/f	Nodular pyogranulomatous dermatitis and panniculitis with necrosis	Negative	
Fel 10	Persian	4/f	Granulomatous dermatitis	*R. erythropolis*	100%
Fel 11	DSH	8/f	Nodular pyogranulomatous panniculitis	Negative	
Fel 12	DSH	2/m	Coalescing pyogranulomatous dermatitis with necrosis	*R. erythropolis*	100%

Breeds: SH, short hair; DSH, domestic short hair; DLH, domestic long hair. Sex: m, male; f, female.

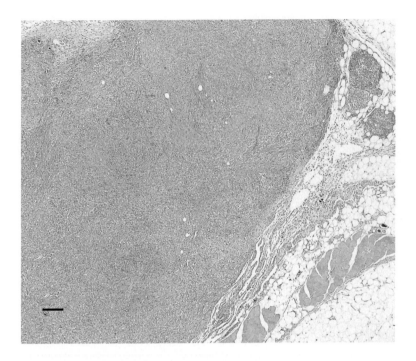

Fig. 5.3.1 Nodular inflammatory lesion in the dermis extending into the subcutis. Small clusters of lymphocytes can be appreciated among a more uniform histiocytic population. H&E; bar = 200 μm.

When analysed by PCR and sequencing, nine samples (75%) had positive PCR reactions with 469-bp amplicons (Fig. 5.3.4); the remaining three samples were negative. The bands varied in intensity from weak ($n = 2$) to strongly positive (4), with three cases being of intermediate intensity. The internal negative controls were negative in all experiments (Fig. 5.3.4). Amplified DNAs from all nine samples had sequences consistent with *R. erythropolis*, sharing between 99% ($n = 5$) and 100% (4) homology.

Control cases (Table 5.3.2)

All neoplastic skin masses from dogs ($n = 3$) yielded an amplicon with 98–99% homology to *R. erythropolis*. All non-inflammatory skin samples from cats ($n =$

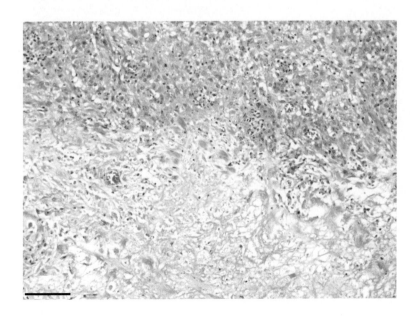

Fig. 5.3.2 Central areas of coagulative necrosis are seen in some of the nodular dermal lesions (bottom half of the figure). H&E; bar = 100 μm.

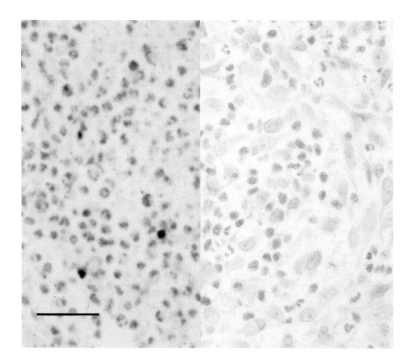

Fig. 5.3.3 Positive control of BCG immuno-histochemistry (left side). The brown coloured cells contain mycobacterial organisms. Nodular lesion from a cat with no recognisable agents by immunohistochemistry (right side). BCG immunohistochemistry. Bar = 30 μm.

3) gave similar results, with amplicons showing 99% homology to *R. erythropolis*. Inflammatory skin biopsies from dogs ($n = 2$) produced amplified products consistent with *Gordona* spp. (1) and *R. erythropolis* (1). The DNA from non-cutaneous tissues produced PCR amplicons of several actinomycetales as specified in Table 5.3.2. The most common bacterial DNA sequence obtained had high homology with *R. erythropolis*. Controls prepared with no added DNA were run in parallel and produced no detectable amplicons.

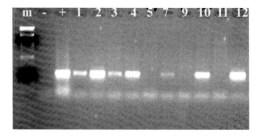

Fig. 5.3.4 Example of PCR amplicon resolution in agarose gel. The first column on the left side corresponds to the molecular weight marker (m). The following two columns correspond to controls (- and +). The numbered columns are from different nodular lesions. The amplicons of 469 bp are present at different concentrations (bright central bands).

Discussion

The initial purpose of this work was to characterise the specific aetiology of pyogranulomatous/granulomatous cutaneous lesions negative for bacterial organisms by acid-fast staining and anti-BCG immunohistochemistry.[23] Histologically, these lesions were similar to acid-fast-positive nodules with reported PCR amplicons consistent with *Mycobacterium* spp.[3,4,10] Considering the higher sensitivity of the PCR technique compared with histochemical and immunohistochemical methods, the study was undertaken under the hypothesis that some of the acid-fast-negative and BCG-negative lesions might be positive for *Mycobacterium* spp. by PCR.

Despite the use of generic primers for *Mycobacterium* spp.,[24] our results documented amplification of *R. erythropolis* DNA, a saprophyte that occasionally functions as an opportunistic pathogen in feline nodular skin lesions.[8,10,25] *R. erythropolis* DNA and DNA from other actinomycetes, such as *Gordona* sp., and *Mycobacterium sphagni,* were also identified in control samples from skin and internal tissues. The presence of DNA of saprophytic organisms in both nodular skin lesions and controls strongly suggests pre- or post-embedding sample contamination. The specific source of the contamination could not be found and persisted despite the adherence to protocols used to decrease the risk

Controls	Species	Tissue	Sequence	Homology
C 1	Feline	Skin (psychogenic alopecia)	*R. erythropolis*	99%
C 2	Feline	Skin (psychogenic alopecia)	*R. erythropolis*	99%
C 3	Feline	Skin (psychogenic alopecia)	*R. erythropolis*	99%
C 4	Canine	Skin (histiocytoma)	*R. erythropolis*	98%
C 5	Canine	Skin (melanocytoma)	*R. erythropolis*	98%
C 6	Canine	Skin (plasmacytoma)	*R. erythropolis*	99%
C 7	Feline	Spleen	*Gordona sp.*	99%
C 8	Feline	Liver	*R. rodochrous*	99%
C 9	Feline	Lung	Negative	…
C 10	Canine	Spleen	Negative	…
C 11	Canine	Liver	*R. erythropolis*	99%
C 12	Canine	Lung	*Mycobacterium sphagni*	98%
C 13	Canine	Skin (allergic dermatitis)	*R. erythropolis*	99%
C 14	Canine	Skin (allergic dermatitis)	*Gordona sp.*	99%

Table 5.3.2 Molecular DNA analysis of control tissues

of environmental contamination.[1,12] Although commercial PCR solutions and reagents have occasionally been reported to contain DNA from contaminant organisms,[20,21] the reagents used in these experiments did not yield PCR products in the experimental negative controls. Only DNA extracted from paraffin-embedded tissues demonstrated the contaminant sequences.

Rhodococcus spp. (family *Nocardioform*, order *Actinomycetes*) are taxonomically related to organisms of the genus *Nocardia* and, to a lesser extent, *Mycobacterium*.[26] They are variably acid-fast, gram-positive, aerobic coccobacilli with mycolic acid in the outer capsule and are described in the literature as causative agents of cutaneous and non-cutaneous infections.[7,8,10,27–29] Based on these similarities, acid-fast stain is not sufficient for an aetiological diagnosis at the species level in cases of actinomycete-induced nodular skin lesions.

Among the rhodococci, *R. equi* is the best-characterised species of the genus. This organism is a common cause of severe internal disease in young foals, producing pyogranulomatous pneumonia and colitis.[30] Sporadic cases in other species have been reported, including dermal infections in cats.[5] *R. equi* was not isolated from any tissue in this study. In humans, other *Rhodococcus* spp. have been reported as causative agents of arthritis/osteomyelitis,[31] subcutaneous abscesses/necrotising tenosynovitis,[27] meningitis,[29,32] deep skin lesions,[7] pulmonary disease[28] and keratitis/endophthalmitis.[25,33] *R. erythropolis* is rarely reported as an infectious agent,[8,10,25] but it has special interest for microbiologists due to its potential use as a decontaminant of biomolecules.[34–36] It has been isolated from soil and marine samples, indicating a high adaptability to extreme environmental conditions.[34,37]

From an array of bacterial genes used for PCR amplification, the 16S rDNA is one of the most used targets. The primary structure of the 16S rRNA gene is composed of segments with highly conserved sequences, spanning hypervariable regions.[38] The gene is phylogenetically conserved among eubacteria and the variable sequences are characteristic of a determined group or species.[17,39] Phylogenetic analysis of 16S rRNA gene sequences has contributed to the classification of mycobacteria[40] and other organisms.[17] Universal or generic eubacterial primers for the 16S rDNA have previously been utilised to detect organisms in paucibacillary infections or organisms that are difficult to culture, such as the case of the agent of canine leproid granuloma.[24] However, at the same time, this approach increases the risk of preferentially detecting closely related sequences of contaminant organisms that are not implicated in the pathogenesis of the process.[1,20] The use of specific primers might be indicated in cases in which a single agent is being investigated, but not as a screening technique for unknown aetiologies.

Contaminant organisms can be reported as aetiological agents by PCR analysis and this occurs more commonly with techniques based on amplification of genes with non-specific bacterial primers.[18] Equally relevant, most mycobacterial organisms possess only one or two copies per genome of the 16S rRNA gene, contrasting with the higher number of gene copies (up to seven) in other eubacterial organisms.[16,41] Consequently, in some specific settings, non-mycobacterial organisms might be preferentially amplified if present as contaminants.[20]

The attempts to eliminate contaminant DNA in similar experimental situations have been counteracted by a considerable decrease in sensitivity.[18,42] Additionally, there are other difficulties inherent to this type of PCR amplification. For example, formalin fixation invariably causes some DNA degradation in the tissue and may limit PCR sensitivity, particularly in paucibacillary mycobacterial infections.[24] Further, the formation of molecular chimeras between DNAs of several organisms has been a complicating factor in some reports, although they were not detected by sequencing in this study.[43] More potential caveats for the PCR characterisation of mycobacterial infections include the intracellular location of the organisms, the presence of a cell wall and the presence of PCR inhibitors in some clinical specimens.[1] The use of multiple controls, including house-keeping genes or internal controls,[44] to rule out inhibition of amplification (false negatives) is strongly recommended for routine PCR analysis for mycobacteria. In our case, house-keeping genes were not utilised due to the continuous amplification of contaminant organisms. For our purposes, the use of unrelated tissues as controls helped to identify the presence of contamination instead of amplification of an aetiological organism.

In paucibacillary infections, such as those produced by *M. tuberculosis,* PCR is generally less sensitive than traditional microbiological culture,[1] and the aetiological characterisation of feline skin nodules has traditionally been challenging.[3] Alternative techniques, such as sequence capture PCR, have been developed to increase the sensitivity of the traditional PCR reaction.[1] Based on our results and the technical barriers described above, the traditional PCR detection of feline cutaneous mycobacterial infections, utilising this particular approach and in paraffin-embedded tissues, may not be more sensitive than histochemical techniques for paucibacillary infections.

Nevertheless, the use of molecular techniques has allowed the recognition and characterisation of some elusive aetiological agents, such as the causative agent of Whipple's disease[45] and the agent of bacillary angiomatosis[46] in humans. The development of new technologies has justified the reconsideration of Koch's postulates for aetiological diagnosis with a series of recently proposed guidelines.[15] As in the case of Koch's postulates, the new principles are intended to serve as a channel for the integration of the molecular techniques as relevant tools in microbiological studies because the simple presence of bacterial DNA obtained during an experimental procedure is not sufficient guarantee of aetiology.[15] Among other conditions, these molecular guidelines indicate the need for the preferential presence of the microbial DNA in lesions, and the establishment of tissue:sequence correlation by demonstrating the specific location of the organisms to areas of tissue pathology.[15]

The discovery of contaminant organisms in fixed tissue samples by PCR analysis may present a significant diagnostic challenge. Differentiation from true aetiological organisms may require the utilisation of complementary techniques like sequence capture PCR, *in situ* hybridisation, or *in situ* PCR.[1]

This study exemplifies the fact that formalin-fixed and paraffin-embedded dermal nodules, negative for acid-fast organisms with special stains, are likely to amplify contaminant DNA when using non-specific primers for PCR, and a variety of controls are necessary to rule out false-positive results.

References

1 Skuce, R.A., Hughes, M.S., Taylor, M.J., Neill, S.D. Detection of pathogenic mycobacteria of veterinary importance. *Methods in Molecular Biology*, 2003; **216**: 201–221.

2 McNeil, M.M., Brown, J.M. The medically important aerobic actinomycetes: epidemiology and microbiology. *Clinical Microbiological Reviews*, 1994; **7**: 357–417.

3 Hughes, M.S., Ball, N.W., Beck, L.A, de Lisle, G.W., Skuce, R.A., Neill, S.D. Determination of the etiology of presumptive feline leprosy by 16S rRNA gene analysis. *Journal of Clinical Microbiology*, 1997; **35**: 2464–2471.

4 Appleyard, G., Clark, E.G. Histologic and genotypic characterization of a novel *Mycobacterium* species found in three cats. *Journal of Clinical Microbiology*, 2002; **40**: 2425–2430.

5 Patel, A. Pyogranulomatous skin disease and cellulitis in a cat caused by *Rhodococcus equi. Journal of Small Animal Practice*, 2002; **43**: 129–132.

6 Reinke, S.I., Ihrke, P.J., Reinke, J.D., *et al.* Actinomycotic mycetoma in a cat. *Journal of the American Veterinary Medical Association*, 1986; **189**: 446–448.

7 Severo, L.C., Petrillo, V.F., Coutinho, L.M. Actinomycetoma caused by *Rhodococcus spp. Mycopathologia*, 1987; **98**: 129–131.

8 Last, R.D., Appleyard, G.D. Canine leproid granuloma: a South African perspective (abstract). *Proceedings of the 18th Annual Congress of the European Society of Veterinary Dermatology/European College of Veterinary Dermatology*, Nice, France, 2002: 242.

9 Weinstock, D.M., Brown, A.E. *Rhodococcus equi*: an emerging pathogen. *Clinical Infectious Diseases*, 2002; **34**: 1379–1385.

10 Foley, J.A., Gross, T.L., Drazenovich, N., Ramiro-Ibanez, F., Anacleto, E. Clinical, pathological and molecular characterization of feline leprosy syndrome in the western USA. In: Hillier, A., Foster, A.P., Kwochka, K.W., eds. *Advances in Veterinary Dermatology*, Vol. 4. Blackwell Publishing, Oxford, 2005: 238–246.

11 Santos-Juanes, J., Galache, C., Martinez-Cordero, A., *et al.* Cutaneous granulomas caused by *Corynebacterium minutissimum* in an HIV-infected man. *Journal of the European Academy of Dermatology and Venereology*, 2002; **16**: 643–645.

12 Hughes, M.S., Skuce, R.A., Beck, L.A., Neill, S.D. Identification of Mycobacteria from animals by restriction enzyme analysis

and direct DNA cycle sequencing of polymerase chain reaction-amplified 16S rRNA gene sequences. *Journal of Clinical Microbiology*, 1993; **31**: 3216–3222.

13 Kirschner, P., Springer, B., Vogel, U., *et al*. Genotypic identification of Mycobacteria by nucleic acid sequence determination: a report of a 2-year experience in a clinical laboratory. *Journal of Clinical Microbiology*, 1993; **31**: 2882–2889.

14 Noordhoek, G.T., van Embden, J.D.A., Kolk, A.H.J. Reliability of nucleic acid amplification for detection of *Mycobacterium tuberculosis*: an international collaborative quality control study among 30 laboratories. *Journal of Clinical Microbiology*, 1996; **34**: 2522–2525.

15 Fredericks, D.N., Relman, D.A. Sequence-based identification of microbial pathogens: a reconsideration of Koch's postulates. *Clinical Microbiological Reviews*, 1996; **9**: 18–33.

16 Sela, S., Clark-Curtis, J.E., Bercovier, H. Characterization and taxonomic implications of the rRNA genes of *Mycobacterium leprae*. *Journal of Bacteriology*, 1989; **171**: 70–73.

17 Laurent, F.J., Provost, F., Boiron, P. Rapid identification of clinically relevant *Nocardia* species to genus level by 16S rRNA gene PCR. *Journal of Clinical Microbiology*, 1999; **37**: 99–102.

18 Corless, C.E., Guiver, M., Borrow, R., Edward-Jones, V., Kacmarski, E.B., Fox, A.J. Contamination and sensitivity issues with a real-time universal 16S rRNA PCR. *Journal of Clinical Microbiology*, 2000; **38**: 1747–1752.

19 Mabilat, C., Desvarenne, S., Panteix, G., *et al*. Routine identification of *Mycobacterium tuberculosis* complex isolates by automated hybridization. *Journal of Clinical Microbiology*, 1994; **32**: 2702–2705.

20 Meier, A., Persing, D.H., Finken, M., Bottger, E.C. Elimination of contaminating DNA within polymerase chain reaction agents: implications for a general approach to detection of uncultured pathogens. *Journal of Clinical Microbiology*, 1993; **31**: 646–652.

21 Maiwald, M., Ditton, H.J., Sonntag, H.G., von Knebel Doeberitz, M. Characterization of contaminating DNA in Taq polymerase which occurs during amplification with a primer set for Legionella 5S rRNA. *Molecular Cell Probe*, 1994; **8**: 11–14.

22 Luna, L.G. *Manual of Histologic Staining Methods of the AFIP*, 3rd edn. *American Registry of Pathology*. McGraw-Hill, Columbus, OH, 1968.

23 Bonenberger, T.E., Ihrke, P.J., Naydan, D.K., Affolter, V.K. Rapid identification of tissue micro-organisms in skin biopsy specimens from domestic animals using polyclonal BCG antibody. *Veterinary Dermatology*, 2001; **12**: 41–47.

24 Hughes, M.S., James, G., Ball, N., *et al*. Identification by 16S rRNA gene analyses of a potential novel mycobacterial species as an etiological agent of canine leproid granuloma syndrome. *Journal of Clinical Microbiology*, 2000; **38**: 953–959.

25 Von Below, H., Wilk, C.M., Schaal, K.P., Naumann, G.O. *Rhodococcus luteus* and *Rhodococcus erythropolis* chronic endophthalmitis after lens implantation. *American Journal of Ophthalmology*, 1991; **15**: 596–597.

26 Ochi, K. Phylogenetic analysis of mycolic-acid containing wall-chemotype IV actinomycetes and allied taxa by partial sequencing of ribosomal protein AT-L30. *International Journal of Systemic Bacteriology*, 1995; **45**: 653–660.

27 Tsukamura, M., Hikosaka, K., Nishimura, K., Hara, S. Severe progressive abscesses and necrotizing tenosynovitis caused by *Rhodococcus auranticus*. *Journal of Clinical Microbiology*, 1988; **26**: 201–205.

28 Osoagbaka, O.U. Evidence for the pathogenic role of *Rhodococcus* spp. in pulmonary diseases. *Journal of Applied Bacteriology*, 1989; **66**: 497–506.

29 DeMarais, P.L., Kocka, F.E. Rhodococcus meningitis in an immunocompetent host. *Clinical Infectious Diseases*, 1995; **20**: 167–169.

30 Hondalus, M.K. Pathogenesis and virulence of *Rhodococcus equi*. *Veterinary Microbiology*, 1997; **56**: 257–268.

31 Broughton, R.A., Wilson, H.D., Goodman, N.L., Hedrick, J.A. Septic arthritis and osteomyelitis caused by an organism of the genus *Rhodococcus*. *Journal of Clinical Microbiology*, 1981; **13**: 209–213.

32 Prinz, G., Ban, E., Fekete, S., Szabo, Z. Meningitis caused by *Gordona aurantica* (*Rhodococcus auranticus*). *Journal of Clinical Microbiology*, 1985; **22**: 472–474.

33 Broadway, D., Duguid, G., Matheson, M., Garner, A., Dart, J. Rhodococcus keratitis. *British Journal of Ophthalmology*, 1998; **82**: 198–199.

34 Poelarends, G.J., Zandstra, M., Bosma, T., *et al*. Haloalkane-utilizing *Rhodococcus* strains isolated from geographically distinct locations possess a highly conserved gene cluster encoding haloalkane metabolism. *Journal of Bacteriology*, 2000; **182**: 2725–2731.

35 Begona Prieto, M., Hidalgo, A., Serra, J.L., Llama, M.J. Degradation of phenol by *Rhodococcus erythropolis* UPV-1 immobilized on Biolite in a packed-bed reactor. *Journal of Biotechnology*, 2002; **97**: 1–11.

36 Castorena, G., Suarez, C., Valdez, I, Amador, G. Fernandez, L., Le Borgne, S. Sulfur-selective desulfurization of dibenzothiopene and diesel oil by newly isolated *Rhodococcus sp.* strains. *FEMS Microbiology Letters*, 2002; **24**: 157–161.

37 Brandao, P.F., Clapp, J.P., Bull, A.T. Discrimination and taxonomy of geographically diverse strains of nitrile-metabolizing actinomycetes using chemometric and molecular sequencing techniques. *Environmental Microbiology*, 2002; **4**: 262–276.

38 Gray, M.W., Sankoff, D., Cedergren, R.J. On the evolutionary descent of organisms and organelles: a global phylogeny based on a highly conserved structural core in small subunit ribosomal RNA. *Nucleic Acids Research*, 1984; **12**: 5837–5852.

39 Marchesi, J.R., Sato, T., Weightman, A.J., *et al*. Design and evaluation of useful bacterium-specific PCR primers that amplify genes coding for bacterial 16S rRNA. *Applied and Environmental Microbiology*, 1998; **64**: 795–799.

40 Boddinghaus, B., Rogall, T., Flohr, T., Blocker, H., Bottger, E.C. Detection and identification of Mycobacteria by amplification of rRNA. *Journal of Clinical Microbiology*, 1990; **28**: 1751–1759.

41 Ninet, B., Monod, M., Emler, S., *et al*. Two different 16S rRNA genes in a mycobacterial strain. *Journal of Clinical Microbiology*, 1996; **34**: 2531–2536.

42 Hughes, M.S., Beck, L.A., Skuce, R.A. Identification and elimination of DNA sequences in Taq DNA polymerase. *Journal of Clinical Microbiology*, 1994; **32**: 2007–2008.

43 Wang, G.C.Y., Wang, Y. Frequency of formation of chimeric molecules as a consequence of PCR coamplification of 16S rRNA genes from mixed bacterial genomes. *Applied and Environmental Microbiology*, 1997; **63**: 4645–4650.

44 Lachnik, J., Ackermann, B., Bhorssen, A., *et al*. Rapid cycle PCR and fluorimetry for detection of mycobacteria. *Journal of Clinical Microbiology*, 2002; **40**: 3364–3373.

45 Relman, D.A., Schmidt, T.M., MacDermott, R.P., Falkow, S. Identification of the uncultured bacillus of Whipple's disease. *New England Journal of Medicine*, 1992; **327**: 293–301.

46 Relman, D.A., Loutit, J.S., Schmidt, T.M., Falkow, S., Tompkins, L.S. The agent of bacillary angiomatosis. An approach to the identification of uncultured pathogens. *New England Journal of Medicine*, 1990; **323**: 1573–1580.

In vivo mRNA expression analysis of *Microsporum canis* secreted subtilisin-like serine proteases in feline dermatophytosis

B.R. Mignon Dr vet med, PhD[1], S.M. Vermout Dr vet med[1], F.D. Brouta Dr vet med, PhD[1], A.F. Nikkels MD, PhD[2], B.J. Losson Dr vet med, PhD[1], F.F. Descamps Dr vet med, PhD[1]

[1] Faculty of Veterinary Medicine, Department of Infectious and Parasitic Diseases, Parasitology and Parasitic Diseases, University of Liège, Liège, Belgium
[2] Faculty of Medicine, Department of Dermatopathology, University of Liège, Liège, Belgium

Summary

Microsporum canis is the main dermatophytic agent in domestic carnivores and the most common zoophilic dermatophyte in man. An *M. canis*-gene family encoding three subtilisin-like serine proteases (SUB1, SUB2 and SUB3) was recently isolated, supporting the potential role of these enzymes in fungal virulence and the host–fungus relationship. In this study, the *in vivo* expression of SUBs was assessed and compared in feline and human *M. canis* dermatophytosis. RT-nested PCRs using specific primers were performed on total RNA extracted from infected hair or scales from naturally infected cats ($n = 4$) and humans (2). The three SUBs were shown to be transcribed in two cats, while mRNAs encoding two SUBs were detected in the other two cats. This strongly suggests that the corresponding proteases are expressed during the invasion of keratinised structures in these animals. Only *SUB1* gene was found to be transcribed in humans. Together, these results provide additional evidence that *M. canis* SUBs could be involved in the cat–fungus relationship as virulence factors, whereas SUB1 could play a significant role in human *M. canis* dermatophytosis.

Introduction

Microsporum canis is the main agent of dermatophytosis in dogs and cats and is also responsible for a frequent zoonosis, whose prevalence is on the rise in many European countries.[1,2] Human infections occur mainly by direct contact with infected cats.[3] This species is considered as the natural host and reservoir for *M. canis*.[1]

Putative attributes which could contribute to *M. canis* virulence include secretion of keratinolytic proteinases.[4–6] These keratinases could provide the fungus with nutrients, by degrading keratin into easily assimilated metabolites, and allow the invasion of keratinised structures.[7,8] Recently, an *M. canis* 31.5-kDa keratinolytic subtilisin-like serine protease (SUB) was isolated and shown to be the major protein secreted by the fungus grown in a minimal medium enriched with cat keratin.[4] The gene encoding this keratinase, called *SUB3*, was isolated, as well

as two other closely related genes, called *SUB1* and *SUB2*.[9] The existence of an *M. canis*-gene family encoding three SUBs could suggest the potentially important role of these enzymes in fungal metabolism and pathogenicity. Indeed, the production of several proteases encoded by a gene family is thought to be related to virulence, as has been shown for aspartic proteases (SAPs) of *Candida albicans* and *Candida tropicalis*.[10] However, the demonstration of the *in vivo* expression of specific microbial proteins constitutes a requisite step towards the demonstration of their implication in pathogenicity.[9,11] In this context, the transcription of all *SUB* genes was demonstrated in hair of experimentally infected guinea pigs.[9] Using the same model, we also demonstrated the immunogenicity of SUB3.[12] However, we recently showed that SUB3, produced as a recombinant protease and used as a subunit vaccine, failed to protect against an experimental *M. canis* infection in guinea pigs.[13]

As a prelude to further investigation of the role of the three SUBs in *M. canis* infection in natural hosts and to their potential use as vaccines in cats, this study was designed to establish their presence in *in vivo* clinical conditions in cats and humans.

Materials and methods

Animals and patients

This study involved four pet cats, and two humans, including one child and one veterinary student, all unrelated (Table 5.4.1). The student was referred, the animals were presented to the Department of Infectious and Parasitic Diseases (Faculty of Veterinary Medicine, University of Liège) with a suspicion of *M. canis* dermatophytosis, and the child was seen by a private dermatologist. All the animals were Wood's light examination-positive. Direct microscopic examination of hair and/or scales from both animals and human patients revealed the presence of fungal arthroconidia and hyphae. Furthermore, *M. canis* was isolated from lesional areas in all cats and humans. None of the cats or humans was treated at the time of the sampling.

Sampling

To study the *in vivo* expression of *M. canis* SUBs, two samples were collected from each case. The first consisted of either Wood's light examination-positive hair (for animals), abnormal broken hair (for the child), or scales (for the veterinary student) taken from a lesional area. The second (control sample) was either Wood's light examination-negative hair, intact hair or scales, respectively, taken from a non-lesional area of the same animal or patient. The samples were placed into sterile 1.5-ml microcentrifuge tubes and immediately frozen in liquid nitrogen. They were stored until use at –80°C to preserve the integrity of RNA until subsequent analysis. The whole study was performed in Belgium within an 8-month period during the years 2002 and 2003.

RNA isolation

For each sample, 10–20 hair fragments or scales were ground under liquid nitrogen using a mortar and pestle, and total RNAs were then extracted using the filamentous fungi protocol of an RNA extraction kit (RNeasy total RNA purification kit, Qiagen). Finally, RNAs were harvested in 60 μl of RNAse-free water. To avoid DNA contaminations, RNAs were treated with RNAse-free DNAse according to the manufacturer's instructions (Promega).

Primer selection

Two specific primer pairs were designed for the amplification by RT-nested PCR of internal fragments of *SUB1*, *SUB2* and *SUB3* mRNAs, on the basis of their nucleotide sequences. These have been described elsewhere.[9] Primer sets for *SUB2*- and *SUB3*-flanked genomic sequences containing introns, while the primer set for *SUB1* did not.

Two specific primer pairs were also designed for the amplification of an internal fragment of *M. canis*

Case no.	Species	Breed or ethnicity	Sex	Age (years)	Infection pattern
I	Cat	Persian	M	2	Weakly inflammatory extensive multifocal chronic dermatophytosis
II	Cat	European	M	1	Alopecic extensive multifocal acute dermatophytosis
III	Cat	European	M	0.5	Alopecic multifocal acute dermatophytosis
IV	Cat	European	ND	1	Alopecic localised acute dermatophytosis
V	Human	Caucasian	M	5	*Tinea capitis* (a single, 3-cm diameter, alopecic, well-demarcated, erythemato-squamous plaque on the scalp)
VI	Human	Caucasian	F	22	*Tinea corporis* (a single, 2-cm diameter, erythematous scaly lesion on arm)

Table 5.4.1 *Microsporum canis*-infected animals and patients used for the *in vivo* analysis of SUB expression

M, male; F, female; ND, not determined.

actin mRNA, which was used as a positive control for *M. canis* RNA extraction and RT-nested PCR. The RT-PCR primers were respectively 5'-CGAACCGT-GAGAAGATGACC-3' and 5'-GAACCACCGATCCA-GACGGAGTA-3', as previously described.[14] Nested PCR primers were designed on the basis of the *M. canis actin* nucleotide sequence and flanked a 67-bp intron.[14] They were 5'-TCCCAGAGCTCCACCCTC-3' and 5'-CGACGATGGGGCGAGAGC-3'.

Reverse transcriptase-polymerase chain reaction (RT-PCR)

RT-PCRs were performed in a PTC 200 thermal cycler (Biozym, Landgraaf, The Netherlands) using a one-step RT-PCR kit (Qiagen). Briefly, 4 µl of each total RNA isolate, 1 µl of both primers specific for *actin*, *SUB1*, *SUB2* and *SUB3* respectively at a 42 µM concentration each, 2 µl of dNTPs at 10 mM each, and 2 µl of one-step RT-PCR enzyme mix were dissolved in a final volume of 50 µl RT-PCR buffer (12.5 mM $MgCl_2$, pH 8.7). The reaction mixtures were incubated at 50°C for 30 min, at 95°C for 15 min, and then subjected to 47 cycles of 1 min at 94°C, 90 s at 55°C and 2 min at 72°C. RT-PCRs were completed by a final elongation step at 72°C for 10 min. Due to the absence of any intron in the *SUB1* nucleotide sequence flanked by *SUB1* RT-PCR primers, an additional control reaction was performed to confirm the amplification of *SUB1* mRNA rather than *SUB1* contaminating genomic DNA. This control was performed by omitting the RT step in a parallel reaction.

Nested PCR

The amplified products from the first RT-PCR step were used as templates in a nested PCR with internal primers specific for *M. canis actin*, *SUB1*, *SUB2* and *SUB3*, respectively. Nested PCRs were performed using the PCR Core System kit (Promega). Five µl of the RT-PCR products, 2 µl of deoxynucleotide mix (containing 10 mM of each dNTP), 1 µl of each sense and antisense oligonucleotide at a concentration of 42 µM, and 2 U of Taq DNA polymerase (Promega) were dissolved in a final volume of 50 µl of PCR buffer (100 mM Tris-HCl, pH 9.0, 500 mM KCl, 15 mM $MgCl_2$, 1% Triton X-100). The reaction mixtures were incubated for 5 min at 94°C, subjected to 30 cycles of 1 min at 94°C, 1 min at 56°C and 1 min at 72°C,

and finally incubated for 10 min at 72°C. The RT-nested PCR products were electrophoresed through 0.8% agarose gel stained with ethidium bromide. The mRNA fragment expected lengths were respectively 282, 388, 1010 and 480 bp for *actin*, *SUB1*, *SUB2* and *SUB3*, while theoretical lengths of *actin*, *SUB1*, *SUB2* and *SUB3* DNA fragments were 349, 388, 1245 and 629 bp, respectively. Reactions were definitively considered as negative when three amplifications failed to give a detectable signal on agarose gel.

Fungal culture, DNA isolation and PCR

Fungal strains from which one or more *SUB* mRNA(s) could not be detected from infected samples were checked by PCR for the presence of the correspondent *SUB* gene(s) in their genomes. For this purpose, these strains were grown for 10 days in liquid Sabouraud medium at 27°C under agitation (150 rpm). Mycelia were harvested on Whatman no. 1 filter paper and rinsed thoroughly with distilled water. Genomic DNAs were then extracted according to the protocol of Girardin and Latgé.[15] Two hundred nanograms of DNA were used as the template for the PCR reactions whose conditions were otherwise identical to those described for nested PCR.

Results

RT-nested PCRs

M. canis actin mRNA was detected in all samples taken from lesional areas (Fig. 5.4.1), indicating that both *M. canis* RNA extraction and RT-nested PCR conditions were successful. The three *SUB* mRNAs were detected in two of four cats (nos I and II). Two *SUB* mRNAs, *SUB1* and *SUB3*, and *SUB1* and *SUB2*, were detected in the two other cats (cat no. III and cat no. IV, respectively). Only *SUB1* mRNA could be detected in samples from both human patients. For *SUB1* reactions, RT-PCR performed in the absence of the RT step did not show any signal after the amplification procedure (data not shown), confirming the amplification of specific *M. canis SUB1* mRNA rather than contaminating genomic DNA. No signal was detected under the same conditions in any of the control samples taken from clinically healthy skin areas (Fig. 5.4.1). Finally, all *SUB* genes for which *in vivo* transcription was not detected were demonstrated to be present in the genomes of the corresponding strains (data not shown).

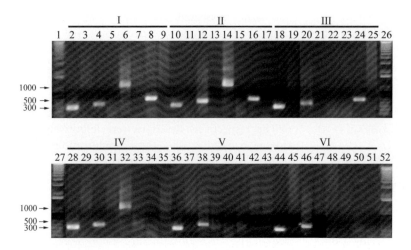

Fig. 5.4.1 Assessment of the *in vivo* production of *M. canis* SUBs. The agarose gel shown results from an assemblage of four different gels performed under the same technical and temporal conditions. Lanes 1, 26, 27 and 52: molecular weight marker (1-kb ladder, Invitrogen). Even lanes: RT-nested PCR products obtained from *M. canis*-infected hair or scales from naturally infected cats and humans, corresponding to internal cDNA fragments of *M. canis actin*, *SUB1*, *SUB2* and *SUB3*, respectively. Odd lanes: RT-nested PCR products obtained from non-infected hair or scales from the same animals or patients. *Actin*, *SUB1*, *SUB2* and *SUB3* internal cDNA fragments were 282, 388, 1010 and 480 bp, respectively. I–VI: case numbers as assigned in Table 5.4.1.

Discussion

Our results demonstrate that in the cat, the natural host for *M. canis*, all *SUB* genes can be transcribed *in vivo*. They suggest strongly that the corresponding encoded proteases are expressed by the fungus during invasion of feline keratinised structures and are involved in the cat–fungus relationship. This is strengthened by the previous *in vivo* immunohistochemical detection of a 31.5-kDa SUB from *M. canis* in naturally infected cats.[16] Indeed, in contrast to RT-PCR, which allows the detection of mRNA, immunohistochemistry is the suitable method for protein detection. However, it was not used in this study, essentially because the quite high homology between SUBs makes it difficult to produce specific non-cross-reactive antibodies.[9] In contrast, the design of highly specific primer pairs is easily performed. Moreover, the production of antibodies directed to specific antigens requires that the targeted antigens are available, which is still not the case for both SUB1 and SUB2. Finally, RT-nested PCR does not suffer from low sensitivity of *in vivo* detection of gene products as happens with classical RT-PCR.[14,17]

Surprisingly, mRNA encoding SUB3 was not detected in one feline sample nor in any of the human samples. Nevertheless, it is the major secreted protein of *M. canis* cultivated *in vitro* in the presence of cat keratin. Furthermore, its keratinolytic activity was demonstrated, suggesting its importance for such a keratinophilic and keratinolytic fungus.[4] Only *SUB1* gene was found to be transcribed in the two human samples. This result should be confirmed using a larger sample size.

The absence of any signal detection for a specific *SUB* mRNA could theoretically reflect two different situations. The first explanation could be a lack of sensitivity of the method. This seems very unlikely because RT-nested PCR appears to be an extremely sensitive method, and experiments were repeated three times. Moreover, *M. canis actin* mRNA, which was shown to be an indicator of fungal viability, was detected in all samples taken from lesional areas, while at least one *SUB* mRNA was detected in all the samples.[14] The second, and most probable, explanation could be a true absence of transcription. This could be related to fungal strain variation. Additionally, the production of peculiar SUBs, or their absence, could be related to fungal adaptation to its host. Indeed, at least two SUBs were shown to be transcribed in the four feline samples. Similarly, in a previous study, Mignon *et al.* detected SUB3 in 10 of 11 naturally infected cats.[16] The *SUB* transcription could also be regulated according to the type of cutaneous structure (hair, stratum corneum) the fungus invades, as shown for *C. albicans* secreted aspartic proteases (SAPs). This pathogenic yeast expresses different SAPs, which are known virulence factors, depending on the type of infection (mucosal or systemic) it causes.[10] However, the fact that *M. canis* SUB1 was detected in both humans, presenting with *Tinea capitis* and *Tinea corporis*, respectively, does not support this theory. Besides a fungal strain variation or a specific adaptation to the host or to the cutaneous structures, the differential expression of proteases, including the *M. canis* SUBs, could be related to the kinetics of infection. Arthroconidia, the most infective fungal form, first adhere to corneocytes and then germinate into hyphae.[18] The latter invade the keratinised areas, such as stratum corneum, hair follicle outer and inner root sheaths, and hair shafts, where they produce ectothrix arthroconidia, completing the fungal life cycle.[19] The infection process and the concurrent modifications of the fungal morphological states could probably affect the protease expression pattern. For example, SUB3 expression seems to be produced by mycelia rather than arthroconidia.[4]

Although these data were obtained from a rather small number of animals and human patients, they are the first dealing with the molecular pathogenesis of dermatophytosis during natural infection. Indeed, they unambiguously demonstrate that mRNA encoding some SUBs are expressed in *in vivo* conditions, strongly suggesting that the corresponding proteases are produced by the fungus during skin invasion. In turn, SUB1 and the three SUBs could play a significant role in human and feline *M. canis* dermatophytosis, respectively. This strengthens the hypothesis that these proteases could be virulence factors involved in cat–fungus relationship. Consequently, additional experiments would be necessary to identify the exact *in vivo* functions of the SUB family. These include the simple role of digesting molecules for nutrient acquisition, the contribution to host tissue adherence and invasion, and the potential role in immunomodulation. Such studies present both fundamental and applied interests. In particular, they could lead to the development of new antifungal strategies, for example, the use of specific SUB inhibitors. In the near future, a similar approach will probably allow the development of new drugs for the treatment of candidiasis, based on protease inhibition. Indeed, it was shown that protection against experimental *C. albicans* infection could be achieved with Pepstatin A, an inhibitor of SAPs.[20,21] Further studies on SUBs could also lead to the development of subunit vaccines against *M. canis* feline dermatophytosis, which remains difficult to eradicate, especially in catteries where the infection can become endemic.[22]

Funding

This work was supported by grant no. 3.4534.01 from Fonds de la Recherche Scientifique Médicale (FRSM). Sandy Vermout is recipient of a studentship of FRIA (Fonds pour la Formation à la Recherche dans l'Industrie et dans l'Agriculture, rue d'Egmont 5, 1000 Bruxelles).

References

1 Scott, D.W., Miller, W.H., Griffin, C.E. Fungal skin diseases. In: *Muller and Kirk's Small Animal Dermatology*, 6th edn. W.B. Saunders, Philadelphia, 2001: 339–361.
2 Lunder, M., Lunder, M. Is *Microsporum canis* infection about to become a serious dermatological problem? *Dermatology*, 1992; **184**: 87–89.
3 De Vroey, C. Epidemiology of ringworm (dermatophytosis). *Seminars in Dermatology*, 1985; **4**: 185–200.
4 Mignon, B., Swinnen, M., Bouchara, J.P., *et al.* Purification and characterization of a 31.5 kDa keratinolytic subtilisin-like serine protease from *Microsporum canis* and evidence of its secretion in naturally infected cats. *Medical Mycology*, 1998; **36**: 395–404.
5 Brouta, F., Descamps, F., Fett, T., Losson, B., Gerday, C., Mignon, B. Purification and characterization of a 43.5 kDa keratinolytic metalloprotease from *Microsporum canis*. *Medical Mycology*, 2001; **39**: 269–275.
6 Brouta, F., Descamps, F., Vermout, S., Monod, M., Losson, B., Mignon, B. Secreted metalloproteases of *Microsporum canis*. *Infection and Immunity*, 2002; **70**: 5676–5683.
7 Apodaca, G., McKerrow, J.H. Regulation of *Trichophyton rubrum* proteolytic activity. *Infection and Immunity*, 1989; **57**: 3081–3090.
8 Apodaca, G., McKerrow, J.H. Purification and characterization of a 27,000-Mr extracellular proteinase from *Trichophyton rubrum*. *Infection and Immunity*, 1989; **57**: 3072–3080.
9 Descamps, F., Brouta, F., Monod, M., *et al.* Isolation of a *Microsporum canis* gene family encoding three subtilisin-like proteases expressed *in vivo*. *Journal of Investigative Dermatology*, 2002; **119**: 830–835.
10 Hube, B., Naglik, J. *Candida albicans* proteinases: resolving the mystery of a gene family. *Microbiology*, 2001; **147**: 1997–2005.
11 Monod, M., Fatih, A., Jaton-Ogay, K., Paris, S., Latgé, J.P. The secreted proteases of pathogenic species of *Aspergillus* and their possible role in virulence. *Canadian Journal of Botany*, 1995; **73** (Suppl. 1): 1081–1086.
12 Descamps, F., Brouta, F., Vermout, S., Monod, M., Losson, B., Mignon, B. Recombinant expression and antigenic properties of a 31.5-kDa keratinolytic subtilisin-like serine protease from *Microsporum canis*. *FEMS Immunology and Medical Microbiology*, 2003; **38**: 29–34.
13 Descamps, F., Brouta, F., Vermout, S., Willame, C., Losson, B., Mignon, B. A recombinant 31.5 kDa keratinase and a crude exoantigen from *Microsporum canis* fail to protect against a homologous experimental infection in guinea pigs. *Veterinary Dermatology*, 2003; **14**: 305–312.
14 Okeke, C.N., Tsuboi, R., Kawai, M., Hiruma, M., Ogawa, H. Isolation of an intron-containing partial sequence of the gene encoding dermatophyte actin (ACT) and detection of a fragment of the transcript by reverse transcription-nested PCR as a means of assessing the viability of dermatophytes in skin scales. *Journal of Clinical Microbiology*, 2001; **39**: 101–106.
15 Girardin, H., Latgé J.P. DNA extraction and quantitation. In: Maresca, B., Kobayashi, G.S., eds. *Molecular Biology of Pathogenic Fungi: A Laboratory Manual*. Telos Press, New York, 1994: 5–9.
16 Mignon, B., Nikkels, A., Piérard, G., Losson, B. The *in vitro* and *in vivo* production of a 31.5 kDa keratinolytic subtilase from *Microsporum canis* and the clinical status in naturally infected cats. *Dermatology*, 1998; **196**: 438–441.

17 Naglik, J.R., Newport, G., White, T.C., *et al. In vivo* analysis of secreted aspartyl proteinase expression in human oral candidiasis. *Infection and Immunity*, 1999; **68**: 2482–2490.

18 Zurita, J., Hay, R.J. Adherence of dermatophyte microconidia and arthroconidia to human keratinocytes *in vitro. Journal of Investigative Dermatology*, 1987; **89**: 529–534.

19 Rashid, A., Hodgins, M.B., Richardson, M.D. An *in vitro* model of dermatophyte invasion of the human hair follicle. *Journal of Medical and Veterinary Mycology*, 1996; **34**: 37–42.

20 De Bernardis, F., Boccanera, M., Adriani, D., Spreghini, E., Santoni, G., Cassone, A. Protective role of antimannan and anti-aspartyl proteinase antibodies in an experimental model of *Candida albicans* vaginitis in rats. *Infection and Immunity*, 1997; **65**: 3399–3405.

21 Fallon, K., Bausch, K., Noonan, J., Huguenel, E., Tamburini, P. Role of aspartic proteases in disseminated *Candida albicans* infection in mice. *Infection and Immunity*, 1997; **65**: 551–556.

22 Moriello, K.A. Management of dermatophyte infections in catteries and multiple-cat households. *Veterinary Clinics of North America: Small Animal Practice*, 1990; **20**: 1457–1474.

Real-time PCR for monitoring cutaneous asymptomatic carriage of *Leishmania* spp. in laboratory mice

G. Marignac Dr med vet[1], G. Fall[2], E. Prina PhD[2], M. Lebastard[2], G. Milon Dr med vet, PhD[2], L. Nicolas PhD[2]

[1] Unité de Parasitologie, École Nationale Vétérinaire d'Alfort, Maisons-Alfort, France
[2] Unité d'Immunophysiologie et Parasitisme Intracellulaire, Institut Pasteur, Paris, France

Summary

It is now known that, in most hosts, *Leishmania* parasitism may remain asymptomatic, which is a serious threat in the context of public and individual health.

Recently, we have developed a real-time PCR assay to quantify the parasitic burden of several *Leishmania* species, based on quantitation of kinetoplastic DNA (kDNA). To determine whether the detected kDNA does assess the presence of live parasites, we have developed an *in vitro* model to monitor the persistence of *Leishmania amazonensis* kDNA in cultured mouse macrophages, after the host leucocytes have been exposed to L-leucine-methyl ester, a leishmanicidal molecule. The detection of kDNA by real-time PCR was correlated with the viability of the parasites in macrophages.

With real-time PCR, we monitored the fate of *Leishmania major* in C57Bl/6 mice following intradermal inoculation of infective metacyclics at low dose (24 hours, 96 hours and weekly for 7 weeks, right ear pinna). We confirmed that *Leishmania* organisms become established in the centre of the inoculated pinna, to a lesser extent at the pinnal border, and in the draining lymph node. We could detect but not quantify the parasite in distant cutaneous sites (left ear pinna, thoracic skin, tail base) and in the femoral bone marrow in some animals. The parasite was detected throughout the experiment in the glabrous skin of the tail base.

The results show that the model could be used for investigating asymptomatic carriage of *Leishmania*. Potential applications of this model are numerous, including evaluation of the efficacy of *Leishmania*-targeting drugs or vaccines in a broader context than merely monitoring of the reduction of the lesions or the prevention of disease.

Introduction

Leishmania spp. cause a large spectrum of diseases in humans and dogs throughout tropical and subtropical areas. Leishmaniases are considered by the World Health Organisation as priority parasitic diseases for research, and development of control tools.[1] Sandflies act as intermediate hosts. Recently, the importance of animal reservoirs, such as dogs and rodents, has been emphasised. Leishmaniasis prevention is complicated by the fact that in mammals the absence of clinical signs does not imply the absence of parasites. In fact, parasites establish dynamic relationships with their host that allow their persistence, often in an asymptomatic manner. Ignorance of this fact has led to serology-based dog culling campaigns that have invariably failed to control visceral leishmaniasis.[2] The detection of asymptomatic dog carriers has many applications. It is an important issue in quarantine facilities in *Leishmania*-free countries.

Asymptomatic carriage also has major implications in epidemiology, pharmacology and in fundamental research, particularly regarding parasite–host interactions and transmission of *Leishmania* spp. Sandfly haematophagia, termed telmophagia, relies on the formation of an intradermal blood lake. One of the authors (G. Milon) formulated the hypothesis that only non-lesional sites would be favourable for the blood meal.[3,4] This would imply that the parasites would also be present in non-lesional skin.

Over several years, a model of infection has been developed in our laboratory that mimics telmophagia closely: low-dose inoculum in a small volume, strict intradermal injection, and use of the infective form of *L. major* found in the sandfly (i.e. metacyclic promastigotes).[3–5]

In order to validate this model, we needed an accurate and sensitive quantification tool. Parasitic load determination in mammalian tissues or organs is currently performed by limiting dilution assay,[6,7] a sensitive but time-consuming method. In addition, this culture-based method requires samples harbouring cultivable parasites; this is a drawback as samples have to be analysed as soon as they are collected. Semi-quantitative polymerase chain reaction (PCR) has been developed to overcome this problem.[8] More recently, quantitative real-time PCR has been shown to allow fast and accurate detection and quantification of *Leishmania* organisms[9–11] or other parasites.[12] This PCR assay amplifies the DNA present in the kinetoplast. Kinetoplastic DNA (kDNA) is composed of minicircles, DNA macromolecules that contain a high number of copies of the same sequences. This explains, in part, the high sensitivity of kDNA-based PCR as developed in our laboratory.[9,10,13]

The aim of the present study was to assess whether *Leishmania* spp. are present in non-lesional skin sites, and how quickly these sites are invaded. We based our experimental model on the hypothesis that *Leishmania* organisms migrate early from the inoculation site, in low numbers and in an asymptomatic manner. In order to pursue this aim, and after validation of the PCR method in our experimental settings, we sought to determine whether the detected parasite DNA originated from live parasites. This was assessed using an *in vitro* model to monitor the persistence of *Leishmania* DNA in cultured mouse macrophages, once the leukocytes had been exposed to leishmanicidal molecules.[14] Asymptomatic carriage of *L. major* early after intradermal inoculation to mice was then explored.

Materials and methods

L. major *DNA quantification*

The parasitic load in various tissues was quantified by real-time PCR with kDNA as target. Real-time PCR was performed with a LightCycler® (Roche Diagnostics) as previously described[9] using primers which amplify a 120-bp DNA fragment from the minicircles of *Leishmania* kDNA. The relative standard curve method was used to quantify parasite DNA. Roughly, the amount of

amplicon present after each PCR cycle is monitored in real time. Increasing amounts of amplicon are reflected by increasing fluorescence from SYBR-Green, a dye that binds double-stranded DNA. The cutting point (C_T) is the cycle at which the second derivative of the quantification curve cuts the y = 0 curve. C_T is inversely proportional to the log of the starting DNA copy number.

The reproducibility of the PCR assay was assessed by measuring interassay variability obtained both for the internal control DNA reference scale and DNA extracted from infected mouse tissue. For the production of the internal control DNA reference scale, *L. major* and *L. amazonensis* promastigotes were cultured *in vitro*, concentrated in phosphate-buffered saline (PBS) and quantified. DNA was then extracted and an internal control DNA reference scale was obtained by successive 10-fold dilutions.

To assess the efficacy of real-time PCR in our experimental settings, we checked that mouse DNA did not interfere with *Leishmania* kDNA by performing quantification of mouse skin DNA extract spiked (or not) with *Leishmania* DNA (data not shown). In order to assess interassay variability, samples obtained at week 7 in the right ear pinna centre (A), border (B) and in the draining lymph nodes, were assayed twice.

The fusion temperature (Tm) specific to the primer we used is 83°C. The presence of a peak at 86–87°C is the sign of a non-specific amplification. The LightCycler software includes any temperature peak obtained to calculate the the cutting point. Thus, we visualised the fusion temperature curves for each sample to validate computer-generated data. The analysis of these peaks also allowed us to determine the lower parasite DNA concentration for which quantification is satisfactory in order to determine the minimal detection level. This is called 'Tm analysis'.

Confirmation that real-time PCR only assesses the presence of living Leishmania parasites

L. amazonensis strain LV79 (MPRO/BR/72/M1841) was used, as an efficient procedure relying on the rapidly acting leishmanicidal *L*-leucine-methyl ester (Leu-O-Me) was available for this megasome-inducing species, but not for *L. major*.[15] Leu-O-Me, which is not toxic for macrophages, is almost 100% active in killing *L. amazonensis*. Propagation, isolation from footpad lesions and purification of LV79 amastigotes have been described previously.[15] Macrophage precursor cells were obtained from the bone marrow of BALB/c mice and cultured in bacteriologic Petri dishes (Greiner, Germany) at 37°C in a humidified atmosphere (5% CO_2, 95% air). Culture medium was RPMI 1640 supplemented with 10% heat-inactivated fetal calf serum (FCS, Dutscher, France), 20% cell-conditioned medium (L929 supernatant) as a source of macrophage colony-stimulating factor (M-CSF), and antibiotics. Six days later, adherent macrophages were recovered and distributed in 24-well tissue culture plates (Tanner, Switzerland) in the same medium supplemented with 3% of L929 supernatant. Fresh medium (non-mitogenic dose) was also added daily to prevent macrophage apoptosis. Twenty-four hours after replating, infection with amastigotes was established with four parasites per macrophage. Parasite-loaded cells were then incubated at 34°C, which is the permissive temperature for the survival and multiplication of LV79 strain amastigotes.[15]

Twenty-four hours after infection, parasite-harbouring macrophage monolayers were treated with 2 mM of the leishmanicidal amino acid ester Leu-O-Me for 45 minutes. Cultures were then placed at 37°C, a temperature that does not permit multiplication of this *Leishmania* strain, therefore the putative residual parasites which had survived the drug killing would die.[14,16] At 1 hour, 24 hours, 48 hours, 72 hours, day 5 and day 7 following the addition of Leu-O-Me, the macrophages were lysed. Total DNA was extracted using the DNeasy Tissue kit® (Qiagen, Courtabœuf, France) as described above.

At each time point following Leu-O-Me exposure, DNA sampling, cell counts (by counting macrophage nuclei as described previously[15–17]) and assays assessing parasite survival were performed in triplicate. Parasite survival was checked by transferring Leu-O-Me-exposed cultures from 37°C to 26°C, allowing live amastigotes to differentiate into promastigotes and to multiply. The presence of motile promastigotes was then monitored microscopically daily for up to 10 days. Both non-treated wells and infected and treated wells were included as controls.

L. major *intradermal delivery to mice and evaluation of their presence in sites distant from the point of delivery*

L. major Friedlin was cultured at 26°C in Hosmem-II medium[18] supplemented with 10% heat-inactivated FC,

100 U/ml penicillin and 100 µg/ml streptomycin (Seromed, Berlin, Germany), until late-log and stationary growth phase promastigotes were obtained. Metacyclic promastigotes were purified on a Ficoll® (Pharmacia, Guyancourt, France) density gradient as described by Späth and Beverley.[19] Ficoll-isolated parasites appeared morphologically homogeneous and actively motile.

Female C57Bl/6 mice (6–8 weeks old) were injected intradermally in the centre of the ventral surface of the right ear pinna with 10^3 *L. major* metacyclics prepared as indicated above. At 24 hours and 96 hours, then weekly until week 7 post-inoculation, four mice were killed for monitoring the distribution of the parasites in the different tissues under study. The following tissues were sampled: inoculated ear pinna centre (sampled with a 6-mm biopsy punch) (Stiefel, Nanterre, France), marginal area of the inoculated ear pinna, retromaxillar draining lymph node, tail skin, haired skin from thorax (6-mm biopsy punch) and femoral bone marrow. The presence of clinical lesions was also assessed by measuring lesion thickness and the weight of the 6-mm biopsies from the ear pinna centre.

Real-time PCR was performed with a LightCycler® (Roche Diagnostics) as previously described[9] using kDNA as a target. The DNA was extracted with the DNeasy tissue kit (Qiagen) as previously described.[9] The optimal elution volume was 200 µl in our conditions. We checked that mouse DNA did not interfere with the *Leishmania* kDNA quantification by performing real-time PCR with mouse skin DNA extract spiked, or not, with *Leishmania* DNA (data not shown). A quantified DNA extract from *L. major* Friedlin promastigotes was used as a reference standard curve.

Results

Validation of L. major *DNA quantification protocol*

The Tm analysis demonstrated that quantification can be performed for crude PCR results above one parasite detected. In our experimental settings, quantification can be considered accurate when the calculated number of parasites by organ is above the following detection limits: 10 parasites/femoral bone marrow sample, 20 parasites/ear pinna sample and 40 parasites/tail sample. Below these thresholds, Tm analysis results can demonstrate the presence of *Leishmania* DNA, but quantification cannot be performed.

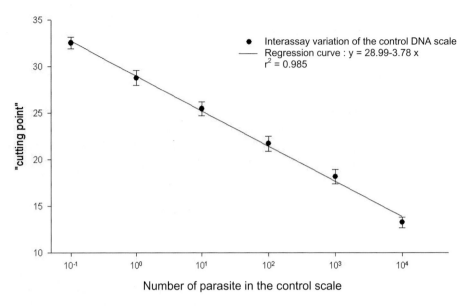

Fig. 5.5.1 Interassay variation of the internal control DNA reference scale (*Leishmania major*). Eight replicates have been used for the 10–1 parasites dilution, and 10 replicates for the other dilutions. Interassay variation of the internal control DNA was between 2% and 4.2%.

Interassay variation of the internal control DNA was between 2% and 4.2% (Fig. 5.5.1). Samples obtained at week 7 in the right ear pinna centre, pinnal border, and in the draining lymph nodes were quantified twice (Table 5.5.1). Tissue interassay variation is higher when the number of parasites quantified is low. Variation is under 7.5% when more than 200 parasites are quantified (crude results), and up to 19% under 200. Some variations were not calculated (mice 2B, 4B, 2C, 3C and 4C) as they were below the quantification threshold.

Evaluation of kDNA as an indicator of the presence of live parasites

In the control wells, the number of infected and treated macrophages remained fairly constant during the experiment (nuclei count).

There was a 100-fold decrease of *Leishmania* kDNA in macrophages exposed to Leu-O-Me, as early as 24 hours post-exposure, while the amount of kDNA in macrophages left unexposed to Leu-O-Me remained stable (Fig. 5.5.2). The decrease of kDNA in drug-exposed macrophages was observed until day 5. In parallel, a replicate of lysates of infected macrophages previously treated with Leu-O-Me was cultured in Hosmem medium to allow the differentiation and multiplication of any live parasites. These later cul-

tures were negative at day 5 and were related to a 4 log decrease of kDNA. At day 7, both PCR and cultures were negative. These results confirm that the presence

Table 5.5.1 interassay variations (*Leishmania major*)

	Mouse 1	Mouse 2	Mouse 3	Mouse 4
Ear centre				
Assay 1	3192.83	871.24	1851.04	82.84
Assay 2	3496.95	938.58	2057.67	108.08
Mean	3345	905	1954	95
Standard deviation	215.05	47.62	146.11	17.85
Percentage	6.4	5.3	7.5	18.7
Pinnal border				
Assay 1	75.48	2.92	201.17	3.46
Assay 2	6169	3.07	159.18	5.68
Mean	69	–	185	–
Standard deviation	9.75	–	22.62	–
Percentage	14.2	–	12.2	–
Lymph node				
Assay 1	316.3	69.64	61.79	143.79
Assay 2	351.11	66.97	45.42	128.92
Mean	334	–	–	–
Standard deviation	24.61	–	–	–
Percentage	7.4	–	–	–

Results obtained at week 7 in the right ear pinna centre, border and in the draining lymph nodes were assayed twice. Results are expressed as parasite/mg of ear tissue and as parasite/lymph node. Some results were below the detection level (mice 2B, 4B, 2C, 3C and 4C).

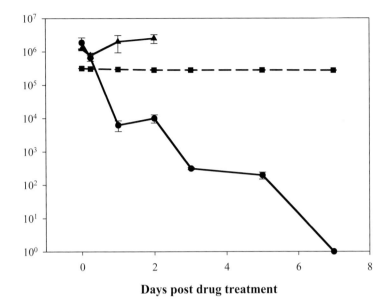

Fig. 5.5.2 Kinetics of *L. amazonensis* kDNA monitored by real-time PCR in mouse-derived M-CSF-dependent macrophages infected with *L. amazonensis* amastigotes and exposed for 45 minutes (closed circles) or not (closed triangles) to Leu-O-Met leishmanicidal ester (2 mM). The macrophage viability after infection and drug exposure was estimated by macrophages nuclei counts (dotted line and square).

Days post drug treatment

of kDNA is positively correlated only with the presence of live parasites.

Evaluation of L. major *presence in different mice tissues following intradermal inoculation of 10^3 metacyclics*

When 10^3 *L. major* Friedlin metacyclic promastigotes were inoculated into the centre of the right ear pinna, the lesions at the site of inoculation were first detectable between week 2 and week 3 in C57 Bl/6 mice and reached around 10^6 per ear at week 4 (Fig. 5.5.3). The thickness of the contralateral left ear, not inoculated, remained constant throughout the experiment and no other clinical signs (skin lesions, emaciation, death, etc.) were observed.

The parasitic loads in the inoculated ear and the draining lymph node, quantified by real-time PCR, are shown in Fig. 5.5.3. The number of parasites in the centre of the ear, after a decrease at day 1 post-inoculation, increased until day 28 (week 4), then remained fairly constant. The number of parasites at the pinnal border of the inoculated ear increased, but reached a plateau approximately 10–100 times below that at the inoculation site (<10^4 parasites per marginal area of the ear) from day 21 to day 42 (week 3 to week 6). An average of 50–100 parasites in the retromaxillary (or submandibular) draining lymph node was detectable

as early as day 1. At day 14, while the inoculated ear remained asymptomatic, parasite counts were high; >10 000 parasites/mg of tissue in the centre and >1000 parasites/mg at the pinnal border.

Detection of parasite kDNA was observed in some mice as soon as day 1 post-inoculation in distant tissues, including the left ear (not inoculated) and the tail skin, and at week 1 in thoracic skin of one animal (Table 5.5.2). At day 4, the tail skin samples from all mice were positive. Most of the femoral bone marrow samples remained negative. These data were qualitative, as the positivity of each sample was determined by the Tm analysis of the fusion curves obtained by real-time PCR.[10]

Discussion

This study was designed to investigate the distribution of *Leishmania* organisms shortly after inoculation and for 6 weeks thereafter in a resistant mouse strain. As far as the inoculated ear centre is concerned, the present results are similar to those found previously with the limiting-dilution assay.[5] We processed the pinnal border and the central part of the ear pinna separately. In the border of inoculated ears (right pinnae), we found 10–100 times fewer parasites, and no peak was observed. This suggests that parasite proliferation or tissue invasion is less important in the skin situated a few

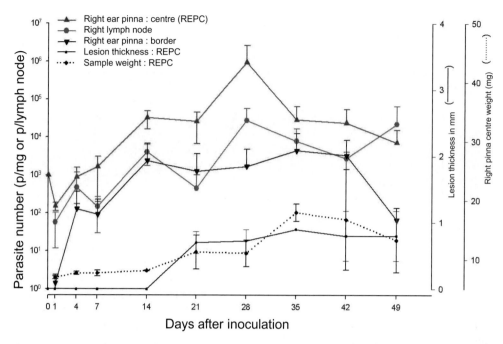

Fig. 5.5.3 Monitoring of the parasitic load in tissues of C57/Bl6 mice after inoculation of 103 *L. major* metacyclic promastigotes (p) into the right ear centre. Parasitic load was estimated by quantitation of *L. major* kDNA using real-time PCR, in the centre (brown triangle) or the pinnal border area (blue inverted triangle) of the inoculated right ear, and in the retromaxillary draining lymph node (green closed circle). Evolution of lesion size of the inoculated ear (dotted line) and evolution of the mean weight of the 6-mm biopsy punch sampled centre of the right ear (dashed line). The data represent mean values ± standard deviation (*n* = 4).

millimetres away from the inoculation site. As reported elsewhere,[5,8] our inoculation protocol aims to mimic a natural infestation (dose, volume, use of infective stage of the parasite) as far as possible. The data obtained here at the inoculation site and the draining lymph node confirm previous studies using similar protocols with either *L. major* in laboratory mice or *L. tropica* in black rats. These are the main site of multiplication of the parasites.[8,13] We have shown that parasites are detectable at the inoculation site, the inoculated pinna border and in the draining lymph node before clinical signs occur.

We have also shown that parasites are detectable early and persistently at various asymptomatic cutaneous sites. It should be noted that the site most consistently positive (from day 4 to week 6 when all samples are positive) is cutaneous and glabrous skin of the tail base. Sandflies feed more easily on glabrous and poorly haired skin due to their small size, feeding habits (telmophagia) and short mouth parts; it is one of our hypotheses that *Leishmania* organisms are probably found in greater number in glabrous skin, an area more favourable for their transmission. Even though our PCR protocol has been proved both previously and in the present study to have a high sensitivity, quantification of such low number of parasite was not possible in the distant sites, but analysis of the fusion

Table 5.5.2 Qualitative detection of *L. major* kinetoplastic DNA by real-time PCR as observed by Tm analysis in C57Bl/6 mice inoculated intradermally in the right ear with 10³ metacyclic promastigotes

Tissue	Time post-inoculation					
	Day 1	Day 4	Week 1	Week 4	Week 5	Week 6
Left ear (centre)	1/4*	1/4	0/4	2/4	0/4	3/4
Left ear (pinna border)	2/4	1/4	1/4	2/4	0/4	2/4
Tail skin	1/3	4/4	4/4	4/4	4/4	4/4
Thoracic skin	0/4	0/4	1/4	1/4	2/4	1/4
Femoral bone marrow	0/4	0/4	0/4	2/4	0/4	1/4

Detection limits by PCR are: 10 parasites/femoral bone marrow, 20 parasites/ear, 40 parasites/piece of tail.
*Number of mice PCR-positive/number of mice analysed.

graphs allowed us to detect the parasite. Enhancing the sensitivity could be achieved by using nested PCR or FRET (fluorescence resonance energy transfer-based PCR). These latter techniques presently have limited application outside the laboratory because of the risk of amplifying contaminated material (nested PCR) and because of cost (FRET mainly) and technological constraints (for both techniques). Thus, enhancing PCR techniques similar to those used in this study should probably be prioritised.

The use of a house-keeping gene would have allowed us to assess the amount of mouse tissue in the sample more accurately and more easily than merely weighing the sample.[11] Because *Leishmania* spp. organisms are eukaryotes, the identification of a suitable house-keeping gene needs to be fully validated.

Validation of the quantification tool

Limiting-dilution assay is a culture-based technique used for the evaluation of *Leishmania* tissue carriage. It is time-consuming and requires samples harbouring parasites that are not only alive, but cultivable. Real-time PCR was used here in order to overcome these drawbacks. We showed that real-time PCR allows detection of low parasite burdens: 10 parasites/femoral bone marrow sample, 20 parasites/ear sample and 40 parasites/tail sample. We also confirmed the findings by Nicolas *et al.*[9,10] that in both our experimental settings, real-time PCR has excellent intra-assay, interassay variations (Table 5.5.1, Fig. 5.5.1). The standard curve designed for quantification of parasites showed linearity over 6 log DNA concentrations (0.1 to 10[4] parasites per reaction) with a correlation coefficient over 0.97 (Fig. 5.5.1). These results show that quantitative real-time PCR is a reliable, accurate and rapid quantification method for *Leishmania* organisms in mouse tissues. The assay performance is likely to be suitable for epidemiological, clinical and pharmacological uses.

The question of whether the kinetoplastic DNA detected by our PCR assay reflects the presence of live parasites was specifically addressed. As RNA is quickly metabolised, reverse transcriptase-PCR (RT-PCR) is used in most models to confirm the viability of the organism or cell to be identified. *Leishmania* spp. minicircle kDNA replication has unusual features, including polycystronic transcription and trans-splicing of pre-mRNA. These early modifications in RNA prevent the use of RT-PCR as a reliable tool to quantify RNA gen-

erated by minicircles. Also, while keeping our highly sensitive tool, we have developed an *in vitro* model to monitor the persistence of *Leishmania* organism DNA in cultured mouse macrophages once they have been exposed to a leishmanicidal agent.

L. amazonensis was used instead of *L. major* in this study. *In vivo*, the effective drugs act slowly and *Leishmania* death takes hours to days to occur. Thus, the accurate assessment of the population of live organisms, dead organisms and undegraded DNA at a given time during the long process of drug action is not possible. On the contrary, using amino acid esters as a leishmanicidal drug in an *in vitro* assay, a 45-minute contact with parasite-harbouring macrophages is sufficient to kill the parasite and the harbouring cell is preserved. In this study we have shown that following leishmanicidal drug treatment, the amount of kDNA from *L. amazonensis* amastigotes rapidly declined and that when kDNA was no longer detected correlated with the time of no surviving amastigotes. The small amount of *Leishmania* kDNA detected at day 5 could reflect the presence of some drug-damaged parasites that had yet to be eliminated but were no longer viable. A further study performed in our laboratory suggested persistence of some parasites not killed by the drug (data not shown). We kept the infected macrophage cultures longer, 1 week after treatment with the drug, and we observed a rise in parasite number. Further studies are necessary to confirm this later finding, but apparently the small signals found at day 5 are very likely assessing the lack of sensitivity of a small number of parasites to the drug that were later switched to re-enter the cell cycle. This would further confirm that only viable parasites are quantified by PCR. Our results are in agreement with those of Jarra and Snounou[20] which showed that only viable *Plasmodium* parasites were detected by PCR and those of Tarleton and Zhang[21] who noted that kDNA of *Trypanosoma cruzi* injected into mouse tissue was detected by PCR only in the 24–48 hours following intramuscular injection.

Perspectives

The presence of parasites in various distant sites early after inoculation, without the presence of clinical signs, has important consequences that should be considered during prevention. Recently, an experimental study on *L. tropica* transmission from the black rat to *Phlebotomus sergenti* has demonstrated that parasite transmission can occur if insects are fed on non-lesional skin.[13]

The apparent lack of symptoms indicates that complex mechanisms involving keratinocytes, the epidermal and dermal leukocytes, the extracellular matrix, and the sandfly saliva[3] are involved in the dynamic relationship that parasites establish with their hosts, allowing their persistence in the tissues. The hypothesis that parasites divert and/or amplify regulatory mechanisms that maintain tissue cells in a non-activable state, so-called homeostasis, is currently being extensively explored. In experimental conditions similar to ours (C57Bl/6 mice inoculated with 1000 metacyclic promastigotes), Belkaid and colleagues have shown that the persistence of 100–10 000 parasites at the inoculation site (once the lesion is healed, 8–10 weeks post-infection) is modulated by CD4[+] CD25[+] regulatory T cells.[22] The absence or inhibition of these leukocytes promotes complete clearance of the parasites, whereas depletion of some T-cells subtypes or cytokines (e.g. IFN-gamma, IL-12) was shown to promote parasite re-expansion coupled to lesion reinitiation.[23] CD4[+] CD25[+] regulatory T cells have been primarily described for their role in the control of the tissue autoreactive T lymphocytes. These CD4[+] CD25[+] regulatory T cells are increased in number after a second parasite inoculation and play a role in the reactivation of quiescent parasites within the primary site.[23] These findings could be highly relevant in clinical settings because re-exposure is frequent in endemic areas.

Our finding that asymptomatic carriage of *Leishmania* spp. can be detected in distant cutaneous sites as early as a few days after inoculation in our model using a kDNA-based PCR technology has broader applications for early, rapid and accurate detection of parasites in tissues.

In most studies performed in dogs and in humans, serological tests show a high degree of cross-reactivity, cannot discriminate between different *Leishmania* species,[10,24] and are less sensitive and specific than PCR.[24–28] PCR is able to detect more asymptomatic carriers[28] when compared with serological studies when used for diagnosis, prevention (animal quarantine, transfusion centres) or epidemiological purposes. Based on our results, it is not necessary to sample the inoculation site to perform a PCR evaluation of a skin biopsy for the detection of asymptomatic carriage. In many circumstances such as quarantine, follow-up of therapy, relapse of disease, pharmacological evaluation of

Leishmania-targeting drugs or vaccines, kDNA-based PCR is more useful than merely monitoring lesion reduction or recurrence of clinical signs. A skin biopsy with a 3-mm biopsy punch is easy to perform under local anaesthesia on most of the body with minimal restraint. Bone marrow aspiration may require sedation and special skills from the practitioner, and has to be performed under strict sterile conditions to prevent septic complications from occurring. Moreover, in a recent epidemiological study of 100 dogs in Majorca, an area of endemic canine leishmaniasis, kDNA-based PCR detected *Leishmania infantum* organisms in 51% of skin samples, as opposed to 17.8% of bone marrow samples and 32% of conjunctival samples.[29]

The growing importance of *L. infantum*-related disorders in dogs and humans makes such a method very interesting.

Acknowledgement

Thanks to Karim Sebastien for mouse handling and counselling. Some of the data have been presented earlier as a poster at the European Congress of Veterinary Dermatology (Tenerife, Spain, September 2003), in CEMI (Institut Pasteur, Paris, February 2002), as a communication in the Congrès du GEDAC (Paris, June 2003), and in front of the Académie Vétérinaire de France with publication of the proceeding in the *Bulletin de Académie Vétérinaire de France*. The entire study presented here is an original publication.

Funding

This study and preliminary studies received financial support from Institut Pasteur and the CNRS (Appel d'offres Puces à ADN co-PI G.Milon/M.Pages/P.Glaser).

References

1 Remme, J.H.F., Blas, E., Chitsulo, L., *et al*. Strategic emphases for tropical diseases research: a TDR perspective. *Trends in Parasitology*, 2002; **18**: 421–426.

2 Courtenay, O., Quinnell, R.J., Garcez, L.M., Shaw, J.J., Dye, C. Infectiousness in a cohort of Brazilian dogs: why culling fails to control visceral leishmaniasis in areas of high transmission. *Journal of Infectious Diseases*, 2002; **186**: 1314–1320.

3 Belkaid, Y., Marignac, G., Milon, G., Pérennité de Leishmania chez ses deux hôtes, impact de leur polymorphisme. In: Milon, G., ed. *Susceptibilité aux Maladies Infectieuses*. Editions Scientifiques et Medicales Elsevier SAS, Paris, 2002: 101–121.

4 Marignac, G., Lebastard, M., Fall, G., Nicolas, L., Milon, G. Ex-

ploration de la dissémination de Leishmania, un parasite délivré et prélevé par le phlébotome au niveau du derme de l'hôté vertébré. *Bulletin de l'Académie Vétérinaire de France*, 2003; **75**: 46–56.

5 Belkaid, Y., Mendez, S., Lira, R., Kadambi, N., Milon, G., Sacks, D.L. A natural model of *Leishmania major* infection reveals a prolonged 'silent' phase of parasite amplification in the skin before the onset of lesion formation and immunity. *Journal of Immunology*, 2000; **165**: 969–977.

6 Buffet, P.A., Sulahian, A., Garin, J.F., Nassar, N., Derouin, F. Culture microtitration: a sensitive method for quantifying *Leishmania infantum* in tissues of infected mice. *Antimicrobial Agents and Chemotherapy*, 1995; **39**: 2167–2168.

7 Leclercq, V., Lebastard, M., Belkaid, Y., Louis, J., Milon, G. The outcome of the parasite process initiated by *Leishmania infantum* in laboratory mice. A tissue-dependent pattern controlled by the Lsh and MHC loci. *Journal of Immunology*, 1996; **157**: 4537–4545.

8 Nicolas, L., Sidjanski, S., Colle, J., Milon, G. *Leishmania major* reaches distant cutaneous sites where it persists transiently while persisting durably in the primary dermal site and its draining lymph node: a study in laboratory mice. *Infection and Immunity*, 2000; **68**: 6561–6566.

9 Nicolas, L., Prina, E., Lang, T., Milon, G. Real-time PCR for detection and quantitation of Leishmania in mouse tissues. *Journal of Clinical Microbiology*, 2002; **40**: 1666–1669.

10 Nicolas, L., Milon, G., Prina, E. Rapid differentiation of Old Word Leishmania species by LightCycler polymerase chain reaction and melting curve analysis. *Journal of Microbiological Methods*, 2002; **51**: 295–299.

11 Bretagne, S., Durand, R., Olivi, M., *et al.* Real-time PCR as a new tool for quantifying *Leishmania infantum* in liver in infected mice. *Clinical and Diagnostic Laboratory Immunology*, 2001; **8**: 828–831.

12 Bell, A.S., Ranford-Cartwright, L.C. Real-time quantitative PCR in parasitology. *Trends in Parasitology*, 2002; **18**: 337–342.

13 Svobodova, M., Votypka, J., Nicolas, L., Volf, P. *Leishmania tropica* in the black rat (*Rattus rattus*): persistence and transmission from an asymptomatic host to sand fly vector *Phlebotomus sergenti*. *Microbes and Infection*, 2003; **5**: 361–364.

14 Rabinovitch, M. Leishmanicidal activity of amino acid and peptide esters. *Parasitology Today*, 1989; **5**: 299–301.

15 Antoine, J.C., Jouanne, C., Ryter, A. Megasomes as the targets of leucine methyl ester in *Leishmania amazonensis* amastigotes. *Parasitology Today*, 1989; **99**: 1–9.

16 Prina, E., Lang, T., Glaichenhaus, N., Antoine, J.C. Presentation of the protective parasite antigen LACK by *Leishmania*-infected macrophages. *Journal of Immunology*, 1996; **156**: 4318–4327.

17 Antoine, J.C., Jouanne, C., Lang, T., Prina, E., de Chastellier, C., Frehel, C. Localization of major histocompatibility complex class II molecules in phagolysosomes of murine macrophages infected with *Leishmania amazonensis*. *Infection and Immunity*,

1991; **59**: 764–775.

18 Berens, R.L., Marr, J.J. An easily prepared defined medium for cultivation of *Leishmania donovani* promastigotes. *Journal of Parasitology*, 1978; **64**: 160–164.

19 Späth, G.F., Beverley, S.M. A lipophosphoglycan-independent method for isolation of infective *Leishmania* metacyclic promastigotes by density gradient centrifugation. *Experimental Parasitology*, 2001; **99**: 97–103.

20 Jarra, W., Snounou, G. Only viable parasites are detected by PCR following clearance of rodent malarial infections by drug treatment or immune responses. *Infection and Immunity*, 1998; **66**: 3783–3787.

21 Tarleton, R.L., Zhang, L. Chagas disease etiology: autoimmunity or parasite persistence? *Parasitology Today*, 1999; **15**: 94–9.

22 Belkaid, Y., Piccirillo, C.A., Mendez, S., Shevach, E.M., Sacks, D.L. CD4⁺CD25⁺ regulatory T cells control *Leishmania major* persistence and immunity. *Nature*, 2002; **420**: 502–507.

23 Mendez, S., Reckling, S.K., Piccirillo, C.A., Sacks, D.L., Belkaid, Y. Role for CD4(+) CD25(+) regulatory T cells in reactivation of persistent leishmaniasis and control of concomitant immunity. *Journal of Experimental Medicine*, 2004; **200**: 201–210.

24 Schulz, A., Mellenthin, K., Schönian, G., Fleisher, B., Drosten, C. Detection, differentiation and quantification of pathogenic *Leishmania* organisms by a fluorescence resonance energy transfer-based real-time PCR assay. *Journal of Clinical Microbiology*, 2003; **41**: 1529–1535.

25 Gangneux, J.P., Menotti, J., Lorenzo, F., *et al.* Prospective value of PCR amplification and sequencing for diagnosis and typing of Old World *Leishmania* infections in an area of nonendemicity. *Journal of Clinical Microbiology*, 2003; **41**: 1419–1422.

26 Cortes, S., Rolão, N., Ramada, J., Campino, L. PCR as a rapid and sensitive tool in the diagnosis of human and canine leishmaniasis using *Leishmania donovani* s.l.-specific kinetoplastid primers. *Transactions of the Royal Society of Tropical Medicine and Hygiene*, 2004; **98**: 12–17.

27 Martin-Sanchez, J., Pineda, J.A., Morillas-Marquez, F., Garcia-Garcia, J.A., Acedo, C., Macias, J. Detection of *Leishmania infantum* kinetoplast DNA in peripheral blood from asymptomatic individuals at risk for parenterally transmitted infections: relationship between polymerase chain reaction results and other Leishmania infection markers. *American Journal of Tropical Medical Hygiene*, 2004; **70**: 545–548.

28 Reale, S., Maxia, L., Vitale, F., Glorioso, N.S., Caracappa, S., Vesco, G. Detection of *Leishmania infantum* in dogs by PCR with lymph node aspirates and blood. *Journal of Clinical Microbiology*, 1999; **37**: 2931–2935.

29 Solano-Gallago, L., Morell, P., Arboix, M., Alberola, J., Ferrer, L. Prevalence of *Leishmania infantum* infection in dogs living in an area of canine leishmaniasis endemicity using PCR on several tissues and serology. *Journal of Clinical Microbiology*, 2001; **39**: 560–563.

Adherence of *Staphylococcus intermedius* to canine corneocytes involves a protein–protein interaction that is sensitive to trypsin, but resistant to cold

C. Simou[1], P.B. Hill[1], P.J. Forsythe[2], K.L. Thoday[1]

[1] The University of Edinburgh, Division of Veterinary Clinical Studies, The Royal (Dick) School of Veterinary Studies, Roslin, Midlothian, Scotland
[2] Veterinary Dermatology Referrals, Dunlop, Ayrshire, Scotland

Summary

The aim of this study was to explore the effect of temperature, storage and trypsin digestion on the adherence of *Staphylococcus intermedius* to canine corneocytes. Sheets of corneocytes were collected from healthy dogs using adhesive tape and stored at –80°C, 4°C and room temperature for 5, 4 and 3 months and 12 days before use and fresh on the day of each experiment. *S. intermedius* from a case of bacterial pyoderma was applied in duplicate to the canine corneocyte-covered tapes using phosphate-buffered saline as negative control. After staining with crystal violet, quantification of adherent bacteria was performed by computerised image analysis. The results indicated that the mechanisms of adherence were not affected by even prolonged storage at cold temperatures. To determine if adherence involved interaction of proteins on the surface of the organism with those on corneocytes, trypsin (a potent broad-spectrum proteinase) was added to the incubation buffers. Adherence of *S. intermedius* to canine corneocytes was completely abolished following incubation of the organism with trypsin at concentrations from 1% to 0.01%, but adherence still occurred at lower concentrations, demonstrating a dose-response phenomenon. These results suggest that a protein receptor on the surface of the organism was digested, eliminating the capacity for adherence. Paradoxically, pretreatment of the corneocytes with trypsin resulted in significant enhancement in adherence of the organism, possibly due to exposure of further underlying binding sites. Our results indicate that the adherence mechanism involves a protein–protein interaction that is sensitive to trypsin, but resistant to cold.

Introduction

Adherence is the measurable union between a bacterium and a substratum and is a prerequisite step in the process of infection. The two interacting components responsible for adherence are the bacterial adhesins on the organism and the receptors on the substratum.[1,2] The capacity to adhere is thought to provide growth advantages for the microorganism, greater toxicity towards the host, and resistance to antimicrobial and antitoxin agents.[1]

A group of adhesins that bind to the extracellular matrix has been described. They are known to bind to fibronectin, collagen, fibrinogen/fibrin, elastin, vitronectin and laminin. Adhesins that bind to the extracellular matrix are termed microbial surface components recognising adhesive matrix molecules (MSCRAMMs).[3] Studies on *Staphylococcus aureus* adherence have shown that its adhesins include fibronectin-binding protein (Fnbp) A and B, protein A, collagen-binding protein and fibrinogen-binding protein.[3–6]

Candidate receptors on animal cells include every constituent of their outer membrane. In the case of corneocytes, the candidate receptors are the constituents of the modified membrane that is composed of a protein–lipid–carbohydrate complex.[7]

Adherence of *Staphylococcus intermedius* to the canine epidermis has been investigated *in vitro* using corneocytes collected from the skin surface of dogs.[8,9] We have previously validated and optimised computerised image analysis for the quantification of bacterial adherence to canine corneocytes. We have shown that *S. intermedius* demonstrated a sigmoid dose-response curve with increasing bacterial concentration, which suggests that *S. intermedius* adheres to canine corneocytes by a specific receptor–ligand interaction. Moreover, *S. intermedius* showed significantly greater adherence to corneocytes of boxers and bull terriers than spaniels and hounds, and also to corneocytes from the head and neck compared with the dorsum. Finally, *S. intermedius* and *Pseudomonas aeruginosa* adhered in greater numbers to canine corneocytes than *S. aureus*, *Streptococcus canis*, *Klebsiella pneumoniae* and *Escherichia coli*.[8]

The aim of this study was to further investigate the specific interaction between *S. intermedius* and canine corneocytes by examining the effect of long-term storage, cold temperatures and trypsin (a broad-spectrum proteinase) on the adherence mechanism.

Materials and methods

Collection of corneocytes

Corneocytes were collected from the ventral abdomen of healthy dogs that had no history or physical signs of skin disease (Table 5.6.1). Initially, the skin sites were prepared by removal of hair with Oster clippers (Oster Professional Products, Tennessee, USA), and removal of surface debris and most indigenous bacteria by serial application of four strips of single adhesive tape (Cellux, Sellotape GB Ltd, Dunstable, UK).[8,10] To collect the corneocytes, a 2 cm² piece of clear double-sided adhesive tape (Tropical Tape 'Super Grip', USA) was used. One side of the tape was mounted onto a clean glass microscope slide (Premium microscope slides, BDH, UK) and the other was applied 10 times to the clean skin surface using the same force on each occasion. The samples were always collected by the same investigator in a standard manner in order to reduce variability.

Staphylococcal suspension

An isolate of *S. intermedius* from a clinical case of canine bacterial pyoderma (M 732, 99) was used. Bacterial

Table 5.6.1 Descriptive data of dogs used for corneocyte collection and the experimental protocols to which they were assigned

Dog no.	Sex	Breed	Age	Experiment
1	FN	Springer spaniel	11 years	Effect of storage and temperature
2	FN	Cross-breed	2 years	
3	F	Cross-breed	7 months	Effect of trypsin on staphylococci
4	M	German shepherd dog	Unknown	
5	M	Lurcher	3 years	
6	F	Labrador retriever-cross	1 years	
7	F	Collie-cross	3 years	
8	F	Collie-cross	6 years	
8	F	Collie-cross	6 years	Effect of trypsin on corneocytes
9	F	Collie-cross	5 years	
10	M	Cross-breed	Unknown	
11	F	Labrador retriever-cross	3 years	
12	F	Collie-cross	3 years	

F, entire female; FN, ovariohysterectomised female; M, entire male.

suspensions were prepared using the technique previously described by Forsythe *et al.*[8] Briefly, for each assay, organisms stored at −70°C on cryobank beads (Mast, Bootle, UK) were inoculated onto horse-blood agar and incubated for 24 hours at 37°C. An individual colony was then subcultured onto horse-blood agar for a further 24 hours. Bacterial colonies were harvested from the agar plate and placed into a sterile tube containing 1 M sterile phosphate-buffered saline (PBS), pH 7.2. The bacteria were washed by vortex mixing for 60 seconds using a Rotamixer (Camlab Ltd, Cambridge, UK) and were then centrifuged for 3 minutes at 3000 rpm using a Centrifugette 4206 centrifuge (Camlab Ltd). The resulting supernatant was discarded, a further 3–4 ml of PBS was added to the tube and the process was repeated. The bacteria were subjected to three washes in total and then resuspended in 1 M PBS by further vortex mixing for at least 2 minutes. Previous studies in our laboratories have established that the optimal concentration of staphylococcal suspensions for adherence studies is 3×10^8 per ml.[8] This density corresponds to an optical density (OD) of 0.289 when measured by a spectrophotometer (Colorimeter 257, Ciba Corning Diagnostics, Halstead, UK) at a wavelength of 600 nm. Therefore, throughout these studies, bacterial suspensions were diluted in PBS to an OD of 0.289.

Adherence assay

For each sample, two duplicate corneocyte-covered slides were used to measure staphylococcal adherence, and one slide was used as a control. The corneocyte-covered slides were placed in moisture chambers consisting of 30×30 cm flat plastic trays with well-fitting lids and lined by a paper towel moistened with water. Then 300 μl of bacterial suspension, or PBS control, was pipetted onto the centre of each piece of corneocyte-covered tape, to form a meniscus. The slide chambers were incubated for 90 minutes at 37°C. Subsequently, all slides were rinsed with 1 M PBS to remove non-adherent bacteria, and finally were stained with 0.5% crystal violet (crystal violet for microscopical staining, 'Gurr' 'Certistain'®, BDH, VWR International Ltd, UK) for 90 seconds.

Quantification of adherence

The quantification of adherent bacteria was performed by means of a computerised image analysis technique as previously validated and used in our laboratories.[8] The same person performed the analysis each time and was blinded to the identity of the samples. Briefly, the analysed fields were selected in a random way by moving the microscope stage in a standard direction and to a standard distance after each image acquisition. A chosen field was rejected if the corneocytes were not confluent, if there were objects other than corneocytes on the field (hair, artefacts), or if it was not possible to bring the entire field into sharp focus.[8]

Previous studies showed that acquisition of 15 fields from each duplicate slide yielded acceptable coefficients of variation of approximately 10%.[8] Therefore, in this study, 15 images of oil-immersion fields (1000×) of each slide were acquired with a JVC TK-C1381 colour video camera attached to a Leica Laburlux S conventional compound microscope (Leica Microsystems UK Ltd, Milton Keynes, UK). Live 24-bit super-VHS colour PAL video was digitised using a Power Macintosh 7100/80 fitted with an AV digitiser (Apple Computer, California, USA). Image acquisition and processing were performed using Object-Image 1.62, a public domain software package, available from the Internet by anonymous FTP from: http://simon.bio.uva.nl/object-image.html.

The software calculated the percentage area covered by staphylococci that were adherent to a confluent layer of corneocytes within a defined area of the captured field. The defined area remained constant throughout the study. For each field the percentage bacterial coverage (termed percentage adherence) was calculated, and the overall percentage adherence figure was determined by calculating the mean of the percentage bacterial coverage of all 15 fields analysed on each slide. The overall percentage adherence was determined by subtracting the percentage adherence of the control slide from the mean of the duplicates.

Effect of storage and temperature

Eighteen corneocyte-covered slides from both dogs 1 and 2 were collected 5 months, 4 months, 3 months and 12 days before the experiments began. Six slides from each date and from each dog were stored at −80°C, 4°C and room temperature (approximately 20°C), respectively, in dark and dry conditions. Another six fresh samples were collected from each dog on the day the adherence assays were performed and used within a maximum of 5 hours. The collected samples were divided into two groups and were processed in two duplicate experiments, which took place on two different days, under identical conditions, to allow the repeatability of the results to be determined.

Effect of trypsin treatment on S. intermedius

Preliminary experiments showed that the enzymatic activity of a 1% and 0.1% solution of trypsin (from bovine pancreas, Type I, Sigma-Aldrich Co., UK) in dilution buffer fell to zero after incubation for 4 hours (data not shown). Hence, all incubations in subsequent experiments were for 4 hours. Further preliminary experiments demonstrated that incubation of S. intermedius with 1% and 0.1% trypsin did not affect the viability of the organism. In addition, S. intermedius did not inhibit or enhance trypsin activity, or produce trypsin or substances with trypsin-like activity (data not shown).

Prior to carrying out the adherence assays, S. intermedius was incubated with tenfold dilutions of trypsin ranging from 1% to 0.000001% for 4 hours. After incubation, the bacteria were washed three times by centrifugation at 6000 rpm for 10 minutes, followed by removal of the supernatant, resuspension in 5–6 ml of 1 M PBS and vortex mixing for 60 seconds. Adherence assays were then performed as described above using corneocytes from dogs 3–8.

Effect of trypsin treatment on canine corneocytes

In these experiments, corneocytes were pretreated with trypsin before adherence assays. Although it was not possible to perform viability assays for canine corneocytes as was performed for *S. intermedius*, trypsin induced no morphological abnormalities in the cells (compared to control slides) that would suggest that adherence assays would be unduly affected. Corneocytes from dogs 8, 9 and 10 were incubated with trypsin at a dilution of 1%, 0.1% and 0.01%, and those from dogs 11 and 12 were used for assays involving trypsin concentrations of 1%, 0.1%, 0.01% and 0.001%. On each slide, 300 µl of trypsin dilution was pipetted onto the surface of a pre-marked area of the corneocytes which were then incubated at 37°C for 4 hours. Samples were then rinsed with PBS to remove the trypsin and 300 µl of a *S. intermedius* suspension was pipetted on the same pre-marked area. After washing and staining, adherence assays were conducted as described.

Statistical analysis

For all experiments, the percentage adherence values at various time points or trypsin concentrations were compared by repeated measures ANOVA. Individual time points or dilutions were compared by Tukey's multiple comparison test. A p value of < 0.05 was considered to be significant in all cases.

Results

Effect of storage and temperature

The effects of storing canine corneocytes at various temperatures and for varying periods of time are shown in Fig. 5.6.1. There was some fluctuation in adherence values over the 5 months in all three groups. When compared by repeated measures ANOVA, this variation was significantly different in samples stored at 4°C ($p = 0.03$) and room temperature ($p = 0.047$) but not at –80°C. However, in none of the groups did subanalysis reveal significant differences between fresh samples and those stored for any period of time under any of the three conditions ($p > 0.05$).

Effect of trypsin treatment on S. intermedius

Treatment of *S. intermedius* with trypsin at concentra-

tions of 1%, 0.1% and 0.01% virtually abolished its adherence to canine corneocytes compared with the negative control (Fig. 5.6.2A) ($p < 0.01$). Adherence returned to normal numbers at concentrations ranging from 0.01% to 0.000001% (Fig. 5.6.2B). Comparison of individual concentrations revealed significant differences ($p < 0.05$) between all values except: 0 vs 0.001%; 0.0001% vs 0.00001% and 0 vs 0.000001%.

Effect of trypsin treatment on canine corneocytes

Trypsin treatment of canine corneocytes resulted in a significant enhancement of adherence compared with the negative control slides (Fig. 5.6.3).

The percentage adherence values among four concentrations differed significantly by repeated measures ANOVA ($p < 0.0001$). (The 0.001% concentration could not be included in the analysis due to missing data points.) Subanalysis revealed that the 1% ($p < 0.05$), 0.1% and 0.01% ($p < 0.001$) concentrations resulted in significantly higher adherence values than the negative control.

Discussion

Surprisingly, storage of corneocytes at –80°C, 4°C or room temperature for up to 5 months did not significantly reduce or increase staphylococcal adherence. The changes in adherence were minimal and the values from the fresh samples were not significantly higher than those from samples stored for 5 months. Hence the receptors on the corneocyte surface are likely to be relatively robust molecules that are not destroyed either by freezing or by prolonged storage at room temperature. This feature of the staphylococcal receptors is useful in that it allows corneocytes to be collected for up to 5 months prior to their use in experimental studies.

In order to further elucidate the nature of these receptors and also the adhesins of *S. intermedius*, we pretreated both the organism and the receptor using trypsin, a broad-spectrum proteinase that can digest surface proteins. Treatment of *S. intermedius* with trypsin did not affect the organism's viability, but it virtually abolished adherence to canine corneocytes when used at concentrations between 1% and 0.01%. At lower concentrations, a dose-response effect could be seen, suggesting that a surface protein critical for

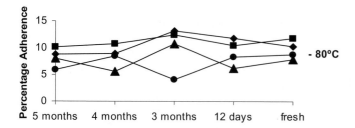

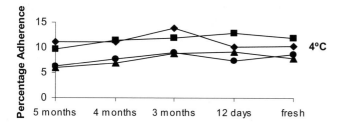

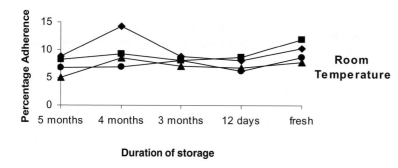

Duration of storage

Fig. 5.6.1 The percentage adherence of *Staphylo-coccus intermedius* to canine corneocytes that had been stored at –80°C, 4°C and room temperature (RT) for 5, 4 and 3 months, and 12 and 0 days. ◆ = experiment 1 (dog 1); ■ = experiment 1 (dog 2); ▲ = experiment 2 (dog 1); ● = experiment 2 (dog 2).

adherence was removed by the higher concentrations. The total abolition of adherence suggests that ancillary non-protein molecules are not involved in the adherence mechanism. The slight enhancement in adherence seen at concentrations of 0.0001% and 0.00001% could suggest that these low concentrations of trypsin were removing coatings on the staphylococcus organism, revealing additional binding sites. However, this speculation requires further study.

Trypsin treatment of other microorganisms has yielded similar effects on adherence. Treatment of *S. aureus* with 0.1 mg/ml trypsin at 37°C resulted in decreased adherence to mucin.[11] Similarly, treatment of *Streptococcus pneumoniae* with 1 mg/ml trypsin at 37°C

blocked its adherence to immobilised fibronectin.[12] The same results were obtained after trypsin treatment of *Streptococcus gordonii*. The adherence of these oral streptococci to human fibrinogen was markedly reduced.[13] In addition, trypsin decreased the adhesion of *S. epidermidis* to immobilised fibronectin.[14] Trypsin treatment of *Malassezia pachydermatis* also reduced the binding ability to canine corneocytes of four of the five strains that were examined.[15]

When canine corneocytes were pretreated with trypsin prior to adherence assays there was a surprising increase in adhesion. This could be due to exposure of surface receptors after the removal of surface proteins that were masking them. It could also be ex-

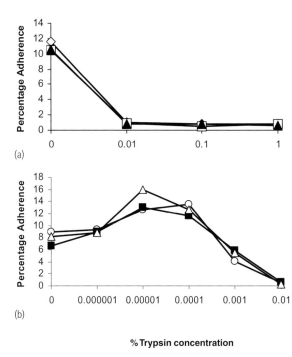

(a)

(b)

% Trypsin concentration

Fig. 5.6.2 Percentage adherence of *Staphylococcus intermedius* after pretreatment with 1%, 0.1%, 0.01% trypsin or buffer alone (a) or 0.01%, 0.001%, 0.0001%, 0.00001% and 0.000001% trypsin or buffer alone (b). ◇ = dog 3; ☐ = dog 4; ▲ = dog 5; ◯ = dog 6; ■ = dog 7; △ = dog 8.

of cytoplasm. It was hypothesised that this may be due to digestion of the membrane-penetrating proteins, resulting in digestion of the keratin fibres and interfilamentous matrix.[17] If this were the case, *S. intermedius* could express greater affinity for these proteins than for the proteins of the envelope. Another possibility is that trypsin treatment removed part of the corneocyte envelope that is covalently bound to lipids. The major lipid constituent of the human stratum corneum is a ceramide,[18] whereas in pigs it is a hydroxyceramide. In the latter species, the lipid envelope is so strong that it co-purifies with the corneocyte envelope.[19] If trypsin removed a part of the cell envelope, it is also possible that the outer lipid layer may be removed. It is possible that the absence of these lipids could facilitate the adherence of *S. intermedius* to the remaining proteins. However, these observations were based on a relatively small number of samples and larger studies would be required to confirm this apparent increase in staphylococcal adherence to trypsinised corneocytes.

In order to minimise variation due to different strains of *S. intermedius*, only one strain was used in this study. Hence, surface molecules and biological behaviour (e.g. possible resistance to trypsin) were directly comparable in every assay. However, it was consequently impossible to draw general conclusions about different strains of *S. intermedius*. Different strains of *S. epidermidis* have been shown to differ in the production of biofilm.[20] In another study, although no difference was detected between the adherence of *S. intermedius* strains that were isolated from pyoderma cases and others isolated from healthy dogs, significant variation was noticed among individual isolates within the groups.[9] Hence, further studies investigating strain differences would be valuable in providing additional

plained by the destruction of the corneocyte envelope and exposure of the underlying cytoplasmic keratin fibres and matrix. When keratinocytes (derived from pig ears) were exposed to 1 mg/ml of trypsin at 37°C for 2 hours, the surface corneosomes were digested.[16] In another study, human corneocytes were treated with 0.4% trypsin at 37°C for 1 hour, resulting in cells free

Fig. 5.6.3 Percentage adherence of *Staphylococcus intermedius* to canine corneocytes that had been pretreated with various concentrations of trypsin. ◆ = dog 8; ■ = dog 9; ▲ = dog 10; ● = dog 11; ✳ = dog 12.

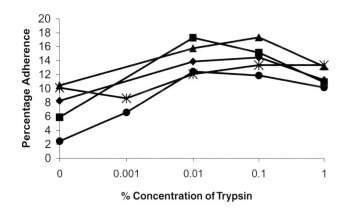

% Concentration of Trypsin

information about adherence mechanisms and how they can be affected by the organism itself.

In summary, these studies provide evidence that adherence of *S. intermedius* to canine corneocytes involves specific protein–protein interactions that are resistant to freezing and long-term storage but sensitive to trypsin. Elucidation of the precise proteins involved could provide molecules that might be amenable to therapeutic targeting.

Acknowledgements

The authors acknowledge members of the Miller Group for various aspects of technical advice and help, Dr Jeremy Brown for help with the microscope facilities, Ms Lorna Hume for bacteriological assistance and Drs Silvia Colombo and Ariane Neuber for access to the corneocytes of some dogs.

Funding

Chrisi Simou was funded by the Triandafillidis Foundation.

References

1 Ofek, I., Doyle, R.J. Principles of bacterial adhesion. In: *Bacterial Adhesion to Cells and Tissues.* Chapman & Hall, New York, 1994: 1–15.

2 Mims, C., Dimmock, N., Nash, A., Stephen, J. Attachment to and entry of microorganisms into the body. In: *Mims' Pathogenesis of Infectious Disease.* Academic Press, London, 1995: 10–17.

3 Joh, D., Wann, E.R., Kreikemeyer, B., Speziale, P., Hook, M. Role of fibronectin-binding MSCRAMMs in bacterial adherence and entry into mammalian cells. *Matrix Biology*, 1999; **18**: 211–223.

4 Aly, R., Levit, S. Adherence of *Staphylococcus aureus* to squamous epithelium: role of fibronectin and teichoic acid. *Reviews of Infectious Diseases*, 1987; **9** (Suppl 4): S341–S350.

5 Foster, T.J., McDevitt, D. Surface-associated proteins of *Staphylococcus aureus*: their possible roles in virulence. *Federation of European Microbiological Societies Microbiology Letters*, 1994; **118**: 199–205.

6 Peacock, S.J., Foster, T.J., Cameron, B.J., Berendt, A.R. Bacterial fibronectin-binding proteins and endothelial cell surface fibronectin mediate adherence of *Staphylococcus aureus* to resting human endothelial cells. *Microbiology*, 1999; **145**: 3477–3486.

7 Matoltsy, A.G. Keratinization. *Journal of Investigative Dermatology*, 1976; **67**: 20–25.

8 Forsythe, P.J., Hill, P.B., Thoday, K.L., Brown, J. Use of computerized image analysis to quantify staphylococcal adhesion to canine corneocytes: does breed and body site have any relevance to the pathogenesis of pyoderma? *Veterinary Dermatology*, 2002; **13**: 29–36.

9 Saijonmaa-Koulumies, L.E., Lloyd, D.H. Adherence of *Staphylococcus intermedius* to canine corneocytes in vitro. *Veterinary Dermatology*, 2002; **13**: 169–176.

10 Lloyd, D.H., Dick, W.D.B., McEwan-Jenkinson, D. Location of the microflora in the skin of cattle. *British Veterinary Journal*, 1979; **135**: 519–526.

11 Shuter, J., Hatcher, V.B., Lowy, F.D. *Staphylococcus aureus* binding to human nasal mucin. *Infection and Immunity*, 1996; **64**: 310–318.

12 Van der Flier, M., Chhun, N., Wizemann, T.M., Min, J., McCarthy, J.B., Tuomanen, E.I. Adherence of *Streptococcus pneumoniae* to immobilized fibronectin. *Infection and Immunity*, 1995; **63**: 4317–4322.

13 Lee, S.Y., Kim, K.K., Choe, S.J. Binding of oral streptococci to human fibrinogen. *Oral Microbiology and Immunology*, 2001; **16**: 88–93.

14 Hussain, M., Heilmann, C., Peters, G., Herrmann, M. Teichoic acid enhances adhesion of *Staphylococcus epidermidis* to immobilized fibronectin. *Microbial Pathogenesis*, 2001; **31**: 261–270.

15 Bond, R., Lloyd, D.H. Factors affecting the adherence of *Malassezia pachydermatis* to canine corneocytes *in vitro*. *Veterinary Dermatology*, 1996; **7**: 49–56.

16 Chapman, S.J., Walsh, A., Jackson, S.M., Friedmann, P.S. Lipids, proteins and corneocyte adhesion. *Archives of Dermatological Research*, 1991; **283**: 167–173.

17 Hirotani, T., Manabe, M., Ogawa, H., Murayama, K., Sugawara, T. Isolation and characterization of horny cell membrane. *Archives of Dermatological Research*, 1982; **274**: 169–177.

18 Wertz, P.W., Madison, K.C., Downing, D.T. Covalently bound lipids of human stratum corneum. *Journal of Investigative Dermatology*, 1989; **92**: 109–111.

19 Swartzendruber, D.C., Kitko, D.J., Wertz, P.W., Madison, K.C., Downing, D.T. Isolation of corneocyte envelopes from porcine epidermis. *Archives of Dermatological Research*, 1988; **280**: 424–429.

20 Hussain, M., Wilcox, M.H., White, P.J. The slime of coagulase-negative staphylococci: biochemistry and relation to adherence. *Federation of European Microbiological Societies Microbiology Reviews*, 1993; **10**: 191–207.

Retrospective histopathological and clinical characterisation of a dermatopathy associated with toxic shock-like syndrome in dogs

F. Ramiro-Ibanez DVM, PhD[1], E.J. Walder VMD[2], T.L. Gross DVM[3]

[1] IDEXX Veterinary Services, West Sacramento, California, USA
[2] An Independent Biopsy Service, Venice, California, USA
[3] IDEXX Veterinary Services and California Dermatopathology Service, West Sacramento, California, USA.

Summary

Staphylococcal toxic shock syndrome in humans is a systemic disease with cutaneous signs initiated by a localised bacterial infection. The offending bacteria generate exotoxins that display superantigen activity. Similar syndromes have been described in animals. Retrospectively, 11 dogs with histopathological lesions closely resembling staphylococcal toxic shock syndrome in humans and the presence of a skin rash, as well as systemic signs, were evaluated. The characteristic dermatopathological finding was superficial dermatitis with epidermal neutrophilic exocytosis and degenerate keratinocytes. Based on information obtained by postal and telephone surveys submitted to the clinicians, the dogs presented with systemic signs and generalised or regionally extensive cutaneous lesions of oedema, erythema, vesicles, pustules and ulcers. Mild anaemia, hypoalbuminaemia, neutrophilia and fever were commonly present. In the only case in which bacterial culture was obtained, pustular lesions yielded a mixed population of coagulase-negative *Staphylococcus* sp. and *Pseudomonas* sp. Cases with delayed antibiotic treatment (cephalexin) were fatal. Until further characterisation and evaluation of the process in dogs, skin biopsies with features of neutrophilic exocytosis and keratinocyte degeneration must warrant consideration of toxic shock-like syndrome.

Introduction

In people, toxic shock syndrome (TSS) is a systemic manifestation of a localised bacterial infection. When caused by gram-positive organisms, typically *Staphylococcus* spp. and *Streptococcus* spp., there is production of bacterial exotoxins with superantigenic activity.[1–4] The syndrome has been associated with the endogenous production of excessive amounts of cytokines, especially tumour necrosis factor (TNF) molecules α and β, and a dominant T helper 1 (Th1) response.[3] Th1 cytokines released after superantigen stimulation are the cause of the systemic signs.[1,3,5] Although immune cells are considered the major source of cytokines, there is also experimental evidence indicating that keratinocytes can overexpress major histocompatibility complex class II (MHC II) molecules and be directly activated by bacterial superantigens to release cytokines.[6,7]

Staphylococcus aureus produces a variety of exotoxins (enterotoxins A, B, C, D, E and G). Toxic shock syndrome toxin-1 (TSST-1) (previously known as enterotoxin F) is the most commonly involved in cases of human TSS.[8–10] Cutaneous or internal infections may be the origin of the disease.[4,8,11] *Staphylococcus*-associated TSS with cutaneous signs was first reported in children in 1978[8] and subsequently described in women in association with the use of superabsorbent tampons.[9,11] The most frequent clinical symptoms of staphylococcal TSS in humans include fever, headache, skin eruption, myalgia and diarrhoea, as well as progression to disseminated intravascular coagulation, acute renal failure and shock.[12–14] The condition has recently been described in a horse with staphylococcal pneumonia.[4] In dogs the most frequent bacterial organism isolated from cases of bacterial pyoderma is *Staphylococcus intermedius*.[15] This bacterium has been shown to produce exotoxins, including TSST-1.[16,17]

In this chapter, we describe a distinct clinical entity in dogs with close similarity, clinically and histopathologically, to staphylococcal TSS in humans.

Materials and methods

Dogs

The cases comprising this study were initially derived from skin biopsies submitted to several diagnostic laboratories in California (IDEXX Veterinary Services, An Independent Biopsy Service, and U.C. Davis Diagnostic Laboratory) for histopathological evaluation, between the years 1996 and 2003. The diagnosis of TSS was based on three basic parameters: (1) the characteristic histological features of the known human condition;[14] (2) the presence of a locally extensive, or widespread skin rash; and (3) systemic signs of disease. In three of the cases (nos 5, 8 and 9), systemic involvement was confirmed via post-mortem examination performed by the referring veterinarian. In the other deceased animals, post-mortem examination was not allowed or pursued. A written clinical survey was submitted to all the clinicians; information was also obtained by telephone. The questionnaire focused on the identification of systemic signs, the characterisation of clinical skin lesions, treatment and final outcome. The submitted information was frequently incomplete and in some cases not obtained by the original referring veterinarian, which is reflected in the lack of uniformity of the parameters obtained. However, in all the cases included in this report, the main criteria initially described (histopathological features of TSS, skin rash and systemic signs) were present.

Tissues

All biopsies were evaluated after routine fixation in 10% formalin, paraffin embedding and processing. Samples were sectioned at 5 μm and stained with haematoxylin and eosin (H&E). All samples were analysed by at least two pathologists.

Results

Eleven dogs with clinicopathological features resembling human staphylococcal TSS were identified. Seven dogs were intact or castrated males, and four dogs were intact or spayed females. Ages ranged from 1.5 to 13 years, with an average of 4.5 years. Large and small breeds were represented; the pug ($n = 3$) and golden retriever (2) were the only breeds with more than one representative (Table 5.7.1).

All dogs had cutaneous lesions. These were generalised in seven dogs and regionally extensive in three dogs. For one case (no. 11) there was no information on clinical distribution of the lesions. Generalised lesions frequently were more severe on the face, ears and legs. When the lesions were regional, the legs and trunk were most commonly involved. The most frequent cutaneous lesions were described as erythema ($n = 11$) and oedema (10), with some dogs presenting vesicles (4), petechiae (3), pustules (3) and ulcers (3) (Table 5.7.2). The evolution to ulcerative dermatitis was not correlated with the severity of the condition or the final outcome. A skin lesion was cultured in only one case (no. 5), yielding coagulase-negative *Staphylococcus* sp. and *Pseudomonas* sp.

The systemic signs were variable, and records were incomplete in some cases. Nine of the dogs were depressed at presentation, and seven had fever. Blood studies revealed hypoalbuminaemia ($n = 9$), mild anaemia (8) and neutrophilia (7) with or without leukocytosis. Other relevant findings included elevation of two or more hepatic enzymes ($n = 6$), thrombocytopenia (5), mild to moderate increase in bilirubin (5) and coagulation abnormalities (3) (Table 5.7.1). In most cases, the initial treatment included a cocktail of antibiotics (in sequence or in combination) and, in three cases, corticosteroids and pentoxyfylline. All the dogs treated with cephalexin ($n = 4$) recovered. One dog recovered with a combination of multiple antibiotics (not including cephalexin) and immunomodulatory agents. Five dogs died despite antibiotic therapy that did not include cephalexin. Another dog died without apparent therapy (no. 11). The overall mortality rate for this limited group was 55%.

Post-mortem analysis was available for three dogs. All three animals had histological features suggestive of disseminated intravascular coagulation (DIC), which included the presence of fibrin thrombi within

Table 5.7.1 Historical, clinical and laboratory data for dogs with staphylococcal TSS-like syndrome

Parameter	1	2	3	4	5	6	7	8	9	10	11
Age (years)/sex	5/M	3/FS	2/MC	5/MC	13/FS	2/MC	6/MC	4/FS	5/F	3/MC	1.5/MC
Breed	GR	BT	LabX	GSHP	WHWT	Pug	GR	Lab	GSDX	Pug	Pug
Fever	+	+	+	+	+	+					
Depression	+	+	+	+	+	+		+		+	+
Anaemia	+	+	+	+	+		+	+	+		
Leukocytosis	+				+	+	+	+			
Neutrophilia	+	+	+	+	+		+	+			
Albumin	↓	N	↓	↓	↓	↓	↓	↓	↓	↓	
Globulin	↓	N	N	N	N	N	↓	N	N		
Thrombocytopenia	+		+				+	+	+		
PT	↑						↑		N		
PTT	↑						N		↑		
ALP	↑	↑	↑	↑	↑		↑	↑	↑		
ALT	N	↑	N	↑	↑		N	N	↑		
AST	N	↑	↑	↑	N		↑		N		
GGT	N		N	N	N				N		
CK	↑			↑	↑						
Bilirubin (total)	↑	N	↑	N	N	N	↑	↑	↑		
Treatment	cx	cx	cx	abc	abc	cx		abc			
Outcome	R	R	R	R	D	R	D	E	D	D	D

M, male; MC, male/castrated; F, female; FS, female/spayed; GR, golden retriever; BT, Boston terrier; Lab, Labrador retriever; GSHP, German short-haired pointer; WHWT, West Highland white terrier; GSD, German shepherd dog; X, cross breed; +, present; N, normal; cx, cephalexin (alone or with others); abc, antibiotic cocktail; R, recovered; D, died; E, euthanasia. Arrows indicate elevation or decrease. Open (blank) cells indicate that information was not recorded.

the capillaries and small vessels of various internal organs (liver, kidney and spleen).

Cutaneous histopathology in this group of dogs is summarised in Table 5.7.3. The dominant pathological feature was a superficial neutrophilic dermatitis with neutrophilic exocytosis, and individual degen- eration of keratinocytes (Fig. 5.7.1). The epidermis was variably hyperplastic and spongiotic (Fig. 5.7.2), and the stratum corneum was occasionally parakeratotic. Degenerate keratinocytes were rounded or angular, hypereosinophilic, and had a hyperchromatic nucleus. They were frequently surrounded by intact or

Table 5.7.2 Cutaneous lesions in dogs with staphylococcal TSS-like syndrome

Lesions	1	2	3	4	5	6	7	8	9	10	11
Pustules	+	+			+						
Ulcers			+	+	+						
Erythema	+	+	+	+	+	+	+	+	+		+
Vesicles				+			+	+			+
Petechiae		+	+								
Papules				+							
Oedema	+	+	+			+	+	+	+	+	+
Distribution	G	G	R	R	G	G	G	G	G		G

G, generalised; R, regional.

Table 5.7.3 Main cutaneous histopathological features in dogs with staphylococcal TSS-like syndrome

Lesion	1	2	3	4	5	6	7	8	9	10	11
Epidermal individual cell degeneration	+	+	+	+	+	+	+	+	+	+	+
Intra-epidermal neutrophils	+	+	+	+	+	+	+	+	+	+	+
Shot-scatter pattern of degenerate keratinocytes	+	+		+		+		+	+	+	+
Panepidermal necrosis				+				+	+	+	
Ulcers				+		+					
Oedema	+	+	+				+	+	+	+	+
Other	F	P	H	H	F				F	F	F

F, folliculitis; P, parakeratosis; H, haemorrhages.

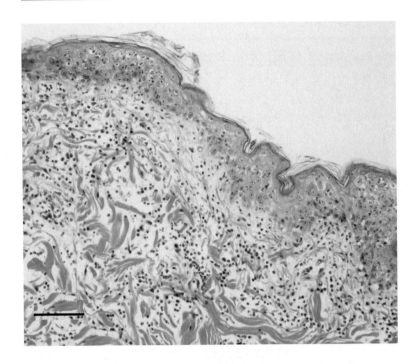

Fig. 5.7.1 Canine staphylococcal TSS-like syndrome. Neutrophils infiltrate the upper dermis and epidermis (exocytosis). A few degenerate keratinocytes (hypereosinophilic cells) are seen within the epidermis. H&E; bar = 100 μm.

degenerated neutrophils (satellitosis) (Figs 5.7.1 and 5.7.3). The degenerate keratinocytes were often distributed in small clusters (scatter-shot pattern) or diffusely throughout the epidermis (Figs 5.7.1 and 5.7.3). The infundibulum of hair follicles was commonly affected. In some cases, lesions evolved to panepidermal necro-

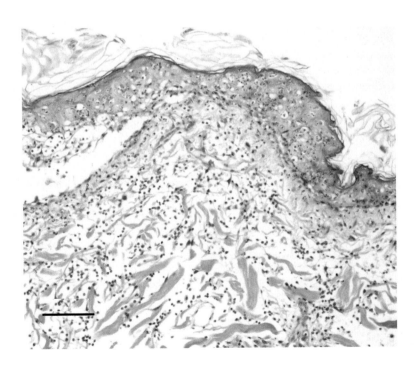

Fig. 5.7.2 Canine staphylococcal TSS-like syndrome. Epidermal hyperplasia and spongiosis. The keratinocytes are separated by clear spaces (oedema). Oedema is also present in the dermis separating the collagen bundles. H&E; bar = 100 μm.

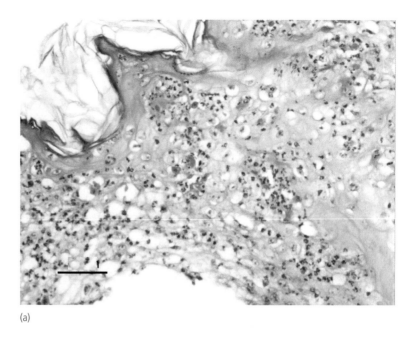

(a)

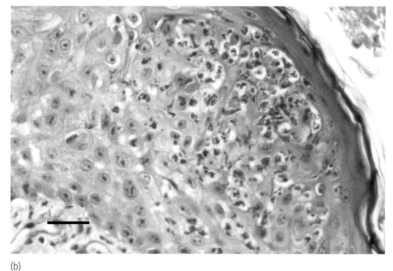

Fig. 5.7.3 Canine staphylococcal TSS-like syndrome. (a) Degenerate keratinocytes in the epidermis (hypereosinophilic cells) are scattered in distribution and often surrounded by neutrophils (satellitosis). H&E; bar = 50 μm. (b) Degenerate keratinocytes are grouped in small clusters (scatter-shot) throughout the epidermis, accompanied by exocytosing neutrophils. H&E; bar = 30 μm.

(b)

sis and ulceration (Figs 5.7.4 and 5.7.5) independently of the final clinical outcome. Neutrophils accumulated in small clusters in the epidermis, or formed degenerate pustules under the stratum corneum (Fig. 5.7.5). Lesions of panepidermal necrosis showed more intense neutrophilic infiltrate. The inflamed superficial dermis was mildly oedematous, and showed vascular dilation and occasional superficial haemorrhage (Fig. 5.7.6). Clear evidence of vasculitis was not present in these cases, although vessels were frequently lined by hypertrophic endothelial cells. The predominant dermal infiltrate was superficial perivascular to interstitial, mild to moderate, and formed by a mixed population of neutrophils, lymphocytes and macrophages (Figs 5.7.1, 5.7.2 and 5.7.5).

Discussion

This work presents 11 field cases of dogs with clinico-pathological features similar to staphylococcal TSS in

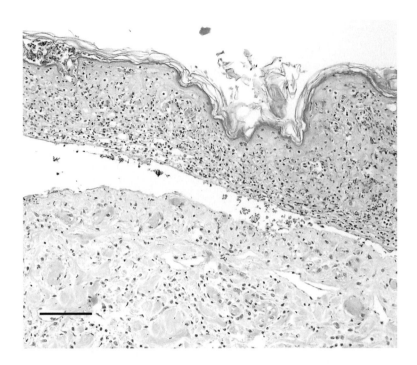

Fig. 5.7.4 Canine staphylococcal TSS-like syndrome. Full thickness epidermal necrosis with dermo-epidermal detachment. The epidermis is replaced by eosinophilic amorphous material and degenerate inflammatory cells. Degenerate neutrophils and cellular debris accumulate under the stratum corneum (micropustules). H&E; bar = 100 μm.

humans.[14] TSS is a systemic disease produced by the release of bacterial exotoxins by some bacterial strains.[2,3,10] In the case of staphylococcal infection, the production of exotoxins has been observed in humans and animals.[8,16,18–21] The most common toxin associated with staphylococcal TSS in humans is TSS toxin-1 (TSST-1), but other exotoxins such as enterotoxins B or C may be implicated.[9,10] These exotoxins have characteristics of superantigens with potential to stimulate large numbers of Th1 cells, particularly CD4+ T cells, without MHC II restriction.[3] The result of the non-restricted stimulation of lymphocytes is the overproduction and

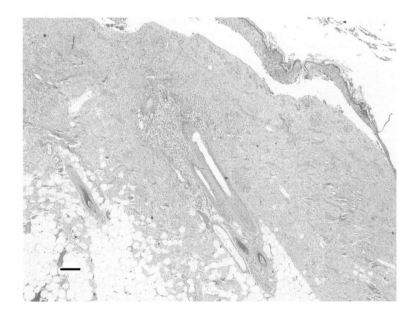

Fig. 5.7.5 Canine staphylococcal TSS-like syndrome. Panepidermal full thickness necrosis with dermo-epidermal splitting. Late stage of evolution of TSS-like induced lesions. There is secondary inflammation surrounding the central follicular unit. H&E; bar = 200 μm.

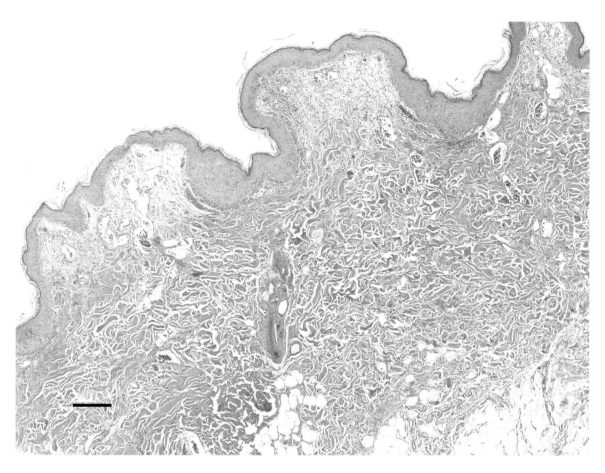

Fig. 5.7.6 Canine staphylococcal TSS-like syndrome. Epidermal hyperplasia, superficial dermal infiltrates, dermal oedema and dermal vascular dilation. H&E; bar = 150 μm.

release of a cascade of Th1-type cytokines, mostly by lymphocytes.[2,3,18,22–25] Keratinocytes and macrophages may be also contributing to the process with additional secretion of cytokines.[7] The most important cytokines produced are TNF-α and TNF-β, interleukin (IL)-1, IL-2, IL-6 and interferon (IFN)-γ, which are considered responsible for the clinical signs in humans.[1,3,9,22,23]

The non-specific stimulation of T cells is preferentially targeted to particular subpopulations of T cells bearing variable β-chain-specific genes in the T-cell receptor (TCR).[3,18,26,27] Therefore, although the stimulus is not restricted by the normal pathways of antigen presentation, there is favoured stimulation of T-cell subpopulations.[2,3] In the case of keratinocytes, the superantigens may directly activate cytokine production after binding to MHC II when overexpressed on their surface.[6,7]

Bacterial colonisation of the skin does not necessarily predispose to TSS, and the host susceptibility to the bacterial exotoxins is apparently determined by the isoform of MHC II proteins, as a result of the different ability of those molecules to present the superantigens to T cells.[3,7,27] This may explain why exotoxin-producing strains can be isolated from sick dogs and people that are not suffering from TSS, as well as from normal individuals.[3,16,17]

Despite the relatively frequent reports of staphylococcal TSS in humans, a similar condition is rarely reported in veterinary medicine. A single case of staphylococcal TSS has been described in a horse, which was initiated by pneumonia.[4] Clinically the horse showed pitting oedema, petechia of the mucosae, and multiple vesicles on the extremities evolving to skin sloughing.[4] This clinical presentation is similar to the dogs in this report and to human cases in the literature.[10,12]

The clinical picture of the dogs in this article, and in cases of human staphylococcal TSS, is different from the previously reported case of staphylococcal TSS in a dog,[28] and from reported cases of canine streptococcal TSS.[29] In these previously reported cases there was regional infection but without characteristic widespread cutaneous lesions of TSS, as seen in humans and in the dogs we report here.

In humans, the criteria for the diagnosis of TSS include fever, low systolic blood pressure, skin rash, and systemic involvement of three or more organic systems; gastrointestinal (vomiting, diarrhoea), musculoskeletal (myalgia, increased CK), mucosae (hyperaemia of mucous membranes), renal (increased BUN and creatinine, pyuria), hepatic (increased AST, bilirubin or ALT), blood (thrombocytopenia) and central nervous system (disorientation).[10] All the dogs in this report had systemic signs and multi-organic involvement. Clinically, they showed depression, cutaneous erythema and oedema, hypoalbuminaemia, neutrophilia, anaemia and fever as the most common signs. Pitting oedema and systemic signs were also described in the reported case of TSS in a horse.[4] Less common signs observed in this study indicating multi-organ involvement included neuromuscular pain, increased CK, vomiting and coagulation abnormalities. The high mortality rate in the dogs described herein (55%) contrasts with the mortality rate in people (around 3%[10]). This difference may reflect a low index of suspicion for TSS in dogs and subsequent delayed treatment. A standardised clinical work-up in suspicious cases may help to define the most prevalent clinical parameters in dogs with staphylococcal TSS.

Bacterial culture and subsequent isolation of bacterial toxins is indicated for a definitive aetiological diagnosis of staphylococcal TSS. Unfortunately, characterisation of bacterial toxins is not done routinely in clinical veterinary medicine, but only sporadically in research settings.[16,17] Production of TSS-1 and other superantigenic staphylococcal toxins has been reported for *S. intermedius*, the most common canine cutaneous staphylococcus.[16,17,20]

The histopathological diagnostic criteria for staphylococcal TSS have been clearly defined in the human literature.[14,30] Hurwitz and Ackerman[14] identify the requisites for diagnosis as: dermal perivascular and interstitial infiltrates with neutrophils and lymphocytes, dermal oedema and vascular dilation, single cell keratinocyte degeneration, spongiosis and neutrophilic epidermal infiltration. Other findings include epidermal microabscesses, eosinophilic infiltrates, superficial haemorrhages, parakeratosis and clustering of degenerate keratinocytes.[14] Confluent epidermal necrosis and vasculopathy have also been described for human staphylococcal TSS.[30] The histopathological constellation of signs in human staphylococcal TSS closely matches the dogs in this study.

Bearing in mind the morphological features observed in the cases described in this study, the main histopathological differential diagnoses in dogs include erythema multiforme (EM) and sterile neutrophilic dermatosis (canine Sweet's-like syndrome). Neutrophils are not the predominant cellular infiltrate in the upper dermis in EM; instead lymphohistiocytic interface dermatitis predominates and lymphocytes, rather than neutrophils, surround the degenerate keratinocytes.[15]

Sterile neutrophilic dermatosis in dogs is a relatively newly recognised condition.[31] In humans it is often produced as a response to drug administration, systemic infections, or internal malignancies.[32] Histopathologically, in humans and dogs, there is a mild to marked neutrophilic infiltrate in the upper dermis, often with dermal oedema, neutrophilic exocytosis and vasculitis.[31,33] In contrast to staphylococcal TSS, single keratinocyte degeneration is generally not reported, although small numbers may be seen in some cases.[34]

In summary, a syndrome resembling human staphylococcal TSS is described in 11 dogs. To the authors' knowledge, a syndrome with these characteristics has not been described previously in dogs. Although isolation of TSS exotoxins was not performed, the condition is considered consistent with staphylococcal TSS based on its close resemblance to the disease in humans. A mortality rate of >50% was found in this small group of dogs, and although not clearly determined by this study, early treatment with cephalexin might have prevented fatal outcome in some cases. Awareness of the existence of this condition in dogs may help to reduce the high mortality rate that is predicted by this report.

References

1 Hackett, S.P., Stevens, D.L. Superantigens associated with staphylococcal and streptococcal toxic shock syndrome are potent inducers of tumor necrosis factor-beta synthesis. *Journal of Infectious Diseases*, 1993; **168**: 232–235.

2   Goodlick, L., Braun, J. Revenge of the microbes. Superantigens of the T and B cell lineage. *American Journal of Pathology,* 1994; **144**: 623–636.

3   Ulrich, R.G. Evolving superantigens of *Staphylococcus aureus. FEMS Immunology and Medical Microbiology,* 2000; **27**: 1–7.

4   Holbrook, T.C., Munday, J.S., Brown, C.A., Glover, B., Schlievert, P.M., Sanchez, S. Toxic shock syndrome in a horse with *Staphylococcus aureus* pneumonia. *Journal of the American Veterinary Medical Association,* 2003; **222**: 620–623.

5   Stevens, D.L., Bryant, A.E., Hackett, S.P., *et al.* Group A streptococcal bacteremia: the role of tumor necrosis factor in shock and organ failure. *Journal of Infectious Diseases,* 1996; **173**: 619–626.

6   Nickoloff, B.J., Mitra, R.S., Green, J., *et al.* Accesory cell function of keratinocytes for superantigens. *Journal of Immunology,* 1993; **150**: 2148–2159.

7   Travers, J.B., Hamid, Q.A., Norris, D.A., *et al.* Epidermal HLA-DR and the enhancement of cutaneous reactivity to superantigen toxins in psoriasis. *Journal of Clinical Investigation,* 1999; **104**: 1181–1189.

8   Vergeront, J.M., Evenson, M.L., Crass, B.A., *et al.* Recovery of staphylococcal enterotoxin F from the breast milk of a woman with toxic shock syndrome. *Journal of Infectious Diseases,* 1982; **146**: 456–459.

9   Jupin, C.S., Anderson, S., Damais, S., Alouf, J.E., Parant, M. Toxic shock syndrome toxin 1 as an inducer of human tumor necrosis factor and γ interferon. *Journal of Experimental Medicine,* 1988; **167**: 752–756.

10 Tolan, R.W., Dhawan, V.K. *Toxic Shock Syndrome.* In: Jaimovich, D., Konop, R., Rauch, D., Steele, R., eds. *eMedicine.* 2003. http://www.emedicine.com/PED/topic2269.htm.

11 Davis, J.P., Chesney, P.J., Wand, P.J., LaVenture, M. Toxic-shock syndrome: epidemiologic features, recurrence, risk factors and prevention. *New England Journal of Medicine,* 1980; **303**: 1429–1435.

12 Todd, J., Fishaut, M., Kapral, F., Welch, T. Toxic shock syndrome associated with phage-group I staphylococci. *Lancet,* 1978; **2**: 1116–1118.

13 Davis, J.P., Osterholm, M.T., Helms, C.M., *et al.* Tri-stage toxic shock syndrome study. II. Clinical and laboratory findings. *Journal of Infectious Diseases,* 1982; **145**: 441–448.

14 Hurwitz, R.M., Ackerman, A.B. Cutaneous pathology of the toxic shock syndrome. *American Journal of Dermatopathology,* 1985; **7**: 563–578.

15 Scott, D.W., Miller, W.H., Griffin, C.E. In: *Muller and Kirk's Small Animal Dermatology.* W.B. Saunders, Philadelphia, 2001: 279–310, 729–740.

16 Burkett, G., Frank, L.A. Comparison of production of *Staphylococcus intermedius* exotoxin among clinically normal dogs, atopic dogs with recurrent pyoderma, and dogs with a single episode of pyoderma. *Journal of the American Veterinary Medical Association,* 1998; **213**: 232–234.

17 Hendricks, A., Schuberth, H.J., Schueler, K., Lloyd, D.H. Frequency of superantigen-producing *Staphylococcus intermedius* isolated from canine pyoderma and proliferation-inducing potential of superantigens in dogs. *Research in Veterinary Science,* 2002; **73**: 273–277.

18 Choi, Y., Kotzin, B., Herron, L., Callahan, J., Marrack, P., Kappler, J. Interaction of *Staphylococcus aureus* toxin 'superantigens' with human T cells. *Proceedings of the National Academy of Sciences (USA),* 1989; **86**: 8941–8943.

19 Lee, P.K., Kreiswirth, B.N., Deringer, J.R., *et al.* Nucleotide sequences and biological properties of toxic shock syndrome toxin 1 from ovine and bovine-associated *Staphylococcus aureus. Journal of Infectious Diseases,* 1992; **165**: 1056–1063.

20 Edwards, V.M., Deringer, J.R., Callantine, S.D., *et al.* Characterization of the canine type C enterotoxin produced by *Staphylococcus intermedius* pyoderma isolates. *Infection and Immunity,* 1997; **65**: 2346–2352.

21 Sanchez, S., Glover, B.M. Prevalence of staphylococcal toxins in equine isolates determined by polymerase chain reaction (abstract). *Abstracts of the General Meeting of the American Society of Microbiology,* 2003; **103**: Z–008.

22 Marrack, P., Blackman, M., Kushnir, E., Kappler, J. The toxicity of staphylococcal enterotoxin B in mice is mediated by T cells. *Journal of Experimental Medicine,* 1990; **171**: 455–464.

23 Miethke, T., Wahl, C., Heeg, K., Echtenacher, B., Krammer, P.H., Wagner, H.T. Cell-mediated lethal shock triggered in mice by the superantigen staphylococcal enterotoxin B: critical role of tumor necrosis factor. *Journal of Experimental Medicine,* 1992; **175**: 91–98.

24 Stiles, B.G., Bavari, S., Krakauer, T., Ulrich, R.G. Toxicity of staphylococcal enterotoxins potentiated by lipopolysaccharide: major histocompatibility complex class II molecule dependency and cytokine release. *Infection and Immunity,* 1993; **61**: 5333–5338.

25 Jardetzky, T.S., Brown, J.H., Gorga, J.C., *et al.* Three-dimensional structure of a human class II histocompatibility molecule complexed with superantigen. *Nature,* 1994; **368**: 711–718.

26 Choi, Y., Lafferty, J.A., Clements, J.R., *et al.* Selective expansion of T cells expressing Vβ2 in toxic shock syndrome. *Journal of Experimental Medicine,* 1990; **172**: 981–984.

27 Herman, A., Croteau, G., Sekaly, R.P., Kappler, J., Marrack, P. HLA-DR alleles differ in their ability to present staphylococcal enterotoxins to T-cells. *Journal of Experimental Medicine,* 1990; **172**: 709–717.

28 Girard, C., Higgins, R. *Staphylococcus intermedius* cellulitis and toxic shock in a dog. *Canadian Veterinary Journal,* 1999; **40**: 501–502.

29 Miller, C.W., Prescott, J.F., Mathews, K.A., *et al.* Streptococcal toxic shock syndrome in dogs. *Journal of the American Veterinary Medical Association,* 1996; **209**: 1421–1426.

30 Vuzevski, V.D., Van Joost, T., Wagenvoort, J.H.T., Michiels-Dey, J.J. Cutaneous pathology in toxic shock syndrome. *International Journal of Dermatology,* 1989; **28**: 94–97.

31 Vitale, C., Gross, T.L. Putative Rimadyl™-induced neutrophilic dermatosis resembling Sweet's syndrome in 2 dogs (abstract). In: *Proceedings of the 15th Annual Meeting of the American Academy of Veterinary Dermatology/American College of Veterinary Dermatology,* Maui, HI, 1998: 69.

32 Cohen, P.R., Kurzrock, R. Sweet's syndrome revisited: a review of disease concepts. *International Journal of Dermatology,* 2003; **42**: 761–778.

33 Malone, J.C., Slone, S.P., Wills-Frank, L.A., *et al.* Vascular inflammation (vasculitis) in Sweet's syndrome: a clinicopathological study of 28 biopsy specimens from 21 patients. *Archives of Dermatology,* 2002; **138**: 345–349.

34 Sitjas, D., Puig, L., Cuatrecasas, M., De Moragas, J.M. Acute febrile neutrophilic dermatosis (Sweet's syndrome). *International Journal of Dermatology,* 1993; **32**: 261–268.

Part 6

Workshops

Canine hypothyroidism

J. Hall[1] (Chairperson), S. Waisglass[2] (Secretary)

[1] Ontario Veterinary College, University of Guelph, Guelph, Ontario, Canada
[2] Doncaster Animal Clinic, Veterinary Dermatology Service, Thornhill, Ontario Canada

Jan Hall *Canada* welcomed the delegates, commenting that the purpose of the workshop was to discuss canine hypothyroidism, its diagnosis, and methods of testing for the disease. She commented that although most veterinarians and dermatologists are 'comfortable' with hypothyroidism, perhaps we are too 'familiar' with it.

Jan Hall Hypothyroidism is considered to be the most common spontaneous endocrinopathy of dogs. I would say that it is also probably one of the most misdiagnosed diseases. When I consider my own referral cases at the University of Guelph, I see many dogs already diagnosed with hypothyroidism prior to referral, with the diagnosis based on results that I question; this is really the issue that we need to deal with. We realise that there are some issues with the accuracy of these diagnostic methods, and their utility in the diagnosis of hypothyroidism.

To start, I would like to discuss the methods that you are using to diagnose hypothyroidism, and what you find to be most successful in your part of the world. We know that the clinical signs of hypothyroidism can be somewhat vague, and we are aware that hypothyroidism can predispose to other diseases. Thus, although we rely on obviously abnormal test results to make a diagnosis, ultimately, we often place the patient on thyroid supplementation, and then judge whether the diagnosis was correct based on the response to supplementation.

Further, I would like to discuss the effect of non-thyroidal factors on thyroid function. We need to remember that many diseases and conditions (such as hyperadrenocorticism, hypoadrenocorticism, and even exocrine pancreatic insufficiency and weight loss) have been shown to affect thyroid function and our ability to try to determine whether a dog is truly hypothyroid. We also know that drug therapy can significantly affect thyroid function in some patients, causing them some patients to appear to be hypothyroid, or actually become truly hypothyroid on occasions.

We will not specifically discuss treatment of hypothyroidism, but I would like to discuss how people are monitoring hypothyroidism. How many people are doing follow-up tests on hypothyroid dogs, and how many are merely monitoring by response to therapy?

The audience was polled as to their methods of diagnosis; nobody utilised response to therapy to make a diagnosis.

Peter Webb *UK* I recommend, at my diagnostic laboratory, that a basal total T4 (TT4) and endogenous canine TSH (cTSH) be used as the first line of attack, although some people are just using a TT4 to make a diagnosis. (Attendees from Germany, Switzerland, Belgium, Sweden, Canada and Ireland were in agreement.)

Sheila Torres *USA* I do that too. However, if a dog is otherwise healthy and is not taking medication that would interfere with thyroid function, and I'm suspicious of hypothyroidism based on clinical signs, I may just start with a TT4 because it's an inexpensive test. And again, I'm assuming that no other factors that can influence the thyroid function are present. In that case, I may not combine it with an endogenous cTSH.

Elisabeth Shultz *Germany*   I may decide, based on the dog's age, whether to run just a TT4 or add a cTSH, but often run just a TT4. The cTSH is also used to differentiate primary from secondary hypothyroidism.

Richard Hertling *Canada*   In my practice, I run a general diagnostic profile with a TT4 and cTSH. (Several attendees confirmed that they were adding a TT4 to a chemistry profile as part of a geriatric screening test.)

Jan Hall   What value do you use to determine that a patient with a low TT4 is indeed hypothyroid?

Peter Webb   The methodology that is used in the test is critical in determining these values in that it will vary greatly between tests. For example, colorimetric T4 will have a completely different reference range than radioimmunoassay and chemiluminescence. And the in-house ELISA kit did not fare well when compared to RIA in a previous study.[1]

Claudia Nett-Mettler *Switzerland*   The in-clinic analyser used at our facility includes a TT4, but the values sometimes appear to be inconsistent with the diagnosis.

Jan Hall   Although some authors have raised questions about the accuracy of in-clinic testing, Peterson reported that if you use the test routinely, and follow the normal range for the test kit, the results are consistent, at least with the kit he evaluated (the IDEXX SNAP T4).[2] He suggested that the test would be appropriate as an initial screen for hypothyroidism, or to monitor therapy.

Peter Webb   Clinical pathology articles that I've read were not very supportive of the in-clinic test.

Elizabeth Hussey *USA*   I rely on a free T4 (FT4) by equilibrium dialysis to make a diagnosis. If the test result is at the lower end of the normal range and I have a high index of suspicion of hypothyroidism, I will go ahead and treat the patient.

Sheila Torres   I would not treat a patient whose test results were within the normal range. The important thing is the method of testing that the laboratory is using. If you rely on that method, results (for normal patients) should be within the normal range. There are many conditions that may cause test results to be in the lower end of the normal range, and I would not treat most of the low-normal patients. I treat patients based on clinical signs and test results that are significantly low.

Jan Hall   Is there a T4 level where one might be comfortable with a diagnosis of hypothyroidism, a grey zone, and then a point where one might be comfortable that the patient is euthyroid? The literature suggests that patients with a level of >25 nmol/L are euthyroid, <20 nmol/L are in the non-diagnostic range, and a level <11 nmol/L should be regarded as probable hypothyroidism. I realise that you are probably going to do another test, but is that the range that is typically being quoted by the laboratories you use? (Most people agreed.)

Peter Webb   Our lab adds to the results an interpretation by our veterinary staff. Regarding the FT4 chemiluminescence test, I don't believe it gives you more information than the TT4; however, the FT4 by equilibrium dialysis is a good second-line test. (Most people were interpreting their own thyroid tests rather than following the laboratory assessment.)

Jan Hall   Do members of the audience have FT4 by equilibrium dialysis or chemiluminescence, or both, available? It seems like most people do not know how the tests are performed in their labs. None of the other attendees seem to believe that chemiluminescence is as good a test as the FT4 by equilibrium dialysis.

Jan Hall asked Peter Webb to explain the methodology of FT4 by equilibrium dialysis.

Peter Webb   FT4 by equilibrium dialysis involves passing the serum across an electric gradient through a membrane to eliminate 'extraneous factors'. It is very time-consuming, as it takes 24 hours to run, needs to be performed in a water bath, and, there are many potential pitfalls. It is very important to have good technique. The analogue techniques are radioimmunoassay or chemiluminescence, and although they claim to measure FT4, they are probably measuring TT4.

Elizabeth Hussey   I use FT4 by equilibrium dialysis as my first-line test. Although the laboratory I use will not run FT4 by equilibrium dialysis without running a TT4, I look at the FT4 by equilibrium dialysis more closely. This test has been considered to be the 'gold standard' test in the past.

Sheila Torres   This is probably true, if you listen to what endocrinologists like Duncan Ferguson and Richard Nelson are saying. FT4 by equilibrium dialysis is less affected by disease and drugs, but we must be aware that it is still affected by those factors.

Jan Hall   I have been running FT4 and TT4 together at the Ontario Veterinary College for the last 4 years and can't remember a situation where my FT4 by equilibrium dialysis and TT4 were discordant.

Peter Webb   There may be a difference in the patients seen at a referral institution compared to the patients in the general population.

Sheila Torres   In the future, we should start to establish normal ranges based on the breed, as this is very important. For example, we know that sight hounds have normal thyroid levels that are lower, and sometimes significantly lower, compared to other breeds. It would be wonderful if we could have breed-related normal levels.

Peter Webb   I agree that a diagnosis of hypothyroidism in sight hounds is very, very difficult.

Jan Hall   This raises another issue that was presented at the 2003 Forum of the ACVIM, concerning the effect of weight loss on thyroid function.[3] They showed that the dogs that typically tended to be very thin, or dogs that dramatically lost weight for any reason, had significantly lower basal T4 than dogs that were somewhat overweight. They suggested that dogs that tend to be thin have a lower basal metabolic rate, and do not need as much thyroid stimulation.

Peter, how do you establish a normal range for your lab?

Peter Webb   Extensive testing, basically.

Jan Hall   But do you have specific breed-related data for these normal animals that come in?

Peter Webb   Unfortunately not. It's very difficult to get 200 normal animals.

Stephen Waisglass *Canada*   There are patients that come to our facility who are on thyroid supplementation because of a lab report that stated that even though the blood tests are within normal ranges, the patient should be placed on thyroid supplementation because the levels are too low for this age of dog. Are there any comments about age-related levels and whether age makes a difference?

Nicolette Salmon Hillbertz *Sweden*   Have there been any studies to check thyroid levels in the first 2 years of age in the dog?

Sheila Torres   I think there was a study performed that showed that thyroid levels are higher when dogs are much younger, and they decrease as they get older. In my experience (and it has been reported also), it's very unusual for a dog to have a diagnosis of primary hypothyroidism when they are younger than 2 years of age.

Jan Hall   Is anyone routinely testing dogs less than 2 years old? Certain breeds perhaps? What about other breeds? Are there breeds in other countries where you are noticing a higher incidence of hypothyroidism, and you may choose to follow more frequently than others?

Golden retrievers (**Richard Hertling**; **Rebecca Frey**, *Sweden*), golden retriever and yellow Labrador retrievers (**Elisabeth Schulz**), dobermans (**Sheila Torres**), Hovawarts (**Ursula Mayer**, *Germany*).

Jan Hall   How many people still perform a TSH stimulation test? (Three people in the audience still do TSH stimulation testing.)

Claudia Nett-Mettler   I use the human product, but it is quite expensive. Therefore it is only done if the other tests are in the grey zone.

Martin Bucksch *Germany*   I use the industrial grade product. In order to avoid anaphylactic reactions, I inject it subcutaneously.

Jan Hall   How often are you using it?

Martin Buksch   Every 2 weeks or so.

Jan Hall   Are you still using cTSH?

Martin Buksch   We don't use cTSH anymore. There was a study in Germany where they found that endogenous TSH is oftentimes within the normal range, even though the patient is hypothyroid, including primary hypothyroidism.

Jan Hall   Would anybody else like to comment on the usefulness of cTSH? Some people believe that it is completely useless.

Sheila Torres   I think that the cTSH test should not be used as the sole test, but can be used in conjunction with TT4 or FT4 by equilibrium dialysis. However, I don't use it routinely.

Jan Hall   What percentage of dogs that are hypothyroid would have a normal cTSH, in your experience?

Sheila Torres   About 25%.

Jan Hall   I think that's what it says in the literature; 25% of dogs that are hypothyroid have a normal cTSH.

Sheila Torres   It was reported in one study that cTSH seems to be less affected than TT4, and even possibly FT4, by drugs and diseases. So, if you have any reasons to test a dog that is on a medication that can affect the thyroid function test, a cTSH test should be included.

Peter Webb   We offer cTSH testing with TT4 testing and not alone. We see about 20% false negatives and about 1% false positives.

Jan Hall   I think everybody is now in agreement here that we don't use cTSH by itself, but it is a useful tool in conjunction with TT4 or FT4, preferably an FT4 by equilibrium dialysis. At the Ontario Veterinary College, we routinely run an FT4 by equilibrium dialysis along with TT4 (because I wanted to compare the FT4 and the TT4 together), and a cTSH. Although the literature tends to suggest that the FT4 by equilibrium dialysis is the better test, I am not absolutely convinced of that.

Sheila Torres   I agree with you, and still offer the TT4 despite the fact that the literature states that the FT4 is the better test. I agree with you that I don't see many cases where there is a significant difference.

Jan Hall   Once again this may be because, as Peter said, as referral specialists we are seeing a different population of patients. What are those of you in general practice doing?

Elizabeth Hussey   I primarily run a TT4 and an FT4 by equilibrium dialysis. I'm sort of on the fence. I don't run the cTSH routinely. I used to run the cTSH on every case, but it increased the costs, and it never changed what I would have done with just the TT4 and FT4 by equilibrium dialysis.

Stephen Waisglass   What about running the TT4 and cTSH and using an FT4 by equilibrium dialysis to 'break the tie' in the case of discordant results?

Sheila Torres   Although I would do that, the TT4 by solid-phase radioimmunoassay (RIA) is affected by the presence of T4 autoantibodies, and the FT4 by equilibrium dialysis is not. It is possible that if you have a hypothyroid dog with high levels of antibodies, the TT4 will be normal. And so measuring the FT4 by equilibrium dialysis rather than TT4 by RIA is preferable.

Jan Hall   There are thyroglobulin autoantibodies, as well as anti-T3 and anti-T4 antibodies. The literature tends to suggest that 20 or 30% of patients don't have antibodies even though they are supposed to have lymphocytic thyroiditis. How significant are they? The literature tends to suggest that thyroglobulin autoantibodies are perhaps the most important. Is everybody in agreement with that statement? How many people are measuring thyroglobulin antibodies?

Peter Webb   Generally a tertiary line of investigation. Perhaps it is performed more often in younger animals with a low TT4, or predisposed breeds and sight hounds.

Elisabeth Schulz   I am following thyroglobulin autoantibodies as well as T3 and T4 autoantibodies in Labrador retrievers.

Sheila Torres   Measuring thyroglobulin autoantibodies is part of a panel in many universities. The OFA (Orthopedic Foundation for Animals) thyroid registry uses the thyroglobulin autoantibody test. We all know that the test just means that the pet has inflammation of the thyroid gland but does not necessarily mean that the patient is hypothyroid. As the disease progresses very slowly, it could be years before the patient shows clinical signs. But because it's a genetic disease, if it's positive, the dog shouldn't be bred.

Jan Hall   Is there any equivalent to a thyroid registry in Europe, where breeders can have their dogs checked for their potential for hypothyroidism? (There was no response from the audience.)

Claudia Nett-Mettler   When I was at the university in Zurich, we were looking into thyroid antibodies in various breeds of dogs that were clinically healthy. We had quite a number of dogs with positive tests, i.e. they had thyroid antibodies. These dogs were followed over 2 years or so and were clinically normal.

Peter Webb   Anti-T3 and anti-T4, while academically interesting, don't have much effect on diagnosis.

Jan Hall   The only time to consider anti-T3 or anti-T4 antibodies is when you have animals with thyroid results that are either very, very low or are very, very high (depending on methodology).

Martin Buksch   Is this for FT4 or just TT4?

Peter Webb   It's only TT4 that is affected, not FT4 by equilibrium dialysis. The reason is methodology. Since the FT4 is passed through a membrane, you won't get the same interference of antibodies as you do with a TT4.

Stephen Waisglass   We were able to demonstrate a number of years ago that, in a case where the TT4 results were extremely high at 795 nmol/L (ref. range: 15–58 nmol/L) due to interference by anti-T4 antibodies, the FT4 by chemiluminescence was affected as well, but FT4 by equilibrium dialysis was not.

Jan Hall   One of the Canadian laboratories likes to run the whole panel including autoantibodies in order to get 'the big picture' as they say. They may interpret results as 'the pet is becoming hypothyroid'. One point that comes out of this workshop very strongly is that you have to be clear as to what methodology your lab is using for the tests that you request.

Martin Buksch   What do you do if you have a patient with low thyroid values (e.g. 11 nmol/L) but no other clinical signs or biochemical abnormalities?

Jan Hall   I was referring to a 2001 article by Robert Kempainnen.[4] They were the values he used. Typically, I like to see results at 5 or 6 nmol/L before I am really concerned that the dog is hypothyroid. However, I've seen sight hounds with these levels that are clinically normal. I am personally not a great fan in looking for this disease unless I have symptoms that make me want to look there. There are certainly veterinarians who, when presented with the difficult pyoderma or other skin problems, start to look. Typically in my practice, I need a reason to consider hypothyroidism, and if TT4 comes out at a low level, I then run a cTSH, and perhaps an FT4. What do other people do?

Sheila Torres   I agree 100% with you. In order to diagnose hypothyroidism, look at more than the results of thyroid hormone tests. The clinical signs should be there plus the test results, that's extremely important. Otherwise, you will be diagnosing hypothyroidism all the time.

Jan Hall   Unfortunately, I believe this is happening too often. I have always maintained that hypothyroidism would not be diagnosed as much, and not as many dogs would be treated for it, if there were significant negative effects from thyroid medication. Does anybody do the TRH response test? I see there is nobody performing this test.

Rebecca Frey   If we are saying that hypothyroidism is over-diagnosed, and that there are false positive and false negative results with the cTSH test, and you have a dog that has low TT4 results, how do you make a diagnosis?

Sheila Torres   All of the tests have false positive and false negatives. You have to have some signs of the disease present. Test results should not be well within the normal range in an affected dog. If they are abnormal (e.g. low TT4) and the dog is otherwise healthy, and there is nothing else that may have caused the TT4 value to be abnormally low (such as concurrent drugs),

I think it's OK to do a treatment trial. It's just important to be very critical. If clinical signs are present, as you supplement the dog you're always going to see a positive response in the beginning. However, in the euthyroid patient, the response becomes static and the dog doesn't continue to improve – at least that has been my experience.

Stephen Waisglass Although we are concerned about the false positive and false negative results in each test, one would expect that if all of the tests concur and point toward hypothyroidism, it would be unlikely that the dog is euthyroid.

Sheila Torres I agree.

Jan Hall If you consider recent studies that have looked at dogs with clinical signs that were consistent with hypothyroidism, only about 30% were confirmed by testing to be truly hypothyroid. Is response to therapy ever justified?

Sheila Torres If the clinical signs are due to hypothyroidism, there should be a significant improvement. If there is not, stop the medication. Be very critical when doing a treatment trial.

Jan Hall The reality with hypothyroidism is that the answers are not always clear-cut. It is important that we make sure that our clients accept the fact that the thyroid gland is very labile, and that drugs can affect results; sulfonamides may produce clinical hypothyroidism. Other drugs will lower thyroid levels, such as corticosteroids and phenobarbital, and there are questions as to whether potassium bromide might slightly lower thyroid levels (some studies suggest it might, others don't). We should approach hypothyroidism from the point of view that there are sometimes no clear-cut answers and we may need to serially test dogs if we are not sure, rather than treat them.

Martin Buksch If you see a patient on a referral basis that you don't feel is hypothyroid, but is already being treated with thyroid supplementation, for how long must the thyroid supplementation be discontinued before thyroid function can be evaluated?

Jan Hall We see many dogs already on thyroid supplementation. In fact, I am often surprised to see the number of pruritic, atopic dogs presented on thyroid medication. I usually do not discontinue the thyroid supplementation. If a dog has received thyroid treatment for 6 months to a year, the thyroid gland has shrunken as a result of the supplementation. Nuclear imaging can be performed to demonstrate how small the gland gets on therapy. By the time you take the dog off therapy, and wait 2–3 months, the gland may be so atrophic that it still may not have recovered. Retesting at this time produces borderline values. Thus, for animals already on supplementation, I may advise the client that I don't believe the results are significant, but I might perform a 4–6-hour post-pill test to make sure the thyroid levels are adequate. The dilemma is trying to determine what is best for the patient. It may be better to keep the patient on thyroid supplementation because there are few side effects, as long as the levels are acceptable

Martin Buksch Are you saying that by supplementing you can cause irreversible damage?

Sheila Torres A study in 1989 did show a trend, but I'm not sure anybody knows.

Jan Hall I think the important thing that has come out of this workshop is that clients are informed that although there are tests for the disease, these tests are not infallible. They are not as clear-cut as we would like. I personally think we should retest suspect thyroid dogs a lot more before treating them presumptively.

References

1 Lurye, J.C., Behrend, E.M., Kemppainen, R.J. Evaluation of an in-house enzyme linked immunosorbent assay for quantitative measurement of serum total thyroxine concentration in dogs and cats. *Journal of the American Veterinary Medical Association,* 2002; **221**: 243–249.
2 Peterson, M.E., DeMarco, C.L., Sheldon, K.M. Total thyroxine testing: comparison of an in house kit with radioimmuno- and chemiluminescent assays. *Journal of Veterinary Internal Medicine,* 2003; **17**: 396.
3 Daminet, S., Jeusette, I., Duchateau, L., Diez, M., Van de Maele, I., De Rick, A. Evaluation of thyroid function in obese dogs and in dogs undergoing a weight loss protocol. *Journal of Veterinary Medicine A. Physiology Pathology Clinical Medicine,* 2003; **50**: 213–218.
4 Kempainnen, R.J., Behrend, E.N. Diagnosis of canine hypothyroidism: perspectives from a testing laboratory. *Veterinary Clinics of North America: Small Animal Practice,* 2001; **31**: 951–962.

Leishmaniasis and other arthropod-vectored diseases

Z. Alhaidari[1] (Chairperson), C. Rivierre[2] (Secretary)

[1] Clinique Vétérinaire, Roquefort les Pins, France
[2] Marseille, France

New approaches for evaluating and controlling immunodeficiency in canine leishmaniasis (L. Ferrer)

Luis Ferrer *Spain*   Canine leishmaniasis is a very complex disease, and before sharing results and explaining our approach to research on canine leishmaniasis, we need to define the problems. The main problems to consider are: some infected dogs remain free of clinical signs whereas others develop a severe life-threatening disease; and some affected dogs respond to conventional therapy whereas others do not. We do not understand why this happens. In the literature, the general explanation given is that the immune response differs between dogs, and that different types of immune responses lead to different outcomes.

However, we still face three major problems which constitute the three lines of our research: first, we do not understand in detail the immune response in leishmaniasis; second, we cannot evaluate or predict the immune response (many tests are needed to be able to do this and predict the outcome of the disease in a single patient); and third, we also need tools to modulate the immune response and direct it in the direction that we think is better for the patient.

Much information about the immune response in leishmaniasis already exists. We know that this disease is a consequence of an infection and an inadequate Th1-specific immune response. Affected dogs have both a general and a specific depression of cell-mediated immunity. We also know a lot about the immunopathologic mechanisms that are involved in the disease, and that cause lesions and clinical signs. Finally, we know that clinically affected dogs are immunodeficient in the acute phase of the disease. Indeed, to define a patient with immunodeficiency, at least two of the following four criteria have to be fulfilled: recurrent and/or chronic course of infection; infection with common non-pathogenic (opportunistic) or unusual infectious agents; severe and often atypical infectious disease manifestation; delayed, incomplete, or lack of response to antimicrobial therapy. All of these criteria are present in canine leishmaniasis, therefore it can be considered that patients with leishmaniasis are immunodeficient.

This may explain the typical deep pyoderma that we see in dogs with leishmaniasis. Mixed infections with several microorganisms are also quite common in this disease, because there is a specific deficiency in the immune response and a general depression of the T-cell response.

Our group has focused on evaluating the immune response in leishmaniasis from a very practical point of view. Specifically, we are considering the best tools that we can offer to the clinician to evaluate the immune status of a patient. We already have a good system to evaluate the humoral immune response. The humoral response can be monitored through protein electrophoresis and specific antibody titres (using laboratory tests such as ELISA, immunofluorescence and

Western blots). We probably need more sophisticated ways to evaluate the B-cell system, but in general, these tests give an approximate idea of B-cell reactivity in a patient. However, we do not have good methods for evaluating the T-cell response, which is more relevant in this disease. The T-cell response can be monitored by assessing the number and functionality of T cells. Ideally, one should combine these two approaches in a single patient. Recently, studies have demonstrated that evaluation of the number of T cells (CD3+, CD4+, CD8+) is a useful approach to define the immune status of a dog. We know that in a normal dog, CD4+ T cells constitute approximately 45% of the circulating lymphocytes, and about 23% are CD8+ T cells. The normal CD4/CD8 ratio is 2:1. In canine leishmaniasis there is a well-documented reduction in the number of circulating CD4+ cells, and therefore a reduction of the CD4/CD8 ratio (< 1.5:1). The reduction in CD4+ T cells shows good correlation with clinical signs and infectivity (higher infectivity is associated with a lower CD4+ count). General practitioners should keep in mind that normal dogs have approximately 1000 CD4+ cells per microlitre in their blood (the total number of lymphocytes is 2300 cells per microlitre). In the very acute phase, diseased dogs only have 400–800 CD4+ cells per microlitre. In the early stages of treatment, there is an increase in the number of CD4+ T cells for the first 2–3 months, followed by a very slow decrease back to within the normal range after 6–9 months. In research studies, CD3+, CD4+ and CD8+ are usually evaluated. However, in practice, the use of only one of these parameters is useful (usually CD4+). The same criteria are used in human AIDS patients to evaluate their response to antiviral therapy.

At the present time, three tests are available to evaluate T-cell function in leishmaniasis: the leishmanin skin test (LST) involves the intradermal injection of leishmania antigen and is very easy to perform; the lymphocyte proliferation assay (LPA) evaluates the response of blood lymphocytes when they are incubated with different mitogens (including leishmania antigen) and is much more complicated; and the interferon-gamma (IFN-γ) bioassay which evaluates the production of IFN-γ after stimulation of T cells with various antigens (including leishmania antigen), and it is also more complicated. Unfortunately, there is a lack of good tests to assay canine cytokines.

We have evaluated the three assays in leishmaniasis. The assays were performed on 56 healthy dogs living in an endemic area. Of these 56 dogs, 48 were considered infected with leishmaniasis by PCR. All three tests were performed for each dog and we found that the LST is probably the most sensitive one with 37 positive results, followed by the IFN-γ bioassay which was positive in 32 dogs. These two tests are very different, and only the LST can be used in clinical practice. The LPA appears to be less sensitive with only 16 positive results.

Finally, there are the questions of whether we can modulate the immune response, and how can the course of the immune response be changed? Older classic, non-specific immunomodulators (such as levamisole, cimetidine and bacterial products) have been demonstrated to be poorly effective. On the other hand, newer generation immunomodulators (such as cytokines and anti-cytokine antibodies) are not yet marketed for use in the dog and are unlikely to be on the market for the next 10–15 years. A major problem with these products is their toxicity, which restricts their use to experimental conditions, and they are therefore not very appealing to drug companies. What we probably need is a product that stimulates T-cell responses in dogs that could be used in various diseases (such as demodicosis, relapsing pyoderma, etc.). Finally, a recent new approach focuses on the hormone prolactin which has a potentiating effect on T-cell-mediated immune responses in mice. Several prolactin-releasing drugs are marketed and could be used as immunomodulators.

To conclude, I think that we should focus on developing drugs that induce immune responses that are not absolutely specific for one particular disease.

Emmanouil Papadogiannakis *Greece* If the CD4/CD8 ratio of a dog with leishmaniasis has normalised, is it appropriate to discontinue treatment?

Luis Ferrer There is no scientific evidence to answer this question. When the ratio has normalised, we usually continue therapy for a few more months, before deciding to discontinue the treatment.

Polymerase chain reaction (PCR) and serology in the diagnosis of leishmaniasis (G. Marignac)

Genivieve Marignac *France* Serology involves the evaluation of the body's immune response to infection by assessing the presence of circulating antibodies against the parasite. The PCR detects the parasite itself by amplification of the parasite DNA. *Leishmania* organisms are kinetoplastidea, and the kinetoplast of these organisms contains much DNA. Consequently, there are two structures that carry DNA in the cell, which has some importance when PCR is performed.

Both of these diagnostic tools have disadvantages. Serology can be negative if no antibody is present; for example, if the parasite is no longer present, or if the host does not react to the presence of the parasite. On the other hand, a positive PCR does not mean that the parasite detected is responsible for the disease.

The basic PCR technique can be briefly described as follows: a DNA sequence that is known from gene banks (called a primer) is mixed with DNA polymerase and with the purified DNA from the test sample. Exponential amplification of the DNA occurs, and electrophoresis reveals what sequence has been amplified. Real-time quantitative PCR refers to another type of PCR in which a fluorescent stain is added to the mix. Each time there is amplification, the fluorescence can be measured and allows quantification of the amplification.

PCRs are not all identical. The choice of the primer is very important. In leishmaniasis, there is also a difference depending on the origin of the DNA, either genomic or kinetoplastic. In the kinetoplast, the DNA sequences are repeated within minicircles (for example, a gene on a minicircle can be present 3000× in one parasite). Therefore, if a kinetoplastic primer is used, the sensitivity of the test will be better than if genomic DNA is used. Another important point to consider is the choice of the organ to sample. As *Leishmania* are intramacrophagic parasites, it is best to sample organs with many macrophages, such as skin (skin scraping), eye conjunctiva (conjunctival swab), or lymph node. Blood is not a good choice, as there are relatively low numbers of circulating macrophages.

The sensitivity and specificity of PCR are difficult to assess from the literature, because all tests are run differently. In most studies, the specificity of PCR is close to 100%. An advantage of PCR is that it allows the differentiation of species, and detects which strain of *Leishmania* is causing an infection. This is very important in humans because of drug resistance of some strains of the parasite. Thus, PCR allows the clinician to select the appropriate drug.

The sensitivity of PCR varies between 50 and 90%, depending on the PCR technique (many of these stud-

ies used blood as samples) and also on the gold standard of the study (culture, serology, etc.). The sensitivity can be improved by several techniques that are currently used in experimental settings.

In conclusion, PCR can allow early detection of the parasite (as early as 1 day after infection), and can detect asymptomatic carriers. Therefore, the results should always be interpreted in the light of clinical signs.

Leishmaniasis in cats: a continuing enigma (P. Bourdeau)

Patrick Bourdeau *France*   For a long time, leishmaniasis was not considered to be a disease affecting cats. In the past, several arguments against the existence of leishmaniasis in cats were presented; for example, the failure of experimental inoculation, and negative results of surveys. More recently, arguments that support its existence have appeared, such as successful inoculation which was achieved in 1984. Several serological surveys of leishmaniasis in cats have been performed. Leishmaniasis has been described in Algeria, Egypt, Iraq, Jordan, Portugal, Spain, France, Switzerland, Ile de la Réunion, USA, Argentina and Venezuela. This accounts for a total of 198 published cases, 30 of which are isolated cases and 168 cases were from general surveys. Approximately 50% of these cats were clinically affected and 50% were asymptomatic cats.

There is little information available regarding the epidemiology of leishmaniasis in cats. The age of affected cats is often not described, although Pernisi reported in 2002 that 35% of the cats were less than 1 year old. There is apparently no sex, breed or haircoat predilection, and both domestic and stray cats can be affected.

In people, an association between leishmaniasis and HIV infection is frequently seen in Southern Europe, where antibodies against *Leishmania* are found in 50% of HIV-positive people. Is leishmaniasis in cats related to some underlying diseases? At first, several reported cases were negative for FeLV and FIV. However, one case was found positive in 1993, and in 2002, about 70% of FIV-positive cats had positive serology for leishmaniasis. However, FIV infection is not a prerequisite for the development of leishmaniasis. There are also some reports of concurrent leishmaniasis in cats with demodicosis, ringworm, toxoplasmosis, eosinophilic granuloma complex, pemphigus foliaceus, and in association with administration of some drugs (such as corticosteroids).

The following *Leishmania* spp. have been described in cats: *L. infantum* in Europe, Vietnam, Ile de la Réunion; *L. venezuelensis* in Venezuela, for which the cat is a regular host; *L. tropica* in Iraq and Jordan.

The clinical signs of leishmaniasis in cats are diverse. Similar to dogs, 50% of affected cats present with general clinical signs that include weight loss, anorexia, fever, and occasionally kidney failure. Skin lesions are frequently noted, with ulcers being the most frequent dermatological sign and present in more than 50% of cases. Ulcers mainly affect the face (ears, lips, tongue), but they can be disseminated over the entire body. Nodules are also frequently seen, affecting approximately 50% of cases. We do not know whether they are oriental sores (infection with *L. tropica* responsible for cutaneous leishmaniasis), or inoculation sores. Nodules can be single or multiple, and may appear all at once or progressively over a period of time. They are generally small (< 1 cm), occasionally large (> 3 cm), and affect mainly the ears, nose, lips, eyelids and the extremities. Lymphadenopathy is another frequent clinical finding, occurring in 30% of cases. The following manifestations of leishmaniasis in cats are also mentioned in the literature: bronchopneumonia, digestive signs, stomatitis, enlarged spleen and liver, and ocular signs (uveitis).

In summary, about 50% of the cases in research are asymptomatic cats. Cutaneous forms frequently exist and involve all the different *Leishmania* spp. True visceral forms also exist (reported from Ile de la Réunion and Spain), as well as the classical generalised leishmaniasis (systemic, cutaneous), and the ocular form. The problem we face is distinguishing between *Leishmania* spp. that are found in the skin; is it cutaneous leishmaniasis, or is it visceral leishmaniasis with skin tropism?

The diagnosis relies on clinical signs and laboratory testing. Haematology reveals a non-regenerative anaemia, leukopenia, monocytosis and leukocytosis. Hyperproteinaemia can be present, but is usually less severe than in dogs. The FIV and FelV status, as well as liver and kidney function, should be assessed. Serology can be performed with immunofluorescent antibody (IFA) testing (positivity is above 80 IU), which remains the test of reference, although low titres are usually found (20–40 IU). There is little data on ELISA and Western blot. Serum agglutination tests have been abandoned. At this time, IFA and PCR appear to be the recommended tests to perform. Cytology from smears and histopathology of biopsies (from ulcers, lymph nodes or bone marrow) may also be performed. Immunohistochemistry might be interesting to confirm the presence of *Leishmania* spp. in skin biopsy samples.

There is little data available regarding the treatment of feline leishmaniasis, as reports of treatment of only 11 cases are documented. Most cases were euthanised without treatment, or they died spontaneously. Surgical treatment may be possible in some cases. Anecdotally, the following drugs have been reported to lead to improvement in cats: pentamidine, ketoconazole and allopurinol; glucantime and ketoconazole; ketoconazole alone; fluconazole, allopurinol and IFN-α; and allopurinol and prednisolone. Treatment failure has been reported with clotrimazole, topical paromycin, metronidazole and spiramycin.

In conclusion, leishmaniasis surely exists in cats, but these animals are quite resistant to this infection. Many infections spontaneously resolve, or the cats remain indefinitely asymptomatic. The cat is not important in the epidemiology of the disease.

Zeineb Ailhadari *France*   I have never seen a single case. Who in the audience has seen a cat with leishmaniasis?

Luis Ferrer   I have seen one case.

Emmanouil Papadogiannakis   I have seen one case.

Lyme borreliosis: does it exist in dogs? (C. Von Tcharner)

Claudia Von Tcharner *Switzerland*   The infective agent of Lyme disease is *Borrelia burgdorferi*, a gram-negative spirochaete. Lyme borreliosis is transmitted by ticks: *Ixodes ricinus* in Europe; *Ixodes scapularis* in the eastern part of the USA; and *Ixodes pacificus* in the western part of the USA. The spirochaete is transmitted only after 24–48 hours of tick attachment. If the tick is immediately removed, no infection will develop.

In people, the disease starts with skin lesions, called erythema migrans. Tumour-like lesions (pseudolymphocytomas) can also occur. Lyme borreliosis exists in dogs, but the main clinical signs are arthritis or endocarditis. The diagnosis of Lyme borreliosis should be made based on the following criteria: a dog living in a tick-endemic area, history of a tick bite, typical clinical signs (mainly lameness), laboratory testing using ELISA or indirect immunofluorescence, culture (which is extremely difficult) or PCR, and rapid response to antibiotics.

The presence of skin lesions is variable. Hot spot-like skin lesions, usually present behind the ear, were first thought to be due to borreliosis. However, histopathology of these lesions revealed diffuse lymphocyte infiltration with some plasma cells and macrophages, but *Borrelia* spp. organisms could never be found.

Since no *Borrelia* DNA was found in the intact skin sampled near tick bites, there is no proof that *Borre-lia* spp. organisms are responsible for the skin lesions described. To my mind, these hot spot-like lesions are probably due to the tick bite itself, and not due to *Borrelia* spp. organisms themselves.

Patrick Bourdeau   If skin lesions exist and are due to the organism (meaning the organism is observed in the lesions), then these lesions should be present at the location of the tick bite. Since *Ixodes ricinus* bites exclusively on the head, the skin lesions should be found exclusively on the head.

Parasites and antiparasitic drugs

R.S. Mueller[1] (Chairperson), M. Shipstone[2] (Secretary)

[1] Ludwig-Maximilians University, Munich, Germany
[2] Dermatology for Animals, Brisbane, Australia

Ralf Mueller *Germany* presented two studies conducted by Patrick Bordeau. The first detailed a study on selamectin spot-on formulation (Revolution®, Pfizer Animal Health, New York, USA) for the control of ectoparasites in mice. The two parasites studied were *Myobia musculi* and *Myocoptes musculinus*.

Ectoparasites in small rodents are one of the most common problems resulting in presentation of the pet to a veterinarian. Many products are used to treat ectoparasites in small rodents, without scientific evidence of efficacy in these species. This study was designed to establish such efficacy. The reported distribution of selamectin following application is via surface spread, absorption and distribution via the bloodstream with subsequent re-excretion. Selamectin also accumulates in the sebaceous glands. Although the toxic dose in rodents is quite high, the low body weight means that this toxic dose may be applied unless the quantity to be used is precisely measured. Selamectin was applied twice at 30-day intervals comparing two doses: 12 mg/kg and 24 mg/kg. A preliminary study was conducted to establish a practical dosing regimen. Two drops of 6% selamectin solution were applied to a cotton bud (Q tip) and this was then rubbed on the back of an average 5-g weight mouse. This provided a dose which was approximately equivalent to 12 mg/kg. A pilot study showed that a dose of 48 mg/kg produced no adverse effects. The second phase of the study used 550 mice (all with confirmed ectaparasitic infestations) of 8 different strains in 2 separate rooms. Mice in one room were treated with two drops of a 6% selamectin solution (12 mg/kg), the mice in the other room were treated with two drops of a 12% selamectin solution (24 mg/kg). One cage in each room was left as an untreated control for the first month. The control cages were treated for the first time with the second application, 1 month after the initial treatment. Treatment was repeated after 1 month on all mice. The study was blinded, such that the investigators assessing parasite numbers (on tape preparations), and those assessing clinical scores, were unaware of the treatment group. The lesions were scored on a scale of 1–5 where: 1 = no lesion on any animal in an individual cage, and 5 = lesions on several animals in the cage. No signs of toxicity were noted in any of the treated animals. Interestingly, when the treatment groups were combined, the clinical score did not change in the mice of either treatment group. However, when the different strains of mice were separated, differences in clinical scores were present. Mite numbers were determined by adhesive tape strips at 0, 2, 4 and 8 weeks. Both dose rates gave good efficacy at week 8, although efficacy is seen much earlier at the 24 mg/kg dose rate. Egg production was reduced by 95% by day 90 and most eggs found at this stage were empty. However, some eggs may still be viable and thus allow the development of a new generation of parasites. There did not appear to be any relationship between the clinical score and parasite numbers. It was thought that other factors, independent of parasitism, were important in the development of pruritus and the behaviour of these mice. In summary, there appears to be a strain difference rather than a dose difference, in improvement of the clinical scores. Further, both dose rates are effective in parasite control, but two applications may be insufficient to guarantee elimination of all viable eggs and thus re-infestation is possible.

The second study by Patrick Bourdeau investigated diffusion of the spot-on and spray formulations of fipronil (Frontline®, Merial, France) in the hair coat of the dog. Spot-on formulations are very popular and easier to apply than sprays.

The first part of the study was to validate a method of evaluating the insecticidal activity of fipronil on the hair coat, and then to compare the efficacy of fipronil following spot-on and spray application. Three dogs were treated with the spot-on formulation, and one with the spray. The spot-on was applied according to label directions on the back of the neck. The spray was applied evenly over the entire body. At various time points from day 0 (pretreatment) to day 70, hair was collected by clipping 20 cm² from different areas of the body. Hair was stored in plastic bags and frozen until all samples were collected and then tested together for their flea insecticidal activity. Ten newly emerged fleas were placed in individual containers, to which a 125-mg aliquot of hair from each sampling period was added. The containers were then placed in an incubator and flea mortality was measured at 1, 6, 12, 24 hours. All tests were performed in duplicate and minimal variability was noted between the two samples. The spot-on formulation showed rapid 100% mortality from samples collected from the back within 2 days of application. This contrasted with samples collected from the side of the thorax where 100% mortality was not reached until 20–30 days post application. However, the spray formulation showed rapid 100% mortality from all sites. Similar results were seen after 37 days, indicating the spot-on formulation did not diffuse evenly over the body, and the spray formulation had a sustained effect. The poor efficacy of the spot-on was due to inadequate insecticide concentration in this *in vitro* test model. In summary, it would appear that the spray formulation was more efficacious as it was evenly applied, while the spot-on formulation did not diffuse as widely as previously thought. It was our hypothesis that fleas were killed when using the spot-on formulation because their movement over the body brought them into contact with the fipronil, rather than as a result

of even diffusion of the active ingredient over the entire body surface.

Ralf Mueller commented on the difference in the incidence of flea allergy dermatitis (FAD), which he found to be high in Melbourne, Australia, but close to non-existent in Fort Collins, Colorado (1600 m elevation and very low relative humidity). He also noted that it was much more difficult dealing with FAD 20 years ago than it is today. The audience was then asked about the incidence of FAD in their practices. Practitioners from Spain (Barcelona), Argentina, UK, Germany, Brazil, South Africa and southern California all reported FAD as a common disease. Those from Colorado, Sweden and Spain (Madrid) found the incidence to be low.

In summary, most did not have problems in treating FAD, but there was a significant variation in the incidence of the disease depending on the practice location.

The audience was then surveyed about which products were used. Carbamates and organophosphates were not used by anyone. Fipronil was used by approximately 60% of the audience, imidacloprid by 30%, lufenuron by 30%, nitenpyram by 25% and pyrethrin by 25% of attendees. Selemectin was not used by anyone. Only 15% used products according to the label recommendations, whilst 85% used them more frequently.

Ralf Mueller commented on potential insecticide resistance with the use of single products versus the use of two products with different modes of action (insect growth inhibitor with adulticides), the so-called 'integrated flea control'.

Mike Shipstone *Australia* asked about recommended frequency of application of products by the audience. Imidacloprid and fipronil spot-on were applied every 2 weeks by 10%, and every 3 weeks by 90%, while fipronil spray was applied every 2 weeks by 20% of the audience.

Hans Koch *Germany* reported on a survey he conducted in his clinic which found that 80% of owners had their pets in their own beds. He then raised the question as to whether this information should be considered with respect to potential adverse effects for in-contact humans.

Ralf Mueller said that he asked if the clients had children. In many instances the clients with children will request a product that minimises the risk of potential chemical contact for their children. He then asked how many in the audience will modify their advice, and not use the externally applied active ingredients, if the pet lives in a house with young children? (Most of the audience agreed.)

Hans Koch asked if anybody in the audience had experienced problems from pharmaceutical companies because of warnings they gave owners regarding human exposure to insecticides. He had been warned by an industry representative not to continue with such advice. However, he still felt it important to give such advice, particularly with products that are known to cause problems for exposed people (i.e. organophosphates, permethrin, etc.). He emphasised the need to know all the potential side effects of any product being recommended for use on animals, in such close-contact situations. For this reason, he was a strong advocate for products taken orally, as they carry less risk for potential contamination. Some products may persist for a long time in indoor environments, and may cause long-term effects that may become apparent after only 15–20 years. He gave the example of Rachel Carson's book *Silent Spring*, which detailed the long-term effects of DDT. He emphasised that it was his opinion that it is the responsibility of the veterinarian to be fully aware of the potential side effects, the half-life and the accumulation of products they are dispensing.

Rene van den Bos *Netherlands* thought it important, and in the interest of both industry and veterinarians, to keep in close contact when talking about effects of products that are used, especially with respect to ectoparasiticides. Any adverse effects should be reported back to the industry. For any product registered anywhere in the world, extensive safety studies are usually performed to recognise any side effects and report these on the label. However, after release of a product for commercial use, further side effects may become known and need to be reported to the company which is then obliged to report these adverse events back to the regulatory authorities.

Ralf Mueller agreed about the importance of reporting any unexpected adverse effect. In his experience, the companies involved had been extremely cooperative in the few cases where he thought an adverse reaction had occurred. He asked how many participants had seen any adverse effects with any of the newer products other than local alopecia and/or inflammation.

Ann Evans *USA* saw an English bulldog that had been treated topically with selamectin. The dog had a long history of allergic skin disease. Roughly 10 days after treatment, it began to slough the skin on its back and side. Interestingly, it spared all of its clinically affected areas (facial folds, external ear canals), but looked like a severe burn in the expected diffusion area of the product. If she had biopsied the affected skin, she would have expected to see a TEN-like reaction pattern.

Ralf Mueller had seen diarrhoea for 24 hours postoral lufenuron dosing in three German shepherd dogs. This adverse reaction had occurred again with subsequent dosing of the drug.

Hans Koch commented that we need to be very careful about attributing an adverse reaction to a product, as application of a product and the perceived adverse reaction may not always be linked.

George Doering *USA* indicated that he clipped a small (4 cm^2) area on the back of cats' necks prior to application of fipronil. He noticed that the product seemed to fill the entire area and appeared to come in much closer contact with the skin, rather than becoming trapped in the hair coat.

Ann Evans asked if it is a problem if a company tested the efficacy of a product without clipping the hair, and if we then clipped the hair coat and had increased penetration of the product and delivery of a higher dose.

Ralf Mueller commented that most of the companies conduct high-dose application studies during product development that should take into account this effect, and thus he would not personally be worried about that. However, if any adverse effect was seen, it should be taken into consideration.

Demodicosis

This was seen as a common problem by nearly all of the audience. Diagnosis was made via deep skin scraping in most cases. Trichograms were used by nine participants, of whom six found them to be better than skin scrapes, particularly when sampling from the feet. Two people found trichograms to be equivalent to skin scrapings, and one person felt that trichograms were less effective than skin scrapings.

Ralf Mueller previously found the trichogram to be less effective, but had recently changed his technique following discussions with **Luc Beco** (*Belgium*). He now plucks an area of similar size to the area he would normally cover with a scraping, and examines all the collected hair roots. This technique is also used by **Kerstin Bergvall** (*Sweden*).

There are two broad categories of demodicosis; juvenile- and adult-onset. The relative incidence of each category seen by the audience was questioned. The consensus was that approximately 25% of patients have adult-onset demodicosis. The audience was asked how many times they find underlying disease in the adult-onset cases.

Ann Evans commonly found iatrogenic hyperadrenocorticism due to administration of glucocorticoids.

Ralf Mueller was unable to find an underlying disease in roughly 30% of cases, but had a number of dogs where initial investigation did not identify an underlying cause, but 12 months later the classic signs of an underlying disease manifested. He had seen this in cases with hyperadrenocorticism, lymphoma and hypothyroidism.

George Doering found underlying disease in <50% of the adult-onset cases, despite thorough investigation.

Hans Koch regularly looked at faecal samples for 5 consecutive days, and in a large percentage of cases found intestinal parasitism. He believed that intestinal parasitism may be a factor.

Ralf Mueller asked what other tests people were performing to look for underlying disease.

Hans Koch recommended complete blood count, serum biochemistry profile, faecal examination and urinalysis (he found some patients with chronic urinary tract infection).

Ralf Mueller asked if anyone investigates for diseases other than hyperadrenocorticism, hypothyroidism, neoplasia, iatrogenic causes, or intestinal parasitism. None of the participants went beyond evaluating the above. He then raised the question of who investigated for hypothyroidism initially, and who was worried about euthyroid sick syndrome.

Cathy Curtis *UK* commented that she now had recombinant human TSH available and used this test for the diagnosis of hypothyroidism.

Ralf Mueller did not have a TSH stimulation test available and did not rely on TSH assays, so he normally began treatment with antibiotics for 4 weeks and started the miticidal therapy before investigating thyroid function after about 6 weeks of therapy.

Kerstin Bergvall *Sweden* looked for hyperadrenocorticism first, either iatrogenic (most common) or spontaneous. The next most common underlying disease would be neoplasia, and then hypothyroidism.

Ralf Mueller asked how many participants had problems with treating individual cases on some occasions. Most participants responded positively. Then the question was posed which treatment was used regularly. Amitraz was used as the first choice of treatment by the veterinarians from the UK, but only because of the legal requirement in that country to do so. No other participant used this as their first choice. The most common first-line product used was ivermectin, while one participant used milbemycin; none used moxedectin or doramectin.

Hans Koch had a case of severe, adult-onset generalised demodicosis (*D. canis*) in an Old English sheepdog. The owner was unwilling to clip the dog, and he treated with amitraz with no improvement. Investigation for underlying disease failed to identify a cause. The dog was supplemented with vitamin E and essential fatty acids, and the diet was changed, with no effect. Finally, one side of the chin and one side of the chest (the most severely affected locations) were treated with calcipotriol (Davamex®, Curaderm®), which is normally used in humans with psoriasis. Calcipotriol has an effect on the proliferation and differentiation of epidermal cells. It was applied to the one side of the body once a day for 6 weeks in conjunction with amitraz (previously used with no effect) and led to marked improvement in the treated areas. The product may be altering sebum and affecting the proliferation of juvenile mites. He stated that with these very preliminary findings, this medication may be useful in future refractory cases in combination with an antiparasiticide to change the micro-environment of the mite. The product is available as a cream or lotion; the lotion was used in this case.

Ralf Mueller asked how many participants used a concentration of amitraz that was different to the label recommendation.

Martin Briggs *South Africa* started with the label recommendation and increased incrementally to end with a maximum concentration of 700 ppm.

Ralf Mueller further inquired what side effects of amitraz were seen.

Cathy Curtis saw haemorrhagic diarrhoea in some dogs, and hyperglycaemia, particularly when used in a diabetic dog.

Ralf Mueller stated that in this case there would be a clear medical reason not to use amitraz and legally use other systemic products. When he used amitraz, lethargy for a day or two after application was the most common side effect.

He then asked, how many participants used this product in the clinic only (only one member of the audience). The reason for his question was he had one owner with an asthmatic reaction, and another owner who had been hospitalised intermittently due to severe migraines of no apparent cause, but the migraines had started after amitraz use on her dog with demodicosis. The migraine headaches never returned once the amitraz was discontinued (when the dog's demodicosis was cured).

Cathy Curtis stated that veterinarians should also be concerned with allowing a diabetic owner to use this product.

Kerstin Bergvall commented that veterinarians should also be concerned about staff administering the product and should ensure that staff are not exposed to this product excessively.

Ralf Mueller commented that staff routinely using the product should be protected with the necessary safety equipment such as gloves, gowns, mask, etc. and that dipping should only be performed in a well-ventilated area. He then asked how many of those using ivermectin administered the bovine injectable formulation orally?

George Doering used the equine oral formulation and felt it to be more effective than the bovine product.

Ralf Mueller asked about the application frequency. Ivermectin was administered every second day by two participants, and everybody else used the product daily.

He then commented that ivermectin should be effective when given every other day due to its long half-life, even at the 300 µg/kg dose. However, he thought that owner compliance would decrease with every second day administration. He recommends daily administration as it is much easier to remember a daily task, whereas with alternate day dosing the product may only be used every 3 or 4 days.

Anne Evans commented on the daily administration. Accumulation within the tissues may be needed to achieve sufficient concentration to kill the parasite. With administration every second day it may take longer to be effective.

Ralf Mueller proceeded to ask the related question about the dose rates used. Many people administering ivermectin every other day used a higher dose (400 or 600 µg/kg) and so would achieve the same dose over time.

Michael Shipstone once plotted the theoretical dose achieved in a steady-state using a half-life of 1.8 days. The steady state was reached at around 6 weeks and at that point the actual dose received was around 1200 µg/kg.

Ralf Mueller once saw a case of a West Highland white terrier that developed ataxia after approximately 10 weeks of therapy with ivermectin. For this reason, he always recommends that owners continue to monitor the dog for adverse effects (lethargy, ataxia, dilated pupils, etc.) even after long periods on therapy. In a study he and others published in 1999, they reported occasional adverse effects in non-collie, non-herding breed dogs. In one case, a Samoyed was dosed with 100 µg/kg and was comatose for 24 hours.

Hans Koch asked whether any participants used a new test that is available to identify dogs susceptible to toxicity. (Nobody used it at this time.)

Ralf Mueller stated that the test identifies whether an individual has the genes which code for P-glycoprotein (a drug efflux pump). Those deficient in the gene are susceptible to the toxic effects of ivermectin. He asked the question if we should routinely test for the presence of the gene. For the past 15 years he had identified susceptible animals by gradual daily increases of ivermectin according to the following schedule: 50, 100, 150, 200, 300 µg/kg once daily, then continued with 300 µg/kg once daily for the duration of treatment. This allowed identification of those that were susceptible before a lethal dose was reached. The P-glycoprotein test would alleviate the need for this build-up, but one of these methods should be used. In no practice should an animal be started at 300 or 600 µg/kg without previous testing or gradual dose increases.

Ralf Mueller asked how many participants used a maintenance dose of 300 µg/kg once daily. Most (75%) of the audience used this dose, while the rest used a dose of up to 600 µg/kg once daily. In a number of cases, 300 µg/kg was used initially with insufficient response, with an adequate response seen after the dose was increased to 600 µg/kg once daily.

The reason for Ralf Mueller's question was the controversy about the correct dose which seemed to be related to the geographic location of the practice. Practitioners from the south-eastern US seemed to have significantly more problems with demodicosis and need higher doses compared to Colorado, and even Australia, where he rarely had to use a dose higher than 300 µg/kg once daily to achieve a response.

Kerstin Bergvall usually started with 300 µg/kg, but occasionally administers up to 400 µg/kg.

Ralf Mueller asked what the group thought of the success rate. Most participants estimated the success rate for juvenile-onset generalised demodicosis to be 70–80%, and most considered the success rate of adult-onset demodicosis to be similar.

Ralf Mueller commented that, in his recent review, it was only ivermectin that worked as well in adult-onset cases as in juvenile-onset cases. However, only 16 cases could be included in this comparison. He mentioned the need to go further and treat a larger number of dogs with adult-onset demodicosis and re-evaluate the success rate. He then asked what dose of milbemycin participants used when this was the selected drug.

Kerstin Bergvall used 1 mg/kg once daily with good results.

Ralf Mueller mentioned that the Swedish studies evaluating milbemycin oxime for the treatment of canine demodicosis were performed with a large number of dogs and achieved good results with the low dose of 1 mg/kg. He had not found similar results, nor had other dermatologists in the United States and Australia. When he used it at this low dose, the animals seemed to clear, but then relapsed quickly once the drug was discontinued. The relapse rate was dramatically lower when the 2 mg/kg dose was used. He speculated that this may be due to climate or differences in strains of demodectic mites.

Ralf Mueller then asked the audience about moxidectin, its dose and frequency of administration. Two participants used the product.

Martin Briggs used it at 400 µg/kg orally once weekly.

Ralf Mueller occasionally used it. He mentioned the problem of anaphylactoid reactions seen with subcutaneous administration. These didn't seem to be prominent with oral administration based on current studies.

Vitamin E was originally used by a Brazilian dermatologist who treated three groups of dogs with generalised demodicosis with vitamin E alone, vitamin E in combination with amitraz, and amitraz alone. All groups went into remission, although the combination group recovered fastest. This study was never duplicated elsewhere. The major question was whether the fact that previously neglected dogs entered the laboratory and then were well fed and cared for may have had a significant impact on the results. Another study could not identify significant differences of vitamin E levels in the serum of dogs with demodicosis, compared to normal dogs. In personal communication with **Craig Griffin** about the study, he had the clinical impression that only one dog had benefited significantly from the vitamin E supplementation. A number of the participants use vitamin E as a supplement or adjunctive therapy.

Hans Koch regularly supplements with essential fatty acids and believes that many dogs benefit.

Ralf Mueller commented on the effect of fatty acids on the immune response in humans and mice, and the possibility that they may affect the cell-mediated immune response. Further studies are needed to investigate this in dogs with demodicosis.

Anti-fungal therapy

D.J. DeBoer[1] (Chairperson), D.N. Carlotti[2] (Secretary)

[1] University of Wisconsin, Madison, Wisconsin, USA
[2] Cabinet de Dermatologie Vétérinaire, Bordeaux-Mérignac, France

Doug DeBoer *USA* I would like to first express my appreciation to Janssen Animal Health for generously sponsoring this workshop. Amongst many fungal diseases, dermatophytosis and *Malassezia* dermatitis are important for veterinary dermatologists. Over the last 10–15 years there has been a real explosion in our knowledge about treating dermatophytosis. This workshop will deal mainly with therapy of dermatophytosis.

Relation between the chemical structure and the effect of azole compounds (K. Vlaminck)

Kathleen Vlaminck *Belgium* Dermatomycosis requires a multi-faceted approach including treatment of the animal (topical or systemic), treatment of the environment (including humans, if affected) and hygienic measures. Azole compounds form a major group of chemical structures, generating agents capable of meeting the needs and requirements for treatment of dermatomycosis and other fungal diseases. Historically, in human medicine, the first broad-spectrum topical antifungals were produced in 1967 (e.g. miconazole, enilconazole). They were followed in 1970 by the first broad-spectrum oral azole anti-fungal, ketoconazole. The triazoles were introduced in the eighties, e.g. itraconazole. In veterinary medicine, miconazole was introduced in 1977 (Surolan®), enilconazole in 1980 (Imaverol®/Imaveral®), ketoconazole in 1983

(Ketofungol®), enilconazole for the treatment of the environment in 1986 (Clinafarm®) and itraconazole in 2003/2004 (Itrafungol®). These subsequent introductions reflect progress in chemical development of the azole nucleus, resulting in higher bioavailability, broader spectrum of activity, higher potency (against systemic fungi, dermatophytes and yeasts) and increased fungal specificity (with a higher safety profile). Miconazole has an imidazole nucleus, a dichlorophenyl group, and its proper branching is responsible for its action on fungi and gram-positive bacteria. Enilconazole has its own branching, which allows it to be used in a vapour phase. It is also lipophilic, with a residual activity of a few days. The introduction of a dioxalane group increases the bioavailability, hence the systemic effect and a broader spectrum. Changing the imidazole group into a triazole group (three nitrogen atoms) increases the potency and specificity. For instance, itraconazole has a more specific activity on dermatophytes and is lipophilic. Fluconazole is also very lipophilic. Propiconazole is used in plant protection. Posaconazole is water-soluble and has side effects. Fluconazole has two triazole groups and is very hydrophilic. It is used in human medicine for the treatment of superficial mycoses; however, resistance has developed (particularly by *Candida* spp.). Voriconazole is very water-soluble.

It becomes obvious that there are many possible chemical variations based on the basic azole nucleus, and additional variations are possible. The main clinical needs and objectives should influence future developments (duration of action, spectrum, etc.).

Doug DeBoer In systemic therapy, what are our clinical objectives that are not being met, or that could be better met through the miracle of drug formulation and chemistry?

Charles Chen *Taiwan* Once a week administration.

Doug DeBoer One desirable thing would be infrequent administration. Do we know if all triazoles accumulate in the epidermis of all species?

Kathleen Vlaminck Trials have been done in several laboratory animals, dogs and cats. There is a tremendous accumulation of itraconazole in the epidermis, and in sebaceous glands above all. In fact, intermittent therapy is possible with itraconazole (alternate weeks) but not once a week administration. In contrast, fluconazole is hydrophilic and does not accumulate, whereas posaconazole is comparable to itraconazole.

Abdo Kallasy *Lebanon* What about vaccination?

Kathleen Vlaminck Vaccination is still in an early stage of development as a prophylactic measure. It can be useful as a therapeutic measure but there are restrictions for its use. In catteries or kennels, a multi-faceted approach may include vaccination.

Doug DeBoer One of the other needs we have, which hopefully can be solved some day, is for more active systemic drugs for treatment of some of the deep mycoses, for example phaeohyphomycosis or dermatophytic mycetoma, for which we still depend largely on surgical excision. Do you see a possibility that by altering these molecules we will have better therapy for deep mycoses?

Kathleen Vlaminck According to our chemical research department, there is a chance.

Helen Globus *USA* We need more safe and effective antiseptics for the environment, at least in the US, since people are very overwhelmed when they're told to bleach everything.

Kathleen Vlaminck Enilconazole is not approved

by the FDA in the US, as it is in Canada and Europe. We have two formulations; Imaverol® for animals and Clinafarm® (foggers and solution) for the environment that are usable in catteries (and also in poultry houses for aspergillosis).

Ljiljana Pinter *Croatia* What is your opinion about combination therapy, i.e. combined topical, systemic and environmental treatment?

Kathleen Vlaminck Topical treatment of the animal is used alone or with systemic therapy, for example in groups of animals or in severe cases, but disinfection of the environment is essential in all cases. Topical treatments include shampoos (miconazole, chlorhexidine) and the off-label use of enilconazole in cats (which is done in many countries without any problems).

Doug DeBoer Is there a difference in the formulations of Imaverol® and Clinafarm®?

Kathleen Vlaminck Imaverol® can be used in the environment but I would not recommend the use of Clinafarm® in animals because the formulation contains surfactants which could be irritant.

Doug DeBoer That is interesting, as many veterinarians in the US do this, since there is no other option.

Bernard Mignon *Belgium* Could we use topical enilconazole twice monthly instead of twice weekly, not only for financial reasons, but also for obvious practical reasons? Is there a chance to see improved topical formulations, or are your efforts concentrated on systemic drugs only?

Kathleen Vlaminck Washing cats is not simple! Currently there is no plan to further develop any topicals.

Abdo Kallasy Can we treat with systemic drugs only, i.e. without topicals?

Kathleen Vlaminck It depends on the kinetics of the active ingredient. If there is good distribution and residual activity in the skin and hair, you may treat only systemically. You may do this with itraconazole, whereas ketoconazole and griseofulvin are less appropriate.

Inhibition of the growth of dermatophytes by chlorhexidine and miconazole (N. Perrins and R. Bond)

Natalie Perrins *UK*   We have previously demonstrated the synergistic effect of chlorhexidine and miconazole against ten isolates of *M. canis in vitro*. The aim of the present study was to determine whether chlorhexidine (CH) and miconazole (MC) had a synergistic effect against other dermatophyte species of veterinary importance.

Minimum inhibitory concentrations (MICs) of CH, MC, and both together were determined for nine isolates of *T. mentagrophytes* (TM), nine isolates of *T. erinacei* (TE) and four isolates of *M. persicolor* (MP) using an agar dilution technique. Miconazole and CH were dissolved in dimethylsulfoxide and serial two-fold dilutions added to Sabouraud's dextrose agar in a 1:1 ratio. The CH concentrations tested ranged from 100 to 3.12 μg/ml. The MC concentrations tested ranged from 3.12 to 0.024 μg/ml. The MC/CH concentrations ranged from 3.12 to 0.012 μg/ml. A stab inoculation technique was used and growth was assessed after 7 days. The MIC was determined as the lowest concentration at which no mycelial growth was evident, provided that growth was seen on the control plate. Fractional inhibitory concentration indices (FIC index) were calculated to assess the interaction of the two drugs. A FIC index of < 0.5 was defined as synergy, 0.5–1.0 as additivity, 1.0–4.0 as indifference, and > 4.0 as antagonism.

The mean MICs (μg/ml) for CH, MC, and both drugs combined are presented in Table 6.4.1. In this study, a synergistic effect was noted for only one isolate of TE and one isolate of MP. An additive effect was demonstrated for 12 isolates (5 TM, 6 TE, 1 MP), and indifference was noted in 8 isolates (4 TM, 2 TE, 2 MP).

Whilst the results of this preliminary study require verification, there was little evidence of a synergistic

interaction between CH and MC against the dermatophyte species tested. This is in contrast to that found previously with *M. canis*. The *T. erinacei* isolated had a significantly higher MIC for miconazole and the drug combination, when compared to *T. mentagrophytes* and *M. persicolor*. This study indicates that there are species differences in dermatophyte susceptibility to anti-fungal drugs, both alone and in combination. Further studies are required to evaluate the clinical relevance of this.

Doug DeBoer   Dermatophytosis is not always caused by *Microsporum canis* and there may be different optimal protocols to treat dermatophytosis caused by different species, for example *Trichophyton* spp. What are our needs for topical therapy and are our needs met by current products?

Helen Globus   We need better disinfectants for the environment.

Luc Béco *Belgium*   We do need better vehicles such as spot-on or foam formulations.

Helen Globus   We also need something usable on furniture and carpets.

Jacques Fontaine *Belgium*   There is a lack of proof of efficacy of the treatment of the environment. We need trials on the prevention of spreading.

Charles Chen   It depends on the environment; for example, in Taiwan there is no carpet.

Efficacy of commercial vaccines (B. Mignon)

Bernard Mignon *Belgium*   Control of dermatophytosis is problematic. It is a contagious disease, with environmental contamination. Treatment is lengthy, expensive and time-consuming. Vaccines could play a role. Commercial vaccines have been developed for cattle, horses, cats and fur-bearing animals. They are attenuated or inactivated. They are not available everywhere. Ringvac® is an effective attenuated vaccine for cattle and is no longer available in Belgium. Insol® Trichophyton is an inactivated vaccine for cattle. Fel-O-Vax MC-K® was developed for cats but is not available any more. Insol® Dermatophyton is licensed for

Table 6.4.1 Mean MICs (μg/ml) for CH, MC and both drugs combined: comparison with *T. mentagrophytes, T. erinacei* and *M. persicolor*

Agents	*T. mentagrophytes*	*T. erinacei*	*M. persicolor*
CH	28.75 ± 3.12	38.89 ± 6.97	38.75 ± 5.73
MC	0.49 ± 0.07	$1.39 \pm 0.16**$	0.35 ± 0.06
CH + MC	0.47 ± 0.09	$0.99 \pm 0.19*$	0.30 ± 0.08

MIC, minimum inhibitory concentration; CH, chlorhexidine; MC, miconazole.
$*p < 0.05$; $**p < 0.01$.

horses, dogs and cats, but the target species is the horse. There is a lack of published scientific data about the efficacy of these commercial vaccines.

I would like to present the preliminary results of a controlled blinded study to evaluate the preventative and curative efficacy of a commercial vaccine against *T. verrucosum* in field conditions in naturally infected cattle. Seventeen heifers of < 1 year of age were selected; eight of them were naturally infected with *T. verrucosum* at the experimental farm of Liège University. We used an inactivated commercial vaccine containing several strains of *Trichophyton* (including *T. verrucosum*) and marketed for both preventative and curative use. A clinical evaluation was done by a single examiner. The extent of cutaneous lesions was expressed as a percentage of the body surface using a grid diagram, and the severity of alopecia and scaling was expressed as a subjective mean score in individual animals, and in each group. A mycological evaluation was performed by myself and was based on microscopic examination of scales and hair, fungal cultures being less reliable with *T. verrucosum*. Heifers were randomly allocated into two clinically equivalent groups (vaccinated animals and controls). The animals were kept together in the same pen during the whole study. Vaccination was performed in the first group using the protocol recommended by the manufacturer. The animals were evaluated every 2 weeks for 5 months.

Non-infected animals did not develop any infection in either group, and no conclusion could be made as far as the preventative effect of the vaccine is concerned.

There was no significant difference between vaccinated and control-affected heifers. All animals were cured after 5 months. In this study the vaccine was not able to demonstrate any preventative or curative effect.

However, vaccines are marketed and used in practice, and they might be useful. So the question of the efficacy and safety of vaccines against dermatophytosis in cattle, horses, cats and fur-bearing animals remains unresolved.

Jacques Fontaine I have not been very happy with Dermatophyton® in cats since many of the cats remain culture-positive. However, in a group of 200 horses in Brussels, it accelerated time to cure, but did not decrease the number of affected horses.

Ross Bond *UK* Insol D®, an inactivated vaccine, was not effective in either groups of cows or ceremonial horses in London.

Doug DeBoer In the literature, killed or inactivated vaccines typically are not very effective at inducing an immune response. Live or live-attenuated vaccines are generally more effective in this regard. Is there any recent report of the efficacy of live vaccines?

Luc Béco Two papers were published in Germany about treatment with vaccines, but in one of them there was only a 'suspicion' of dermatophytosis and no control group.

Jacques Fontaine There are vaccines in Russia for human beings, particularly children. I don't know if they are killed vaccines.

Ross Bond The Ringvac® vaccine was considered as effective in cattle in tough conditions (non-disinfected pens) in London.

Doug DeBoer The inactivated Fel-O-Vax MC-K® vaccine (*M. canis*-based) was not particularly effective for either prophylaxis or therapy. I wonder if live vaccines intended for horses and cattle have been used in cats, because there is cross-reactivity between dermatophyte species.

Bernard Mignon Insol® Dermatophyton is marketed in Belgium for horses, dogs and cats, but it does not seem to be very effective in carnivores.

Charles Chen What are your own data on vaccination?

Doug DeBoer We presented some data about a modified-attenuated vaccine from *M. canis* in cats. We were not able to demonstrate prophylactic activity and the development of that vaccine for cats was not pursued. A similar vaccine was developed for fur-bearing animals in Scandinavia.

Marie Christensen *Sweden* Ringvac® is marketed in Scandinavia.

Audience *Germany* Some owners would not accept live vaccines as a prophylaxis, particularly on a yearly basis.

Doug DeBoer There is regulatory concern over the potential use of a live spore vaccine in a home environment, particularly if there are immunosuppressed persons in the household.

Bernard Mignon The ideal would be the development of a non-attenuated vaccine, such as a subunit vaccine, but it is difficult.

Clinical presentation of unusual cases (J. Fontaine)

Jacques Fontaine I would like to share with you some practical aspects of the treatment of dermatophytosis. I have been able to use the human formulation of itraconazole for several months, and more recently the veterinary formulation which is going to be launched soon. The recommended dose is 5 mg/kg once daily on an alternate-week basis, for at least 3 weeks.

Case 1 concerns 11 indoor short-haired cats, all infected with *M. canis* for a long time. Previous treatments were not effective, with regular recurrence of infection. Mean age of the cats was 7.5 years, and there were 5 females and 6 males. Clinical signs were variable; only two cats did not have lesions. All cats were culture-positive. Treatment included intermittent itraconazole as indicated above, and enilconazole in the environment at day 0 and day 7. No topical treatment was possible. At day 35, almost all lesions had disappeared, with alopecia still present in six cats and a positive culture in one cat, surprisingly without lesions. At day 56, clinical healing was achieved in all cats and all cultures were negative.

Case 2 is a Persian cat with dermatophytosis, living with a less affected Chartreux. Contagion occurred in all humans living in the household. The Persian cat had been treated with ketoconazole and lufenuron. *Microporum canis* was identified by fungal culture. The Persian cat was clipped. Treatment of both animals included itraconazole as indicated above, topical enilconazole twice a week, and enilconazole at day 0 and day 7 in the environment. At day 35 there was a clear clinical improvement in both cats which were still positive on Wood's lamp, trichogram and culture. Both FeLV and FIV testing were negative in the two cats. At day 60, the Chartreux was clinically normal and culture-negative, but the Persian cat was still affected with one lesion on the tail. At day 90 the Persian was still positive (Wood's lamp, trichogram, culture) with the same area affected. Resistance to itraconazole was suspected and the sys-temic treatment was changed to terbinafine (25 mg once daily). At day 120 the cat was clinically normal but positive on Wood's lamp, trichogram and culture. Sensitivity testing showed sensitivity to itraconazole, terbinafine and posaconazole. Itraconazole was given again. The animal remained clinically normal but positive on Wood's lamp, trichogram and culture, until 9 months after the first visit. The other cat remained negative.

Charles Chen I have had good results with fluconazole in similar situations in Yorkshire terriers.

Chiara Tieghi *Italy* Regular clipping again and continuous therapy could be considered.

Jacques Fontaine Pharmacokinetics indicates that continuous therapy is not necessary.

David Duclos *USA* Perhaps lifelong treatment should be considered if humans were not affected any more.

Doug DeBoer Do we know if azole-resistant strains of *Microsporum canis* exist, or does failure of absorption exist pharmacologically?

Kathleen Vlaminck Resistance is theoretically possible but this is probably not what happened in this case; the strain was not resistant. Other factors may be involved and we don't know what they are.

Jacques Fontaine Maybe we should take skin biopsies to evaluate the cutaneous concentration of itraconazole.

Ross Bond Perhaps a higher dose would be more effective, as a higher dose of antibiotics is sometimes used by clinicians to treat canine deep pyoderma. Pharmacokinetics is perhaps not the same in all animals and some individuals will require higher doses. What about griseofulvin?

Jacques Fontaine Why do such cases occur mainly in Persian cats (and not in all long-haired cats)?

Luc Béco And why no self-cure?

Bernard Mignon How did you do your direct examination and culturing?

Jacques Fontaine   We picked up fluorescent hairs on the tail for direct examination and used a toothbrush for culturing.

Bernard Mignon   Positive cultures performed with toothbrushes may only reflect a mechanical carriage.

Doug DeBoer   We could theorise that there is some sort of genetically determined failure of development of cell-mediated immunity in these Persian cats. In typical cases of ringworm, the combination of anti-fungal therapy in concert with immunological response will provide the ultimate cure.

Claude Favrot *Switzerland*   These Persian cats could also have an accelerated epidermal turnover, and require a continuous treatment.

Kathleen Vlaminck   We did some studies and there is no difference between Persian and European cats.

Bernard Mignon   And there are normal Persian cats that will respond well to classical treatment.

Doug DeBoer   Thanks to everybody and particularly to the presenters. Thanks also to Janssen Animal Health for sponsoring this session.

References

1 Perrins, N., Bond, R. Synergistic inhibition of the growth *in vitro* of *Microsporum canis* by miconazole and chlorhexidine. *Veterinary Dermatology*, 2003; **14**: 99–102.

New developments in dermatopathological diagnosis

E. Clark[1] (Chairperson), A. Yu[2] (Secretary)

[1] Department of Veterinary Pathology, Western College of Veterinary Medicine, University of Saskatchewan, Saskatoon, Canada.
[2] Dept. of Clinical Studies, Ontario Veterinary College, University of Guelph, Guelph, Ontario, Canada

Application of PCR technology in small animal infectious diseases (J. Foley)

Janet Foley *USA*   Polymerase chain reaction (PCR) has been developed because it is a fast and efficient diagnostic test. A further impetus for the development of PCR has been the inability to make any progress with traditional bacterial microbiological culture techniques for atypical organisms (e.g. feline leprosy and canine leproid mycobacterial infections).

Our alternatives at this time include:

(1) Gross visualisation and microscopy; low sensitivity and specificity (PCR can be overly sensitive depending on the investigator).
(2) Special stains; often not as sensitive as PCR.
(3) Culture; many organisms do not grow *in vitro*.
(4) Immunofluorescent antibodies; they only document previous exposure, not current infection.

PCR carries many advantages over traditional techniques. It is often very sensitive, detecting as few as ten copies of the original nucleic acid. However, in some diseases, such as mycobacterial infections, PCR lacks sensitivity due to the resistance of the glycolic acid cell wall of mycobacteria to extraction. In general, nucleic acids correlate well with an active infection. Note, however, that PCR may remain positive post-antibiotic therapy while the remnant DNA is still present, even though there is no viable pathogen.

Although the procedure is not difficult or expensive to perform, controlling false positives due to contamination (negative controls must be incorporated), interpreting findings, and most importantly, choosing good primers (proprietary assays should not be trusted and only tested assays should be used) warrants a significant amount of training. Be careful of recently published PCR assays that haven't been proven, as they may detect unrelated organisms, even though closely related organisms do not cross-react. The following is a 'cook book' of PCR chemistry.

- Step 1: Extract DNA from sample (there are also PCRs for RNA as well)
  Blood, skin, faeces, and sputum samples:
  - Each tissue has optimal chemistries for extraction.
  - Blood has issues with haemoglobin and inhibitors.
  - Faeces is similarly difficult to extract.
  - Skin and sputum, although they need to be digested, are easily extracted.
  Digest extra protein, remove inhibitors, and isolate and precipitate DNA. Fix DNA to membrane in a column or silica tube (Qiagen® Kit, Valencia, CA, USA).
- Step 2: Add DNA to the PCR mix
  Taq (Thermus aquaticus) polymerase originates from thermal vents (72°C). Polymerisation is best performed at higher temperatures, whereas mam-

malian DNA polymerases work at 37°C. Deoxyribo-nucleotide triphosphates (dNTPs) are the raw un-linked bases (GCTA) that can be added and attach to the new DNA strand that PCR is generating. Primers, double-stranded DNA followed by single-stranded DNA, are the signals to stimulate *Taq* polymerases to start making/filling in the double-stranded DNA. Magnesium is required by *Taq* polymerase.

The DNAs are sticky acids that exist in double strands in their natural stable form. If there is a single-stranded DNA, in a test tube for example, it will quickly anneal to any complementary strand that is available so that it can move to its stable double-stranded form.

- Step 3: PCR recursive cycling (hot – cool – warm – repeat)

  Add sample to master-mix in a separate proce-dures room to minimise contamination, and an-chor tubes to eliminate spillage. Denature dou-ble-stranded DNA (95°C). A high temperature is needed for double-stranded DNA to be converted to two single-stranded DNAs. Allow primers to an-neal to single-stranded regions (low 50°Cs). Allow *Taq* to polymerise central area between two prim-ers (72°C). Each cycle doubles the amount of target DNA; 25–30 cycles will generate millions of copies of the target DNA.

- Step 4: Running and interpreting PCR

  Positive and negative controls are included in the agarose gel (seaweed matrix) along with test samples and size markers. To read the gel, ethidium bromide is added; it intercolates into DNA and then reflects UV. Finally, the bands can also be sequenced. Main-tain photo record and annotate result on photo or digitise in computer.

Designing a primer is extremely important. First, it must anneal at 50°C. Secondly, selection of prim-ers requires prior knowledge about the target and its sequence comparison. To increase your chance of finding an organism, select sequences with homolo-gous regions with related organisms. For example, to detect all strains of *Anaplasma*, choose forward and reverse primers in the yellow region (Fig. 6.5.1). To increase the specificity of the PCR test, be certain to choose sequences that are discriminate from various organisms. For example, choosing primers in the blue region poses a risk that some *Anaplasma* strains will be selected, but not all (Fig. 6.5.1). Ultimately, we

want to amplify a region that differentiates the target from other organisms with minimal cross-reaction by verifying the discriminating regions. Sometimes a good primer fit cannot be found; if so, looking at a different gene may help. Software programs deter-mine whether the primers are going to work (correct length and chemistry) with PCR. Luckily, traditional PCR primers cost only $15, therefore you can run a number of them to test.

New organisms may be found by using universal primer sites that anneal to sequences in areas that all known eubacterial species conserve, e.g. 16S gene *S. pneumoniae* (16S RNA). The 16S RNA has areas of conserved sequences (e.g. the hairpin turns) amongst all known bacteria, which are located between variable regions. The variable regions are then sequenced and allow for production of a more specific PCR design.

The specificity of PCR is defined by no other patho-gens that are likely to be amplified, whereas sensitivity is equated to the number of related infections detected, and thus the number of DNA molecules detected.

In conclusion, there are good and bad PCRs. They are not panaceas, but PCRs are extremely useful. With a good assay (based on appropriate extraction, high-quality primer sites and good laboratory technique), we can have very sensitive and specific diagnostic tests for the nucleic acids of specific pathogens in target tis-sues.

Emily Walder *USA* What samples are appropriate for evaluation?

Janet Foley We are not as fussy about sample quality, unlike other diagnostic techniques. Fresh, frozen, for-malin-fixed and -embedded, imprints or blood smears are suitable. Worst-case scenario is a false negative.

Marianne Heimann *Belgium* Can PCR discriminate between vaccine antigens and real disease?

Janet Foley Ideally, there should be a marker inher-ent within the product that allows you to discrimi-nate the engineered product from the natural prod-uct. Unfortunately, this is not common. Most of the time, if the vaccine strain is different, we can design PCRs that will discriminate vaccine strain from field strains, such as that for FIV. It costs $25 each direc-tion per sequence. It takes good information about the vaccine strain. With bacterins however, such as

```
                                    4251                                          4300
A phag (AF412827)   (77)   AGGACATCGTTCAGTTTGCCAATGCTGTGAATATTTCTTACCCTAAAATT
A phag (AF512493)   (83)   AAGATATCGTTCAGTTTGCTAAGGCCGTGGAGATTTCTCATCCTACTATT
A phag (AY112690)   (83)   AGGACATCGTTCAGTTTGCTAAGGCGGTGGAGATCTCTTACCCTAGTATC
A phag (AY137510)   (4250) AAGATATCGTTCAGTTTGCTAAGGCCAGTGGAGATTTCTCATTCCGATATT
A phag (AY151054)   (1170) AGGACATCGTTCAGTTTGCTAAGGCGGTGGAGATCTCTTACCCTAGTATC
A phag (AY176527)   (77)   AGGATATCGTTCAGTTTGCTAAGGCGGTTGGGGTTTCTCATCCTAATATT
A phag (AY253529)   (40)   AGGACATCGTTCAGTTTGCTAAGGCGGTGGAGATTTCTCATTCCGGCATT
       Consensus    (4251) AGGACATCGTTCAGTTTGCTAAGGCGGTGGAGATTTCTCATCCTA TATT
A phag (AY176527)   (211)  --AAGACAGCACAGTGTAGCGGGTTGA---ATG-------------CCG
A phag (AY253529)   (187)  GAAAGTGGCTGTGTGTGCTGGAACTAACGGGAATACCACAACCAAGCCC
A phag (AF412827)   (127)  GATGAGCAGGTTTGTAATAAAAA---TCATACAGTGTT-----------
A phag (AF512493)   (133)  GATGGGAAGATTTGTAAGACTAA---GGATGGTGCTTCGAGCGGAGACAA
A phag (AY112690)   (133)  GATGGGAGGTTTGTAGTGGAAA---GCATGCGGCGCTTGCAGCAAACAA
A phag (AY137510)   (4300) GATGGGAAGATTTGTAGGACGAAGCGGAAGGCTGGTGACAGTAGCGGCAC
A phag (AY151054)   (1220) GATGGGAAGGTTTGTAGTGGAAA---GCATGCGGCGCTTGCAGCAAACAC
A phag (AY176527)   (127)  GATAAGAAGGTTTGTAATGGTAA---GCACA-AGCACAGG----A----C
A phag (AY253529)   (90)   GGTAAGAAGGTTTGTGTGACGAA---GAAGGGGACAAACAGTAGCAATTT
       Consensus    (4301) GATGGGAAGGTTTGTA TA  AA   GCATGC GC       A ACAC
                                    4351                                          4400
A phag (AF412827)   (162)  GAATACGGGGAAAGGGACAACCTTTAATCCAGATCCCAAGACAACCGAAG
A phag (AF512493)   (180)  GTATGGTAAATACGCTGCTGAGTCAGATAGGGATGGTTCAAGCAACTATG
A phag (AY112690)   (180)  GAACGCGGGGAAAAAGTACGCGGTTGAGCCTGCGAACGGCGGAACAGACG
A phag (AY137510)   (4350) CTATGCCAAGTATGGGGAAGAAACGGATAA--TAA-TACTAGCGGTCAAA
A phag (AY151054)   (1267) GAACGCGGAGAAAAAGTACGCGGTTGAGCCTGCGAACGGCGGAACAGACG
A phag (AY176527)   (165)  AGAGGATGGAAGTCCGACAGATTTTGAGGCGGTGCCAAA---AACTAAC-
A phag (AY253529)   (137)  ATATGCCGTTTATGCTGAGAGGACGGATAACGTAGCTACAGCGGGGAGG
       Consensus    (4351) G ATGC G GAA G G A G G TTGAT C G    A  AGAAC GA G
                                    4401                                          4450
A phag (AF412827)   (212)  ATAATACAGCGCAGTGCAGTGGGTTGA---ACA-------------CGA
A phag (AF512493)   (230)  GTAATGTAGCGCTTTGCGGCGCTGCTG---GTAATAGTAGTAATA--CTG
A phag (AY112690)   (230)  GGAGCACGTCGCAGTGTAGTGGTTTGA---GTAA---TGGTAGT--GCGG
A phag (AY137510)   (4397) GTACGGTTGCGGTTTGTGGAGAGAAGG-CTGGA----CACAAC---GCCA
A phag (AY151054)   (1317) GGAGCACGTCGCAGTGTAGTGGTTTGA---GTAA---TGGTAGT--GCGG
```

Fig. 6.5.1 Multiple sequence alignment from several horses and people positive for *Anaplasma phagocytophyllum* that is colour-coded. Yellow = bases are EXACTLY the same; blue = similarities exist; clear = no similarities.

Lyme bacteria, there is no difference, therefore you need to do Western blot testing.

PCR-based detection and quantification of canine *Leishmania* infections in formalin-fixed and paraffin-embedded skin biopsies (M. Welle, C. Brachelente, N. Müller)

Monika Welle *Switzerland* Leishmaniasis is a non-pruritic cutaneous and systemic disease frequently seen in the Mediterranean, parts of north and east Africa, India, China, Central and South America and sometimes in other areas of the world. The cutaneous lesions most often involve the muzzle, periorbital region and pinnae; clinically the most common finding is an exfoliative dermatitis with silvery-white, adherent scales and alopecia (Fig. 6.5.2). Peripheral lymphadenopathy is common.

Diagnostic methods

Most frequently, histopathological findings in canine cutaneous leishmaniasis consist of a nodular dermatitis (Fig. 6.5.3) but if organisms are rare it is a diagnostic challenge for the pathologists to make the diagnosis of leishmaniasis with only the haematoxylin and eosin (H&E) stain. In particular, if few organisms are present, they need to be distinguished from nuclear debris. Often special stains or other diagnostic methods are needed to confirm the diagnosis. Leishmaniasis may also present with a perivascular to diffuse dermatitis, making the diagnosis based on histology even more difficult. *Leishmania* organisms stain positive with Giemsa, but based on our experience, the sensitivity is poor. Immunohistochemistry (IHC) is another diagnostic method to demonstrate *Leishmania* (Fig. 6.5.4). However, if only small numbers of organisms are present, speculation may arise as to whether a true IHC-positive reaction exists or whether it is simply a precipitation of the coloured dye.

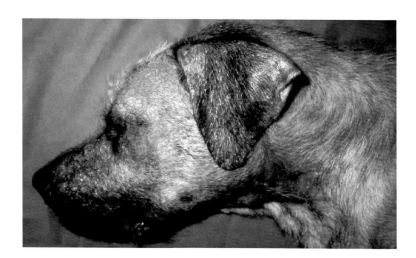

Fig. 6.5.2 Typical case of leishmaniasis in a dog. Note alopecia, and silvery adherent scales involving the pinna and muzzle.

Other diagnostic tests, such as serology and intradermal testing, also have drawbacks as the clinician has to be contacted to initiate these tests.

As the treatment for leishmaniasis is quite different to the treatment for many other nodular, perivascular and diffuse dermatoses, PCR from paraffin-embedded tissue sections was developed to provide a more rapid and definitive diagnosis from samples already submitted.

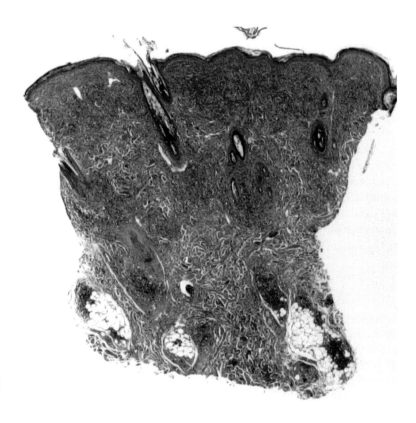

Fig. 6.5.3 Nodular dermatitis from a patient with leishmaniasis (H&E) .

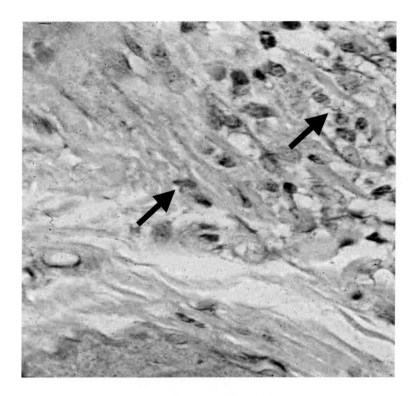

Fig. 6.5.4 Immunohistochemical positive precipitation from a patient with leishmaniasis. Note pink colour stain of organisms (arrows).

DNA extraction from paraffin-embedded tissue

The technique only requires one or two 4-μm sections of a tissue block. However, formalin-fixation of tissue may lead to destruction of the DNA, which may affect the efficiency of a diagnostic PCR. Furthermore, amplification reaction inhibitors residing in the extracted DNA have been identified as potential factors that may hamper PCR-based analysis of histological specimens. Consequently, standardised testing of such samples and minimisation of false-negative results relies on including suitable control measures which monitor the degradation status of, and inhibitory components within, respective DNA preparations.

PCR analysis

Previously described primers from highly repetitive sequences of Old World cutaneous and visceral leishmaniasis are used, that result in an amplicon of 260 bp.[1] To evaluate samples for possible DNA degradation due to previous formalin-fixation of the biopsy sample, a 'universal' α-actin gene-specific PCR was introduced as a first analytic step. Equally important, especially when dealing with paraffin-embedded tissue, false-negative results caused by inhibitory compounds must also be ruled out. To exclude these in the PCR tests, we developed a recombinant internal DNA positive-control and included this in the reaction tube. This control is a PCR construct of a plasmid fragment and the *Leishmania* reverse and forward primers. In Fig. 6.5.5 and Table 6.5.1, possible results of PCR reactions and their interpretation are demonstrated.

Quantitative PCR for leishmaniasis

Additionally we developed a quantitative PCR for *Leishmania* from paraffin-embedded tissue in order to be able to correlate the number of organisms with other findings in retrospective studies. Quantitative PCR is comparable to conventional PCR, but the amount of the amplification product is measured after each cycle, and not only at the end of a complete PCR run. Several fluorescence techniques can be applied for the quantification of the PCR products. In our approach, SYBRGreen I (a double-stranded DNA-binding dye that emits fluorescence directly dependent on the amount of DNA that is

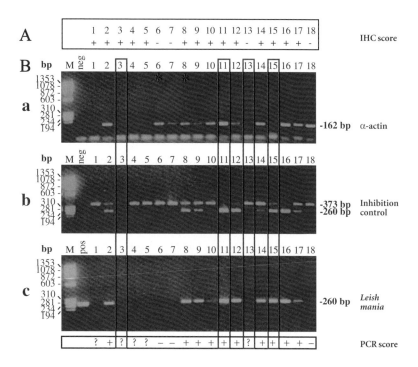

Fig. 6.5.5 PCR gel with 162-bp positive control, 373-bp negative control, 260-bp amplicon of *Leishmania*. Interpretation of results is provided in Table 6.5.1.

Table 6.5.1 Interpretation of PCR gel for *Leishmania* in Fig. 6.5.5

Lane (sample)	Positive control (162 bp)	Inhibition control (373 bp)	*Leishmania* (260 bp)	Interpretation
8	Amplification	Amplification	Amplification	Positive
6	Amplification	Amplification	No amplification	Negative
3	No amplification	No amplification	No amplification	Uncertain result, since positive control and inhibition control are negative
11	Amplification	No amplification	Strong amplification	Positive result indicating a high number of *Leishmania* using up PCR primers before getting to inhibition control
13	No amplification	Amplification	No amplification	Uncertain result, since positive control is negative
15	No amplification	Weak amplification	Strong amplification	Positive result indicating a high number of *Leishmania*

present), was used. Fluorescence emission was measured by the LightCycler Instrument, a thermal cycler with a fluorescence detection system. The data analysis software package plots the fluorescence versus the cycle number in a graph, and thus determines the threshold cycle (Ct value), which is the first cycle above background. In order to obtain absolute quantification of the *Leishmania*, the Ct value is then compared to external standards which have been amplified in the same PCR run and are plotted on a logarithmic graph (Fig. 6.5.6).

In summary, a reliable detection method for *Leishmania* in paraffin-embedded tissue has been established. Furthermore, paraffin-embedded tissue can also be used for quantification of the organisms. This

can thus be an important tool for retrospective studies.

David Shearer *UK*   I often receive cases where four to six biopsy samples are submitted, and perhaps only in one sample are organisms seen, or are positive with IHC. Will PCR detect *Leishmania* in the other samples that were negative on routine staining and IHC, especially if a nodular dermatitis is present?

Monika Welle   PCR will only be positive if *Leishmania* is present in the sample. However, the method is very sensitive and thus samples which are negative on histology or IHC may be positive if PCR is applied. For

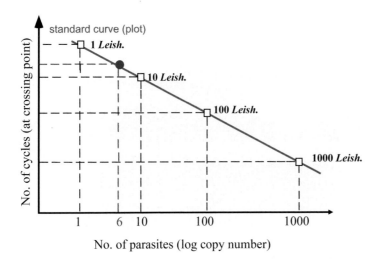

Fig. 6.5.6 Use of external standards for PCR-based quantitation of *Leishmania*. The blue line coming from the y-axis indicates the threshold cycle of the unknown sample.

example, a feline biopsy with findings consistent with pemphigus was found to be positive for *Leishmania* with PCR and also serology. This prompted a review of the sample which still revealed no histological evidence of *Leishmania*.

David Shearer   Is the evaluation of *Leishmania* via PCR available commercially?

Monika Welle   It is not commercial yet, but you can send samples to my lab.

Alessandra Fondati *Italy*   I note that the presence of parasites does not directly correlate to disease. Positive findings need to be assessed in light of clinical signs and serologic and laboratory.

Monika Welle   I agree, however a positive finding on PCR from tissue samples may help support further diagnostic evaluation of the patient for leishmaniasis, e.g. serologic testing.

Francesco Abramo *Italy*   If only a positive PCR is detected without skin signs, do you treat?

Alessandra Fondati   This is classified as infection without the presence of disease. I do not treat if clinical findings do not support condition.

Ultrastructural study of cutaneous lesions in feline eosinophilic granuloma complex (A. Fondati)

Alessandra Fondati   I would like to present the results of a study that we have performed that was recently published.[2]

Flame figures were originally observed by Dr Wells, over 30 years ago, in Wells' syndrome, and defined as 'dermal flame-like extensions of a brightly eosinophilic material adherent to collagen'. The term flame figure has been adopted later in veterinary dermatopathology to describe similar lesions in the feline eosinophilic granuloma complex (EGC). Flame figures in cats have been classically considered to be composed of degenerating collagen and degranulating eosinophils.

However, despite this classical report of the presence of collagen degeneration, there was some evidence to suggest otherwise. Two histopathological studies of EGC lesions demonstrated, with trichromic stains, that normally stained collagen fibres were present in the middle of both flame figures and the large dermal accumulations of eosinophilic to partly basophilic debris, which may be observed sometimes in cats and which are referred to as 'collagen degeneration' (Fig. 6.5.7). In addition, electron microscopic studies of flame figures in Wells' syndrome showed that they were composed of normal collagen bundles surrounded by degranulating (cytolytic) eosinophils and free eosinophil granules.

Therefore, with this background, it was decided to investigate the ultrastructure of flame figures in feline

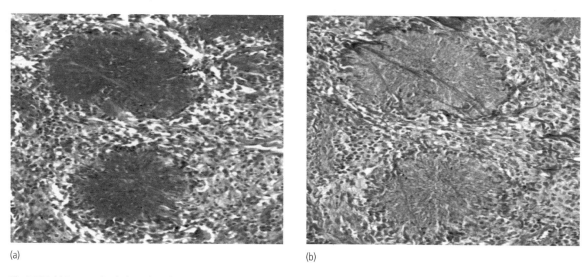

(a)   (b)

Fig. 6.5.7 (a) An example of a large dermal accumulation of eosinophilic to partly basophilic debris, which may be observed sometimes in cats and referred to as 'collagen degeneration' (H&E). (b) Blue collagen fibres are visible in the middle of these accumulations (Gallego trichromic stain).

EGC lesions, including collagen fibre and fibril morphology and eosinophil degranulation pathways.

Materials and methods

This electron microscopic study was performed on eight cats with a clinical and pathological diagnosis of EGC, and two normal cats as controls. Collagen fibres and fibrils morphology in flame figures was studied, and 40–44 fibril cross-striations were measured in each sample.

Eosinophil morphology was also studied. Eosinophils were classified as resting (cells with normal morphology) and degranulating. Two degranulation morphologies were described; eosinophilic cytolysis (ECL) and piecemeal degranulation (PMD). These represent the two most common mechanisms of eosinophil granule content release *in vivo* in humans. Eosinophilic cytolysis is characterised by chromatolysis and loss of plasma membrane integrity, whereas PMD (a progressive release of eosinophil granule content through transporting vesicles) is characterised by the presence of partially to completely empty granules in viable cells.

Results and discussion

In flame figures, collagen fibres were partially disrupted by intense oedema, cellular debris and free eosinophil granules. Collagen fibrils had a normal morphology both on transverse and longitudinal sections and the periodicity of cross-striation was regular. In summary, there was no ultrastructural evidence of collagen degeneration (Fig. 6.5.8), at least according to what is reported as typical of collagen degeneration in EM studies in humans. Veterinary dermatopathology describes collagen in these samples as 'degenerating', 'collagenolysis', 'necrobiotic' and 'necrolytic', demonstrating the lack of clarity and definition of such terms in both histopathology and electron micrography. Granule proteins which are able to directly induce oedema are likely to contribute to this oedema, which may persist as long as free granule proteins persist in the skin; this may be as long as 6 weeks in humans. This might explain the aspect of indurated papules, suggestive of chronic oedema, which is commonly observed clinically in feline EGC lesions.

In flame figures, all the eosinophils were degranulating via ECL (Fig. 6.5.9) or PMD (Fig. 6.5.10). There were no resting eosinophils. In six out of eight samples, ECL was the predominant mode of degranulation. In addition, some macrophages with phagolysosomes containing a material similar to eosinophil granule cores were observed. Macrophages were also found to contain a core-like material in the phagolysosomes. This finding suggests that eosinophil granule proteins incite the granulomatous reaction, rather than the degeneration of collagen. Granule proteins persist in

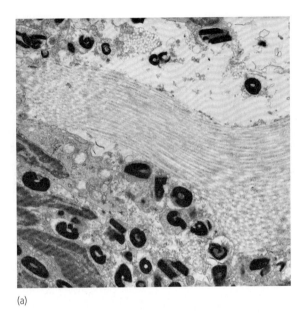

(a)

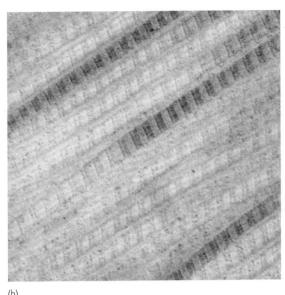

(b)

Fig. 6.5.8 (a) Electron microscopic appearance of a flame figure. Note the collagen band surrounded by prominent oedema, eosinophilic granules and cellular debris. The oedema leads to partial dispersion of collagen fibres. (b) Electron microscopic appearance of flame figure at higher magnification. On transverse sections, the collagen fibrils appeared uniform in diameter with regular profiles; and on longitudinal sections they were found to have regular periodicity (mean 43.08–61.24 nm) of cross-striations.

the skin for weeks, and as they are poorly soluble at physiological pH, they might precipitate and act as a foreign body able to cause the granuloma formation (if present in large quantities). In this way, macrophages may neutralise the cytotoxic potential of extracellular granule proteins and free granules.

In summary, the findings indicated that feline flame figures, analogous to human flame figures, comprise undamaged collagen fibrils and partially dispersed collagen fibres surrounded by degranulating eosinophils. Apparently, eosinophils play a primary effector role in flame figure formation. Eosinophils recruited to the skin might adhere onto collagen fibres, and activate

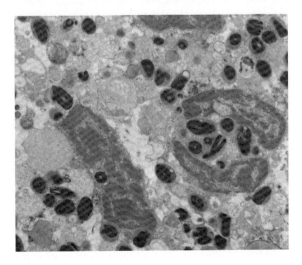

Fig. 6.5.9 Typical image of ECL, with nuclear remnants, cellular debris and clusters of free eosinophil granules.

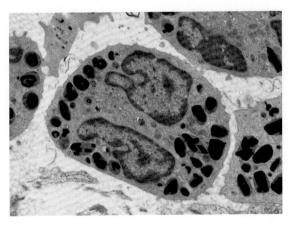

Fig. 6.5.10 Piecemeal degranulated eosinophil. A viable cell with partly empty specific granules.

and release their granule contents, mainly via ECL. In fact, in humans, adhesion is essential for eosinophil activation and degranulation (especially for ECL). This progression is essentially what we see in EGC lesions on light microscopic examination.

Maja Suter *Switzerland*   You mentioned that you don't have a definition for degeneration. You do not have any ultrastructural changes in collagen, and there is no degeneration, and there are different diameter collagen fibres; however, there are many other defects that lead to eosinophilic 'mush' that have a functional deficiency, and we assume that collagen is not in its normal state, but we do not see anything with EM.

Alessandra Fondati   The feline EGC collagen does not have the classical appearance of collagen necrobiosis described in human dermatopathology. For instance, in lesions of granuloma annulare or necrobiosis lipoidica, collagen is classified as necrobiotic whereby there is a loss of definition, and the collagen is more compact. This is not seen in our flame figures, as the EM collagen fibrils are of regular diameter and cross-striations, and there is no evidence of functional collagen abnormalities in EGC; this is more of an inflammatory disease causing collagen alteration as opposed to collagen degeneration. There is no evidence of damage to this collagen, therefore we should abandon the use of the word 'degeneration' as there is no alteration of nucleated cells.

Emily Walder   Are the collagen bundles in flame figures the same size as those in normal surrounding tissue, or are they possibly unravelling?

Alessandra Fondati   They are the same size as normal adjacent collagen bundles.

Emily Walder   Why do the eosinophils stick to the collagen?

Alessandra Fondati   In human studies, eosinophil adhesion to collagen fibres is mediated by integrin binding of fibronectin which is located outside the collagen fibres. This mechanism is important for eosinophil survival and activation/degranulation.

Emily Walder   Why is it so focal?

Alessandra Fondati   There is something there, but I do not know what is causing the localisation of eosinophils.

New developments in canine alopecia: cyclic flank with interface dermatitis (E. Mauldin)

Elizabeth Mauldin *USA*   There are a group of non-inflammatory alopecic disorders in dogs that overlap histopathologically, although clinically they are quite different. They include: curly-coated alopecia (Chesapeake Bay retriever, Irish water spaniel), cyclic flank alopecia (CFA) and cyclic flank alopecia with interface dermatitis.

The typical lesions of CFA are present in a hyperpigmented arcuate pattern with minimal to no inflammation (Fig. 6.5.11a and b). In contrast, CFA with interface dermatitis in boxers[3] (there is one reported case in a Bouvier) has annular areas of crusting within the hyperpigmented alopecic regions (Fig. 6.5.12a). The crusted lesions were once thought to be pyoderma until further histopathological evaluations were performed, revealing a true interface dermatitis with blurring of the dermal–epidermal junction with vacuolar changes and pigmentary incontinence (Fig. 6.5.12b), along with the infundibular hyperkeratosis (witches foot) (Fig. 6.5.11b) that is characteristic of CFA. Interestingly, CFA with interface dermatitis and exfoliative cutaneous lupus erythematosus of German short-haired pointers (where necrotic keratinocytes and a true lymphocytic interface dermatitis are present) are clinically distinct; however, their histological features are similar.

Thus far, we have seen ten boxers with CFA since January 2004 at the University of Pennsylvania, and four cases with interface dermatitis have been documented. Perhaps the low number is indicative of the clinical knowledge of this condition, and cases may be treated empirically without pursuing biopsies. Dr Credille at Texas A&M University Dermatopathology Service finds one of every eight to nine cases of CFA submitted has interface dermatitis.

Clinicians are treating CFA with interface dermatitis similarly to CFA, by either benign neglect with cyclical spontaneous recurrence, or with a combination of tetracycline/niacinamide for the interface dermatitis, and melatonin for the alopecia.

The pathogenesis of this condition is speculative at this point and includes: solar exposure, fixed drug eruption, abnormal response to a bacterial infection, or some other unknown mechanism.

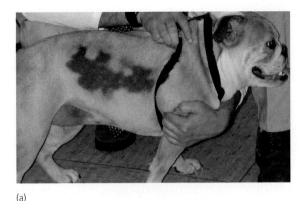

(a)

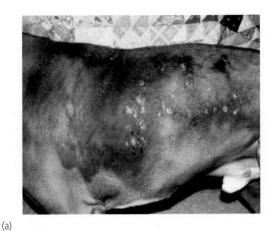

(a)

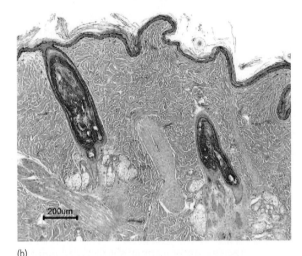

(b)

Fig. 6.5.11 (a) Classic clinical lesions of cyclic flank alopecia in an English bulldog. (b) Classic histopathological lesion of cyclic flank alopecia which lacks interface dermatitis. Note the characteristic infundibular hyperberatosis (witches foot).

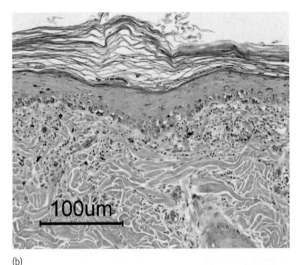

(b)

Fig. 6.5.12 (a) Cyclic flank alopecia with interface dermatitis in a boxer. Note annular areas of crusting within the alopecic hyperpigmented skin lesions. (Courtesy of Dr W. Miller, Cornell University, Cornell, NY, USA.) (b) Histological lesions of cyclic flank alopecia with interface dermatitis.

Audience   Where do you biopsy these cases?

Elizabeth Mauldin   The interface dermatitis has been found in crusted lesions.

David Shearer   Has anyone seen this condition in Europe? (None noted thus far in many boxer biopsies.)

Elizabeth Mauldin   We have only started seeing these cases in the past 2 years.

Emily Walder   It is rare in southern California, thus it is unlikely that the condition is solar-induced.

Ted Clark *Canada*   There was one case of CFA with interface dermatitis positively diagnosed from Canada (included in the paper), where solar/actinic conditions are rarely diagnosed, thus making solar damage less likely as an aetiopathogenesis.

David Shearer   A number of biopsies from boxers with CFA have small areas of lymphoid perivascular dermatitis within the deep dermis and subcutis with 50–60 lymphocytes around blood vessels. Has anyone else ever seen this pattern? (No response.)

References

1 Piarroux, R., Fontes, M., Perasso, R., *et al.* Phylogenetic relationships between Old World Leishmania strains revealed by analysis of a repetitive DNA sequence. *Molecular and Biochemical Parasitology*, 1995; **73**: 249–252.

2 Bardagí, M., Fondati, A., Fondevila, D., Ferrer, L. Ultrastructural study of cutaneous lesions in feline eosinophilic granuloma complex. *Veterinary Dermatology*, 2003; **14**: 297–303.

3 Rachid, M.A., Demaula, C.D., Scott, D.W., Miller, W.H., Senter, D.A., Myers, S. Concurrent follicular dysplasia and interface dermatitis in Boxer dogs. *Veterinary Dermatology*, 2003; **14**: 159–166.

Pseudomonas otitis

T.J. Nuttall (Chairperson), H.C. McArdle (Secretary)

The University of Liverpool, Faculty of Veterinary Science, Liverpool, UK

Tim Nuttall *UK* *Pseudomonas* and other gram-negative rod bacteria are uncommon inhabitants of the healthy ear canal and middle ear. *Pseudomonas* otitis is, however, one of the most challenging clinical problems that we see. There are a number of reasons for this: antibiotic resistance is very common; treatment is often time-consuming and expensive (for example, my cases routinely cost €1500–€2000 and short-cuts often turn out to be even more expensive); and the infections commonly recur. Recurrence is often associated with: inappropriate antibiotic use; failure to thoroughly clean the ears; failure to treat for long enough; failure to manage chronic pathological changes; otitis media; and failure to detect and control primary and predisposing causes.

We are very fortunate to have three world leaders in this field with us today. Prof. David Lloyd from the Royal Veterinary College in the UK will discuss resistance mechanisms and trends, minimum inhibitory concentration (MIC) data versus Kirby-Bauer (K-B) discs, and nosocomial infections; Dr Didier Carlotti from France will discuss antibiotic options and delivery; and Dr Lynette Cole from The Ohio State University in the US will discuss ear cleaning and ear cleaners, and the role of Tris-EDTA.

Resistance mechanisms and assessment of antimicrobial resistance in *Pseudomonas aeruginosa* (D.H. Lloyd)

David Lloyd *UK* *Pseudomonas* spp. are ubiquitous organisms which colonise many clinical environments and tend to persist in hospitals where exchanges can occur between patients and environmental habitats. Normal individuals are resistant to infection but immunocompromised patients, particularly those treated with antibiotics to which the pseudomonads are resistant, are susceptible to these infections. Such treatment promotes infection with resistant strains of *Pseudomonas aeruginosa* and selects for resistance. Recurrent or extensive hospital infections tend to be associated with more virulent strains of *Pseudomonas* that become established in hospital or farm premises.

Ps. aeruginosa depends on four broad mechanisms for its resistance to antimicrobials: (1) low cell wall permeability; (2) a large genome with the capacity to express a wide range of resistance mechanisms; (3) chromosomal mutations leading to changes in the regulation of resistance genes; and (4) acquisition of resistance genes from other organisms. Amongst clinical isolates, correlation has been shown between resistance to antibiotics and biocides, indicating that their use can promote resistance to either class of antimicrobials.

Increased resistance to antimicrobials amongst clinical isolates of *Ps. aeruginosa* has been reported amongst urinary tract isolates from Canada between 1984 and 1998. However, a report from Michigan State University Animal Health Diagnostic Laboratory found no consistent trends in specimens from canine skin and ears over the period 1992–1997. In Europe, studies in

Glasgow examined canine and feline bacterial isolates between 1989 and 1997, and showed a rising trend in multidrug resistance in *Pseudomonas* spp. from a veterinary community practice, but not from a veterinary small animal hospital.

We have examined sensitivity of *Ps. aeruginosa* from canine infections (predominantly skin and ears) to enrofloxacin and marbofloxacin and contrasted frequencies in 1992, 1995 and 2003 using both disc and broth macrodilution tube assay techniques. In 1992, 79% of 19 isolates showed disc sensitivity to enrofloxacin, whereas in 1995 only 45% of 49 isolates were sensitive; 90% of isolates were sensitive to marbofloxacin in 1995. In 2003, of 41 canine isolates, 14.6% were sensitive to enrofloxacin and 85% were sensitive to marbofloxacin (chi-squared test, $p < 0.001$). These data indicate a substantial decrease in sensitivity to enrofloxacin since the antibiotic became available in the UK. Low levels of sensitivity to enrofloxacin have also been reported in Spain, where a study of 23 isolates of *Ps. aeruginosa* from canine chronic otitis externa found only 52% sensitive to enrofloxacin, whereas 91% were sensitive to marbofloxacin. In Croatia, isolates of *Ps. aeruginosa*, predominantly from the skin and ears of dogs visiting the University of Zagreb clinic during the years 1993–2000, were nearly all (93%) sensitive to ciprofloxacin and marbofloxacin, whilst 71% were sensitive to enrofloxacin. The authors related this to extensive veterinary use of enrofloxacin, whereas marbofloxacin was not available, and ciprofloxacin was used very rarely in veterinary practice.

There seems to be a convincing trend towards increasing resistance to enrofloxacin amongst isolates from chronic otitis cases, and studies have indicated that this resistance is associated with mutation of the *gyrA* gene coupled with up-regulation of efflux pump activity.

It is difficult to compare the different studies of antimicrobial resistance in *Pseudomonas* owing to differences between sources of isolates and the sampling and sensitivity test methods used. For instance, there is evidence that isolates from the middle ear and those from the horizontal ear canal of dogs with otitis media differ in sensitivity. In addition, disc sensitivity tests do not necessarily correlate with dilution methods. The significance of elevated levels of resistance to antibiotics (as indicated by the disc sensitivity test), is that empirical selection of antibiotic for systemic therapy in chronic otitis is unwise. However, where topical

therapy is planned, sensitivities assessed with systemic treatment in mind are misleading, as much higher levels of antibiotic can be achieved and these will commonly exceed the resistance levels of the infecting bacteria. Nevertheless, the observation that antibiotic resistance levels in *Ps. aeruginosa* are rising is a warning that needs to be heeded. We need to develop rational policies of antibiotic prescription and use which will help to reduce the selection of resistant strains.

Evidence that resistance to biocides may be correlated with antibiotic resistance in clinical isolates of *Ps. aeruginosa* (recent data showing that methods used for assessment of antimicrobial synergy between EDTA and antibiotics have been flawed), show that we still have a lot to learn about handling these very interesting organisms.

Pseudomonas are common in the environment wherever there is moisture. Nosocomial infections, as for methicillin-resistant *Staphylococcus aureus* (MRSA), are therefore a concern for hospitalised patients. Antibiotic usage selects for resistant strains of *Pseudomonas*; resistance to enrofloxacin, for example, develops within a few passages in culture. Furthermore, when *Pseudomonas aeruginosa* organisms are stressed, they can exhibit a phenotypic switch to rough small colony variants (RSCV). This is a transient switch, but RSCV are much more resistant, and the roughness of the colonies may enhance attachment. This change can be influenced by antibiotics and other environmental stresses, e.g. reduced nutrients. It is regulated by the *PvrR* regulator gene, which could prove a target to control *Pseudomonas* in the future. Avirulent oropharyngeal flora has also been shown to provide promoters that can enhance antibiotic efflux via an interaction known as quorum sensing.

Aiden Foster *UK*   Could you clarify whether the isolates of *Pseudomonas* were from referral and outside cases?

David Lloyd   I think that the majority of samples were from referral practice, with others received from first-opinion practices.

Giovanni Ghibaudo *Italy*   Fluoroquinolones appear to be more efficacious *in vivo* than *in vitro,* so how accurate are disc sensitivity data? We often use higher doses, especially with topical medication, than are present on the discs, leading to an increased efficacy and apparently more sensitive *Pseudomonas* strains than K-B disc data would suggest.

David Lloyd   Topical therapy allows one to attain much greater concentrations at the site of infection than is possible with systemic medication. *In vitro* sensitivity data are therefore potentially misleading when applied to topical therapy. The MIC data can allow you to calculate whether the MIC is exceeded at the site of infection, but the response to topical antibiotic treatment often relies on assessing clearance of the bacteria by cytology and repeated culture.

Tim Nuttall   Could you comment on steps to avoid nosocomial infections?

David Lloyd   Good hygiene, as for management of MRSA infections, is of paramount importance. Barrier nursing should be established for animals with suspected or confirmed infections with antibiotic-resistant organisms. Asymptomatic carriage is uncommon, but environmental reservoirs could be a source of infections. *Pseudomonas* are, however, very susceptible to drying, which is a simple way to control them.

Pseudomonas otitis in the dog: antibiotic options and delivery (D.N. Carlotti)

Antibiotic options

Didier Carlotti *France*   At the present time, the usable antibiotics are: (a) aminoglycosides (gentamicin, tobramycin and amikacin); (b) veterinary fluoroquinolones (marbofloxacin and enrofloxacin); (c) polypeptides (polymyxin B and colistin); (d) penicillins active against *Pseudomonas* species (ticarcillin and piperacillin); and (e) third-generation cephalosporins (ceftazidime).

Several studies have investigated the antibacterial susceptibility pattern of *Pseudomonas* strains. Clearly, the most efficacious antibiotics are polymyxin B and tobramycin, followed by marbofloxacin and ceftazidime, then gentamicin and ticarcillin. Susceptibility to neomycin and enrofloxacin was low in many studies.

It is well documented that ciprofloxacin has greater activity against *Ps. aeruginosa* than enrofloxacin. The susceptibility breakpoint for enrofloxacin is, however, lower and different methods may have been used in these studies. Ciprofloxacin appears to be better than

enrofloxacin for systemic administration in *Pseudomonas* otitis externa, but this question is still controversial.

We have used injectable colistin in a few cases. We have also tested six *Ps. aeruginosa* strains with cefoperazone, a third-generation veterinary cephalosporin used to treat bovine mastitis, but only two were sensitive.

Antibiotic delivery

Classically, topical therapy is always indicated in otitis externa or media. However, systemic therapy is indicated when: (a) severe otitis externa is present; (b) marked proliferative changes are present; (c) otitis media is present; (d) owners cannot administer topical treatments; and (e) topical adverse reactions are suspected.

In my opinion, in most cases of erythematous ceruminous otitis externa, systemic antibiotic therapy is useless, as bacteria are present only in the external ear canal and cerumen. Topical treatment is therefore sufficient in these instances. However, in cases of suppurative otitis externa, pus in the ear canal is abundant and above all, otitis media is possible. Even if organisms present in the external ear canal are easier to reach with topical therapy, particularly after cleaning, systemic antibiotic therapy can be useful to reach the deep ceruminous glands of the external ear canal and the middle ear. Obviously the selection of a systemic antibiotic must be based upon bacteriological culture and sensitivity testing.

Can systemic antimicrobial therapy be effective on its own in a certain number of cases? To our knowledge, the only study regarding this matter was presented at a meeting in Belgium in 1996 and at WCVD3 in Edinburgh but was never published. In summary, 54 dogs with suppurative otitis externa (from which at least one strain of *Pseudomonas* was isolated in 43.8% of the ears), were treated with oral marbofloxacin at 5 mg/kg once daily for 21 days (short-treatment). Some dogs continued on this treatment, depending on the clinical outcome on day 21, for a total of 42 days (long-treatment). The only associated treatment was cleansing of the external ear canal with saline solution. The dogs were evaluated at day 0 and after 7, 21 and 35 (short-treatment) and additionally at 42 and 56 days (long-treatment). Efficacy was assessed as the change in the main clinical scores (suppuration, pain and ulcerations); 27.8% of dogs were considered cured, 5.6% had a clear improvement, 37% a partial improvement and 29.6% were failures. Only three dogs suffered mild adverse effects related to treatment (mainly vomiting), and treatment had to be discontinued in only one case (on day 35).

Further studies are needed to evaluate the efficacy of antibiotics given orally in association with topical antiseptics or antibacterial preparations (whether the antibiotics administered topically and systemically are the same or not).

Paul Bloom *USA* What about using systemic glucocorticoids?

Didier Carlotti Immunosuppression is a worry, but they are useful to decrease hyperplasia.

Paul Bloom I use short-term glucocorticoids to reduce pain and decrease hyperplasia.

Jan Hall *Canada* Minimum inhibitory concentrations are used to predict the use of fluoroquinolones, but I find them to be of no clinical benefit. I find a dose of ciprofloxacin of 23 mg/kg is much better. Initially I do cytology, then use glucocorticoids first (1–2 mg/kg once daily if severe, or topical if mild). Two weeks later, I perform a culture and sensitivity to select antibiotics. I do not use topical antibiotics, but instead try to get the dog to 'self-cure' following glucocorticoid therapy to correct hyperplastic changes in the ear canal and addressing the underlying problem if present. Serial use of topical antibiotics can lead to *Pseudomonas* infections, and what started as a mild ear problem can, after the use of several topical antibiotics, become a severe problem (i.e. we create the problem).

David Lloyd Antibiotics are delivered at a much higher dose when given topically, so sensitivity testing and MICs are less necessary. Glucocorticoids and cleaning are the main treatments to correct hyperplastic and inflammatory changes and remove purulent debris. Also, *Pseudomonas* is sometimes sensitive to oxytetracycline, which is often overlooked.

Jan Hall Glucocorticoid use for *Pseudomonas* infections of the skin or ears does not seem to cause systemic problems or disseminated infections. Fluoroquinolones can, however, affect other organisms, e.g. *E. coli*.

David Lloyd We do disrupt other flora in the environment by using antibiotics.

Aiden Foster What is the feeling about using marbofloxacin at a 2 mg/kg compared to the 5 mg/kg dose?

Didier Carlotti Concentration-dependent antibiotics work best at high doses for deep pyoderma.

Lynette Cole *USA* Marbofloxacin and enrofloxacin have flexible dosing schedules (flexible dosing ranges are on data sheets in the USA only) so I use the higher doses. Susceptibility patterns are based on plasma levels, so I use topical antibiotics even when they appear resistant *in vitro* since a much higher dose is achieved when applied topically.

Jan Hall There is a 'must use antibiotics' dogma. If instead we change the ear canal by cleaning and drying it, the *Pseudomonas* will die.

Babette Baddaky-Taugboel *Norway* In Norway, where we only have enrofloxacin, we see resistant *Pseudomonas* in cases of unilateral otitis externa that have had lots of antibiotics. What about surgery to try to open the ear canal and make the ear environment drier? Also topical treatment becomes more difficult because these dogs are in pain.

Didier Carlotti The success of surgery depends on the surgeon! We consider surgery as a last resort really.

Paul Bloom Do you use just systemic colistin?

Didier Carlotti Colistin and Epi-Otic®.

David Lloyd In response to Dr Baddaky-Taugboel, I treat severe cases medically instead of surgically. I recommend using injectable antibiotics topically, glucocorticoids to open up the ear canal, and cleaning and drying the ear canal.

Ewa Sevelius *Sweden* I see a poor response in American cocker spaniels with hyperplastic ear canals.

Jan Hall Dr Rod Rosychuck's work suggests that this condition could be due to either a hypersensitivity reaction to fatty acids in the ear canal, idiopathic seborrhoea (keratinisation disorder) leading to an increase in turnover of epidermal cells in the skin and the ear canal, or due to another immune-mediated or hypersensitivity condition.

Christophe Rème *France*   Ciprofloxacin appears to be more effective *in vitro* and *in vivo*, but enrofloxacin is metabolised to ciprofloxacin in the body.

Lynette Cole   The bioavailability of ciprofloxacin in the dog is 40% but that of enrofloxacin is 100%, so much higher doses of ciprofloxacin are needed.

Paul Bloom   For ciprofloxacin, I use double the enrofloxacin dose, i.e. 20 mg/kg ciprofloxacin, or higher still.

Ear cleaning, ear cleaners and the role of Tris-EDTA (L.K. Cole)

Otic flushing

Lynette Cole   Most cases of *Pseudomonas* otitis require a deep ear flush in order to clean the ear of purulent exudate. Otic flushing is expensive, but is very important when dealing with *Pseudomonas* otitis externa. Exudate and purulent material is irritating and can lead to ulceration, hide foreign bodies and masses, act as a growth medium for bacteria and yeasts, reduce contact between topical medication and the epithelium, inactivate topical medication, and prevent evaluation of the tympanic membrane.

For a deep ear flush, the animal is anaesthetised and endotracheally intubated. Swabs are taken from the horizontal ear canal for cytology and bacterial culture and susceptibility testing (C/S). The ear canal is soaked with a ceruminolytic ear cleanser, flushed with a bulb syringe, and then an 8-French polypropylene urinary catheter attached to a 12-ml syringe passed through an otoscopic cone. Some ceruminolytic agents may be ototoxic. If the tympanic membrane is not intact, repeated flushing of the middle ear with saline should be performed to remove the ear cleanser. If the tympanic membrane is not intact, samples for cytology and bacterial C/S are obtained from the middle ear cavity. If the tympanic membrane is intact, appears abnormal, and otitis media is suspected, a myringotomy is needed to obtain samples for cytology and bacterial C/S.

Glucocorticoids are used appropriately, both topically and systemically, with a blood screen in older dogs in case of diabetes mellitus. Radiographs are taken before the flush in chronic cases of disease (i.e. 6 months, or longer, duration of the otitis externa). When changes in the tympanic bullae are found (lysis and/or sclerosis) surgical treatment is offered if medical treatment is not working well.

Possible complications of ear flushing and myringotomy are Horner's syndrome, facial nerve paralysis, vestibular disturbances and deafness. Owners should sign a consent form prior to the procedure.

Ear cleaning/drying agents

Once the ear has been flushed, at-home cleaning is performed using a cleaning/drying agent containing acids, to dry the ear canal. Ear cleaners are used for the long-term management of *Pseudomonas* otitis to help prevent recurrence. There are good *in vivo* data for the activity of Epi-Otic® against *Malassezia*, *Staphylococcus* and *Pseudomonas*. When Epi-Otic® was used twice daily as the only treatment for 1–2 weeks in cases with a first infection, or a recurrent (but not chronic) otitis, the results were: 61% infection-free after 1 week and 68% infection-free after 2 weeks. After 2 weeks, all ears were negative for *Pseudomonas* (4 initially infected), 83% were negative for *Staphylococcus* (12 ears initially infected), and 72.7% negative for *Malassezia* (22 ears initially infected). There was also a decrease in exudation, stenosis and erythema within the first week.

The role of Tris-EDTA

Exposure of gram-negative bacteria to Tris-EDTA damages the cell surfaces, resulting in leakage of cellular contents and increased permeability of the cell to antibiotics. *In vitro*, *Pseudomonas* organisms are lysed in the presence of Tris-EDTA. Tris enhances the effects of the EDTA. Products containing Tris-EDTA have been used topically prior to the application of a topical antibiotic for the treatment of *Pseudomonas* otitis externa. The MIC of enrofloxacin is decreased when *Pseudomonas* organisms have been exposed to Tris-EDTA for 5 minutes.

Tris-EDTA (tromethamine + EDTA) is used in all my cases of *Pseudomonas* otitis. There are no data on ototoxicity, so care must be taken if otitis media is present. Tris-EDTA can be used twice daily after ear cleaning, followed 15 minutes later by a topical antibiotic solution (this allows time for the Tris-EDTA to chelate the bacteria). Alternatively the antibiotic can be mixed with the Tris-EDTA. The topical antibiotic solution is not selected on the basis of sensitivity testing owing to the much higher concentrations achieved with topical treatment.

Questions that remain to be answered include: should we use Tris-EDTA once or twice daily; what is the optimum time to apply antibiotics after application of Tris-EDTA; is concurrent administration of antibiotics and Tris-EDTA better; and is it necessary to use antibiotics at all?

Giovanni Ghibaudo   In Italy we use Tris-EDTA with or without chlorhexidine in bacterial otitis externa. There appears to be a synergistic action between Tris-EDTA and chlorhexidine (at 0.15% concentration this is not ototoxic).

Lynette Cole   Have you published this?

Giovanni Ghibaudo   There is a poster at this meeting comparing Autodine® (Tris-EDTA with chlorhexidine) with Tris-EDTA and sterile saline. We think it is a very interesting combination.

Lynette Cole   I use an ear cleaner, then Tris-EDTA, then either Baytril otic® or Baytril® injection (enrofloxacin) with a vehicle, polymyxin B or tobramycin (all given topically).

Carol Beckenridge *UK*   I am a general practitioner in the UK and see *Pseudomonas* problems. One particular case had surgery creating a skin tunnel which developed a *Pseudomonas* and MRSA infection. I use acetic acid, Tris and buffer for problem ears.

David Lloyd   I like that approach. Tris chelates the cell wall, causing it to be degraded. We can then avoid using antibiotics and maybe use other antimicrobials instead, thus reducing the appearance of resistant bacteria into the environment. By keeping the environment clean and dry we can increase the susceptibility of the bacteria as well.

Beth McDonald *Australia*   I see *Pseudomonas* infections in referred cases and I am concerned that Epi-Otic® twice daily would lead to maceration of the ear canal.

Lynette Cole   Over-treating topically can lead to an excess of exudates, even after pus is no longer being produced. This exudate contains epithelial cells only (without infection), so I monitor this cytologically. If there are no bacteria present, I reduce topical treatment to once daily or every alternate day.

Jan Hall   Cytology is important alongside clinical signs. We are under pressure to eliminate infection. In chronic cases, what is our end-point aim? Should we aim for a completely sterile ear canal?

Eva Paulssen *Sweden*   What about bacteriophage usage?

David Lloyd   Experiments have been done in the UK with bacteriophages, which seem to show that they kill *Pseudomonas*, but it is difficult to do trials in clinically affected animals.

Tim Nuttall   Could the panel indicate how they use sensitivity data to select antibiotics?

Lynette Cole   Systemic treatment is based on sensitivity testing (Kirby-Bauer). Topical treatment is not based on sensitivity testing because a much higher dose is administered.

David Lloyd   I culture to see what is there and use sensitivity testing (MIC) for systemic treatment. Topical treatment with a fluoroquinolone means a high concentration reaches the site. Kirby-Bauer testing is not a guide to susceptibility with topical treatment.

Didier Carlotti   I perform culture and sensitivity if I see rods on cytology.

Ewa Sevelius   Can you use any preparation for topical treatment?

Lynette Cole   I use products labelled for ocular use as most ear preparations have corticosteroids in them.

David Robson *Australia*   I rarely culture ears because a Kirby-Bauer sensitivity test is no use. I only culture if I get no response to treatment. In otitis media, I use topical treatment alone. I anaesthetise the dog weekly and instil Baytril® injection into the middle ear.

Jan Hall   Do you use glucocorticoids as well?

David Robson   Yes.

Jan Hall   Maybe you should try just glucocorticoids instead of glucocorticoids and Baytril® topically.

Tim Nuttall   This has been a fascinating and enor-mously rewarding workshop. We have, unfortunately, raised more questions than we have answered but that is the nature of these complex and difficult problems. With luck and hard work, some of these problems may have been answered by the next world congress. I would like to thank our speakers for their excellent presentations, the audience for their lively participa-tion and Vétoquinol for their sponsorship.

Neoplastic and paraneoplastic skin diseases

F. Abramo[1] (Chairperson), J.R. Rest[2] (Secretary)

[1] Dipartimento di Patologia Animale, Pisa, Italy
[2] Swaffham Prior, Cambridge, UK

Francesca Abramo *Italy* This workshop will cover neoplastic-like diseases, paraneoplastic syndromes and neoplasms. I will introduce three mini-talks presented by Joan Rest, Elizabeth Mauldin and Marianne Heimann. The first topic on mast cell proliferations focuses on species comparisons with emphasis on young animals that may develop multiple masses of mast cells with lymphatic spread, yet they experience self-cure. The topic raises the question of what is hyperplasia, and what is neoplasia? The second presentation introduces paraneoplastic syndromes. These are cutaneous manifestations of internal malignancy. A single tumour type may have different cutaneous skin manifestations. For example, a pancreatic tumour may be associated with superficial necrolytic dermatitis or paraneoplastic alopecia. The third presentation introduces neoplastic-like lesions, classified by the World Health Organization as hamartomas and tumour-like lesions. These single to multifocal lesions usually develop slowly, but can cause discomfort or induce inflammation. One of the most common, fibroadnexal hamartoma, is frequently detected on the legs and digits. Another more rare hamartoma is angiomatosis, which affects blood vessels.

Mast cell proliferations (J.R. Rest)

Joan Rest *UK* Mast cells originate in the bone marrow and are distributed throughout the body, particularly in subepithelial and perivascular locations, and in lymph nodes. They normally travel in lymphatics and

blood vessels, and they have roles in allergy and protection from bacteria. Different subtypes have functional diversity. Apart from neoplastic mast cell proliferations, single or multiple proliferations of mast cells in young animals may be diffuse or nodular in the dermis, with or without dermatological clinical signs such as pruritus, and with or without eosinophils. Benign proliferations are often locally 'invasive' and the cells normally move around the body in the circulation. Neoplasia (cancer) is a genetic disease, with malignancy characterised by invasion and metastasis. However, some cases of non-neoplastic human mastocytosis have genetic mutations of c-KIT, the stem cell factor receptor. Therefore, mutations do not explain the cause of disease and their prognostic significance is uncertain. However, it is known that skin mast cell proliferations have an imbalance in mast cell proliferation and apoptosis, with increased Ki67 proliferation markers and decreased TUNEL apoptosis.

In one dog with mastocytosis, a single type of proliferation with multiple masses throughout the skin and subcutaneous tissues was recorded. The dog was without clinical illness and the masses spontaneously resolved.

Mastocytosis in cats is recorded as multiple nodules in kittens, and as an adult-onset familial disease in Sphinx and Devon Rex cats. The former is not pruritic and often regresses. The latter is not characterised by nodular lesions, it is usually pruritic, and it waxes and wanes, suggesting that a better name would be 'mast cell-rich papular dermatitis'. The adult Siamese also develops histiocytic-type nodules, which may be single or multiple, and may regress.

In humans, mastocytosis is relatively benign and indolent. As in cats, some lesions regress (particularly in children), some remain stable, and others are slowly progressive.

Mastocytosis may be associated with genetic abnormalities, but these abnormalities may not be relevant to prognosis. From a diagnostic point of view, the breed may be important, but clinical signs and stage may be less relevant than age of onset. The histopathologic type may be relevant. Ultimately, the important factor is the well-being of the individual animal and not necessarily its cure. As in humans, this may best be achieved by avoiding mast cell secretory stimuli (such as allergens, trauma and sunlight), together with antipruritic and symptomatic treatment.

Thelma Lee Gross *USA*   I have also seen cases in Labrador retrievers. One Labrador retriever which had multiple mast cell proliferations as a puppy, had massive internal organ involvement at 18 months of age.

Joan Rest   I have seen this in kittens, with recurrence of multiple mast cell growths later in life. In children, these proliferations may be present in internal organs but they are not necessarily a sign of malignant disease.

Anthony Chadwick *UK*   In the clinical case quoted by Joan Rest, follow-up was for 2 years and, to my knowledge, the dog is still fit and well.

Rick Last *South Africa*   How do we differentiate between well-differentiated neoplasia and mastocytosis. Is it only by age?

Joan Rest   If there are multiple lesions in young dogs, they are probably not neoplastic. Although neoplasia is due to genetic alteration, there may also be genetic alterations in mastocytosis. The diagnosis of mastocytosis is sometimes made to try to keep these dogs away from oncologists who give immunosuppressants.

Emily Walder *USA*   I agree with these comments. One of the criteria for histologic differentiation is that a tumour is a solid discrete mass. Mastocytosis mass-type lesions do not look like a typical tumour; they are either diffuse or plaque-like.

Joan Rest   Very benign mastocytomas tend to be diffuse, except for one well-circumscribed type which occurs in the superficial dermis with epidermotropism. This may be a fundamentally different mast cell type. Luis Ferrer may have done some work on this.

Judith Nimmo *Australia*   We have mentioned Labrador retrievers. Young Shar peis in Australia sometimes have diffuse nodular mastocytosis. Multiple metastatic neoplastic lesions may be diffuse, but the mast cell population is usually more pleomorphic. In my experience, mast cell tumours have a Grenz zone, but metastatic lesions do not have a Grenz zone.

Joan Rest   Boxers often have mast cell proliferations on their ears. These are probably inflammatory and not a primary proliferation.

Luis Ferrer *Spain*   There is not always a sharp distinction between neoplasia and hyperplasia. It is not always possible to differentiate the two on the basis of genetic alteration, as this may be present in both mast cell tumours and mastocytosis. There are more genetic mutations in neoplasia, with progression in some cases. Hyperplasia may be explained by an increase in stem cell factor, and mast cells that survive longer.

Claudia Von Tscharner *Switzerland*   Histiocytic mast cell tumours have recently been shown by Verena Affolter to have histiocyte markers, and are now classified as histiocytic tumours.

Francesca Abramo   What about eosinophils in mast cell tumours and mastocytosis; are there any differences?

Joan Rest   Tumours almost always have eosinophils, sometimes with a band of eosinophils around the margins. In my experience, non-neoplastic proliferations may have fewer eosinophils. In the cat, proliferations which are probably inflammatory (rather than hyperplastic) and mast cell-rich, have many eosinophils. The eosinophils may indicate which are more likely to be pruritic, or primarily inflammatory.

Paraneoplastic alopecic disorders in the cat (E. A. Mauldin)

Elizabeth Mauldin *USA*   Thymoma-associated dermatosis is characterised by clinical features of hyperkeratosis and matted hair. One complex case was in a Siamese cat with failure to respond to thymectomy and was thus given adjunctive treatment with IgG, 4 weeks after surgery. Histopathologic features included parakeratosis, hyperkeratosis, interface dermatitis, keratinocyte necrosis, mural folliculitis and loss of sebaceous glands. Erythema multiforme could not be ruled out as a differential diagnosis. The cat is alive, but is now diabetic.

A second case of thymoma was a 9-year-old Domestic Short Hair with periorbital and perianal ulcerative dermatitis, scaling, and bilateral ulceration of the external ear canals. The histopathology was indistinguishable from erythema multiforme.

The third thymoma case, again in a Siamese cat, had clinical hyperkeratosis and alopecia. Histopathologically, there was both an interface pattern and acantholysis with pustule formation.

The clinical features of pancreatic paraneoplastic alopecia include shiny skin. Histopathologically, the epidermis can be hyperplastic, but there is profound and diffuse follicular atrophy. Paraneoplastic syndromes often have *Malassezia* overgrowth, so they are pruritic.

Marianne Heimann *Belgium*   Evaluation of the patient for systemic disease is often needed to make the diagnosis.

Claudia von Tscharner   Why has thymoma-associated skin lost its sebaceous glands?

Elizabeth Mauldin   I don't know, but this is probably part of the mural folliculitis.

Judith Nimmo   Do sebaceous glands regenerate?

Elizabeth Mauldin   I don't know. It may be helpful to rebiopsy these cats.

Monika Welle *Switzerland*   We saw a case with more parakeratosis than hyperkeratosis. This was associated with liver disease.

Elizabeth Mauldin   I have also seen a case with parakeratosis, but it was associated with a pancreatic tumour.

Anthony Chadwick   What is the pathogenesis of thy-

moma-related skin disease? Is it related to T-cell destruction of sebaceous glands?

Elizabeth Mauldin   This is not known. Thymoma has an epithelial component so perhaps there is cross-reactivity with keratinocytes.

Emily Walder   In people, thymomas are associated with abnormal subsets of T cells.

Elizabeth Mauldin   It is strange that they only attack the epidermis and not other epithelial surfaces.

Emily Walder   They have been recorded as attacking the intestine in humans.

Francesca Abramo   There are sometimes nodules of fat necrosis associated with pancreatic tumours. Is this a paraneoplastic syndrome?

Emily Walder   This is due to the normal activity of the gland and is therefore endocrine in nature, and it should not be defined as a paraneoplastic syndrome.

Feline apocrine gland hamartoma resembling human syringocystadenoma papilliferum (M. Heimann)

Marianne Heimann   Two young European cats, aged 8 months and 1 year, one male and one female, presented with skin plaques that were unilateral, irregular, alopecic and exudative. One lesion was on the temporal area of the head, the other on the flank. One had a rough surface with hyperkeratosis and hyperpigmentation, the other was exudative. Both had been present for 2 months. One cat was lost to follow-up, but the lesion in the other cat recurred 3 months after surgical excision. The lesions may have been congenital. They did not exhibit aggressive behaviour. They were composed of well-differentiated epithelium without malignant features.

The folliculo-apocrine unit has three types of epithelia; the first is continuous with the infundibular epithelium of the follicle, the second is the ductal epithelium, and the third is apocrine secretory epithelium. The tumour, located in the superficial dermis, is characterised by coalescent tubular to papillary apocrine gland proliferations opening either within dilated infundibula, or directly to the surface.

In humans, syringocystadenoma papilliferum is classified with apocrine hamartoma, apocrine naevus and supernumerary nipples. About 90% of lesions occur on the head and neck, but they may occur in the inguinal region, chest, or the axillary and genital areas. They may arise at any age, or be present at birth. Complete surgical excision appears to be curative.

Emily Walder Thelma Lee Gross and I have seen a few of these which we did not know how to classify. In humans, does the congenital multiple-type have the same plaque-like appearance?

Marianne Heimann I am not sure.

Joan Rest Julie Yager and I have each seen a case of multiple sweat gland proliferations in young cats.

Food allergy: hydrolysed vs limited-antigen diets

H.A. Jackson[1] (Chairperson), R.A. Garfield[2] (Secretary)

[1] Department of Clinical Sciences, North Carolina State University, Raleigh, North Carolina, USA
[2] Animal Dermatology Referral Clinic,, Dallas, Texas, USA

Hilary Jackson *USA*   How many of those in attendance are performing diet trials to diagnose food allergy in companion animals, and for how long are these trials conducted? (All attendees were performing diet trials for the diagnosis of food allergy ranging from 6 weeks to 12 weeks in length.)

Craig Griffin *USA*   I will re-evaluate patients 4 weeks after starting the diet trial and, if improvement is noted, I will continue for 8 weeks or longer. During the initial part of the food trial, I treat secondary infections and use antihistamines and shampoo therapy as necessary.

Ed Rosser *USA*   I begin a food trial and concurrent aggressive symptomatic treatment with prednisone and antibiotics, as necessary, for 3 weeks and re-evaluate at 4 weeks. If pruritus is still present, I will repeat aggressive symptomatic treatment for 3 weeks and again re-evaluate at 8 weeks, continuing in this manner. In my opinion, food trials are best performed during the winter months where the only environmental antigen that patients are exposed to (in Michigan, USA) is the house dust mite.

Other respondents stated that they clear infections prior to the food trial and use no other treatments during the food trial.

Genevieve Marignac *France*   In Europe we do not appreciate the sharp seasonal fluctuations that Ed Rosser describes.

Reid Garfield *USA* and **Craig Griffin**   Up to 80% of their allergic patients have non-seasonal disease and therefore diagnostic food testing is usually performed at a time where atopic dermatitis may also be active.

Many respondents expressed difficulty in getting their clients to continue with the diet trial and to strictly adhere to the restricted diet. Most routinely had their clients avoid all other treats, table food, masking medications (used for oral drug administration, e.g. peanut butter, meats, cheese), and flavoured medications such as found in heartworm prophylactics.

Ed Rosser   I additionally ask my clients to isolate the dog in a separate room away from the family at meal time.

Craig Griffin   I recommend that when dogs are walked they be muzzled to prevent accidental ingestion of food during walks.

During a general discussion it was agreed that cat food must be kept away and even the dog's access to the cat's litter box must be avoided. Additionally, cats must be kept indoors exclusively and the owner must be willing to rinse dishes, or put them away, after each meal to prevent accidental exposure to other food ingredients.

Jesper Orum *Denmark* Farm dogs must be kept away from the stables due to ingestion of allergens in cow or horse manure.

The discussion then turned to confirming a food allergy with dietary provocation.

Genevieve Marignac Exacerbation with diet provocation is more important than judging improvement with dietary restriction. I challenge with the previous diet (no treats) initially, and symptoms often flare within a few days if food allergy is present.

Craig Griffin Provocation is important since seasonal fluctuations due to atopic dermatitis may cause symptoms to wax and wane, confusing apparent improvement with dietary restriction. In addition, gastrointestinal symptoms must also be monitored during the challenge. Some dogs will have a recurrence or increase in borborygmus, flatulence, or a decline in stool quality. Increased number of bowel movements of four or more daily is suggestive of food allergy.

Helen Globus *USA* Choosing which food to use for the challenge can be difficult because of the large numbers of food types to which the animals have previously been exposed.

While some respondents challenged with the previously fed diet only, others re-introduced the previous diet and all treats and table food at one time.

Michael Hannigan *Canada* I introduce the previous diet first, followed by one single treat every 14 days.

Claudia Nett-Mettler *Switzerland* Challenging cats is difficult, as many owners have often rotated their cat through a large selection of foods.

Ed Rosser The last previously fed diet on which the cat was symptomatic would be sufficient.

Diagnosis and management of 22 dogs with adverse food reactions (A. Loeffler)

Annette Loeffler *UK* We previously reported and published a retrospective evaluation of 63 dogs with allergic disease seen at the Royal Veterinary College in London, UK.[1] In all cases, a strict diet trial with a chicken hydrolysate diet (Hills prescription diet z/d ULTRA allergen free, Hills Pet Nutrition Ltd, Kansas, USA) was recommended. In these 63 dogs, 46 clients fed the diet exclusively as directed. Seventeen clients (27%) failed to comply with instructions. In ten of these cases, owner compliance was an issue. Four dogs found the diet unpalatable, one dog was euthanised due to an unrelated disease, one dog developed diarrhoea, and one client refused to challenge the dog with its previous diet to confirm the diagnosis. Similar studies in which home-cooked diets were used have reported a drop-out rate of between 27 and 52% in one study,[2] and between 32 and 41.7% in another study.[3] Of those dogs completing the diet trial in our study, nine (19.6%) were diagnosed with adverse food reaction only, nine (19.6%) had adverse food reaction and concurrent atopic dermatitis, and four (8.8%) had adverse food reaction concurrent with another pruritic disease.

Twenty-two dogs were followed for 3–9 months after diagnosis. Nine dogs were still eating a chicken hydrolysate diet. Eleven dogs were receiving an alternative limited-antigen diet, and two were no longer on dietary restriction. Offending foodstuffs were identified as chicken (one dog) and other limited-antigen diets (three dogs).

Sixteen owners mentioned cost factors with regard to a long-term diet choice.

The failure rate (unable to complete the diet trial) in this study was favourable (27%) when compared to the previously reported 47% for home-cooked diets.[3] The percentage of allergic dogs diagnosed with an adverse food reaction in this study (19.6%) is similar to previous reports.

Kimberly Coyner *USA* Of the dogs diagnosed concurrently with food allergy and atopic dermatitis, how many could be satisfactorily controlled with the diet alone?

Annette Loeffler Approximately 50%. The dogs with food allergy had increased daily defecation rates.

Anna Jackson *UK* Would stabilising these patients' diets have improved GI symptoms, even without adverse reactions to food?

Craig Griffin Fibre may increase bowel movements. The home-cooked yam and pinto bean diet I use may cause dogs to defecate five to six times per day. I consider dogs on maintenance diets with more than three bowel movements per day to be abnormal. In addition, owners often believe that the yam and pinto bean diet will increase flatulence, but this is not usually the case.

Hilary Jackson Is immunological cross-reactivity between different proteins clinically important? I have a clinical impression that intolerance to chicken clinically spans the poultry group.

Craig Griffin and Rusty Muse *USA* Some patients sensitised to chicken will react to hydrolysed chicken (Hill's Z/D), and some do not. We have the same observation for soy-allergic patients on hydrolysed soy diets. Venison may also share allergens with beef.

Phil Roudebush *USA* Dogs sensitised to chicken are reacting to chicken serum albumin, which is not present in the z/d chicken hydrolysate diets.

Michael Hannigan I have had success using buffalo meat even in beef-allergic patients.

Hilary Jackson Do you consider the carbohydrate component of the diet important in selecting a diet for a food trial?

Craig Griffin The carbohydrate component contains small amounts of protein that can act as a food allergen. Ten per cent of patients with food allergy cannot be controlled on commercial diets and must be fed home-cooked restricted-allergen diets in the long term.

Hilary Jackson We are assuming that food allergy in dogs and cats is IgE-mediated. If mediated by T cells, the hydrolysed proteins may still be presented to the immune system and provoke a clinical reaction. It is also possible that the carbohydrates can act as allergens.

Jesper Orum Should we measure allergen-specific IgE to guide the choice of diet?

Hilary Jackson There is currently no evidence to support this. In people, the predictability of serum allergen-specific IgE concentrations varies between allergens and with the age of the individual. In dogs there is evidence that recent oral exposure may influence the serum allergen-specific IgE concentration, but we know nothing about other factors. Commercially available tests are not standardised with serum from known allergic patients.

Genevieve Marignac Some pet foods are labelled 'allergen free', which is misleading.

Phil Roudebush Most (90%) of chicken-sensitised dogs do not react to chicken hydrolysate diets. This meets regulatory requirements, but does not preclude any clinical allergy to chicken.

Craig Griffin We do not know what the specific antigens in food are that cause food allergy.

David Lloyd *UK* If we don't know what the allergens are, how do we create a reliable test for them? The discussion here today is anecdotal and we need good prospective studies to understand food allergy in dogs and cats. We should look at the gut before and after challenge.

Claudia Nett-Mettler I use a horse-meat and potato diet, and if the patients do not lose weight, I feel the clients are not compliant with the diet.

Others responded that they felt many of their patients lose weight due to the elimination of other treats. Oil may also be added to increase the caloric content.

Hilary Jackson Weight loss may also be due to the discontinuation of prednisone in some cases.

Hilary Jackson Do people have a preference for canned food over dry food for food trials? And could the difference in processing affect the antigenicity of the protein?

Phil Roudebush Different parts of the animal species are used in canned food compared to dry food and these differences are more likely to be important than the different processing, as both forms are cooked.

Hilary Jackson Has anyone found storage mites in dry food to be a problem?

Phil Roudebush   The mite content of the original ingredients (grains) are more likely to be the source of storage mite contamination than storage of the bag of food in the home.

Genevieve Marignac   We looked at food left open in catteries for 3 months and it did not contain storage mites.

References

1 Loeffler, A., Lloyd, D.H., Bond, R., Kim, J.Y., Pfeiffer, D.U. Dietary trials with a commercial chicken hydrolysate diet in 63 pruritic dogs. *Veterinary Record*, 2004; **157**: 519–522.
2 Chesney, C.J. Food sensitivity in the dog, a quantitative study. *Journal of Small Animal Practice*, 2002; **43**: 203–207.
3 Kunkle, G., Horner. S. Validity of skin testing for diagnosis of food allergy in dogs. *Journal of the American Veterinary Association*, 2002; **200**: 677–680.

New forms of therapy for atopic dermatitis

C.E. Griffin[1] (Chairperson), G. Marignac[2] (Secretary)

[1] Animal Dermatology Clinic, San Diego, California, USA
[2] École Nationale Vétérinaire d'Alfort, Paris, France

Craig Griffin *USA* I have invited some people to share with us their work in treating, or trying to improve the treatment of, atopic dermatitis (AD). We are going to begin with Dr Carlotti's work on interferon-omega (IFN-ω). I thought this would be interesting data and stimulate others to share their experience with interferons.

Didier-Noël Carlotti *France* This is part of the free communication presented at this meeting. This is a very preliminary study. Interferons (IFNs) are regulatory proteins divided into type I (α [alpha], β [beta], ω [omega] and τ [tau]), and type II (γ [gamma]). Their immunomodulatory effects may be exemplified by IFN-γ for instance, which shows: inhibition of IL-4-induced IgE synthesis; inhibition of expression of Fcγ receptors; and inhibition of superoxide production by circulating monocytes. These effects may explain why IFN-γ has been used successfully in man to treat atopic dermatitis (AD), as reported in double-blinded placebo-controlled clinical studies. There are grounds to try IFN-γ in canine AD. The presentation given in this congress by Toshiro Iwasaki also shows some beneficial effect in treating AD dogs with IFN-γ. In addition, type I IFNs and IFN-ω have several actions including: antiviral activity; inhibition of cell proliferation; promotion of T-cell differentiation; activation of effector cells including T cells, NK cells and macrophages; effect on synthesis of various cytokines by decreasing the synthesis of pro-inflammatory interleukin (IL)-1, IL-8, and TNF-α; and increasing anti-inflammatory cytokines IL-10 and TGF-β. This suggested that IFN-ω might be beneficial in allergic disease.

This preliminary study was designed to assess if a commercial recombinant IFN-ω (Virbagen® Omega, Virbac, France), may reduce clinical signs in canine AD. Three investigators performed this prospective, non-comparative study in dogs with AD. All cases met Willemse's criteria for the diagnosis of AD, had positive intradermal tests, had parasitic diseases and adverse food reactions excluded, and microbial infection controlled, prior to entering the study. Treatment with IFN-ω at 1 million IU/kg given subcutaneously three times weekly for 3 weeks was administered. Concurrent treatment was restricted to a non-medicated shampoo (Sebocalm®, Virbac, France), antiseptic ear cleaner (Epi-Otic®, Virbac, France) and flea control. Each visit (day 0 [inclusion day and first treatment], day 7, day 21 and day 42) included general and dermatological examination, as well as ear and skin cytology. Clinical signs were assessed by LICAD (lesion index for canine atopic dermatitis) and PICAD (pruritus index for canine atopic dermatitis) index, which are derived from the previously published CADESI scale.

Eighteen dogs were included in the study. A significant reduction in LICAD and PICAD indexes was obtained at day 7, 12 and 42, when compared to day 0 results. There were no discrepancies between the two indexes in each dog. This is the first evaluation of IFN-ω in canine AD. We used high doses and high frequency, which may be impractical in clinical practice due to cost and practicability. The route of administration (subcutaneous injection) might be difficult for the average owner. This treatment resulted in very impressive results in some dogs. Tolerance was good with only one dog developing an erythematous rash that resulted in discontinuation of therapy. Another dog experienced mild gastrointestinal signs that did not cause termination of treatment. It is likely that IFN-ω activity is only short term. Last, but not least, this product, especially at the doses used in this study, is prohibitively expensive. For instance, the cost for a 35-kg Labrador retriever was €1500. The good clinical results obtained here provide grounds for further studies to confirm our results. There is a need to find an effective protocol using doses lower than the antiviral doses we used, in order to decrease the cost. Induction and maintenance phases should be evaluated. During induction phase, IFN-ω should be compared to a reference product, for instance cyclosporine, and during maintenance, the reduction of recurrence of microbial infection (bacterial or fungal) should be assessed.

Has anybody from the audience used IFN in AD?

Jorg Defen *Switzerland*   You said that the IFN-ω has a short-term action. Can you comment on that?

Didier-Noël Carlotti   After the study we continued to evaluate the dogs. Clinical signs recurred soon after day 42 of the study, keeping in mind that the dogs' last treatment was on day 18.

Jorg Defen   Is it possible to use IFN-ω with antibiotics and food changes?

Didier-Noël Carlotti   Our study design did not assess this question in particular, but why not? Yes.

Craig Griffin   This study has shown some efficacy, now further studies are needed to evaluate the product for practical use. I would also point out that IFN-α is used orally in cats and dogs, and also at extremely low doses. For example, cats are given 30–60 IU orally once daily. In the stomach, IFNs are rapidly destroyed, so low doses have to be absorbed from the oral cavity, and these low doses and an alternative route of administration should be evaluated. I would like to ask if the animals from your study were put on allergen-specific

immunotherapy (ASIT)? If yes, did you feel they responded to ASIT?

Didier-Noël Carlotti   They did not receive ASIT during the study, but later some did go on ASIT and responded.

Craig Griffin   There is a human AD study[1] where they used IFN-γ with ASIT. They had four groups: (1) house dust mites ASIT only; (2) IFN-γ only; (3) both ASIT and IFN-γ combined at the same time; and (4) a control group. That small pilot study showed that the only group that had a decrease in clinical scores was the combination therapy group.

Didier-Noël Carlotti   We should perhaps try to use IFN-γ in combination with ASIT in dogs. This seems to be a very good suggestion.

Christophe Rème *France*   Tim Nuttall presented a study at this congress that showed that IFN-γ is found in lesional skin of dogs with AD. He proposed that IFN-γ was correlated with maintenance of AD. How can you explain the gap between the two facts?

Geneviève Marignac *France*   Both in clinical or *in vitro* studies, discrepancies are commonly observed regarding cytokines levels, their presence, their activity, etc. Explanations include: variation in cytokine local concentration; presence or absence of other cytokines; cellular/tissue activity; etc. Basically anything can be seen and happen with cytokines.

Didier-Noël Carlotti   IFN-γ and IFN-ω do not exactly share the same activity. Nevertheless, they have given apparently similar clinical results in the dog.

Craig Griffin   Christophe Rème will now begin the discussion on house dust mites by presenting results on the *in vitro* efficacy of permethrin and pyriproxyfen on the house dust mite *Dermatophagoides farinae*.

Christophe Rème   A large volume of evidence in the literature underlines the importance of house dust mites for triggering AD in dogs. A recent study[2] demonstrated that if good in-house control with acaricidal products is performed, significant alleviation of clinical signs is obtained in atopic dogs. We therefore decided to look at whether a widely available commercial in-house anti-flea product (Indorex, Virbac, UK) could also have significant activity on house dust mites under well-controlled environmental conditions *in vitro*.

The design of the study was simple. First, dust mites (in their rearing medium) were poured onto experimental units previously sprayed with test and control products. Then, at various intervals in time (2, 4, 8 and 12 weeks) mites and eggs were extracted and counted using reference methods. All procedures complied with French official guidelines (AFNOR G 39-01) and the tests were performed in a specialised pest laboratory (TEC, France) under Good Experimental Practice rules. We used *Dermatophagoides farinae* because, worldwide, it is the most common allergen in atopic dogs. The *D. farinae* strain used in this study originates from INRA (Institut National de la Recherche Agronomique, France) and was reared in the laboratory since 1997. The strain had no previous contact with any pesticide. The mites were raised in specialised premises under standard conditions (weekly renewed food, 24°C, 75% relative humidity and isolation). Basically, mites were cultured in Petri dishes turned upside-down. A polystyrene disk was placed at the bottom of the dishes on which rearing medium was poured. The top of the Petri dish prevented mite dispersion while some air-flow was permitted by an aeration grid. The units were allocated to four treatment groups: (1) treatment-free (control group); (2) vehicle only (vehicle group); (3) vehicle and pyriproxyfen (IGR group); and (4) vehicle, IGR, permethrin and piperonyl butoxide (treatment group). The product was sprayed on the disk using a precise standardised method (5-second pulses for a 1 m² surface at a distance of 50 cm) to deliver pyriproxyfen (PPF) at 1.25 mg/m² and permethrin at 64.4 mg/m² (the recommended anti-flea label dose). Three hundred mobile mites (± 5%) were inoculated to each experimental unit (density of 5000 mites/m²). The method for mite counting differentiated the mobile forms (larvae, nymphs and adults) from the eggs. When the Petri dish was placed on a heated plate (40°C), the nymphs and adults tended to move upward and stick to an adhesive disk placed above the rearing unit. Under the microscope, the eight-legged nymphs and adults were differentiated from the six-legged larvae, and the total number of mites on the whole adhesive disk surface was recorded. The eggs were counted directly from the Petri dish by use of a special transparent sectored disk. The experiment was replicated four times in the four treatment groups at the four different time intervals (2, 4, 8 and 12 weeks), i.e. a total of 64 experimental units were examined in this study.

In the control and vehicle groups, there was exponential mite growth (adult and nymphal counts) over 12 weeks (valid growth conditions, no acaricidal effect of the vehicle). In the treatment group, immediate killing was evidenced by the absence of mobile forms from 2 to 12 weeks post-exposure. In the IGR group, adult and nymphal counts decreased regularly from week 4, while no mites could be detected at week 12, which reflected the natural kinetics of adult deaths and the absence of population renewal. Larval counts yielded similar results. The egg count outcome was also similar, except that egg numbers decreased significantly at week 4 only in the treatment group (lag time), since acaricidal drugs are not active on eggs but only on emerging larvae.

The most interesting finding in this study was that pyriproxyfen proved to be an acarine growth regulator in addition to being an insect growth regulator (wider scope of 'Arthropod Growth Regulator'?). Shall we use an IGR then in the homes of dogs with AD in order to get significant control of house dust mites?

Craig Griffin Thank you very much, Dr Rème. I propose that we continue on the house dust mite presentations unless there are specific questions with these products. Dr Rème has given us a good introduction and, controlling house dust mites (HDM) could be of interest, especially in Europe where atopic dogs commonly are sensitised only to house dust mites. In the USA, the situation is different. For instance, in southern California, only about 5% of our atopic dogs are sensitised to house dust mites alone. But, even in southern California, we realise that some animals do benefit from HDM control. The results of the previously mentioned study[2] are very exciting, but it is also important to consider the dog antigen. The major allergen is different for atopic dogs than humans. Dogs seem to react primarily to a high molecular weight allergen. Very few dogs are reactive to Der p1, Der p2, Der f1 or Der f2 (low molecular weight allergens) which are the major allergens in humans. Those specific antigens are often used to detect the presence of mites in various dust samples. We also know that there is a lot of cross-reactivity. I refer for instance to the presentation by Anna Jackson at this congress describing the prevalence and characterisation of HDM and HDM allergens collected from the bedding, skin and hair coat of dogs in south-west England. In their sampling, there were actually no *D. farinae* mites found, and 8 of 68 samples had *D. pteronyssinus*. *D. pteronyssinus* and *D. farinae* allergen were detected in 54% and 5.9% respectively.

Killing these mites is an important step, but the antigens remain in the environment and remain as a triggering factor. Antigen denaturation is also mandatory, especially if other sources of allergen (i.e. dandruff, fibres, pollens) besides house dust mites and storage mites are present. In the study by Swinnen and Vroom[2] with house dust mite atopic dogs, at least 50% of dogs respond well if house dust mites are controlled, but it could take as long as 4 months to obtain negative house dust mite detection. A small study was performed 12 years ago by Dr Rosenkrantz and myself with the sodium polyborate ingredient in Flea Busters flea powder. Is that product available in Europe?

Didier-Noël Carlotti   Yes, at least in Germany.

Craig Griffin   This study showed that borate did significantly reduce house dust mites when applied to all beds, upholstered furniture and carpets. Recently, a research study was performed by Arlian that evaluated disodium octaborate tetrahydrate (DOT). This study was funded by the company that developed a water-miscible borate product for flea and dust mite control. Pieces of carpet were inoculated with *D. farinae* and *D. pteronyssinus*. One set was treated with DOT in water spray, one set was left untreated, and one set was treated with an equivalent water spray without DOT. Mites were counted 2, 4 and 8 weeks after treatment.

The results for *D. pteronyssinus* mites/gram counts were: (1) 885 at 2 weeks, 93 at 4 weeks, and 10 at 8 weeks for DOT-treated; (2) 2293 at 2 weeks, 109 993 at 4 weeks, and 82 987 at 8 weeks for untreated; and (3) 12 528 at 2 weeks, 166 580 at 4 weeks, and 32 260 at 8 weeks for water-treated. The results for *D. farinae* mite/gram were: (1) 17 555 at 2 weeks; 14 486 at 4 weeks; and 1106 at 8 weeks for DOT-treated; (2) 32 171 at 2 weeks, 64 651 at 4 weeks, and 70 793 at 8 weeks for untreated; 32 8111 at 2 weeks, 98 101 at 4 weeks, and 70 273 at 8 weeks for water-treated.

House dust mites, especially *D. pteronyssinus*, need humidity, and when moisture is elevated, the *D. pteronyssinus* proliferation rate significantly increased. In this study, DOT was very effective against *D. pteronyssinus* (10 mites/gram at week 8) but apparently less active against *D. farinae*, though still significant reductions to 1100 mites/gram at week 8. An independent study on DOT[3] showed a significant residual effect. They followed DOT activity on mite levels every 2 months for 6 months in 93 private homes which were randomised into three groups, similar to the study by Arlian. By 2 months, the active group was significantly less (*p* <0.001), but by 6 months only the carpet had significantly lower mite levels, though both carpet and sofa had lower mite allergen levels.

Products are coming out that claim not only to kill mites, but to destroy allergens as well. In 2000, the company that produces Ecology Work® anti-allergen solution had an *in vitro* study done to evaluate the denaturing effect of the anti-allergen solution (AAS) contained in their product, and compared to tannic acid (Allersearch® ADS) and benzoyl benzoate (Allercare® Johnson). They assessed Der p1, Der f1, Can f1 (canine major allergen for humans), Fel d1 (feline) and Bla g1 (cockroach) after these products had been applied to dry and liquid samples containing the allergens. They reported only some effect for benzyl benzoate against Can f1 and Der p1, and that tannic acid had very good denaturing effect on Fel d1, Can f1, Der p1 and Der f1 in dry samples but not liquid phase, and their product had good denaturing effect on all five allergens evaluated, both in liquid and dry phase. One of the concerns with this study is that the allergens evaluated, particularly Der p1 and Der f1, are not important in the dog. Therefore one must be cautious in interpreting results of such studies for the dog.

In 2003, Bob Esch from Greer Laboratory did a study to evaluate an anti-allergen spray (Aveho Biosciences, USA), which contains the AAS, on canine house dust mite allergens. An ELISA-inhibition potency assay was performed in duplicates in wells coated with reference *D. farinae* allergen. A 40–75% reduction was found with 1:2, 1:4 and 1:8 dilutions, i.e. that was concentration-dependent. When more diluted, AAS had no effect. According to Greer, tannic acid had no effect on canine house dust mite allergens, and AAS is the first product that they looked at that lowers canine house dust mite allergens. However, Dr Esch believes that a 99% reduction in environmental allergenic load would be required to obtain relevant clinical results. So, AAS apparently does denature relevant canine house dust mite allergens, but not to a degree, at least with one treatment, sufficient to obtain clinical results.

In conclusion, killing mites is only one part of the puzzle. If we want fast results, allergen denaturation is also needed, particularly if one considers that there are other potential sources in the dog's environment that are producing cross-reactive allergens. Destroying these latter sources could be of importance. Considering that in the south-west of England where the study presented by Anna Jackson showed that in homes where no *D. farinae* could be detected, some dogs had *D. farinae* allergens on their coats.

I would like to open the floor for questions related to house dust mites and their control.

Lars Mecklenburg *Germany*   Based on the presentation of Dr Bieber from the first day of the congress (where he describes the hypothesis in human atopic dermatitis that people eventually develop stage III and they develop autoimmunity), then avoidance of allergen may not work if we consider that dogs who have very bad atopic dermatitis manifestations could also suffer from a type of autoimmunity. I am thinking in particular of the very bad German shepherd dogs, where nothing helps. This idea that autoimmunity could be involved in severe cases of AD is, I think, probably appropriate in most severe canine cases of AD, and then avoidance would not work.

Craig Griffin   What I understood from his presentation was that the key was to prevent people from reaching stage III. That is why they recommended cleansing and trying to control the bacteria and prevent the patients from reaching stage III. The idea is that if the antigens are not there, you never get to stage III.

Lars Mecklenburg   Yes that is right, but what if you get the referral very late, there is probably no point in avoiding the allergen once the dog has reached stage III. That is my question.

Craig Griffin   If we look at Swinnen and Vroom's paper, half of her house dust mite-positive dogs responded to house dust mite control.

Lars Mecklenburg   How old were they, that is the point.

Craig Griffin   We don't know how severe their disease

was, nor if they reached stage III, or even if stage III is applicable to dogs at this point. If some dogs do reach stage III, then that might explain why some dogs don't respond. If this is true, that would confirm how important it is to treat early in the disease. How many people are using HDM control in their practice? (Approximately five people.) How do you feel about it? In my practice (south-west USA), we have prescribed a fair amount of house dust mite control. I do not have actual numbers at this time, just clinical impressions. Despite the fact that I have observed some individual cases where improvement was amazing, overall I certainly have not seen 50% responding. These impressions may reflect that I only have about 5% of dogs that are purely HDM sensitised.

Didier-Noël Carlotti   I have not used it very much, perhaps I should.

Pascal Prelaud *France*   I have used it indirectly where families have atopic children and do a lot of house dust mite control, but I still see very allergic dogs in these families.

Craig Griffin   That is interesting as I have some clients who continue to use house dust mite control because a family member has improved, but the dog has not. This may be because the dog allergen is significantly different; however, I am not sure of the exact reason for this observation.

John Birley *Australia*   In humans, oral hyposensitisation is effective and widely used now. I was wondering what would happen if we fed house dust mites to dogs, as a way to induce oral tolerance in dogs.

Craig Griffin   In humans, there have been studies looking at giving allergen-specific immunotherapy orally versus subcutaneously.

Didier-Noël Carlotti   Sublingually?

Genevieve Marignac   This might be a problem in dogs, as in humans there is some evidence that the oral route is not effective as opposed to the sublingual route which is effective. Giving immunotherapy by the sublingual route in the dog may be difficult. Also, the level of protein used is very high compared to that used for subcutaneous injections. The price, of course, would be a problem if it were used at the dose used in humans;

the price would increase by 10–50 times. Nevertheless, we have no idea of what would be the right dosage in the dog.

Craig Griffin   There is another area to consider. How many of you think that when very good flea control is used, some of the atopic dogs are doing significantly better? I have certainly seen that. I always thought that was from the flea control. I am wondering, considering the work Christophe Rème just presented, how much of this effect may be from topical anti-flea products actually treating house dust mites, at least on the dog's bedding and where the dog is spending time?

Didier-Noël Carlotti   I have seen a lot of dogs with classical atopic dermatitis signs and flea allergy dermatitis and, undoubtedly, some of these dogs respond to good flea control and the atopic signs are eliminated, or at least decrease significantly. Perhaps it is not from only killing fleas; perhaps it is not from decreasing the threshold effect, but also from lowering the allergic load from mites.

Daniela Delius *Germany*   What do you think of treatment with Frontline® (Merial, France)? I have thought it may help atopic dogs and this may have been from effects on dust mites or other allergens.

Craig Griffin   My impression was that anything that kills HDM and fleas might be working by more than one process. I do not know of any precise data on Frontline® for house dust mites, but we know it kills other mites. Christophe, do you have any idea on other insecticides that can be used to kill house dust mites?

Christophe Rème   *In vitro* studies reported in the literature suggest that methoprene could be effective against house dust mites, although at high concentration (1–5%). The question is: when one applies a spot-on flea control product containing methoprene to the dog, is there enough methoprene that can spread and be effective in the environment against dust mites?

Liora Waldman *Israel*   In Israel, organophosphates are used against cockroaches and they kill so many things I would think they would be effective on HDM. My question was: has anyone tried to use fibres indicated for asthmatic kids, such as GoreTex™ or covers for beds that are used?

Craig Griffin   Has anybody used those? I am aware of a recent study that shows that they are not so effective in people.[4] I am not sure that we know how effective they are in dogs. Anyway, if you control mites in the dog bedding, do you still get the mites where the dog is having the most exposure to mites? I am not sure we know that yet.

Audience *Switzerland*   I am wondering how many times per year we should treat the environment? Secondly, what are the possible side effects for the young children that are rolling on the floor?

Craig Griffin   Yes, this is certainly an excellent point. I cannot comment on all of the products. I know that DOT claims a full year of efficacy for fleas, with some studies showing more efficacy than that. The study by Codina *et al.*[3] showed 6 months efficacy on HDM in carpets, not the bed. Another polyborate has been available for many years, from Flea Busters™, the company that marketed it, who have treated thousands of houses all over the USA. The safety profile was phenomenal. The California Environmental Protection Agency has approved it as a safe product for flea control. But, treating a house for fleas is not the same as treating a house for HDM. Against HDM, all the beds, sofas and furniture have to be treated, while for fleas, only the floors are treated. I do think that this has to be taken into consideration.

Terill Eckert *Germany*   Regarding the safety of tetraborate in children, that question was raised to me by people who wanted to treat their house against fleas but were concerned for their children's health. Two toxicologists told me that tetraborate is apparently less toxic than table salt. After I found out, I had to convince these owners to use tetraborate by drinking a glass of water with a tablespoon of tetraborate!

Craig Griffin   That is one dedicated study! Let's move on to other aspects of AD treatment with some unpublished data on the addition of storage mites to HDM immunotherapy in dogs, presented by Geneviève Marignac from Alfort Veterinary School in France.

Geneviève Marignac   My presentation will consist of retrospective comments on three cases. In Alfort we added the following storage mites to our intradermal testing (IDT) panel in 1999: *Acarus siro* (As),

Lepidoglyphus destructor (Ld), *Glyciphagus domesticus* (Gd), *Tyrophagus putrescentiae* (Tp), and a storage mites mix marketed by the Stallergènes (Antony, France). We first evaluated these allergens by IDT and did not use them in ASIT. After a while I had some dogs that were positive to storage mites, but hyposensitised only to HDM. One day, a student asked me the reason why, and I answered that I was still evaluating these allergens. Hearing that, and considering that her dog was a failure on ASIT with only HDM, the owner insisted that we would introduce storage mites to her dog's treatment.

I report here on three dogs: a 9-year-old Yorkshire terrier, a 7-year-old Labrador retriever and a 3-year-old pit bull. They had chronic relapsing pruritic dermatitis that did not respond to flea control or food elimination. Treatment of secondary infections was only partially effective, while glucocorticoids were effective only as long as they were administered. In these three dogs, IDT were positive for both storage mites and HDM. The Labrador retriever was positive for *D. farinae* and *Tyrophagus putrescentiae* only. In this dog, other mites were negative or weakly positive. In the other dogs, all mites were more or less positive. They had all received ASIT containing one or both HDM. The ASIT for the Yorkshire terrier also contained cereal-mix pollen. After 14 months to 3 years, the efficacy of ASIT in these three dogs was very poor, despite very good owner compliance. In particular, glucocorticoids still had to be used repetitively to control their pruritus.

Thus, in all three dogs, ASIT composition was modified by the addition of one (*Tyrophagus putrescentiae* in the Labrador retriever) or three storage mites (both other dogs), based on the IDT results. After 1 year with the new ASIT, all owners assessed improvement of >75% in their dog's pruritus and clinical signs. This being a retrospective assessment, no CADESI or PICAD assessment has been performed. Orally administered treatments were dramatically reduced or discontinued in all three dogs. Secondary infections did not recur, except occasional episodes of otitis externa that were still present. After 18 months to 3 years of follow-up, there were no more signs of skin disease. Two of these dogs were quite elderly, and their atopic dermatitis had been attended to by our department for many years. My conclusion is that spontaneous cure is possible, but over the 3–5 years prior to the final ASIT (with storage mites included), the dermatological conditions of these dogs had worsened, despite very observant owners.

Cross-reactions between house dust mites and storage mites are probably common. This is indicated, for instance, by the fact that most atopic dogs are more or less positive to all mites, both HDM and storage mites. However, the actual extent of these cross-reactions is unknown in the dog at this time. For instance, from these three cases, the Labrador was positive only to two mites. Current explanations for this cross-reactivity include difference in dog's exposure to environmental mites, and differences in the allergen content of various mites extracts. The cases presented here are only anecdotal, but may indicate that the importance of storage mites in canine atopic dermatitis should not be underestimated.

Craig Griffin These cases give some evidence that storage mites may play a role. I think that these mites are more readily available for testing in Europe than in North America.

Pascal Prélaud Since I have been using these mites, I have had problems with the reproducibility of storage mite allergens between each batch. Once *D. farinae* and *D. pteronyssinus* extracts are produced, they are biologically standardised. However, we have to use crude extracts of storage mites that are not biologically standardised. For me, we don't have reproducible results for both intradermal and *in vitro* testing. So, before using them for treatment, we should aim at a better standardisation.

Craig Griffin Do you believe that storage mites play a role in atopic dermatitis?

Pascal Prélaud Yes.

Ralf Mueller We performed a study some years ago using various concentrations of both storage mites and HDM. We did IDT in about 20 normal dogs and 25–30 atopic dogs. Our results were similar to what Richard Halliwell has published: there was no difference between normal and atopic dogs regarding the incidence of sensitisation to mites. Regarding the concentration, nothing could really be concluded, except that the stronger the extract used, the more likely we would get a reaction. Another point is that nobody really knows to which mites, and to what extent, dogs are really exposed. There is a recent study in England showing that there is no *D. farinae* found in houses, while the majority of dogs are IDT-positive to *D. farinae* extracts. How do we make sense of this? What about recommendations made by some dermatologists to owners whose dog are sensitised to mites that they should freeze their food, feed canned food, and so on? We do not know if these mites are really present in dog's food or their environment, and we don't know where or how dogs are sensitised. I totally agree with you in that we should use these storage mites, as we are already empirically doing when we use HDM mites in allergy testing and ASIT. Nevertheless, we should now try to put more science in our use of mite extracts in testing and treating dogs.

Craig Griffin   About the study, you said that the HDM and the storage mites reacted with the same incidence in both normal and atopic dogs. Then you said that one should be careful about storage mites, but I am sure that you included *D. farinae* and *D. pteronyssinus* in this.

Ralf Mueller   My point was that we have to be really careful to use allergy testing only in atopic dogs, and then interpret test results only in the light of the dog's history and exposure to a given allergen.

Didier-Noël Carlotti   Cross-reactivity certainly does exist. In a retrospective study published by E. Bensignor and myself[5] on mite sensitivity, we found that only a few dogs reacted only to storage mites. This has also been shown in a Japanese study. So the same cross-reactivity exists in Japan as well. My second point is that ASIT with storage mites has given rise to much debate on the VetDerm list. I only have a few dogs that have been hyposensitised just to storage mites, and the results are highly variable. If there was a study that shows that dogs undergoing storage mites ASIT monotherapy do get better we would be very happy to use these extracts. My third point is that I wonder if dogs have storage mites around them? There is a study that shows that there are no storage mites in dry dog food when the bag is closed.[6] But as soon as it is opened, mites multiply. They were able to demonstrate a considerable number of mites after a few days in those bags.

Geneviève Marignac   During the workshop on food allergy that took place yesterday, three people said that

they have not been able to demonstrate mites in dry dog food, even after the bag was opened for some time. It is interesting that yesterday we all agreed that mites are not a problem in dry dog food and here we have an opposite point of view. I wanted also to comment on Ralph's study. Patrick Bourdeau in Nantes is testing dogs with *Blomia tropicalis* extracts. Apparently, this mite does not occur in Europe at all. In the west of France, he is finding that a lot of dogs are positive for this mite. As a final comment, in a retrospective study made on 52 IDT performed in Alfort, we find that the allergen dogs most commonly react to is *D. farinae* (94%), then *Acarus siro* with as high as 67% of dogs positive. *D. pteronyssinus* is only in the third position with 56%. Other storage mites were positive in 39–50% of dogs. So sensitisation to storage mites is far from being an anecdotal phenomenon.

Craig Griffin   There are studies showing *Blomia tropicalis* is important in human allergy and prevalent in tropical and subtropical climates.[7,8] So these mites are found, and we should pay more attention to them. We are now going to move on to Dr Pascal Prélaud's presentation on immunotherapy.

Pascal Prelaud   For allergen-specific immunotherapy (ASIT), there are questions regarding the dosage, time interval between injections, protocols to follow, etc. I am going to present to you very preliminary results of an ASIT study comparing the commonly used protocol (named low-dose protocol) to a protocol using very high dosages of allergens, over 1 year. I wanted to assess the long-term efficacy of ASIT. This is the reason why we did not use lesional or clinical scores. My opinion is that in a protocol assessing a monotherapy for a short term, comparison of clinical scores can be used. For a long-term treatment, involving several treatments, clinical signs are not suitable to assess efficacy. So we used medication scores and compared them. For instance, one point was attributed to each shampoo, or 1 day of antibiotics use. The use of glucocorticoids was assessed as 1–2 points depending on the dosage, and topical steroids were attributed one point. Cyclosporin A was not used in any of these dogs. All the animals were more than 2 years old, all with non-seasonal atopic dermatitis, and all positive with IDT to *D. farinae,* or to both *D. farinae* and *D. pteronyssinus*. As we used medication scores, we did not have any washout period.

Three practitioners performed the study; two in Paris (E. Bensignor and P. Prélaud) and one in the French Alps

(D. Groux). Allergens used for ASIT are alum-precipitated (Allerbio, France), biologically standardised (IR: reactivity indices). After an 11-week induction period, the 'classic' protocol consisted of an injection of 10 IR once a month, for a total amount of 115 IR after 1 year. In the high-dose protocol, 600 IR were administered in 1 year as the induction period was shorter (8 weeks) and 25 IR were injected every 2 weeks. No side effects were noted in either group. Six dogs have been included in the high-dose protocol and five in the low-dose protocol. Results were assessed by adding the total medication scores during each 3- or 6-month period during the study. For each dog, we then compared the total medication scores of the first 6 months of ASIT to the second 6 months, and also the first 3 months to the last 3 months, and generated percentage of lowering of the medication score interpreted as improvement scores.

With the first assessment method, we obtained a 39% (low-dose) and 35% (high-dose) reduction in the medication score. With the second method, a 57% reduction with the lower-dose and, to my surprise, the result with the higher dosage was much less at 28% reduction. With so few dogs included, it is impossible to statistically compare the results. Anyway, we can conclude that using a higher concentration of HDM allergens in ASIT does not improve the result after 1 year. The good surprise was that no side effect was observed, even with the highly concentrated allergen extract used in the high-dose protocol (50 IR/ml).

In conclusion, I think that I will stop using the high-dose protocol as it does not seem to be effective, and is much more expensive. I think that we really need double-blinded studies to be performed in the dog in order to assess what we are really doing during ASIT. We have been using this treatment for half a century now, and, for instance, we all respect an induction period. What is the rationale behind that? The only answer I could find was that we have been applying human protocols to veterinary medicine. There are reports of human patients having severe side effects, including death when too high a dosage was injected without an induction period. But such side effects are not encountered in dogs, so why keep this habit of the induction period? Why not start using the 1-ml dosage once a month directly?

Craig Griffin Thank you for this very interesting preliminary study. Concerning your final point, my clinical impression is that if a dog has not improved after 6 months of ASIT, I decrease the dosage I am giving

to them because some will then respond favourably. About 70% of the dogs I am treating will never get to, or not stay on, the higher dosage. Some years ago, there was an unpublished study presented that compared the 'classical' protocol to a low-dose,[9] and it found the low-dose to have better results. I think that high-dose is going in the wrong direction, and we should be aiming at lowering the doses.

Didier-Noël Carlotti In America, you are using aqueous extracts for ASIT, while in Europe we used aluminium or calcium phosphate suspension. This makes a big difference.

Audience In your study, you base your ASIT treatment on IDT results, or *in vitro* results, and which *in vitro* results? This makes a huge difference.

Pascal Prélaud IDT tests were used at all times in this study. With regards to *in vitro* testing, there are a lot of different labs with many different tests. My opinion is that if you add IDT results to *in vitro* results, you are just increasing your chance of getting positive results. By the way, the same observation applies in medicine in general.

Craig Griffin A review of the literature shows that the same ASIT results were obtained when the allergens included were based on IDT or on *in vitro* tests.[10] The key is that you use allergens for which the dog you are treating is specifically sensitised.

Ralf Mueller We conducted a clinical study that will be published in the *Veterinary Record* where we used two vials (2 ml) instead of one vial in some dogs with numerous reactions on IDT. When we compared their clinical outcome, we found no differences compared to dogs that received the standard protocol, even when we only compared those dogs undergoing the standard protocol that had the same number of positive allergens on IDT than the dogs receiving two vials. I think that this is consistent with the results you have just presented. We all know dogs are doing very well on a small dose, and get itchy again if the dose is increased.

Craig Griffin Yes, excessive amount of allergen is the most common reason for ASIT side effects.

Ralf Mueller An interesting question is whether we

achieve more by giving a lot of allergens in a short time and then stopping, or by giving smaller amounts over a longer time? Do we make the immune system very 'nervous' by repeatedly injecting allergens in the body? Or should we start with low doses from the beginning? I don't know!

Craig Griffin Ralph Mueller is going to talk to us about rush immunotherapy and another study using bacterial DNA in ASIT.

Ralf Mueller In human rush immunotherapy, the induction period is decreased to 1 day in order to achieve ASIT in a shorter period of time. Such protocols mean that a large dose of antigen is administered in a short period. To explore the feasibility and efficacy of rush immunotherapy in the dog, we conducted a double-blinded randomised study and compared conventional immunotherapy induction. The results of this study have been reported at this congress.[11]

The second type of study we performed was to combine bacterial DNA in a liposome complex with allergen extracts. Bacterial DNA sequences bind to antigen-presenting cells. There is a lot of evidence showing that their presence induces a down-regulation of the Th2 response. Now there is also some evidence that they down-regulate Th1 responses to some extent, particularly in the allergic patient. Studies have been done in ragweed-allergic patients using bacterial DNA combined with allergen extract. Our study has been reported at this congress as well.[12]

Craig Griffin Thank you very much for these very interesting studies. It seems that immunotherapy is a very complex treatment. I am sorry that we don't have time to comment further on the subject, but we don't know what a combination of several of these therapies (bacterial DNA, interferon, cyclosporin A, and so on) might achieve. For instance in humans, a placebo-controlled blinded study used the antihistamine terfenadine during the induction phase of immunotherapy for bee stings.[13] After 3 years of ASIT, the patients were challenged with bee stings or venom. They found that the people who had been concurrently treated with antihistamine had less systemic reactions. We have to begin to look at what combination therapies do, because we don't really know what is happening.

Ralf Mueller Such studies are really interesting because I am sure that in 99% of AD case, we use combination therapies. (The audience agrees!)

Craig Griffin Thanks very much to all of you for attending this workshop and for your participation.

References

1 Noh, G., Lee, K.Y. Pilot study of IFN-gamma-induced specific hyposensitization for house dust mites in atopic dermatitis: IFN-gamma-induced immune deviation as a new therapeutic concept for atopic dermatitis. *Cytokine,* 2000; **12**: 472–476.
2 Swinnen, C., Vroom, M. The clinical effect of environmental control of house dust mites in 60 house dust mite-sensitive dogs. *Veterinary Dermatology,* 2004; **15**: 31–36.
3 Codina, R., Lockey R.F., Diwadkar R., Mobley, L.L., Godfrey, S. Disodium octaborate tetrahydrate (DOT) application and vacuum cleaning, a combined strategy to control house dust mites. *Allergy,* 2003; **58**: 318–324.
4 Woodcock, A., Forster, L., Matthews, E., *et al.* Control of exposure to mite allergen and allergen-impermeable bed covers for adults with asthma. *New England Journal of Medicine,* 2003; **349**: 225–236.
5 Bensignor, E., Carlotti, D.N. Sensitivity patterns to house dust mites and forage mites in atopic dogs/150 cases. *Veterinary Dermatology,* 2002; **13**: 37–42.
6 Brazís, P., Pérez, E., García, O., Puigdemont, A. Presencia de ácaros de almacenamiento en dietas secas para perros. *Consulta Difus Vet,* 2004; **111**: 87–89.
7 Medeiros, M. Jr, Figueiredo, J.P., Almeida, M.C., *et al.* Association between mite allergen (Der p 1, Der f 1, Blo t 5) levels and microscopic identification of mites or skin prick test results in asthmatic subjects. *International Archives of Allergy and Immunology,* 2002; **129**: 237–241.
8 Arlian, L.G., Bernstein, D., Bernstein, I.L., *et al.* Prevalence of dust mites in the homes of people with asthma living in eight different geographic areas of the United States. *Journal of Allergy Clinical Immunology,* 1992; **90**: 292–300.
9 Wagner, R. A retrospective survey of hyposensitization therapy using low concentrations of alum-precipitated allergens (abstract). *Proceedings of the 15th Annual Congress of the European Society for Veterinary Dermatology and European College of Veterinary Dermatology, Maastricht,* 1998.
10 Griffin, C., Hillier, A. The ACVD task force on canine atopic dermatitis (XXIV): allergen-specific immunotherapy. *Veterinary Immunology and Immunopathology,* 2001; **81**: 363–383.
11 Mueller, R.S., Fieseler, K.V., Zabel, S., Rosychuk, R.A.W. Conventional and rush immunotherapy in canine atopic dermatitis (abstract). *Veterinary Dermatology,* 2004; **15** (Suppl. 1): 4.
12 Mueller, R.S., Veir, K., Fieseler, K.V., Dow, S. Use of immunostimulatory bacterial DNA sequences in allergen-specific immunotherapy of canine atopic dermatitis (abstract). *Veterinary Dermatology,* 2004; **15** (Suppl. 1): 32.
13 Muller, U., Hari, Y., Berchtold, E. Premedication with antihistamines may enhance efficacy of specific-allergen immunotherapy. *Journal of Allergy and Clinical Immunology,* 2001; **107**: 81–86.

Equine allergic disease

M. M. Sloet van Oldruitenborgh-Oosterbaan[1] (Chairperson), D.C. Knottenbelt[2] (Secretary)

[1] University of Utrecht, Utrecht, The Netherlands
[2] University of Liverpool, Liverpool, UK

Marianne Sloet *The Netherlands* I am very pleased that this workshop is taking place to discuss the important issue of allergy testing using blood and intradermal methods in horses presented with a variety of 'allergic conditions'.

Our main speakers are Derek Knottenbelt from Liverpool, Wayne Rosenkrantz from California and Stephen White from California. They are willing to present some data and their own personal impressions of the value of the testing, and the limitations and benefits that they have encountered with the various testing modalities. I will also describe my own research findings and I hope that this will stimulate active discussion. I also hope that everyone present will join in with us to ensure that we make progress in our understanding of tests and their relative values.

Allergic disease manifests clinically in many ways; wheals, wheals that ooze serum, or various degrees of focal or generalised pruritus. In all of these states, it is frequently very difficult to identify an underlying cause; usually an exhaustive history and a detailed clinical examination may be all that can be used. Imagine then, two horses with a similar clinical presentation of pruritus; without further information, both could easily be diagnosed with *Culicoides* hypersensitivity or 'sweet itch'. However, one was presented in summer with no history of any problems in winter. By contrast, the other presented in the middle of winter having been inside all the time. So perhaps we could justifiably 'assume' that the first horse has 'sweet itch', but the other is most unlikely to have the same condition. The second horse is more likely to be atopic, although they have a very similar clinical appearance. These two cases demonstrate the importance of a good signalment and an accurate and full clinical history.

We are easily drawn to the major clinical sign and it is similarly easy to draw the wrong conclusions without fully considering the history. If a case is presented with rounded alopecic lesions and the history reveals that they have been present for more than 6 months, then dermatophytosis is extremely unlikely and an alternative diagnosis should be considered; perhaps the animal has occult sarcoid or alopecia areata lesions.

A full clinical examination is essential in every case and the results of this (and the history) should be written down carefully and accurately. The extent of the clinical examination may vary, depending on the findings. Sometimes, a rectal examination can be helpful in dermatological examinations, e.g. in lymphosarcoma. Four years ago, at the British Equine Veterinary Association Congress, I described several cases in which rectal examination provided significant diagnostic information for skin disease, and so I consider that it can be justified as a routine part of the investigative protocol. Lameness examinations may be much less significant overall, but it remains unwise to ignore any body system, as some conditions have a polysystemic clinical presentation.

Additional laboratory support can be used of course. Most of us are familiar with biopsy techniques, trichogram examinations, and bacterial and fungal cultures. The value of good laboratory support for routine microbiology, cytology, and for histology of biopsy specimens cannot be overstated.

In the horse there are currently two ways of testing for allergic disease conditions.

1. Intradermal testing

At the University of Utrecht we investigated the possible value of this method but we were not happy with it. In Utrecht, Ton Willemse has been working for 30 years to establish threshold values for allergens in the dog. His work has been published, and he helped us to attempt to extrapolate his findings to the horse. We used 15 healthy research horses and we performed allergy testing using standard intradermal protocols. Regrettably, we could not determine threshold values for our allergens. For example, one horse reacted at 1:100 dilution and another reacted to the 1:1000 dilution. It is entirely possible that a total of 15 horses was insufficient, or that we did not have the correct allergens, but we assumed that the protocols were correct and that the tests were performed fairly and properly.

We then undertook a second study to establish the basic pathophysiology that followed the intradermal injection of an allergen. We set out to investigate the pathological relationship between the macroscopic (clinical) effects and the pathological (histological) changes. The results of this trial have been submitted for publication to *Veterinary Dermatology*. Initially, we performed a pilot study to compare shaving, clipping, or chemical depilation of the hair at the site of the test. We also set out to establish the best biopsy size for the injection sites. We found that clipping was the most reliable way of preparing the skin; the other methods resulted in detectable cutaneous inflammation at the site within 12–24 hours so that there is histological evidence of dermal changes without having injected anything at all. Further, we found that two small biopsies heal more quickly than one larger one. We gave five injections of each substance and took repeated biopsies over a period of time. A 5-cm gap should be left between each injection site to avoid the risk that the wheals will interfere with each other.

Therefore, we clipped the horses 24 hours before the intradermal test was to be performed and we marked the injection sites. Prior to the test, all horses were sedated with detomidine (Domosedan®) intravenously.

We accept that xylazine may be a better alternative for a short-term procedure, but it is not licensed for use in horses in the Netherlands and we felt that detomidine had no influence at all on the test. We used saline as a negative control, and histamine as a positive control.

Following the injections, we repeatedly evaluated the sites clinically and at each of these evaluations we performed two biopsies; one biopsy sample from each site was fixed in buffered formol saline, and the other was frozen. Sequential biopsies were taken to try to establish the progression of the inflammatory pathology at the site; this was graded on a scale of 0–5. In this way we assessed and biopsied five wheals from saline, five wheals from histamine, five wheals from compound 48/80 and five from each test substance. There were no detectable problems with pain or non-healing at the biopsy sites. The wounds healed within 14 days. Specimens were subjected to routine histological preparation and examination and also for immunohistochemistry.

Broadly, we could not always demonstrate a relationship between macroscopic response and microscopic pathology. For example, one gelding had a clear macroscopic wheal 15 minutes after injection, but neither inflammation nor oedema could be seen microscopically. At 48 hours, a wheal was still present but it was a little smaller. However, at this stage it had an inflammation score that was reasonably high, and CD8 staining confirmed that most of the cells at the site were lymphocytes. Therefore we recognised that there was not always a clear relationship between the visible appearance, the measured size of the response, and the pathological changes in the skin. Interestingly, after 8 hours, this same horse had a significant wheal and an inflammation score on the biopsy of 1, and this is the same horse where the wheal was much smaller but the inflammation score much higher at 48 hours. This illustrates that the histological dermal changes are not related to what we see and what we measure grossly. I considered this to be very disappointing; I had hoped to find a close relationship.

The conclusions from this study were that the microscopic alterations develop later than the macroscopic findings and that the macroscopic findings after 24 hours no longer correlate to changes occurring within the skin; in our study the clinical and pathological relationship was closest between 15 minutes and 4 hours.

This year we performed a third study to test whether Greer Laboratory's *Culicoides* antigen was usable in the Netherlands, and whether it is possible to test a horse in the winter when clinical signs are absent. We were able to recruit ten pairs of horses; one horse from each pair had a known *Culicoides* hypersensitivity and the other did not. Each pair had, for at least the previous 2 years, the same pasture, feeding and hay. In this way we had pairs of horses with one affected and one non-affected control. I did not look at age, breed or sex. In this way we hoped to check whether this allergen could help us to establish a diagnosis in winter so all horses were tested in March, and one person performed all the tests. We injected 0.1 ml of allergen because the more commonly used 0.05-ml volume does not appear to work well in our experience. We used two different histamine concentrations and three different dilutions of the *Culicoides* antigen. Before the test, we clipped the horse over the neck region. The various injections were made intradermally at each marked site.

We took readings after 0.5, 4, 24 and 48 hours. We felt this was necessary in winter as the horses have long hair. Currently we only have preliminary results. Disappointingly, in six pairs, the control reacted the same or more than the affected. Further, we could not tell whether the 1:1000 always reacted more than the 1:10 000 or 1:25 000 dilutions. In three pairs, the affected patient reacted more than the control, while in one pair the control reacted more than the affected patient, i.e. the patient did not react at all. There may be different explanations for these equivocal results; they may reflect that the *Culicoides* species represented in the antigen solution are not the correct ones for the Netherlands (perhaps a different species is involved), or the antibody concentration is too low after winter. It is clear that we still have a problem. We intend to repeat this study in September in the season when there are clinical signs.

2. Serum allergy testing

Allergy testing using serum is the second method available to us. I personally have little experience with this method. In Europe there are two tests available; one in Belgium, and one in France. In response to a request for clinical information, both labs provided information on how to sample and how much blood should be sent and, very importantly, what it costs. Neither provided any scientific evidence for sensitivity or specificity. Most of the cases that have been referred to us have already been tested. In my experience it may be just as effective and much cheaper to toss a coin!

The serum samples from horses are tested with anti-IgE antibodies used to test for IgE in other species of animals. A recent workshop on this subject in Germany in Essen failed to clarify the value of the testing. In Utrecht, we prefer intradermal testing for research but not for patients and we do not do any blood tests because we do not think it is worth the money.

I asked Danny Scott to present his findings at this workshop, but regrettably he was not able to attend this meeting. However, he was kind enough to send his results based on 40 intradermal allergy tests in horses between 1979 and 2001 where he had a true follow-up. Overall, he had 60% success with immunotherapy where success was defined as both full recovery and any detectable improvement. It is not entirely clear what other management measures were taken apart from the immunotherapy procedures, or to limit the exposure to known or suggested allergens. Again, like us, some of the patients referred to him have already had blood tests in practice before referral. In his hands, he had the same findings as us that in no instance did the tests results explain the problem. So he also remains sceptical of serum allergy testing.

Wayne Rosenkrantz *USA* On the issue of the species of *Culicoides*, do you have a feel what are the most important indigenous species in your area?

Marianne Sloet No, this would be a significant and helpful factor of course, but there are few entomologists who are either able or willing to do the identification work. I have not done that yet because I thought I would do it the other way round, as the expectation was that *Culicoides* sp. have common antigens such that the allergy test would work even if my species were a little bit different from the American species.

Wayne Rosenkrantz I know the Greer allergen is specifically *Culicoides variipennis*. There were also other sources that were available for a short period of time. The other species available was *Culicoides nubeculosus*, which I thought was more of a common species in Europe. If this antigen is still available you might want to consider further studies and compare the two different antigens side by side.

Marianne Sloet I did try to get the older allergen that was available in the UK but this is not available any more to my knowledge.

Seth Bornstein *Sweden* What was the reaction of a histamine positive control?

Marianne Sloet They were normally between 15 and 30 mm in diameter, and the controls were negative.

Seth Bornstein Did you get the same type of reaction in any animal?

Marianne Sloet If the reaction to the histamine was not as expected, then the horse would have been excluded from the study. Fortunately, all ten pairs of horses reacted normally to the histamine and so were justifiably included in the study. As there is some controversy over which dilution of histamine gives the best positive control, and in order to maximise the chances of a good response, we used two concentrations of histamine.

Janet Littlewood *UK* A few years ago I performed intradermal tests in a few ponies, which belonged to the Animal Health Trust, Newmarket, UK, that had clinical signs of *Culicoides* hypersensitivity. I tested them with both the Greer antigen and a crude extract preparation from local indigenous trapped flies that was made by Ken Baker. These gave larger and more reliable results than the Greer antigen. I did not have the opportunity to do negative controls because of Home Office regulations but I think it is likely that there is a potential problem if the wrong species is used. I also had thought that there ought to be enough common antigens for a meaningful test result to be achievable.

Gabriela Kolm *Austria* We performed a study using *Culicoides variipennis* (kindly provided by Greer) some years ago that is published in the *Equine Veterinary Journal*. We also had no positive reactions in truly *Culicoides* hypersensitive horses. Recently I have discussed the problem with Greer and they informed me that there had been problems with that extract because it was very old. Thus, it does not seem to be the species, but the old extract. Of course, there is a publication by Fadok in the nineties performed in Florida, where the extract seemed to work very well. When we got the extract it was already 8 years old. Now we have got the *C. nubeculosus* extract, and tested a lot of many non-affected horses that were all negative. We also tested horses affected by *Culicoides* hypersensitivity, which developed strong positive skin reactions upon intra-dermal injection with the *C. nubeculosus* extract. So it seems to be fine, and we will now perform a study with the new extract.

Marianne Sloet Thank you for this new and helpful information.

Gabriela Kolm I think it is now commercially available and the Greer people told me the new extract is the European species, so the Americans also get the *C. nubeculosus* species now.

Derek Knotttenbelt *UK* I think this discussion highlights my big concern. What do you test for? Which horses must you test, and which antigen must you use under particular circumstances?

Clearly there are significant variations in species sensitivities in local populations of horses and, given the pathophysiology of hypersensitivity responses, this is hardly surprising. The main questions relate to the sensitivity and specificity of the skin and blood testing methods. Often the clinical signs are characteristic, and this is especially true for *Culicoides* hypersensitivity, so there is often little added value from the test under these conditions. Michael Burrell has used allergen neutralisation methods with some success; intradermal serial dilutions of a proven significant antigen are made to establish a neutral point, i.e. one that does not react. In general however, the question must be asked, 'Will the results alter what you do?'

I approached this problem from a slightly different perspective by performing a study on horses that have already been tested (either intradermally or by blood sampling, or both) prior to referral. Most of the horses are presented for 'unexplained' (idiopathic) persistent pruritus of proven 'non-insect' origin, urticaria, or uncontrollable insect hypersensitivity in a few cases. A large majority of these had already been subjected to exhaustive investigation culminating in a diagnosis of 'supposed allergy or hypersensitivity'. We included also cases of 'suggested' food hypersensitivity, which included horses showing persistent urticarial or pruritic responses (or diarrhoea) or combinations of these signs when exposed to various foods. Many of these were apparently related to exposure to cereal foods and other graminicid plants. The results of the testing procedures were included in the referral information.

I have reviewed records from 73 such horses. I recognise that this is a small number and that we did not undertake allergy testing, either by blood or skin test. My immediate thoughts were: 'Why is this horse being presented to me when it has already been subjected to the full range of investigative technology?'

These cases identify that there is a significant problem with the test and possibly with the treatment. Where the test fails to identify the significant causative allergen, subsequent use of 'other' allergens for desensitisation would probably not resolve the issue. Most of the ELISA tests identify a panel of putative allergens, but the test cannot hope to be exhaustive. In some cases there are up to 40 or more of the 150–200 allergens to which the horse is variously sensitive; some are strongly positive while others are moderately or slightly positive. The difficulty of establishing what should be included in the desensitisation process is the crux of the matter. Failure to include the one allergen that causes the problem will probably result in failure of the treatment protocol.

We then have to resort to 'simple' clinical or historical information. The standard procedure for management of *Culicoides* hypersensitivity (for which clinical and historical information is probably easily recognised) is to avoid contact with the allergen. If this can be achieved and the clinical signs resolve, then the diagnosis can be assumed to be correct. This procedure may create a management problem, but it is usually relatively cheap! The client wants an answer and is usually satisfied when they know what the problem is, even if treatment is not either possible or affordable. The same applies to feed sensitivities. Significantly though, these appear to cause more urticaria and less pruritus. I have a clinical impression that food hypersensitivities do exist in horses and there are horses that will have food-induced urticaria and/or pruritus, particularly to carbohydrate feeds, and even in small amounts. We just identify a diet they can tolerate that doesn't bring them up in lumps or doesn't make them pruritic. In my experience, that works at a fraction of the cost, time and trouble.

Peter Webb *UK*   In the dog, we have already recognised which allergens are important, such as pollens. It is unlikely that the horse is going to be sensitive to different pollen allergens from the dog. Those are the ones that are predominant.

Derek Knotttenbelt   Why should horses react to the same panel of allergens as the dog? Dogs and cats aren't

the same, as I understand it, so why should dogs and horses be the same?

Peter Webb   Because they are airborne. I think that work has already been done in the dog, so you should be able to pick the same panels for the horse. The allergens are the same. The problem comes with fungi.

Derek Knotttenbelt   So far we have no apparent consistency between the results of the clinical tests and the reports that the clients get. In small animals it is probably relatively easy to identify the allergens because you have dogs and cats in a relatively confined environment.

The concept of having four fungi you can avoid doesn't help me with the horse. How does the client avoid it when they do not know where it is and how the horse is exposed to it?

Janet Littlewood *UK*   I am depressed that you are so negative about it. There is not one single good case report in the literature of food allergic horses. I haven't brought my data with me but when Sue Patterson and I were working together we looked at pruritic and urticarial horses and found none of them improved with anything you mentioned. I think that urticarial reactions are more often due to the amount of feed given, but it does not behave like a true food allergy such as we recognise in other species. These horses can be given concentrated food but less of it and they seem to have less urticaria. This is not the same thing as an adverse food reaction. It may be that the threshold of their immune system is affected by their nutrition, at least that is my working hypothesis. I think that it is related to nutrition and how fit the horse is. I know in humans, stress will affect the manifestation of urticaria and allergy to feeds.

Participant   I am like everybody else who has spoken so far. I have yet to see any convincing data about the validation of serological testing in the horse or any species. After performing an elimination diet and seeing no improvement, I do intradermal testing and find it really helpful for the client to see what their pet is allergic to. The horse didn't evolve to live in stables. How do you avoid fungus? You turn it out in a field and you manage it as a horse that is not stabled. Many that I have seen have so-called indoor reactions, so they react to dust mites, for example, that you find in an indoor environment. If you convince clients on how to change management, you can improve them enormously; I have not used much therapy because management changes work very well.

Participant The allergens I have used are pollens where I can't do very much about controlling the environment. However, many of these horses are multiple allergic, just like cats and dogs. Even if they have *Culicoides* hypersensitivity, they may still have other hypersensitivities.

Marianne Sloet I think what this is highlighting for me is we need a better understanding of what the pathology is, and of what the processes are at work.

Stephen White *USA* The discussion over the last 10 minutes has been about the growing pains of equine allergy that we went through in small animals 15 years ago and, in fact, are still going through. I am more selective in what I subject to skin testing in horses. I want to be sure before I spend the client's money that I have eliminated parasite allergy as best I can. I live in an area which has a temperate climate and does not have the swings of climatic temperature of other parts of the world, but we do see some seasonal variation and horses that are quite pruritic in the summer and less so in the winter. I always want to differentiate between the truly atopic horse and the one with a likely parasite allergy. I don't usually jump in with skin testing or blood testing until I am sure the owners have done the best they can to eliminate parasites.

I have seen two horses in the last 25 years that had a food allergy whereby we saw improvement when we took a food away; both of these had pruritus. It is difficult to convince owners not to feed alfalfa if that is what they have been feeding their horses all their lives. Once the alfalfa is withdrawn, the pruritus goes away; re-introduction causes the signs to recur. I have not seen urticaria associated with food. I know of only one case in the literature by Dawn Logas, which I think was urticarial pruritus but only if it was fed a certain food and exercised.[1]

There are 18 cases in the last 6 years that we have skin tested and blood tested. There are a number of different breeds with the thoroughbred the predominant breed: I always thought the quarter horses would be over-represented. I am not sure that these 18 horses all had the same disease but I am assuming they gave a

reaction to an allergen based on the history. They were all about 5 or 6 years of age when they started and it was about 1–1.5 years later that they were presented to us. Ten patients had chronic urticaria, five had pruritus, two had both, and one horse had allergic airway disease. I am not convinced that this is the same disease that affects the skin, but then I am not convinced in the asthmatic dog or cat either.

Eight cases had intradermal testing, six had a serum test and four had both skin and intradermal tests. Selection of tests to be used was based on the owners' resources and preferences, and the temperament of the horse. My preference would be to do both tests because I would like to maximise the amount of information; the two tests together can identify a wider range of allergens and may provide correlative information.

Let us consider a horse that has positive reactions to almost every allergen. As Derek said, what does it mean? We must assume that it means something if we can interpret it on the basis of the history and if we have ruled everything else out. I think you can have classic animals that have seasonal changes that are not related to ectoparasites. You can have semi-classic animals that aren't necessarily seasonal but again you have to rule out parasites. Then you have other horses that you just don't know what else to do.

Positive reactions of course depend on what you want to call it. You can use a 1+ or 4+ scale; we take a positive to be more than half of the difference between the diameters of the positive and negative control, so it is something around 2+. For blood tests, if the laboratory marked it positive, then I considered it positive. Some laboratory sheets just give gradations from 1 to 100; I arbitrarily took 80–100 as positive.

These allergens (house dust, *D. farinae*, Bermuda grass, privet, Johnson grass, yellow dock, pigweed, alfalfa, black ant, housefly) are the ones that were positive in more than two-thirds of the horses. It is interesting, but I don't know how relevant it is to science or to life, but house dust was at the top of the list for these horses. I think that house dust is a melange of stuff; farm dust is also a melange and there are probably all sorts of cross-reactions. The rest of these are various grasses, and insects including black ants and houseflies. Interestingly *Culicoides* didn't appear in this series although we've been testing for this for a long time. This means one of two things. Either we were not testing for the specific species or we had done a reasonably good job of eliminating the *Culicoides* horses by parasite control measures. I am not sure if that is self-congratulatory or just lucky. The same thing happens to some extent with serum test allergens (*Aspergillus*, ragweed, cocklebur, mulberry, stable fly, *Penicillium*, Bermuda grass, orchard grass, yellow dock, Russian thistle, olive, *Mucor*, pine shavings), although stable flies (a mix of species) were commonly represented. Bermuda grass and yellow dock are the only two allergens that consistently showed up and rated as positive allergens in two-thirds of the horses.

We have to bear in mind that when we are looking at skin tests and serum tests, we are testing for different things. In the skin test you are presumably looking at the reaction of the mast cells and in the serum tests we are presumably looking at equine IgE in the blood stream.

For the four cases that had both tests, how did these compare? For one thing one of them was blood tested before it came in and we never got the full sheet. We just received the information that it was positive to three different allergens based on the blood test. Not all allergens are included in both tests. However, the best correlation between blood testing and skin tests was between weeds and grasses; it was poor with trees and insects and worse with moulds. I do have a problem with fungi and moulds because they are ubiquitous; you could burn down the barn and turn the horses out to pasture. The other thing, however, is some of the horses were out in the pasture and not in barns, but were coming up with mould allergies. You must remember that moulds are everywhere but probably worse inside; you can't escape moulds just because you are living outside.

Interestingly, most dogs subjected to skin testing undergo immunotherapy. By contrast, in horses only half of the owners decided to attempt immunotherapy. Many horse owners are satisfied with a diagnosis alone; their reluctance to undertake the treatment is not seemingly related to any disinclination to inject the horse, but rather due to the long-term effort that is required. The mean duration of immunotherapy was usually 2 years; the longest being about 4 or 5 years. The latter owners obviously felt this helped the animal.

Although these are small numbers, our success rate seems reasonable. Five horses were treated over a mean of 11 months and of these, four horses improved. I based this on comments made in the records and on the basis of owners calling up and continuing the treatment. If the horse wasn't getting better, the client would probably not seek to continue the treatment, although clearly we have to be careful how we interpret this. One horse was lost to follow-up. It is hard to say, but I felt that this particular horse improved and then was sold. One horse again has only been on treatment for 2 months. Overall we can say that based on this extraordinarily small, statistically insignificant group of horses, perhaps 50% will get better.

By coincidence, the day after I received an email from Marianne asking me to look at my experiences, the horse that has been on allergens the longest actually came in and the owner said the allergies are doing fine but remarked that the insects were picking up and that she was having more problems. She wanted to know if there was a similar insect therapy.

Wayne Rosenkrantz   Do you remember which labs you were using?

Stephen White   It was mainly Spectrum labs. Two later cases were tested at Greer, but it was mainly Spectrum.

Luc Beco   Has any one used Heska Laboratory for allergy in horses?

Marianne Sloet   I have not. It is unfortunate that Wendy Lorch is not here as she has done some testing.

Participant   We evaluate a lot of small animal tests with Heska. I think the technology is interesting. The biggest problem in small animals is that we have a higher level of false-negative reactions because of the specificity of the test when compared to skin testing.

Participant   What criteria do you have for a false negative? How can you say it is a false negative and that the horse is not atopic? The skin test could be positive on a negative horse. The skin test is only used for immunotherapy and I personally do not use that for diagnosis.

Stephen White   That certainly identifies some of the problems; how many horses are going to react? A couple of horses were urticarial and a couple were pruritic. At least one of those, if I remember correctly, was urticarial and it said in the record that it was not pruritic.

Tony Yu *USA*   Were there pollen or environmental allergies?

Stephen White   The horses that improved were mostly pollen allergic, but then again most of them were positive, to house dust and insects. I think there are a lot of cross-reactions between insects and other arthropods.

We really need to take horses that are atopic and skin test positive, and non-selectively choose the top ten allergens in our experience and put them on immunotherapy with these allergens, and see how many get better. There is no doubt that this happens in studies in cats and dogs. In fact, 20 years ago, if you had any allergic reactions in dogs and they were simply given the top ten allergens, a significant number got better. We don't actually know, but we assume that 50% got better. Maybe horses would get better if we simply take house dust, house dust mite, and a couple of pollens and injected them!

Participant   How quickly do you see an improvement in horses?

Stephen White   We tell owners not to expect an improvement before 6–12 months. Most of our cases started to improve within 6 months. In one case the owner couldn't believe how much better the horse was in the first 6 months. This horse had already been on parasite control. We generally advise, just as in small animals, that a response may not be seen for the first 12 months; occasional horses get better quicker. There is much variability.

If I had a horse that had a totally negative skin test and totally negative blood test, I guess I would revisit the allergy first. We don't usually do a food elimination diet because I was so disappointed with owner compliance and return. That is probably my prejudice, although I know I will never make the diagnosis if I am not looking for the disease. I'm not going to find it if I don't look for it. If I had an animal that was totally negative, a diet change is probably one of the things I would look at, just like for a horse that had failed immunotherapy. The problem with the totally positive case is how many of these allergens do you put in a solution? With the dog you can have about 20 different allergens and still have a reasonable success. If you have 15 pollens, do you try to choose the ones that are genetically the closest? I don't know.

Wayne Rosenkrantz   Stephen has mirrored some of our experiences. Being from the same state, we are going to have somewhat similar results, although southern California is a little more temperate and has a more consistent climate than northern California.

In the majority of cases, I see a combination of allergies. They include insect and environmental allergens and, although mould reactions in southern California are not that prominent, they are sometimes involved. This mirrors what we see in small animals from the same region. I think there is definitely a geographical factor, because when I do the same allergy tests on horses or small animals in other areas like Hawaii, which is very moist and humid, my mould reactions are much higher. Similarly when I go to the dry arid regions like Las Vegas, I hardly ever see mould reactions. There seems little doubt that location is going to influence what you see. I think that summation of effect and the threshold phenomenon are just as important as they are in small animal allergies. It is important to perform insect control and control secondary infections, as these can add to the summation effect in horses and push them above their allergic threshold and produce clinical lesions. The concept of a cure simply from immunotherapy is probably somewhat unrealistic. I think we have to think about managing the allergic horse as we think about managing the allergic dog. It is a multi-therapeutic approach.

With reference to food as the cause of urticaria or pruritus, we need some documented data, but this is lacking in the current literature. Most cases have not been properly challenged to document the food hypersensitivity. In my 20 years of dermatology, I can think of only one horse that actually was likely to have had food hypersensitivity as the cause of its pruritus. I also believe it is important to consider that horses, just like in small animals, can have multiple allergies, and that some horses with food hypersensitivities will often also have environmental and insect hypersensitivities. The majority of food allergy cases that I see in small animals have concurrent environmental hypersensitivities.

In 1992 I looked at ten pruritic horses and attempted immunotherapy. We had to eliminate concurrent disease and establish that the horses were otherwise normal. I had to exclude 30–35% of the horses that were supposedly normal in the eyes of the owner, because after my historical and physical evaluations I determined that many of these cases were not normal. Many owners often consider occasional hives, mild folliculitis, alopecia, or mild pruritus as still being normal. There is a wide interpretation of what is considered normal by both owners and investigators. Furthermore, there have been some well-controlled studies that show that subclinical forms of airway disease exist in the horse that do not manifest clinically with COPD, or reactive airway disease, unless they are evaluated with more extensive bronchiolar alveolar testing and lavage. So, I think that normal horses are not easy to identify.

When evaluating these ten pruritic horses, an excellent result was defined as included no other therapy apart from the immunotherapy. However, insect control measures were used consistently prior to, and throughout, the study. We considered that a good result was one in which the horse was permitted to be on antihistamines. Hydroxyzine is the most effective one in our view.

In 1996 Valerie Fadok presented some comparative information between atopic and insect-sensitive horses. She had five out of seven (72%) purely atopic horses that had greater than 50% improvement with immunotherapy. She then compared this to a group of horses with both atopic disease and insect allergies. In this group 7 out of 13 (54%) had greater than 50% improvement. In her last group she looked at horses with insect allergy only. In this group, three out of four (75%) had greater than 50% improvement. I performed a double-blinded controlled study to evaluate immunotherapy in both insect and environmental allergic horses and published it in *Advances in Veterinary Dermatology* in 1998. Sixty-four per cent of the horses that were treated with immunotherapy showed a 50% or greater improvement, compared to only 23% improvement in the placebo group. This was a significant difference between the two groups.

In previous studies where I have looked at normal horses and compared those to horses that had clinical disease, the general consensus was that normal horses will show reactions on intradermal testing, but the degree of reactivity and the number of reactions were much lower. Interestingly, in our study, deer fly, horse fly, yellow dock, black fly, mosquito, fleas and firebrush all showed higher reactions in clinical and normal horses. Stephen White's results showed yellow dock and pigweed which were also some of our higher false positive reactions. We also saw more Russian thistle reactions in normal horses. In a more recent review, I looked at horses that had been on immunotherapy for 2 years or longer for either recurrent urticaria or pruritus, or a combination of the two. There were relatively equal numbers in each of these groups. Overall we had 30 cases, with 4 cases dropping out. The 26 cases completing the 2-year follow-up study showed 67% with good to excellent responses. This result is consistent with other studies performed over the last couple of decades. This also corresponds roughly to the canine immunotherapy success that we see in our practices. Derek Knottenbelt made a valid comment yesterday that when you are handling these cases as a specialist, you are inevitably managing all aspects of their disease, in addition to the immunotherapy. For example, insect control may have been increased in some cases over what they may have been doing previously. However, many of the cases I see on referral are already on excellent insect control programmes. In addition, the horses in this most recent study were also required to keep consistent insect control.

I think intradermal testing is valuable, but I don't rely on it as an ultimate diagnostic test. I think it is best viewed as a diagnostic aid. It should be used to help in the selection of allergens for immunotherapy and to help with avoidance when feasible.

I am currently looking into the role of storage mites in allergic skin disease in the horse. We have been performing intradermal tests to some of the more common storage mites. One thought that I have is that a lot of the house dust mite reactions we see in the horse may actually be cross-reacting with storage mites. I believe that these insects share some common epitopes and that cross-reactions are likely. We have performed Western blot analysis in small animals and I was amazed when we saw such similar protein fractionations with black fly and black ant associated with flea and house dust mites. In small animals we try to select allergens that we feel fit the clinical history the best. We do the same thing in the equine cases and I believe that is going to increase the effectiveness of immunotherapy. Just like in small animals, 'cook-booking' your immunotherapy in the horse doesn't work as well as adjusting your injections based on clinical disease. You need to adjust your antigen dosing and frequency on a case-by-case basis. There is no doubt that immunotherapy is effective in many cases; the symptoms abate when the horse receives their immunotherapy injections.

Babette Baddaky *Norway* This year I have started to use the Heska test for horses. There are two panels, an insect panel and a 24-allergen panel, and so far we have had many blood samples from horses with clinically recognisable 'sweet itch'. We have compared the tests and the clinical signs in 30 or 40 horses overall and they match really well with the insect panel. As expected, they come up positive to *Culicoides* and some other insects too. Clearly these may be cross-reactivities. We want to collect samples from ten insect hypersensitive horses and ten normal horses and then repeat this test on both groups. Another thing that I noticed was that when we started testing in the early season at the beginning of May (insects are quite late because of the cold in Scandinavian countries), the insects started coming up, and the horses that have had hypersensitivity in the past year start itching very quickly. If you take a sample immediately, you do not get a positive reaction. If you wait 3 or 4 weeks, then they will be positive.

Wayne Rosenkrantz   The timing of the testing process has been looked at in small animals, but I don't think anyone has studied this in the horse, so it is a very valid point.

I would like to start working more with Heska; perhaps doing some serum *in vitro* testing on horses. My experience with some of the other labs, including Spectrum and Biomedical labs in the USA, has not been overly impressive. I had a recent case that was initially completely negative on the *in vitro* testing but we had a very good skin test. I would not necessarily expect serum testing and skin testing to always match. They are two different tests looking at two different things, but you certainly would like to see some positives on the *in vitro* serum tests in these clinically affected horses.

Participant   Have you had a negative test in an animal with clinical signs?

Wayne Rosenkrantz   I have certainly had some tests that have been unimpressive in horses with clinical disease. Just as we see in small animals, not all cases will test positive. However, it is pretty rare to get a negative test in clinically affected horses, assuming proper drug withdrawal and testing concentrations are correct. We also feel we have screened our cases based on history and physical findings, and we are limiting our testing to those horses we truly believe are allergic animals.

I would encourage those of you who will be doing intradermal testing to review the recent publication by Dan Morris in *Veterinary Dermatology* that determined recommended insect allergen testing concentrations. Over the years we have become better at determining the required testing titration. By following the recommended dilutions for testing you are going to minimise false reactions on intradermal testing.

Participant   Your 67% success is an excellent response. What do you do with the ones that don't improve? How do you manage them? I agree with you completely that you have to manage the problem, not necessarily fix it. What do you do with horses where immunotherapy doesn't seem to help?

Wayne Rosenkrantz   Cases that are failures on immunotherapy are going to be managed in a variety of ways. Unfortunately I have to use a lot of glucocorticoids in most refractory cases. For the most part, horses tolerate glucocorticoids very well, and I have a lot of horses that have been given glucocorticoids most of their lives. The dose may have to be adjusted seasonally and from year to year. I have cases that have been managed with alternate-day prednisolone, and others on dexamethasone two or three times a week, for many years. This is certainly not optimal but there are cases where no other therapy works. Sometimes we can reduce the dose of glucocorticoids by using antihistamines. I do think they have sparing effects on the amount of glucocorticoids that are needed to alleviate the symptoms. I have been less impressed with fatty acid supplementation, but on occasion will include it as an adjunctive therapy. In some cases we continue immunotherapy because we think it too has a sparing effect on the glucocorticoids required. I have also used pentoxifylline in some of our urticaria and pruritic horses. My clinical impression is that it is occasionally beneficial in some of the urticaria horses, but less so in the pruritic horses.

Participant   Has anyone followed recurrent urticarial horses longitudinally more than a year or two?

Wayne Rosenkrantz   I haven't followed all cases long-term, but in some cases it seems the urticaria lasts a year or two and then the problem subsides or goes into remission. I often wonder whether this is related to whether the causative allergen is no longer in the environment, or at least at a reduced level? If the horse is on immunotherapy we often claim success, but one could certainly argue that some of these cases may be improving based on reduced allergen exposure.

We usually tell clients that 50% of horses on immunotherapy will have improvement in their urticaria. We tell them it may take 6–12 months before the horse will show optimal improvement. When using glucocorticoids for urticaria, dexamethasone seems to work the best and it is an inexpensive drug. Often we use dexamethasone for short periods of time on a decreasing or lowest controllable dose. We try to use it every other day, or every 3 days, for maintenance. There is a possible risk of laminitis in some horses, although I truly think it is minimal. In the few cases that it has occurred, I often wonder whether it was just a result of the chronic disease I was treating as opposed to a side effect from the dexamethasone.

Marianne Sloet   I would like to thank the speakers and the audience for attending this workshop.

References

1 Logas, D., Kunkle, G., Calderwood-Mays, M., Frank, L. Cholinergic pruritus in a horse. *Journal of the American Veterinary Medical Association,* 1992; **201**: 90–91.

Genodermatosis: alopecia and hypotrichoses

M. Paradis[1] (Chairperson), R. Cerundolo[2] (Secretary)

[1] University of Montreal, Quebec, Canada.
[2] University of Pennsylvania, Philadelphia, PA, USA

Manon Paradis *Canada* welcomed the participants and gave an overview of the topics to be covered by the speakers and invited everyone to participate in the discussion after each presentation.

Canine pattern alopecia (E. Walder)

Emily Walder *USA*   Canine pattern alopecia (CPA) does not refer to an alopecia with a precise anatomical distribution. It is a breed-specific folliculopathy, very similar, but not identical, to human androgenetic alopecia (human pattern baldness). The term used in veterinary medicine is not perfect and a better name should probably be used.

According to the textbook *Small Animal Dermatology*,[1] there are five coat types in dogs. One of them is 'short/fine' and the most representative breeds are: dachshund, smooth chihuahua, greyhound, Italian greyhound, whippet, Boston terrier and Manchester terrier. All the breeds in which CPA has been reported belong to this group.

CPA maybe an excessive reaction to artificial selection pressure that favours the fine delicate coat sought by breeders who often attempt to manipulate the appearance of a dog without considering possible genetic damage. One of the characteristic clinical features is the tardive onset of alopecia, as affected dogs are born with a normal hair coat and then they lose it around 6–9 months of age. The affected dogs of various breeds have been subdivided into several groups.[1] In the first group, male dachshunds are usually affected on the pinnae, although I have also seen it in females. In the second group, affected areas are the ventral neck, chest, abdomen and/or thighs, and females are usually affected. In a third group are greyhounds, in which the caudal thighs are affected. This syndrome is different from the lateral thighs syndrome which seems to be a specific entity called 'greyhound thigh alopecia'.

CPA is not a systemic disorder, as affected dogs have normal endocrine function. The pathogenesis in dogs is not known. In men there is an androgen receptor dysfunction. The condition affects dogs at an early age and with an equal sex distribution, while men are affected at middle age; this makes it less likely that an androgen receptor dysfunction is present in dogs.

Histologically, there is a gradual decrease in size of the folliculosebaceous unit. During this process, normal follicular cycling (anagen-catagen-telogen) occurs, and it is still possible to distinguish among anagen, catagen and telogen hair follicles. When the follicles become very small it is difficult to say if they are in telogen, or if they are tiny follicles with small anagen bulbs. In men, telogen arrest eventually occurs. It is difficult to confirm the stage of the hair follicles in dogs as too few cases have been seen, and proliferation markers have not been used.

Secondary features are keratin accumulation in the small follicles and infundibular melanin clumping caused by shrinkage following apoptosis. Melanin subsequently drops out and accumulates in macrophages.

The epidermis is generally unremarkable except for hyperpigmentation. Dermal collagen is normal. In early cases, abnormal features can only be appreciated if a section from affected skin is compared with sections from normal skin.

In the early stage of the disease, the anagen follicles are smaller, narrower and have bulbs that are located more superficially in the dermis than normal. Anagen follicles are normally recognised by a glycogenated outer root sheath epithelium in the inferior segment, and a large dermal papilla in the deep dermis surrounded by the epithelial bulb. Melanin is often present in both the bulb and papilla. Later in the disease, hair follicles are severely attenuated and have tiny follicular papillae that are located in the mid-dermis. Follicular papillae are distinguished from secondary hair germs by their densely hyperchromatic nuclei and lack of recognisable cytoplasm. In the late stage of the disease, it is often difficult to say if there are telogen hairs or extremely attenuated anagen hair follicles. The first event in the catagen phase is the cessation of melanogenesis and the arrest of mitotic activity in the papilla; if the follicular papilla contains melanin, this might suggest a diminutive anagen follicle, but proliferation markers would be needed to confirm this. At low magnification, CPA might look like an endocrinopathy, so clinicopathologic correlation is critical.

Wayne Rosenkrantz *USA*   These are frustrating cases. It would be fascinating and extremely useful to biopsy some dogs of the predisposed breeds prior to onset of disease, and then do serial biopsies during their life. This could allow a better understanding of the pathogenesis.

Emily Walder   The biopsy is often received from dogs in a late stage of the disease.

Wayne Rosenkrantz   Miniaturisation of the hair follicle is still a controversial aspect of this condition, as there are pathologists who do not believe this would occur in dogs.

Lars Mecklenburg *Germany*   I am not convinced that miniaturisation of anagen hair follicles occurs in CPA. It is difficult to rule out a cycling disorder and the use of proliferation markers or semi-thin sections should allow a better understanding of the hair cycle stage.

Emily Walder   I agree that in order to confirm that attenuated anagen follicles are present it would be ideal to use proliferation markers such as Ki67 to prove that the cells of the follicular papillae are cycling. This would allow a better understanding of the pathomechanism of alopecia.

Ed Rosser *USA*   In this syndrome, a central endocrine disorder has been ruled out, but the involvement of an abnormality in a hormone receptor on the hair follicle is still debatable. A similar syndrome occurs in greyhounds on the lateral-posterior thighs during their period of athletic racing activity. Approximately 90% of these alopecic greyhound dogs grow back the hair when they end their racing activity, as we have observed in retired racing greyhounds used as blood donors at Michigan State University.

Wayne Rosenkrantz   The role of the hair follicle receptors may be relevant. Occasional cases have responded to melatonin which modulates the sex hormones.

Emily Walder   In dachshunds and chihuahuas, the hair loss might be irreversible.

Wayne Rosenkrantz   I have noticed that in severe cases the alopecia is irreversible, but in mild cases they may be melatonin responsive.

Manon Paradis   The ventral type of CPA is more common than the bald-pinna type. The ventral type affects both sexes, and boxers (who also have a fine coat, and are not typically listed as a predisposed breed in the literature) are also commonly affected. Spontaneous hair regrowth in CPA is unlikely to occur, although it has been observed in a case of the bald-pinna type. Over 50% of dogs with the ventral type respond to melatonin administration. Experience with melatonin in the bald-pinna type is limited, but it has been said to be effective in some cases.

Emily Walder   The boxer has a fine coat but I have not recognised the disease in this breed.

Ed Rosser   At Michigan State University, minoxidil was evaluated for its ability to stimulate hair growth, specifically at the sites of topical administration. Unfortunately, the drug was systemically absorbed through the skin, and hair regrowth occurred at sites distant from the site of topical application (i.e. hair grew on the noses of these dogs after application over the dorsal shoulder region in dogs with a generalised alopecia). Therefore, caution should be used when minoxidil is applied topically in dogs as the cutaneously absorbed blood concentration could be very high and result in cardiomyopathy.

Rosario Cerundolo *USA*   In human androgenetic alopecia, other drugs, apart from minoxidil, are routinely used, such as finasteride. It stops the conversion of testosterone to dihydrotestosterone by inhibiting the enzyme 5α-reductase. It is routinely used in dogs with benign prostatic hyperplasia and it might be useful in dogs with CPA. The use of topical anti-androgens such as cyproterone could also be useful in these dogs.

Manon Paradis   I know of anecdotal cases of CPA that responded to finasteride without any adverse effect.

Emily Walder and Lars Mecklenburg   Should there be concern about possible adverse effects in women handling the finasteride tablets, especially if they are broken?

Fernando Ramiro-Ibanez *USA*   Is there any study on decreased perfusion of the skin in this condition?

Emily Walder   Although minoxidil is a drug causing vasodilation, it does not automatically mean the disease is the result of an impaired cutaneous perfusion.

Ed Rosser   CPA looks very different to an ischaemic vasculopathy on the pinnae of dogs when examined histologically.

Post-clipping alopecia (E. Walder)

Emily Walder   Post-clipping alopecia (PCA) is still a very confusing disease for many veterinarians. A prolonged lack of hair regrowth after close clipping is a fairly common presenting complaint. The large majority of cases have histological evidence of an endocrine dermatopathy, usually hyperadrenocorticism. No breed specificity has been reported other than that associated with the various endocrinopathies.

True PCA is a specific, uncommon syndrome. It usually affects northern breeds which have guard hairs and thick undercoats, such as the Siberian husky, Alaskan malamute, Samoyed, American Eskimo dog. True plush-coated dogs such as pomeranians and chow chows, which lack guard hairs, are also reported to be predisposed to true PCA. No underlying endocrinopathy is present and the hair regrows in 6–12 months, which is a longer period of time than the 3-month average recently documented in Labrador retrievers.

It has been proposed that these breeds normally have a hair follicle cycle with a prolonged catagen phase, which possibly developed as an energy-saving device in extremely cold climates so they do not have to shed and regrow their coat.

Histologically, there is catagen arrest with some telogen hair follicles. The hair shafts are retained and few flame follicles or dysplastic follicles are seen. There are no significant abnormalities of the epidermis, sebaceous glands, or dermal collagen. Biopsies from non-alopecic skin, although rarely submitted to the pathologist, may show similar features.

A retrospective study of 40 skin biopsies from Siberian huskies, submitted for unrelated skin diseases or skin tumours between 2002 and 2004, was performed to determine if there really is a catagen predominance. This included as many cases as possible from states other than California, and from all seasons of the year. There were four cases each from malamutes, Samoyeds and American Eskimo dogs. Normal beagle dogs have a 50:50 of anagen/telogen ratio histologically, but in Siberian huskies, many sections revealed an increased proportion (up to 30%) of unremarkable catagen follicles. All sections also contained anagen follicles and some of these were of full size and depth.

In conclusion, catagen arrest does not appear to be normal for northern-breed dogs, regardless of climate or time of year. Thus, PCA does appear to represent a breed-related folliculopathy of undetermined aetiology, and it is not an iatrogenic disorder.

More biopsies from clinically normal skin of affected dogs are needed to assess possible causes, such as subclinical follicular dysplasia which becomes manifest when they are shaved, or thermal factors such as decreased temperature caused by shaving. Their undercoat would normally be expected to keep a high temperature at the skin level.

Wayne Rosenkrantz   I believe they might have some

form of follicular dysplasia which is hormonally modulated at the hair follicle receptor site. Histology of skin specimens of the contralateral site, at the same location, makes it very difficult to distinguish the haired site from the shaved site. It is likely that shaving will manifest the disorder and PCA is just a sign that there is another problem affecting the hair follicle.

Ed Rosser   I recommend that sled dogs are never shaved, unless it is absolutely necessary, as it can take over a year for the hair to grow back. These dogs also have unique behaviour, as they prefer to stay outside exclusively when the first snow falls and it is hard to force them to go inside their dog houses unless it is a very wet and rainy day. If they are shaved during the winter months they can get frost-bitten over any areas that have been shaved as they will continue to stay outside during the freezing temperatures. In addition, I have noticed shaved areas on sled dogs during the summer months that fail to regrow, and they are predisposed to sunburn and actinic keratosis.

Fernando Ramiro-Ibanez   Are the characteristic hair follicles seen histologically in telogen arrest or catagen arrest, and how would you differentiate them histologically?

Emily Walder   In catagen phase, the hair bulb disintegrates via apoptosis, so the entire hair shaft becomes encased in what was the isthmus outer root sheath of the follicle. These keratinocytes are not glycogenated or basaloid, but instead are cuboidal with pink cytoplasm; there is a slightly increased amount of amorphous tricholemmal keratin around the hair shaft, and the dermal papilla is still readily recognisable but separate from the bottom of the follicle. In telogen phase, apoptosis progresses and there is loss of large pink keratinocytes, and the follicles become narrow and are only a few cell layers thick. At the base of the telogen follicle there is a cluster of hair germ cells, and it is often difficult to identify the follicular papillae. An example of telogen arrest is seen in dogs with hyperadrenocorticism.

Lars Mecklenburg   Depending on the plane of the sections, it may be difficult to morphologically differentiate late-catagen phase from telogen phase. It does not make sense to have an arrest in the catagen phase where there is active remodelling of the lower portion of hair follicles. Instead an arrest in telogen would be plausible. The geographic region where the dogs live might play an important role in this condition.

Wayne Rosenkrantz   I believe there are variations in this syndrome according to the geographic area as I have seen differences between biopsies from dogs with PCA from the northern latitudes and those from southern California. Thus, photoperiod and environmental temperature might play a role in dogs.

Ed Rosser   In sled dogs, there is a dramatic change in the hair coat during the summer months when all of the undercoat is shed and they take on the outward appearance of German shepherd dogs, thus suggesting changes in the coat occur according to the season. The histological features may vary depending on the time of year that the skin biopsies are examined.

Emily Walder   If they are genetically meant to live in an environment with prolonged darkness and low temperature, it may be that they become abnormal when they are moved to a different environment.

Anti-androgenic drug for the treatment of pomeranians with alopecia (M. Nagata)

Masahiko Nagata *Japan*   As castration is often an effective treatment for alopecia X, and as androgens play a role in the pathogenesis of hair loss in this disorder, we evaluated the efficacy of osaterone acetate, an oral anti-androgen licensed in Japan for the treatment of canine benign prostatic hyperplasia, for treatment of pomeranians with alopecia X. Thirteen cases were recruited. All dogs received osaterone acetate at 0.25–0.50 mg/kg once daily (the manufacturer's recommended dose) for 7 consecutive days. The duration of therapy was only 1 week as osaterone efficacy should last for 5–6 months. The response to the treatment was considered excellent if there was truncal hair regrowth, good if incomplete hair regrowth, fair if there was only partial hair regrowth, and poor if no hair regrowth was noted. Seven of 13 dogs showed clinical improvement (1 excellent and 6 good), 3 cases had partial hair regrowth, and in the other 3 cases there was no hair regrowth. No adverse effects to the therapy were detected. These results suggest that alopecia might be caused by the activity of androgens at the level of the hair follicle. This condition resembles the human androgenetic alopecia. In man, anti-an-drogens (such as finasteride) promote hair regrowth by blocking the conversion of testosterone to dihy-drotestosterone. Repeated treatments with osaterone acetate might lead to better results in those dogs in which the hair regrowth was not very good.

Manon Paradis   I have used finasteride for the treatment of alopecia X. I have successfully treated a kees-hond, although the duration of the therapy has been quite long before having hair regrowth.

Ed Rosser   I am still in favour of castration as the first therapeutic approach for these dogs, although I have noticed that after an initial hair regrowth, hair loss can occur again. In one pomeranian, hair loss re-occurred after 7.5 years.

Manon Paradis   I agree that castration works in probably 50% of dogs with alopecia X and, according to the participants, melatonin works in probably 25–30% of alopecic dogs.

Rosario Cerundolo   Trilostane is another drug used in pomeranians and miniature poodles with alopecia X (a few participants agreed on its efficacy), although it should be kept in mind that adverse effects such as hypoadrenocorticism could occur. Pomeranians and miniature poodles might be slightly different from other breeds as an increased urinary cortisol/creati-nine ratio has been found in affected dogs, thus suggesting an abnormal pituitary-adrenal axis function resembling a hyperadrenocorticism-like condition.

Astrid Thelen *Germany*   I believe that alopecia X is just an aesthetic condition and some owners accept it.

David Senter *USA*   I have seen four dogs with insu-lin-resistant diabetes with high levels of 17-OHP and progesterone with classical clinical signs of alopecia X, and these dogs did not have Cushing's disease. This suggests that some dogs might develop, or have con-current, other hormonal diseases, thus early treatment should be recommended.

Ed Rosser   I have noticed that some dogs develop sec-ondary pyoderma. Perhaps these cases do not only have alopecia X, but also a concurrent underlying hormonal disease. One of the first names given to this syndrome, 'pseudo-Cushing's syndrome', suggests that abnormal adrenal function could be likely.

Manon Paradis   I have seen two dogs which devel-oped hyperadrenocorticism after a number of years; this could be an end-stage of alopecia X in rare cases.

Emily Walder   Let me comment on the histological differences between alopecia X and hyperadrenocorti-cism. In plush-coat dogs with hyperadrenocorticism, there is often catagen arrest instead of having telogen arrest, so it is important to look histologically at other adnexa l structures such as sebaceous gland atrophy and dermal atrophy to distinguish them from those with true alopecia X.

Manon Paradis   Thank you to the speakers and par-ticularly the audience for their participation in the dis-cussion.

References

1 Scott, D.W., Miller, W.H., Griffin, C.E. *Muller & Kirk's Small Animal Dermatology*, 6th edn. Philadelphia: W.B. Saunders, 2001.

Therapy of recurrent pyoderma and use of immunostimulants

L. Saijonmaa-Koulumies[1] (Chairperson), C.F. Curtis[2] (Secretary)

[1] Veterinary Clinic Mevet, Helsinki, Finland
[2] Dermatology Referral Service, Ware, Herts, UK

Leena Saijonmaa-Koulumies *Finland* Pyoderma is a common problem in dogs. It can occur as a result of primary immunodeficiency, be idiopathic in nature or, most commonly, it is secondary to some underlying or concurrent disease such as a hypersensitivity disorder, ectoparasitic infestation or an endocrinopathy. Individual cases vary considerably with respect to the depth and severity of infection, and the clinical appearance of the disease, but many cases have one thing in common: a high rate of recurrence despite repeated courses of therapy with seemingly 'appropriate' antibiotics.

Staphylococcus intermedius is the most important pathogen and is believed to be responsible for more than 90% of cases of canine pyoderma. This bacterium is a resident member of the canine microbial flora at the mucosae in most healthy dogs. From there it is seeded onto the host's skin during grooming. When conditions are favourable to the bacteria, they start to proliferate on the skin and this may lead to clinical infection. Occasionally, gram-negative bacterial species, such as *Escherichia coli, Proteus* spp. and *Pseudomonas aeruginosa,* are involved in deep infections as secondary invaders. Recent studies have also reported the detection of methicillin-resistant staphylococci (MRS), such as *Staphylococcus aureus* (MRSA) and *S. schleiferi*, in recurrent and refractory cases of canine pyoderma. This is alarming because methicillin resistance implies resistance to all beta-lactam-based antibiotics, including cephalosporins. In humans, MRSA is a cause of great concern, particularly in hospitals where it may be passed on to many patients via nosocomial infections. Heavy empirical use of broad-spectrum antibiotics has been implicated as a potential contributory factor for this infection in both humans and animals, emphasising the importance of performing bacterial culture, bacterial species identification and sensitivity testing in difficult and refractory cases of canine pyoderma.

Antibiotics are the cornerstone of treatment for canine pyoderma. The selected drug must be effective against the target pathogen, it must be capable of penetrating to the site of the infection, and it must be administered at the correct dose to reach adequate serum and tissue concentrations. The course of treatment must also be continued for a sufficient period of time to ensure cure, instead of transient remission. Whenever possible, underlying/concurrent disease, which may be predisposing the individual to infection, must be identified and treated. However, despite these practices, pyoderma recurrence rates are high, prompting clinicians to prescribe repeated courses of antibiotics. One of the main problems with repeated and heavy use of antibiotics is the appearance of resistant and multi-resistant strains of bacteria. In canine studies, it has been shown that staphylococci resistant to multiple antibiotics are more commonly isolated from cases of recurrent and deep pyoderma which have been treated repeatedly with a variety of different drugs. Resistance to narrow-spectrum antibiotics, such as lincosamides and macrolides, appears to develop relatively quickly. With extremely low or negligible resistance rates for cephalosporins, clavulanate-potentiated amoxicillin and fluoroquinolones, it is clear why clinicians and dermatologists frequently select drugs from these classes for empirical treatment. However, should they be our first-line choice of antibiotic? Do we know what the long-term 'collateral damage' might be? Should we encourage sensitivity testing in all cases of recurrent pyoderma instead of empirical use of cephalexin, and try to administer narrow-spectrum antibiotics whenever possible? What about drug dosage? Optimal dosing strategies for difficult cases appear to be lacking, although there are some anecdotal reports which suggest that higher than recommended dosages could be more efficient in some difficult cases of pyoderma. What about pulse therapy? Does it constitute good veterinary practice, and when and how should it be used? What are its benefits compared to a standard antibiotic protocol, and is it safe? Do bacterins and other immunomodulators offer us any additional benefits, given that the majority of the reports on such preparations are anecdotal and involve small numbers of dogs? Are these products likely to be more useful to us in the future?

Some of these points will be discussed as a group, but we will also hear short presentations from five speakers who will cover the topics of drug selection, pulse therapy, antibiotic resistance, bacterin therapy and immunomodulators, in the hope that we all leave feeling better able to tackle this common but often challenging disease.

Antimicrobial therapy: which antibiotic, why, and how? (D.J. DeBoer)

Doug DeBoer *USA*   There isn't one correct answer to the first part of this question, so we can hopefully generate some discussion. Whether dealing with a superficial or deep recurrent pyoderma, even if it is associated with a specific immunological effect, we have to choose an antibiotic. I would like to make a statement that we should be using cephalexin, 'period'. Important reasons for advocating its use include susceptibility of 100% (or nearly so) of *S. intermedius* isolates, and a failure of emergence of resistant strains with chronic or repeated use even in individual cases, as illustrated in literature studies showing the pattern of emergence of resistance of *S. intermedius* from canine skin during the period 1981–1986. Despite a reduction in the percentage of isolates susceptible to drugs like trimetho-

prim-sulpha and chloramphenicol in these studies, 100% of isolates were sensitive to cephalexin and there was no reduction in the percentage of isolates that were sensitive over time. Additional benefits are that, in most countries of the world, it has a moderate cost, a relative lack of toxicity, and no reports of adverse effects on neutrophil function, in contrast to some other antibiotics.

The next question relating to the best antibiotic protocol to use for recurrent disease has not been researched in dogs or man. A few days ago at this conference, Didier Carlotti presented his findings from a placebo-controlled study investigating the use of a 'weekend' pulse cephalexin regimen. Most clinicians appear to advocate some type of intermittent or 'pulse' therapy protocol in favour of a low-dose maintenance protocol. As the latter may be more likely to induce antimicrobial resistance, the former is somewhat safer in that regard.

The use of topical therapy for the treatment of recurrent pyoderma should also not be overlooked. In my experience, localised pyoderma in particular is amenable to this form of therapy. I have not found any of the chlorhexidine products to be particularly good and they do not prevent relapses. I prefer to use mupirocin ointment (Bactoderm®, USA/Bactroban®, UK) as this is effective against staphylococci.

I therefore have two relevant questions for discussion regarding antibiotics for canine recurrent staphylococcal infections:

(1) Is it really true that *S. intermedius* occasionally develops true resistance to cephalexin? Looking back over my own microbiology laboratory's data from the past 11 years, not one strain of cephalexin-resistant *S. intermedius* has been cultured from canine skin, although a few resistant strains have been cultured from canine ears. Has anyone documented resistant strains from dogs with pyoderma, and does resistance really exist or is it a myth?
(2) In the case of staphylococcal skin infections NOT caused by *S. intermedius*, i.e. *S. aureus* or *S. schleiferi*, which antibiotic choices are possible? The latter organism has been isolated most frequently from dogs receiving antimicrobials, and is often methicillin-resistant. So what antibiotic choices do we have?

Leena Saijonmaa-Koulumies   When you do a sensitivity test and you discover that the organism is sensitive, for example to a lincosamide or macrolide antibiotic as well as to cephalexin, what do you do?

Doug DeBoer   I tend to pick cephalexin anyway because I'm usually dealing with a recurrent pyoderma. In my experience, you can use erythromycin or lincomycin perhaps the first or second time you treat the pyoderma, but by the third or fourth time you reliably have a strain that is resistant to that antibiotic. So rather than starting with one and switching around, I start with cephalexin. Am I right to do that?

Leena Saijonmaa-Koulumies   Well, the concern is that you could induce resistance in other species of bacteria, e.g. *E. coli*, etc.

Doug DeBoer   Yes, you mean it could spread as a result of the use of broad-spectrum antibiotics?

Leena Saijonmaa-Koulumies   Yes.

Cathy Curtis *UK*   Could we just have a show of hands to see who uses cephalexin as a first-line antimicrobial? (Approximately 50% of the audience raised their hands.)

Doug DeBoer   So a lot of hands there. Anyone who doesn't use it for recurrent pyoderma? Any brave souls? (Approximately 33% of hands raised.)

Guillermina Manigot *Argentina*   Sometimes I will use a different drug if the patient is intolerant.

Doug DeBoer   Is your choice based upon the specific organism isolated?

Guillermina Manigot   Yes.

Alan Bell *New Zealand*   Doug, could you just describe your protocol for using mupirocin for the treatment of recurrent localised pyoderma?

Doug DeBoer   What we have done is to start using it twice daily. Typically, if it is going to work, it will prevent relapse when used at this frequency. After approximately 2 weeks we will reduce to once daily for 2 weeks, and then use it on an alternate-day basis. In my experience, it needs to be applied at least every other

day to be effective. I have not been able to use it once weekly for example, with good effect.

Alan Bell   Over what period of time have you used it, and have you encountered any problems with resistance; *S. aureus* can become resistant to this drug?

Doug DeBoer   The longest case I have followed is approximately 18–24 months, as unfortunately referral cases are often difficult to follow long-term. I have not seen resistance develop, although it may occur. This does not mean that it hasn't but if it did, I have not heard about it. I would like to say again though that only a few cases are suitable for this form of therapy; the disease needs to be very localised and predictable. If it is more generalised, then it's not a very practical form of therapy.

Candace Sousa *USA*   I think we need to be more clear about our definition of recurrent pyoderma. For example, can a dog that develops the disease in January of one year and December of the next be defined as having recurrent pyoderma in the same way as a dog that develops disease in January and then again in February? In my practice, which is a referral practice, most cases were not so much 'recurrent' as a failure to cure, as they had not been treated appropriately. So, I agree with Doug that using cephalexin as a first-line choice works very well. It's just that the referring practitioners may have only been treating for 10–14 days. When you use cephalexin, quite a few dogs will vomit, so I'm excited by the prospect that in the US we will soon have a once-daily tablet containing cefpodoxime (Simplicef®, Pfizer, USA), which may help us to overcome some of these problems. Hence, our definition of what is recurrent pyoderma, the significance of duration of treatment, and owner compliance, are issues to keep in mind when we discuss this topic.

Use of cephalexin intermittent therapy to prevent recurrent pyoderma in dogs with underlying allergic dermatitis: a double-blind placebo-controlled trial (E. Guaguère, C. Rème, A. Mondon and C. Salomon)

Christophe Rème *France*   Recurrent pyoderma may be a challenge in some dogs despite intensive efforts to control underlying dermatoses. The aim of this study, which spanned over a 2-year period, was to investigate the value of using strategic intermittent systemic antibiotic therapy to prevent the recurrence of superficial pyoderma in allergic dogs.

Dogs included in the study were presented with folliculitis and had shown more than three relapses of superficial pyoderma in the year before, despite adequate periods of antibiotic therapy (product, dose, duration), identification and stringent management of underlying allergy (parasiticides, elimination diets, immunotherapy) and exclusion of other causes. The 72 dogs were given cephalexin (Rilexine®, Virbac, France) at a dose of 15 mg/kg twice daily orally, until 10 days post-resolution of clinical signs. The dogs were then randomly allocated to one of two 18-week preventive regimen groups and received either cephalexin or similar placebo tablets for 3 consecutive days a week. Anti-allergenic therapy was maintained over the study period while use of other antibiotic treatments and medicated shampoo were forbidden.

The majority of dogs in the placebo group (20/34, 58.8%) relapsed within 18 weeks post-resolution, while few relapses were recorded in the cephalexin intermittent-therapy group (5/38, 13%). The median time to relapse was significantly lower in the placebo group (log-rank test, $p < 0.0001$). The administration of treatment (cephalexin) and underlying food hypersensitivity were both found to be significant prognostic factors for pyoderma relapse. However, with regard to the food-hypersensitive dogs, the data may have been influenced by the inevitable variability in degree of owner compliance associated with feeding a restricted diet for a protracted period of time. Breed, sex, age, number of previous relapses and presence of co-housed animals were not significant prognostic factors (multivariate logistic regression analysis). The *S. intermedius* strains isolated from animals that relapsed did not show development of resistance. Few gastrointestinal adverse events were recorded in both groups.

In conclusion, cephalexin pulse therapy 3 days a week for several months appears to significantly reduce the risk of pyoderma relapse in refractory allergic dogs, in addition to specific allergy therapy. Further, this form of therapy did not appear to induce bacterial resistance.

Doug DeBoer   I have a dose question. It seems that it's common practice in Europe to use cephalexin at 15 mg/kg twice daily, whereas in the US we are typically using it at 22–30 mg/kg twice daily. I have seen cases that have failed to cure when they were on dosages lower than 22 mg/kg twice daily, and when I increased the dose, they cured. So, is 15 mg/kg the standard dose used in Europe?

Christophe Rème   In Europe, cephalexin has a veterinary licence, whereas I believe the preparations you have available in the US are medical products? We are obliged to use the label recommended dose of 15 mg/kg twice daily. European dermatologists and practitioners find this effective. Perhaps a difference in the medical and veterinary preparations exists which could explain this?

Guillermina Manigot   I always used to use the higher dose, but recently have been trying the lower dose on some of my patients and have been very pleased with the results; some of them are responding beautifully.

Christophe Rème   I would really like to see the results of a double-blind study to compare a cephalexin product as used in the US, with Rilexine® (cephalexin) at the lower European label dose. I think that prescribing habits do become ingrained and that this is an important factor in dose selection. However, I am unable to support this opinion with any scientific data.

Antimicrobial sensitivity of pathogenic staphylococci in recurrent canine pyoderma (D.H. Lloyd and A. Loeffler)

Annette Loeffler *UK*   *S. intermedius* is the major pathogenic *Staphylococcus* involved in canine pyoderma, and this disease is one of the most common reasons for antimicrobial therapy in small animal practice. High levels of resistance to penicillin (around 80–90%) and to a lesser extent to sulphonamides, macrolides, lincosamides and tetracyclines (15–40%) have been reported in Europe. An increase in the proportion of multi-resistant strains has also been demonstrated, and recurrent therapy has been shown to be associated with acquisition of multi-resistant strains. Unfortunately, national surveillance programmes of antimicrobial resistance in animals generally do not provide data on companion animals, and it is difficult to compare temporal and regional changes within Europe. However, surveillance programmes in Sweden (SVARM) and Norway (NORM-VET) are now reporting annually on the sensitivity of *S. intermedius*. In 2002, a high prevalence of resistance to fusidic acid

(59%) and tetracycline (53%) was reported in Norway, and resistance levels of 8–12% have been reported between 1992 and 2002 in Sweden. Resistance to amoxicillin/clavulanic acid and to cephalexin is very uncommon, despite the use of large quantity of these antimicrobials in small animal practice. However, amongst 692 isolates submitted to the Royal Veterinary College (RVC) laboratories from 2002 to 2003, we found that about 3% were resistant to amoxicillin/clavulanic acid, whereas no resistance was found from 1980 to 1996. Although cephalexin resistance is known in *S. intermedius*, it does not seem to develop readily, and all resistant isolates reported at the RVC are invariably reclassified as *S. aureus* when checked. At this congress, a paper is being presented showing that, during prolonged cephalexin pulse therapy, no change in resistance occurred. This should not be used as a reason for indiscriminate use of this very valuable antibiotic. Where extensive multi-resistance is reported in a single strain to cephalexin, amoxicillin/clavulanic acid, fluoroquinolones and other antibiotics, the correct identification of the bacterium should be checked. This resistance pattern is a hallmark of MRSA.

Although *S. aureus* represents less than 10% of isolates from canine pyoderma in most studies, we have recently identified two cases of recurrent pyoderma in dogs associated with MRSA. In one dog, MRSA was isolated from lesions of superficial pyoderma and acute moist dermatitis, while the other dog had deep pyoderma lesions on the chin. Both cases had responded poorly to antimicrobial therapy and, in both cases, a connection of the owners to a hospital environment was made. Our colleagues in the surgical and internal medicine departments have recorded a total of 12 cases of MRSA in dogs and cats between November 2003 and March 2004, and they were associated with suture problems and wound breakdowns in 40% of the cases. The remaining 60% of these cases had concurrent internal disease. Since 1999, reports of MRSA in various domestic animal species have become more frequent, but the prevalence of this organism amongst pets is unknown. We conducted a survey of mucosal carriage and environmental contamination of this organism amongst in-patients, staff and environmental surfaces, in a small animal referral hospital. We isolated MRSA from 14 of 89 staff, 4 of 45 dogs, 3 of 30 environmental sites, and from none of the cats. Sensitivity to other antimicrobials amongst the 28 isolates followed seven different patterns. The seven isolates from dogs and

the environment had the same pattern of sensitivity. Pulsed-field gel electrophoresis has shown that an epidemic human hospital clone (EMRSA) predominated amongst all of the isolates. Although the isolates originated from intact mucosal sites, MRSA should be considered as a complicating cause of recurrent pyoderma, especially once more data regarding its prevalence become available.

Leena Saijonmaa-Koulumies   How many of you have come across MRSA in your practice? (Only one hand raised in the audience.)

Clinical experiences with a staphylococcal autogenous bacterin (C.F. Curtis, A. Lamport, D.H. Lloyd)

Cathy Curtis   Before I begin, can I ask how many of the audience has any experience with the use of bacterin therapy for recurrent pyoderma? (Approximately 5% raised hands.) I first became interested in autogenous bacterins during my residency at the Royal Veterinary College (RVC). A *S. intermedius*-based autogenous bacterin had been used there for 20–30 years and had been developed under the guidance of Mr Tommy Thomsett, who had adapted a method used for the production of an autogenous vaccine for the treatment of bovine papillomas. Encouraged by the results of an open pilot trial, a blinded controlled study was devised to investigate the efficacy of the bacterin in the control of canine idiopathic recurrent superficial pyoderma. Ten dogs with at least three prior episodes of disease were recruited. All were free of ectoparasitic and fungal disease and had failed to improve on a dietary trial. Those exhibiting signs of pruritus responded completely to antibacterial therapy. Haematological and biochemical parameters were unremarkable and all dogs were euthyroid. *S. intermedius* cultures from lesions were used to produce an autogenous bacterin for each animal. A numerical lesional score was generated for each dog, and dogs were randomly divided into two groups of five each. Both groups received a 4-week course of antibiotics. In addition, group 1 also received concurrent subcutaneous injections of bacterin which continued until week 10 of the study, while group 2 received no additional therapy. All dogs were re-examined and scored for lesions again at weeks 5 and 10. Repeat blood samples to screen for adverse effects were submitted at week 10. Comparison of lesional scores at week 0 and week 5 (Mann-Whitney U test) revealed no significant differences between the groups. At week 10, group 2 lesional scores were significantly greater ($p = 0.05$), and there was a significant increase in the lesional score for dogs in group 2 at week 10, compared with week 5 ($p = 0.029$). No adverse reactions to the bacterin were detected and all ten dogs subsequently received the therapy. At the end of a 9–18-month follow-up period, five of the ten dogs were still receiving bacterin as their owners and veterinary surgeons considered it to be of benefit.

These results suggest that autogenous bacterins may provide an alternative, safe, and effective method for the control of canine idiopathic recurrent pyoderma. However, despite many similar favourable anecdotal reports of their benefits, few veterinarians and dermatologists use these products on a regular basis. The RVC's product is cost-effective when compared with repeated or protracted courses of antibiotics. The current cost is approximately €40 for a 3-month course of therapy. If this therapy is successful, it should continue to be administered at 1–2-week intervals for as long as it is of benefit. In my experience, the most common cause of failure is premature withdrawal of therapy, or attempting to increase the interval between injections to beyond 2 weeks.

Candace Sousa Do you have any thoughts on the method of action of the bacterin?

Cathy Curtis We did actually submit serum samples from each of the study dogs to Doug DeBoer's laboratory to assess their anti-*S. intermedius* IgG and IgE responses. The levels were highly variable and our small sample size made it impossible to draw any conclusions from the data. *In vitro* studies have demonstrated that the *S. aureus*-based bacterin, Staphage Lysate® (Delmont Laboratories, USA), is capable of stimulating proliferation of human T and B lymphocytes, and in laboratory animals, this product has increased the ability of macrophages to inactivate staphylococci. However, to my knowledge, no such studies have been conducted with a *S. intermedius*-based autogenous bacterin.

Candace Sousa Antibody opsonisation of microbes facilitates phagocytosis, so do you think this product could be working via mechanisms other than antibody production? Are these therapies generating a specific antibody response or are they non-specifically stimulating phagocyotis? What are your thoughts?

Cathy Curtis The wide variety of responses to Staphage Lysate® in dogs and laboratory animals suggest it could have a whole range of specific and/or non-specific immunomodulatory actions. I'm afraid it's not possible to answer that question at this time.

Doug DeBoer I think that the evidence we have so far does not favour a mechanism involving bacterins acting via the induction of an increased IgG titre. When we looked at a number of killed strains of *S. intermedius*, there was quite a variation in their lymphocyte-stimulating capabilities and their ability to induce certain target cell lines to produce cytokines. There was a marked variation in the immunomodulatory effects of killed strains, at least *in vitro*. When we look at the results of a study like the one just presented, we have to wonder how much of the patient's response depends on the dog's disease, versus the immunomodulatory effects of the particular bacterial strain(s) used in the bacterin.

Cathy Curtis Ultimately the aim must be to develop a standardised, generic, commercially available bacterin product which contains the relevant bacterial antigens for the treatment of canine disease.

Leena Saijonmaa-Koulumies Have you used this product for the treatment of deep pyoderma?

Cathy Curtis Yes, I recruited two affected English bull terriers to the study initially. However, due to their recurrent relapses, I decided to limit the selection criteria to only dogs with superficial disease. Anecdotally, I have had a few dogs with deep pyoderma that have temporary responses to the autogenous bacterin, but it has generally not been my experience that they respond as well to the product. Dogs with deep pyoderma may have immunological differences which predispose them to this form of the disease in the first place, which may account for the less favourable response.

Immunostimulants; how might they work and how might they help in the future? (A. Hendricks)

Anke Hendricks *UK* Immunostimulant, or immune enhancer, is a broad term used to describe substances that have been found to stimulate one or several functions of the innate or adaptive immune response, and by doing so to help prevent or overcome infectious or neoplastic disease.

Immunostimulants have been used as adjuvants in vaccines for decades, although their important role in directing the immune response, and their modes of action, have only recently been appreciated. Furthermore attempts at using certain drugs and substances with non-specific immunostimulatory effects to help combat infectious and neoplastic disease have met with limited success. Some of those substances with relatively ill-defined mechanisms of action occupy specific therapeutic niches in human medicine, such as contact sensitisers, cimetidine and levamisole. Adjuvants, such as those used in vaccines, are also commonly used, particularly in animal species, despite a number of potential side effects.

In recent years, innate immunity been promoted from a first line of defence only, to a central director and regulator of adaptive immune responses. The current model of immunity (first described in the mid-1990s) hypothesises that an immune response only ensues if antigen-presenting cells (APCs) are activated by a variety of endogenous and exogenous alarm/danger signals from their immediate environment. Activated APCs then increase MHC expression and provide co-stimulatory signals to fully activate T cells and thus initiate an adaptive response. The type of co-stimulatory signals and production of different mediators by the APCs is crucial in determining the nature and extent of the immune response. Thus, the innate immune system has been promoted from a first-line defence system to a central director and orchestrator of the immune response. One important mechanism of detecting danger signals uses conserved pattern recognition receptors (PRR). These PRRs bind to a range of conserved microbial structures and certain host molecules. One large family of PRRs is that of the Toll-like receptors (TLRs). Based on this new understanding, the concept of augmenting and manipulating innate immune responses, and thus indirectly also adaptive responses, by TLR (or other PRR) agonists, is intriguing. Additionally, direct stimulation of adaptive immune responses by APC-independent co-stimulatory signals is conceivable. Both approaches are currently in variable stages of experimental and clinical investigation in people and animals.

Stimulators of adaptive immunity include endogenous cytokines and chemokines that bind to their specific receptors, as well as other substances (certain saponins, tucaresol, thymic peptides and purine analogues) that have a variety of co-stimulatory effects. This generally results in augmented T-cell reactivity to antigens.

Stimulators of innate immunity activate a variety of innate immune cells, particularly APCs, but have no direct effect on T cells. Most of them are microbial components or their derivatives, and act as TLR agonists (CpG motifs, LPS, muramyl peptides, lipid A derivatives, beta-glucans). Some have been used in humans for many years as non-specific immunostimulators (e.g. for the treatment of actinic keratoses or squamous cell carcinoma *in situ*), but we are only now beginning to understand their mode of action. TLR agonists tend to promote Th1-type responses. The imidazoquinolines (imiquimod, resiquimod) are also TLR agonists, whereas α-galactosylceramide is presented by the MHC class I-like molecule CD1d and recognised by natural killer (NK) T cells. Activated NK cells then produce IL-4 and can skew the response of naive T cells towards a Th2-type response. Stimulators of innate immunity potentially have a large number of future clinical applications, both preventative and therapeutic.

1 Disease prevention

(a) Response-defining adjuvants in vaccines against intracellular microbes (e.g. CpG-mediated Th1 response).
(b) Stimulation of innate immunity prior to exposure.

2 Therapy

(a) Immunomodulation by shifting of immune response type
  – Th2-type allergies (e.g. allergen-specific immunotherapy in combination with a Th1 immunostimulant such as resiquimod or CpG).
  – Th1-type autoimmune diseases (e.g. Th2 stimulants such as α-galactosylceramide).
  – Infectious diseases (e.g. leishmaniasis with a Th1 stimulant such as resiquimod or CpG).

(b) Augmentation of immune response in immunocompromised individuals.
(c) Initiation of tumour immunity (e.g. imiquimod).

Whilst some clinical uses are already established (e.g. imiquimod for viral warts and actinic keratoses), most are still experimental. No experimental studies with immunostimulants on classical extracellular bacterial infections have been published to date. Furthermore, some practical issues, such as species-specificity of some of the immunostimulants, and optimal timing of the treatment, need to be considered before using such immunostimulants. A major, currently unresolved concern is that of adverse effects, as have been observed in some murine studies. Stimulation with TLR agonists may actually result in enhanced virulence in those viral infections affecting immune cells. In mice, it has been associated with a reduced toxic shock threshold. It may also lead to acceleration or triggering of Th1-driven autoimmune disease.

In conclusion, evidence is beginning to accumulate for the preventative and therapeutic potential of potent immunostimulators in infectious, immune-mediated and neoplastic disease. These offer exciting opportunities but also the potential for serious adverse effects and extensive clinical trials are needed. I have not mentioned staphylococci specifically during this presentation because, to date, the majority of studies have centred on diseases involving intracellular bacte-

ria, However, as more data is published, we will hopefully be able to extrapolate from it and understand further some of the clinical responses we are observing, for example to the bacterin products in our canine patients. The timing and route of administration of these products are undoubtedly important and I have often wondered how these products work. The efficacy rates for Staphage Lysate® and the autogenous bacterin are fairly similar and both obviously contain staphylococci. Perhaps the peptidoglycan of the bacterial cell wall induces a non-specific immune response via TLRs, as it is a ligand for these receptors? In Europe, some practitioners have traditionally been using killed pox virus preparations and acemannan from aloe vera as immunomodulators. We know from recent studies that such products are effective via the stimulation of PRRs, so at least we can now begin to understand why and how they may be working.

Leena Saijonmaa-Koulumies   We are now at the end of this session and need to close. I wish to thank again our sponsors (Schering Plough), our speakers, and all of you for attending and for your contributions. Thank you very much.

Rodent and rabbit dermatology

S.D. White[1] (Chairperson), S.I.J. Vandenabeele[2] (Secretary)

[1] University of California, Davis, California, USA
[2] University of Ghent, Merelbeke, Belgium

Stephen White *USA* Our session today will cover various topics in rodent and rabbit dermatology.

Bernard Mignon *Belgium* I would like to start with a case presentation. A 2-month-old male guinea pig presents with an irritated eyelid. This animal has been acquired in a pet shop and is the only pet in the household. The owner first noticed the lesions 2 weeks ago. The area was reported to be pruritic prior to the onset of the lesions. The lesions consist of a well-demarcated periorbital alopecia that is spreading peripherally, and an area of alopecia in the concave portion of the ipsilateral pinna. The alopecic lesions are so well demarcated that they cannot be caused by the scratching of the animal. There are areas of erythema, scale, crusts and alopecia in the perigenital area and on one tarsus.

Differential diagnoses are primarily dermatophytosis, which typically starts periorbitally and is commonly seen in young rodents (especially if they come from pet shops), or trixacaric or sarcoptic mange. Other differential diagnoses are pseudomange (*Chiroidiscoides caviae*), lice infestation, or demodicosis. This last disease is less likely. Demodicosis has been described in guinea pigs but I have not seen a case.

A trichogram revealed hyphae and spores. These are often more difficult to visualise in rodents than in cats. A good clearing agent (chlorphenolac or potassium hydroxide) should be used when trying to visualise the fungal elements in the hairs of rodents. Also, one should look closely at broken hairs where fungal elements might be seen more readily. A fungal culture identified the fungal organism as *Trichophyton mentagrophytes*. This is the most common cause of dermatophytosis in the guinea pig and rabbit. *T. mentagrophytes* organisms can be identified in cultures using several criteria; microconidia generally form grape-like clusters, macroconidia (only seen on culture) are sausage-shaped, and typical spiral hyphae may also be present.

Treatment was initiated with itraconazole 10 mg/kg once daily orally for 1 month. This medication was chosen because of its high level of efficacy and the lack of availability of griseofulvin in Belgium. Concurrently, enilconazole 0.2% (Imaverol®, Janssen Pharmaceuticals, Belgium) dips were applied twice weekly for 1 month. Although dermatophytosis can be self-limiting, it is advisable to treat the affected animals to avoid human infections and environmental contamination. Once the lesions were resolved, a second culture was performed. This culture was negative and the therapy was discontinued. This treatment modality is acceptable when treating single animals; for guinea pigs housed together, treatment should be continued for another 2 weeks once the culture is negative.

Natalie Perrins *UK* Did you supplement the diet or think any supplementation was indicated?

Bernard Mignon No, I did not supplement the diet. It is not my experience that a guinea pig with dermatophytosis will respond better to treatment when supplemented with vitamin C.

Stephen White　Vitamin C can be degraded when the food is stored for a long time.

Bernard Mignon　I do recommend feeding oranges because they are a natural source of vitamin C.

Wieland Beck *Germany*　Are there any disadvantages with using griseofulvin as opposed to itraconazole?

Bernard Mignon　Again, the reason for choosing the itraconazole was because griseofulvin is not available in Belgium, not because of any known disadvantages.

Stephen White　How many people in the audience have seen dermatophytosis in the guinea pig?

Everybody in the workshop had seen dermatophytosis in the guinea pig. Some people had seen *Microsporum* dermatophytosis in guinea pigs. Also, people mentioned that the guinea pigs affected with *Microsporum* spp. can fluoresce when examined with the Wood's lamp.

Bernard Mignon　Guinea pigs in the lab always fluoresce under the Wood's lamp when infected with *M. canis*.

Luc Beco *Belgium*　The dose of itraconazole (10 mg/kg) used in this case was double the dosage proposed in cats; what was the reason for the higher dose? Is there any scientific evidence for this higher dose?

Bernard Mignon　I have always used the higher dose, but there is no scientific report indicating that the higher dose is associated with more rapid resolution of clinical signs. No safety studies have been performed with itraconazole in rodents that I am aware of, but I have never seen toxicities. As this drug is available in 100-mg capsules containing 1000 granules, it is harder to administer the precise dose. The drug is available as a liquid for human medicine in some European countries. The liquid formulation is easier to dose.

Marianne Mellgren *Sweden*　I use the 10 mg/kg dose for 3 weeks.

Christina Colonna *Austria*　During the presenta-

tion of the Janssen Animal Health company, it was announced that a veterinary liquid itraconazole formulation will become available in Europe. This formulation could be used on a 1-week-on, 1-week-off regimen for 3 weeks.

Stephen White　The preparation is already available in some countries, and this regimen for dogs and cats is feasible, presumably because itraconazole stays in the stratum corneum long enough to be effective.

Patrick Bourdeau *France*　Itraconazole has a better safety record and is better tolerated than ketoconazole in rodents and rabbits. A safety study was performed in our lab in which 10 mg/kg of ketoconazole was administered daily for 3 months to rabbits and guinea pigs. No adverse reactions were noted, but a slight increase in hepatic enzymes was seen. So itraconazole, which is even safer than ketoconazole, is probably safe at the 10 mg/kg dose. It is in fact enilconazole which can cause problems. This drug is toxic when ingested, and because rodents are meticulous groomers, they are more likely to ingest the drug applied to the skin.

Koji Nishifuji *Japan*　Can someone comment on the administration of terbinafine to treat dermatophytosis in rodents?

Stephen White　There are at least two articles which report that terbinafine was well tolerated in guinea pigs for the treatment of experimental dermatophytosis.[1,2]

Charles Chen *Taiwan*　I use terbinafine at a dose of 10 mg/kg for 2–6 weeks, making a suspension of the terbinafine in water or syrup.

Stephen White　How many people in the audience have used griseofulvin and have you seen toxicity reactions?

Thio Benderson *UK*　I have seen one guinea pig which died 1 week after initiating treatment with griseofulvin.

Luc Beco　I would like to speak about notoedric acariasis in hamsters and rats. Notoedric acariasis in hamsters affects mainly the ears, face, genitalia and tail. The diagnosis can be made by distribution and characterisation of the clinical signs and by performing skin scrapings.

One study[3] compared the efficacy of parenteral ivermectin and oral moxidectin for the treatment of notoedric acariasis in hamsters in a prospective, open, parallel (without cross-over) study. The ivermectin was injected subcutaneously once weekly, while the moxidectin was administered orally once or twice weekly. Each treatment group consisted of ten hamsters. Clinical lesions were graded with a system similar to the CADESI score used for evaluation of clinical signs in atopic dermatitis in dogs. Animals were evaluated weekly for pruritus (pruritus score for each group is the number of pruritic activities during 30 minutes divided by the number of hamsters) and the number of mites (assessed by skin scrapings of ear pinna of each hamster). There was no difference in pruritus, number of mites, or CADESI score between the different groups at 4 or 8 weeks of treatment, although the moxidectin was much easier to administer. In each group, at the end of the study period, some hamsters remained positive for mites on scrapings, indicating that 8 weeks of treatment is sometimes not long enough for complete remission. It can take up to 3 weeks to see clinical improvement with these treatments. One hamster developed necrotic lesions on the ear pinna following ivermectin injection.

Notoedric acariasis in rats clinically resembles the disease in hamsters, except that they can sometimes present with nasal 'horns' (Fig. 6.13.1). Frequently, the mite can be visualised when a skin scraping of this nasal hyperkeratotic lesion is performed. The recommended treatment for notoedric acariasis consists of ivermectin 500 μg/kg administered subcutaneously every 15 days. The oral and pour-on administration remain to be evaluated.

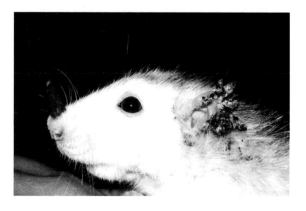

Fig. 6.13.1 Nasal horn in a rat with notoedric acariasis. Note also the lesions on the ear pinna associated with pruritus due to the mite infestation.

Bernard Mignon   I have tried the ivermectin as a pour-on with success.

Luc Beco   Other drugs that could probably be used are doramectin, selamectin and moxidectin. Unfortunately, no studies have been published concerning the administration, safety and doses of these drugs in rats.

Stephen White   How many people in the audience have seen notoedric mange in rodents and how did you treat them?

Bernard Mignon   I have seen an increase in notoedric mange in rats and feel that rats have less severe lesions than hamsters; and rats respond well to selamectin.

Stephen White   Is it easy to find the mites?

Both Drs Mignon and Beco said the mites are very easily found.

Stephen White   I have seen one case in which the owner had skin lesions.

Patrick Bourdeau   In contrast to the highly contagious *Sarcoptes* in dogs and *Notoedres* in cats, *Notoedres* in rats is not often a zoonosis. I have seen only one case in a man.

Stefanie Koebrich *Germany*   Is the reaction of the ivermectin injection due to the ivermectin or is this reaction seen with the injection of other drugs as well?

Luc Beco   I have seen this type of reaction in three cases due to ivermectin and it can probably be seen with injections of other drugs too.

Peter Lemmens *Belgium*   Has anybody tried administering ivermectin orally?

Luc Beco   I have not tried this. (Someone in the workshop had tried ivermectin orally at a dose of 300 μg/kg.)

Wieland Beck   I apply fipronyl (Frontline®, Merial, France) spray once weekly for two treatments when treating ectoparasitoses in rodents.

Luc Beco   Remember not to use fipronyl on rabbits.

Patrick Bourdeau I would like to speak on three topics concerning ectoparasitoses in rodents and rabbits. Acarioses can be divided into classical (or typical) acarioses and atypical acarioses. The latter is more common and can be attributed to the different host reactions. Acarioses are often misdiagnosed and are an emerging problem. *Ornithonyssus bacoti* is an example of an 'old' parasite that has recently emerged as a cause of parasitic disease in rodents and rabbits. Similarly, a recrudescence of sarcoptic mange is being seen in people.

Mites from the family Psorergatidae can cause an infestation in rabbits which presents as an alopecic lesion around the neck. The parasite resembles *Notoedres* mites, but differs in that it has a rounded body, but no anal plaque on the dorsal pad and has no suckers; it has claws that differentiate it from *Notoedres* spp. Treatment with 0.05 ml of 10% pyriproxifen (Cyclio® 10% Spot-on for cats, Virbac, France), which has been shown to be an effective treatment for some acarioses and inhibits ticks' moulting process, had no effect. Ivermectin 0.4 mg/kg injected subcutaneously resulted in slow clinical cure after 3 months. The mites of the family Psorergatidae are *Psorobia* and *Psorergates*. *Psorergates simplex* is found in mice, *Psorergates oettlei* is found in rodents. Both parasites cause intrafollicular cysts necessitating biopsy for definitive diagnosis. The rabbit could be an asymptomatic carrier where the mite is considered to be a surface mite.

Glycyphagid mites were seen in two chipmunks that were housed together. Only one animal developed clinical signs which consisted of alopecia, crusts and mild pruritus on the face, genital area, flank and the base of the tail. Skin scrapings revealed the presence of multiple asegmented, headless mites. A biopsy demonstrated hyperkeratosis and intrafollicular mites. The parasites were identified as nymphal forms of a new Glycyphagid mite, *Sciuropsis*. Treatment was initiated with ivermectin and carbamate dust 5%, without effect. Treatment with pyriproxifen resulted in a slow resolution of clinical signs within 2 months. Since this description, six other cases have been seen, always in chipmunks.

Another parasitosis is caused by the nymphal form of *Acarus farris*, a storage mite that can be found in homes. Sometimes a nymphal form, the hypopode (deutonymph), can cause dermatitis. This has been reported in a gerbil that presented with a progressive pruritus of the tail, head and legs. The hypopode is a life stage between classical nymphal stages I and III. The deutonymph stage can be characterised by the fact that there are no mouth parts or head present. The gastrointestinal tract is rudimentary and this stage can be active or immobile. These deutonymphs are hard to identify due to morphologic convergence of hypopodes forms. A parasitosis caused by deutonymphs of *Acarus farris* has been described in two guinea pigs,[4] and was clinically characterised by pruritus and alopecia of the tail and rump. Diagnosis can be made by skin scrapings; treatment is not difficult.

Some mites cause clinical signs only if the host develops a hypersensitivity to these mites. For example, *Myocoptes musculi* and *Myoptes musculinus*, both fur mites of rodents (mainly mice), may sometimes be found incidentally or as superinfestations. *Radfordia* spp. are mainly found on the head, *Myocoptes* spp. on the trunk, and *Lepora* spp. in the rabbit on the ventral abdomen and dorsum. Diagnosis is straightforward (because of the multitude of mites present) and is made by clear (Scotch) tape preparations, combing and skin scrapings. Parasitoses caused by fur mites are hard to eliminate from rodent colonies. Mice can present with alopecic and crusting lesions on the top of the head and dorsum. Acaricidal treatment in these species can easily result in toxicity reactions because one tends to overdose. Toxicity reactions could be more commonly seen with fipronil (oral toxic dose is 100 mg/kg) or ivermectin (oral toxic dose is 10 mg/kg). While one drop of these drugs is safe in the adult rat, the same dose can already be toxic to the mouse. In one experiment, a swab technique was developed on gerbils. For example if you want to treat a rodent with 12 mg/kg, two drops of selamectin would be placed onto the swab and then onto the dorsum of the affected animal. Five hundred mice with a *Myoptes* or *Myocoptes* infestation were treated using this technique. Once the mice cleared their parasitic infestation, clinical signs were still present and the lesions were much slower to resolve. Other factors such as genetic diversity are important in the response to treatment. An example is mice-associated ulcerative dermatitis (MAUD), which is a dermatosis associated with a hypersensitivity to *Myocoptes* in which the clinical presentation and response to treatment are linked to the presence of two genes.

Finally, infestations with Trombidiforms or Gamasiforms can be seen in rodents. These parasites are hard to identify and such parasitoses can often be overlooked. Recently *Sciuropsosis* was found to be the cause of a dermatosis in a Canadian marmot (*Marmotta vancouverensis*). These animals presented with alopecia in the dorsal lumbar area.

Taina Kivisto *Germany* Have you had any experience with *Straelensia* infestations?

Patrick Bourdeau This is a dog parasite described mainly in France (cases also mentioned in Italy, Spain and Portugal). I have seen biopsies from one case in a dog from Israel, and diagnosed a case in a cat in France.

Vanessa Miller *UK* Is it possible that the slow hair regrowth that is seen in rabbits that are treated for a parasitic infestation is due just to the slow hair growth as opposed to a slow cure of the parasitosis?

Patrick Bourdeau It is possible.

Stephen White How many people have seen demodicosis in hamsters and what treatments are you using? (About one half of the people had seen demodicosis in hamsters.)

Charles Chen Ivermectin orally once daily for a period of time up to 3 months.

Patrick Bourdeau I often change the nutrition first and if no improvement is seen within 2 weeks, I treat with amitraz at half the usual dose.

Liora Waldman *Israel* I have seen a dog with an ulcerative dermatitis in which an *Ornythonyssus bacoti* infestation was diagnosed even though the animal had been treated with selamectin (Revolution®, Pfizer Animal Health, USA) monthly.

Patrick Bourdeau The first nymphal stages and the adults of *Ornythonyssus* spp. bite. A high blood level of acaricidal product is necessary to be effective on these intermittent parasites. This is difficult to attain with macrocyclic lactones. Also, re-infestations can occur from the environment.

Liora Waldman I have seen alopecic squirrel monkeys with a change in coat colour (becoming a golden colour) that were negative on skin scrapings but cleared when treated with ivermectin every 2 weeks and dietary supplementation.

Wieland Beck Can ivermectin be used to treat demodicosis in the hedgehog?

Patrick Bourdeau Ivermectin is probably safe when used in hedgehogs. Selamectin is usually better tolerated and safer, but has a shorter half-life. I have also seen pruritic, crusty hedgehogs with an *Otodectes cynotis* infestation (a parasite normally only seen in carnivores).

Wieland Beck I've seen alopecic hedgehogs caused by demodicosis.

Stephen White I wanted to end this workshop with a few observations. First, skin scrapings at UC Davis are performed with a medical grade spatula instead of blades. These spatulas can be obtained at www.fisherscientific.com. The spatulas are dull enough so that they do not cut but are sharp enough to perform even deep skin scrapings and can be found in the scientific catalogue under number 21-401-20.

Second, I have seen a few cases of old rats that had a facial pruritus and died soon after they were presented for their dermatosis. These rats were then diagnosed with an internal neoplasia. Possibly the facial pruritus in these animals was a paraneoplastic phenomenon. It might be interesting to perform an ultrasound in such animals to rule out internal neoplasias.

Third, it is important to remember that in rabbits and rodents, teeth or eye problems may affect the skin. A chinchilla was seen with an area of alopecia under the eye. The chinchilla was diagnosed with an obstruction of the tear duct due to the bath dust in the cage.

I am indebted to Dr Klaus Earl Loft in Denmark who has informed me of a group of capybaras with partial alopecia. These animals were diagnosed with a dermatophytosis.

I would lastly like to mention that it is important to remember that some rabbits can present with a patchy alopecia during physiologic shedding.

References

1 Petranyi, G., Meingassner, J.G., Mieth, H. Activity of terbinafine in experimental fungal infections of laboratory animals. *Antimicrobial Agents and Chemotherapy*, 1987; **31**: 1558–1561.
2 Mieth, H., Leitner, I., Meingassner, J.G. The efficacy of orally applied terbinafine, itraconazole and fluconazole in models of experimental trichophytoses. *Journal of Medical and Veterinary Mycology*, 1994; **32**: 181–188.
3 Beco, L., Petite, A., Olivry, T. Comparison of subcutaneous ivermectin and oral moxidectin for the treatment of notoedric acariasis in hamsters. *Veterinary Record*, 2001; **149**: 324–327.
4 Linek, M., Bourdeau, P. Alopecia in two guinea pigs due to hypopodes of *Acarus farris*. *Veterinary Dermatolology*, 2004; **15** (Suppl. 1): 69 (Abstract).

Shampoos and topical therapy

K.W. Kwochka[1] (Chairperson), W.S. Rosenkrantz[2] (Secretary)

[1] DVM Pharmaceuticals Inc, Miami, Florida, USA
[2] Animal Dermatology Clinic, Tustin and San Diego, California, USA

Ken Kwochka *USA*   Good afternoon and welcome to the Shampoo and Topical Therapy Workshop. This session is being sponsored by ICF Italy and we would like to thank them for their generous support. My name is Ken Kwochka and I am Vice President of Research and Development for DVM Pharmaceuticals, Miami, Florida, USA. Dr Wayne Rosenkrantz is the Secretary of this workshop. Dr Rosenkrantz is from the Animal Dermatology Clinic in Tustin, California, USA. Wayne and I have decided to make this very informal. We are not going to have formal presentations, but four clinicians and scientists will comment on their work followed by questions and discussion.

The use of topical therapy really exploded in veterinary dermatology about 30 years ago. Dermatologics for Veterinary Medicine (now DVM Pharmaceuticals) and Allerderm (now Virbac) started producing topical products specifically for companion animals, including many different shampoos, rinses and sprays. Over time, other companies have developed similar and unique products. However, the industry seems to have reached a plateau in development at this point in time, and I hope that over the next 5–10 years the specialty will see new drugs and new topical delivery systems for topical and systemic agents.

One of the big problems with topical therapy is owner compliance, since topical therapy is difficult and time-consuming. We also have a problem with a lack of regulation of topical products and their active ingredients. For example, most of the topical products that are available in the United States are not approved by the Food and Drug Administration (FDA). Therefore, many different companies can manufacture and distribute these products. This results in a real problem because without control of the formulation and manufacturing process, the potency, stability, efficacy and safety of the products are not always certain. This presents a dilemma for practitioners trying to decide what to use, especially when there are similar products on the market.

Wayne and I have been fortunate to get some excellent participants who are going to give us informal presentations on work that they have done with tacrolimus, cyclosporine, control of dust mites and topical approach to seborrhoeic skin disease.

Use of topical tacrolimus in veterinary dermatology (J.G. Griffies)

Joel Griffies *USA*   I would like to discuss our work with tacrolimus (Protopic®, Fujisawa Healthcare, Inc., Illinois, USA) in the treatment of discoid lupus erythematosus (DLE) and pemphigus erythematosus (PE).[1]

We explored the use of 0.1% tacrolimus ointment applied topically as a treatment modality for DLE and PE. Discoid lupus erythematosus has been cited as the second most common immune-mediated skin disease of dogs and in most cases it is a relatively benign disease with no systemic involvement. Pemphigus erythematosus is thought to be a variant of DLE and pemphigus foliaceus (PF), or perhaps a milder form of PF. The side effects associated with some of the therapies that have been utilised for these diseases in the past can sometimes be worse than the disease itself. So we thought we would look at using a topical therapeutic agent to treat these diseases.

Tacrolimus is a macrolide that has a mechanism of action almost identical to cyclosporine. It has been estimated to be 10–100 times more potent than cyclosporine. One of the big differences is that this is a drug that is well absorbed through the skin whereas, in many cases, cyclosporine is not. We did an open clinical trial with 12 dogs; 10 with DLE and 2 with PE. We applied topical 0.1% tacrolimus ointment every 12 hours for 8 weeks. After 2 weeks, if there was substantial improvement, we allowed the owners to reduce application to once daily. We evaluated scores every 2 weeks for degree of erythema, crusts, ulceration, erosions, depigmentation, scarring and the distribution of the lesions and areas involved. Clients completed a questionnaire every 2 weeks to assess any perceived adverse effects. We also asked about sunlight exposure, since we know that this aggravates these diseases. We performed complete blood counts (CBCs) and serum chemistries every 2 weeks and we also measured serum tacrolimus levels. In assessment of our results, we called an excellent response a reduction by 2 units in two or more of the parameters that we looked at, and partial responses a reduction by 1 unit in two or more of the parameters. Our results revealed five excellent responses, five partial responses and two with no change. Complete blood counts and serum chemistries were normal, with the exception of those cases that had previous liver enzyme elevations as a result of prior systemic or topical glucocorticoids. We found that, by the end of the study, these dogs' liver enzymes returned to normal as we were able to decrease or discontinue the glucocorticoid therapy. Eight of the ten dogs had a beneficial response and were only on topical tacrolimus by the end of the study. Many were initially on a variety of medications including tetracycline/niacinamide, prednisone, triamcinolone and topical amcinonide.

In addition to this study, we recently reviewed 12 other dogs diagnosed with DLE that were treated with tacrolimus. This was a very loose retrospective analysis of medical records only. Seven out of 12 had positive effects from using tacrolimus. We see a variety of DLE cases; some with mild depigmentation and crusting, and some with more aggressive disease that have erosions and crusts and even recurrent or intermittent

bleeding. My feeling is that topical tacrolimus is a great first-line drug therapy for early and mild DLE. My typical approach is to start with topical tacrolimus as well as tetracycline/niacinamide and then, over time, hopefully decrease, or discontinue, the tetracycline/niacinamide.

Katarina Varjonen *Sweden* Did you have any problems with dogs licking the product off and developing toxicity?

Joel Griffies I meant to mention that. We actually had a lot of questions from owners when we first started the study. What we have done is to try and convince owners to either apply it just before they are going for a walk, feeding the dog, giving a chew toy, or something of that nature. What I like about the preparation of commercially available tacrolimus is that it is in an ointment base. I don't feel that licking the product off is so much of an issue. Even though we know that some dogs will lick after application, it does not seem to affect the results.

Katarina Varjonen Is tacrolimus available everywhere and what is the cost?

Joel Griffies In the United States a 30-g tube of the 0.1% tacrolimus is about $60 to $70. Can I get an idea from the audience of what the cost is elsewhere?

Sue Patterson *UK* About €40 in most of Europe.

Joel Griffies Another use for tacrolimus is in pinnal vasculitis cases. We have had some really nice success, and in many cases as a sole therapy. Both Dr Rosenkrantz and myself have had cases respond positively, although there have been no controlled studies.

Alicia Fernández de Cózar *Spain* Can you comment on safety and blood levels in your cases, and the concern for human toxicity when owners apply the drug to their dogs?

Joel Griffies Tacrolimus has been used topically in thousands of humans for severe allergic eczema and atopic dermatitis. The drug is approved and is safe to use in 10- or 12-month-old children, so I am not very nervous about it. The absorption or blood levels in dogs were difficult to determine. We used a standard therapeutic monitoring assay used in humans. Unfortunately, there was poor correlation with the tacrolimus application, as some dogs that were not treated had positive levels. It was not a very useful assay.

Marie Christensen *Sweden*   Do you have any experience with using tacrolimus for perianal fistulas in German shepherd dogs?

Joel Griffies   We do, and there are publications to support its use. I am routinely using tacrolimus for perianal fistulas. However, it depends on the degree and severity as to whether or not I am using it initially. In really severe cases I start with cyclosporine. As the condition improves, I try to transition them to using tacrolimus. In three or four cases I have been able to eliminate cyclosporine and use tacrolimus for long-term therapy, which owners are thrilled about because it is less expensive.

Wayne Rosenkrantz *USA*   Most of these dogs with perianal fistulas will not let you get close to the lesions because they are often so painful. One of the things that Joel mentioned is starting off with the systemic therapy of cyclosporine in combination with ketoconazole; once the inflammation is calmed and there is less pain, switching over to tacrolimus is often possible. Particularly in the German shepherd dog breed, it has been difficult to consider any kind of topical application initially because of the pain and subsequent aggression when trying to treat the lesions topically.

Ken Kwochka   With no more questions for Joel, I would like to ask Dr Kerstin Bergvall to come up and share her experiences with the use of tacrolimus for plantar fistulation in German shepherd dogs.

Tacrolimus for plantar fistulation in German shepherd dogs (K. Bergvall)

Kerstin Bergvall *Sweden*   We will continue with a discussion of tacrolimus 0.1%. This was an open trial and it was performed in German shepherd dogs that developed plantar or palmar fistulas just proximal to the midtarsal and mid-carpal pads. The first reason for considering tacrolimus therapy was the possibility that there is an immunological aetiology to this condition. Cases have been controlled, after secondary infection has been cleared, with immunomodulating therapies like prednisolone and tetracycline/niacinamide. Another reason

for trying tacrolimus for these cases is that they often relapse, with the redevelopment of secondary bacterial infections and the need for more antibiotic therapy. Antibiotic therapy is of major concern worldwide, so we wanted to try a better way to prevent recurrences. Further, with the successful use of tacrolimus in some German shepherd dogs with perianal fistulas, I thought it would be worth trying with this condition.

We had seven German shepherd dogs that had more than one foot affected because we wanted to have at least one leg untreated to serve as the dog's own control. They had to have had lesions persistently for at least 6 months so that we could minimise the effect of the waxing and waning nature of the condition having any influence on the results of the trial. The dogs also had to be treated with antibiotics after susceptibility testing, until no further response was seen. Lesion severity was recorded in a simple fashion from 0 to 3, where 0 was normal and 3 represented the most severe cases with draining fistulas. We initially clipped the area and kept it clipped during treatment. Owners applied 0.1% tacrolimus twice daily. The dogs wore an Elizabethan collar for 20 minutes after application to prevent them from licking the medication off.

We rechecked the dogs after 3 and 6 weeks of treatment and recorded the lesion severity. After 6 weeks of therapy, the untreated legs were unchanged and the treated legs were much improved. Four of the seven dogs were in complete remission, while three of the dogs had palpable, but not visible, lesions. These dogs have been followed for 2 years. We now let the owners treat all the legs and they have been kept in remission by using tacrolimus intermittently. They use it when they can palpate a lesion coming up, applying tacrolimus twice daily until the lesion resolves. Up until now, no side effects have been reported and we have checked two of the dogs with CBCs, serum chemistries and urinalysis, without any abnormalities found. For me, this is a safe treatment option to prevent recurrences while the secondary infection is controlled. This treatment is steroid-sparing, but more importantly it is antibiotic-sparing. Of course double-blinded controlled studies are needed to confirm these findings.

Ken Kwochka   I would like to make a comment, because Kerstin talked about sparing antibiotic usage. Medical personnel in the Scandinavian countries have done a great job, more so than perhaps other parts of the world, in trying to spare antibiotic usage and decrease the emergence of resistance. Most of the good information that we have in humans concerning methods to decrease antibiotic resistance by the use of topical therapy and better hygiene has come from the Scandinavian countries. We should all embrace the philosophy of reducing antibiotic use to situations and conditions when it is absolutely necessary.

Wayne Rosenkrantz   A few cases that we have had over the years tend to be very resistant to antibiotic therapy. I am interested to get some feedback on how many people have seen these fistulas in German shepherd dogs, or maybe other breeds, and whether there is a consensus that these cases are refractory to antibiotics. How many people have seen or recognised these fistulas? Of those, how many say that they are purely antibiotic-responsive? How many say that you usually have to use some type of anti-inflammatory therapy like glucocorticoids? Has anybody had dogs respond completely to tetracycline/niacinamide?

It sounds like most of you have had similar experiences. In our experience these have been tough to treat, even with glucocorticoids. Some may respond, but when you stop or lower the dosage of the glucocorticoids, lesions re-occur. If we can get as good a response as Kerstin, that would be quite impressive with just topical tacrolimus therapy.

Marie Christensen   I have a lot of German shepherd dogs in my practice. I have used cyclosporine for these lesions and I have seen that they usually go into remission. I generally use it the same way as Kerstin has done with the tacrolimus. There is a product available in Norway called Optimmune (Schering), a topical cyclosporine, that I use.

Ken Kwochka   In what other breeds are people seeing this particular syndrome?

Marie Christensen   Labrador retrievers, pit bull terriers, mastiffs and Bichon mixes. Possibly we could try to remove the proposed anatomical reason for this condition. I do not believe that these breeds are too low in the hocks, and the German shepherd dogs that develop the lesions even in the front legs are not necessarily lower in the carpal areas.

Ken Kwochka   I am going to ask Dr Susan Patterson to talk to us about the use of cyclosporine topically for

sebaceous adenitis. Before she does, I would like to ask Sue to make some comments on what her approach is for acral lick dermatitis and how she uses topical tacrolimus for these lesions.

Susan Patterson *UK*   Acral lick dermatitis cases are almost always allergic but we will usually perform thyroid function tests, biopsy, bacterial and fungal tissue cultures, food trials, and probably skin testing. In some cases, we will have radiography as well as EMGs performed. Once we have the infection under control we will often try tacrolimus topically and we have had some good response. Most breeds like Dobermann pinschers and Labrador retrievers, which I find get really obsessive, can benefit from tacrolimus. I think this tends to make them more comfortable and gets them to leave the lesions alone.

Joel Griffies   Have you gotten any adverse affects or apparent burning sensations when it is applied?

Susan Patterson   Not that I am aware of.

Joel Griffies   A burning reaction is the most common reaction in people treated with tacrolimus, and I had one case with DLE that very briefly seemed to have that response, but it went away.

Susan Patterson   I have used it in the pinnal vasculitis cases that you are talking about, and have seen it irritate some of these cases, but they are quite thin ears. The dogs with acral lick dermatitis have really huge granulomatous lesions and the owners are only applying it to the top of the lesion. We have not seen any reactions at all.

Ken Kwochka   Do they get bandaged after application, or wear an Elizabethan collar?

Susan Patterson   Most of these dogs are in collars anyway because they are ripping their feet to pieces, so they have collars on all the time.

Joel Griffies   Are you able to eliminate the collar over time?

Susan Patterson   Yes, but I have not been using it that long. It was something I reached for in desperation after having gone through everything else.

Ken Kwochka   Do you concurrently use any psychotropic drugs?

Susan Patterson   No, not at all.

Ken Kwochka   We will now let you get back to your original subject.

Topical cyclosporine in sebaceous adenitis (S. Patterson)

Susan Patterson   Twenty cases of canine sebaceous adenitis were treated with topical cyclosporine therapy. Oral cyclosporine is very expensive in the UK and we were looking for a way to reduce the expense, and get some response by using the drug applied topically to the skin. We spoke to Novartis about it and they said it was a waste of time because it is not absorbed through the skin. We thought we would give it a try in any case.

We tried it on two dogs to start out with; one chow chow and one standard poodle. We made up a solution with a cyclosporine concentration of 100 mg/ml. We added 25 ml to 250 ml of water and asked the owners to spray half the dog only. They sprayed either the left side or the right side of the dog and the patients were re-evaluated after 2 weeks. After 2 weeks, these two dogs came back and on one side the hair coat was quite long and luxuriant and the other side was bald. The owners then begged us to use it on the whole dog. When you plucked hairs out of the side that had not been treated, very prominent follicular casts were seen. On the treated side, the follicular casting had disappeared completely and the hairs were almost completely normal.

On the basis of the results in these two dogs, we have been using topical cyclosporine over the last 3 years to treat almost all the cases of sebaceous adenitis that we see. We perform diagnostic tests as already indicated and use the 1:10 dilution topically on the skin. Some of these dogs are on adjunctive antibiotic therapy because of severe secondary infections, and some remain on pulse treatments with antibiotics. We usually follow up the topical therapy with a humectant such as Humilac (Virbac, UK), or an oil-based moisturiser on the skin. We have had no failures so far and have used topical cyclosporine on standard poodles, chow chows, akitas, Staffordshire terriers, springer spaniels and Labrador retrievers. The problem that we have had with long-coated breeds like chow chows and akitas is that as the hair starts to grow

back it gets progressively more difficult to apply the spray. We keep these dogs clipped short, which makes it much easier for the owners to maintain them.

In the first dogs we treated, blood values were normal and serum cyclosporine levels were undetectable. We have been very careful with owners: they wear gloves during application; let the dogs dry for 5–10 minutes after application; and apply the spray late at night to minimise handling the dogs. We have had no side effects associated with topical application, and to date we have had no failures. In many cases, topical therapy can be decreased from daily to twice weekly. If owners stop therapy or relapse occurs during longer treatment intervals, the cyclosporine can simply be restarted or the treatment intervals decreased and the dog will recover.

Wayne Rosenkrantz   The liquid formulation of cyclosporine in the US is in some type of an oil-based emollient like olive oil. It might be worth seeing what the benefits of the vehicle are by itself without the actual cyclosporine. We treat a lot of sebaceous adenitis cases in the US by using topical emollients. These may be propylene glycol, mineral oil, or a variety of different humectants and emollients. The second question relates to expense. Is it a lot less expensive to go this route than to give oral administration of cyclosporine? It seems like a lot of liquid cyclosporine especially in large-breed dogs.

Susan Patterson   Based on clinical presentation, you can often tell if you have a case of sebaceous adenitis. We will send biopsies off and in the 2-week period while we are waiting for biopsy results, we will treat with high doses of essential fatty acids (EFAs) and topical humectants. When these dogs come back they are only slightly better. The striking observation in the dogs on just humectants and oil-based preparations is that the follicular casting does not resolve, so the hair looks better but the cast is still there. We also get hair to grow back, and I have never gotten hair to grow back on a dog with sebaceous adenitis on humectants alone. The remaining hair looks better with humectants, but there is not new hair regrowth, which I do see in the dogs on cyclosporine.

Joel Griffies   Have you rebiopsied any of these cases after therapy, and are there substantial changes? Also, is there variation in response to treatment where you can get some sebaceous adenitis dogs very early in the disease and there are still some sebaceous glands present versus those that are end-stage that have no sebaceous glands?

Susan Patterson We have used it on dogs in all stages, so we have certainly seen some end-stage dogs that have no glands at all and it seems to work well. We have only rebiopsied two dogs, and histologically they still have sebaceous adenitis. It is cheaper for us to treat topically rather then systemically in a big dog like an akita, chow chow, or Labrador retriever. I see very few small dogs with sebaceous adenitis.

Ken Kwochka Do you have a feel for why it is working?

Susan Patterson None.

Ken Kwochka At Ohio State we published one case and then had several additional cases with sebaceous adenitis treated systemically with cyclosporine. They did very well. Cyclosporine was the only drug that we ever used for treatment where dogs grew back normal hair coats. Some of these dogs had no sebaceous glands, and after successful regrowth of hair, still no sebaceous glands were present. I know that Tony Stannard always said, from his observations, he believed that this was not a primary glandular abnormality, but it was a follicular keratinisation defect where the sebaceous gland empties into the hair follicle. He felt that this is more of a follicular keratinisation abnormality and that the sebaceous gland is the secondary bystander. Certainly cyclosporine can improve or normalise the follicular keratinisation process by a number of different mechanisms. I would suspect that is why we see that type of dramatic response topically and systemically even in patients that would be classified as end-stage cases.

Wayne Rosenkrantz These are interesting comments. We have also used systemic cyclosporine to treat a variety of different sebaceous adenitis presentations and I would say that our experiences have been mixed with the poodles, akitas, Samoyeds, German shepherd dogs and the long-coated breeds. Sometimes the responses are fairly impressive. I cannot think of a case that is 100% normal though. On the other hand, the short-coated variation of sebaceous adenitis, as we would recognise in the vizsla or the miniature pinscher, seems to respond much more dramatically to

cyclosporine. Again, we may ask if that is the same disease or a slight variant? Certainly they can have quite a few histologic similarities.

Susan Patterson I would agree that the most dramatic coat improvements have been in short-coated breeds. We treated a Staffordshire terrier with topical therapy. The owners were told that when they sprayed they should not get the drug in the dog's eyes so the owner used a gloved hand over the dog's face. When he came back for his 3-week check there was the impression of his fingers in an alopecic area where the hair failed to grow back.

Ken Kwochka Are there any other uses for topical cyclosporine that have not been discussed?

Susan Patterson I have played with it in some allergic dogs. I have used the same preparation to spray on the ventrum of dogs with atopic dermatitis and it did not work.

Ken Kwochka I would like to ask Dr Christophe Rème to talk about some work on seborrhoea that he has been doing at Virbac.

Antimicrobial efficacy of tar and non-tar antiseborrhoeic shampoos in dogs (C. Rème)

Christophe Rème *France* The problem with seborrhoea arises especially in those cases that are severely greasy and usually require the use of coal tar. The problems with tar are that they are drying, need to be left on to work, and have undesirable colour and odour. A recent concern in some European countries, and in some of the states in the US, is the safety of tars for humans. Virbac decided to design a new shampoo for severe seborrhoeic disorders that does not contain tar and has a new delivery vehicle system.

I would like to present a double-blinded study that I presented last year at the ESVD-ECVD meeting. We compared a tar-based product (Sebolytic/Allerseb-T, Virbac, France) to a non-tar-based product (Sebolytic/Allerseb without tar, Virbac, France). We included 47 dogs in this study. We selected dogs with primary or secondary keratinisation disorders that were free of infections and with no concurrent parasitic disease. We divided these into two groups for treatment; tar-based and non-tar-based shampoo. The animals were treated for 3 weeks at 3-day intervals. The study was double-blinded as we provided the owners with identical bottles and they performed the bathing at home. The clinical signs related to seborrhoea were scored and defined based on a KSD index (keratoseborrhoeic disorder index) which included scaling, greasiness, malodour, and overall skin and coat condition as well as associated signs of pruritus, erythema and excoriations. Each of these was scored on a 0–4 point scale. Dogs included in the study presented with a marked KSD index of >7 in 70% of the dogs. We also performed cytology and about 60% of the dogs had *Malassezia*, with half of these having concurrent cocci. Specifically, *Malassezia* population scores were >2 in 64% of the dogs and cocci population scores were >2 in 32% of the cases. Most of the dogs had underlying atopic disease or some other kind of allergy. The results of the study showed significant reduction of the KSD index in both treatment groups (percentage score reductions of 80–90%) over the 3-week period. There was no statistical difference that could be detected between the two groups. Marked microbial count reduction occurred in both treatment groups. Both products were tolerated very well and appreciated by the owners, but the tar-free product was rated better on appearance, odour and colour. In conclusion, the Sebolytic/Allerseb without tar proved as effective as the Sebolytic/Allerseb-T product in controlling severe KSD signs and associated microbial infection in dogs. This new antiseborrhoeic shampoo combines salicylic acid, zinc gluconate, vitamin B6, linoleic/gamma-linolenic acids, piroctone, olamine and tea tree oil. This unique combination of agents allows for a product that controlled epidermal proliferation and microbial overgrowth in a non-irritating and cosmetically acceptable alternative to coal tar-based products.

Wayne Rosenkrantz   Years ago, people used a product in the US called 'Head and Shoulders', which supposedly has a zinc-based component to it. I do not recall the exact concerns, but I remember there were rumblings about zinc toxicity related to the use of that product. Possibly percutaneous absorption through mucous membranes was a mechanism of the zinc toxicity. I am wondering if you know of any issues with topical zinc toxicity? Maybe Ken can comment on the 'Head and Shoulders' product.

Christophe Rème   I think the ingredient that you refer to in the 'Head and Shoulders' product is zinc pyrithione 1%. It was a product of some concern and potential toxicity in Europe. The zinc in the new Virbac product is not the same and is considered very safe. We performed toxicity studies in cats, which are normally more sensitive than dogs, and had no problems.

Anthony Chadwick *UK*   There was quite a bit of concern with zinc-based products, as some of the previously used zinc products may cause some type of retinal problems in dogs.

Ken Kwochka   A retinal degenerative problem was associated with zinc pyrithione in dogs.

Christophe Rème   We have done some safety studies and I can tell you that these products have been available in Germany, United Kingdom, and in the US. It has been used in a fair number of cases and the zinc used in this product has not been shown to create any problems.

Abdo Kallassy *Lebanon*   You are combining different components to get the antiseborrhoeic effect. So we know that every component has some activity and needs a certain concentration to reach its desired effect. So how are you determining the concentration and duration of time to reach its effect?

Christophe Rème   It depends on some of the ingredients, but usually you use the shampoo at least twice weekly during the first stage of the disease. That is the usual interval between shampoos we tested in a clinical setting, and in real conditions we found this also to be effective. I can give you individual data on each of these ingredients, but what is important is that it worked in real conditions. It would be a never-ending problem if you were to test every ingredient in the shampoo.

Abdo Kallassy   Maybe you should design two shampoos to determine the effects that individual ingredients may have.

Chistophe Rème   Two shampoos are not very practical for veterinarians. It is also an owner compliance issue and it is very important to make it easier for the clients because we know that topical therapy relies very heavily on the compliance of owners to perform the shampoos repeatedly.

Ken Kwochka This is a fascinating discussion because it really brings out some of the challenges of developing topical therapeutic products. This actually explains why most of the topical products that we use in veterinary medicine are not registered by the FDA or other authorities because you would have to study all the individual components, not only by themselves but also in all possible combinations. It means that you would never get these shampoos formulated because the market is not large enough, so no company would have the funds to be able to get a registered product. So Virbac, DVM Pharmaceuticals, and some of the other companies, take what we know about the individual ingredients and then have the formulating chemists make stable formulations, and then test them *in vitro* and *in vivo* to see if we have a product that is safe and effective for the indicated condition(s).

Abdo Kallassy I want to say that maybe one ingredient you have to use twice a week and another once per week. How do you control this?

Ken Kwochka Again that would be very difficult to do without doing all of the individual component studies.

Ken Kwochka Our last presenter is Wayne Rosenkrantz who will present some work he has been doing with a product designed to control house dust mites in the environment and on the pet.

Environmental and topical control of house dust mites and their allergens (W. Rosenkrantz)

Wayne Rosenkrantz As we have heard at this meeting, there have been many papers and discussions on the importance of house dust mites (HDM) in the pathogenesis of allergic skin disease in small animals and the importance of controlling, reducing and avoiding exposure to these common household mites. I have had a strong interest in house dust mite control for many years. Two major agents have been looked at for control of these mites in the environment: borates, and denaturing agents. In 1991, I performed a pilot study to evaluate borates for HDM. In this study I measured treated (six) and untreated (three) homes for HDM levels via the Acarex test that measures guanine (mite faecal product), in six homes. Homes were treated with the standard so-

dium polyborate powder commercially available from Flea Busters. The results showed significant reduction in guanine levels. Guanine has been shown to correlate with concentrations of Der p1 and Der f1. As a result of this study, I have used this product intermittently for HDM control until recently, when more effective products have become available. Other researchers have shown the effectiveness of borates for HDM control.

A study performed by Dr Arlian at Wright State University on the acaricidal efficacy of a commercial product containing disodium octaborate tetrahydrate (DOT) for reducing mite density in carpets showed very effective results. This was a placebo-controlled study with carpet pieces inoculated with *Dermatophagoides farinae* and *D. pteronyssinus*: three replicates with one set treated with DOT, one set untreated and one set treated with water. Post-treatment measurements at 2, 4 and 8 weeks showed marked reduction in total mite counts: 885 to 10, and 17 500 to 1100 mites/gram of dust for *D. farinae and D. pteronyssinus,* respectively. A more recent study showed relevant clinical application of borates when DOT application and vacuum cleaning were combined to control HDM.[2] This was a placebo-controlled 6-month study in 93 homes with active, placebo (water) and negative control groups. Dust was collected pre- and post-treatment every 2 months from carpets and sofas. Measurements of live mites, total mites and mite allergen levels were taken. The DOT and vacuum cleaning killed mites in carpets and sofas for up to 6 months, sofas were less affected. HDM allergen was significantly lower in the carpets and sofas at 6 months post-treatment.

Denaturing agents have also been evaluated for their ability to immediately reduce the HDM allergens that are produced by the mites and their by-products. The most recent product evaluated is a new anti-allergen denaturing agent (Allerase, Aveho Biosciences). This product contains a citric acid derivative with soybean-extracted fatty acids and fatty alcohol surfactants. It has been evaluated clinically and in three more controlled studies. In-home use has shown good clinical responses with reduction of measurable mite allergen from textile surfaces after treatment based on the Mite-T-Fast Test (Aveho Biosciences: validated swipe test with porous sampling pin in association with an immunochromatographic test system that detects Der p2/f2 with sensitivity of 62% and specificity of 94% when compared to an ELISA assay).

There have been three *in vitro* studies to evaluate the Allerase product. The first study performed by IBT Reference Laboratory (P.B. Williams, May 2000) compared the denaturing effects of the anti-allergen solution Allerase, to tannic acid (Allersearch, ADS) and benzyl benzoate (Allercare, SC Johnson) on five protein allergens: Der p1 and Der f1 (dustmites), Can f1 (canine), Fel d1 (feline) and Bla g1 (cockroach). Benzyl benzoate had no denaturing effects on Fel d1 or Der f1, and some effect on Can f1 and Der p1. Tannic acid had good denaturing effects on Fel d1, Can f1, Der p1 and Der f1 in dust samples but was ineffective in liquid samples. Allerase showed good denaturing effects on Fel d1, Can f1, Der p1 and Der f1 in both dust and liquid samples.

The second study was an ELISA inhibition potency assay using Allerase (R. Esch, Greer Labs, May 2003). In this study, freeze-dried *D. farinae* allergen was reconstituted (10 µg/ml) in varying concentrations of Allerase (1:2 to 1:32 dilutions), left overnight and then measured for residual activity of *D. farinae* by standard ELISA assay, by adding this to a mite-sensitive serum. The results showed detectable reduction (50–70%) in HDM allergen when exposed to 1:2 and 1:4 dilutions overnight. The investigator commented on this being the first decrease in HDM allergenicity seen with any product using canine IgE antibodies, and was not used at full strength concentration.

The third study evaluated Allerase treatment of HDM extract applied to kennels of dogs with known HDM allergies (R. Marcella, University of Florida, February 2004). In this study, Allerase was added to HDM extract and allowed to dry overnight in a Petri dish. HDM-sensitive dogs were exposed to both Allerase-treated and saline-treated (placebo) HDM extract applied to kennel floors. The results showed no statistical difference between the groups. However, the researchers commented that the amount of Allerase was too low and the study needed to be repeated with higher concentration and volume of Allerase that would approximate real clinical applications. Other researchers have been evaluating the effects of Allerase (spray and shampoo formulations) as a topical therapy on the dog as a means of eliminating or reducing percutaneous absorption of allergen on the skin surface. This is particularly interesting based on the recent work showing the presence of HDM and their allergens on the dog's coat and in their bedding. Lastly, the Allerase topical and shampoo products have been looked at for environmental mould control and topical use in *Staphylococcus* and *Malassezia* dermatitis with promising results. Are there any questions?

Anthony Chadwick   What allergen is this diagnostic test detecting?

Wayne Rosenkrantz   It is detecting both Der f2 and Der p2, so it is picking up the allergen of two HDM species. It does not pick up Der f1 at all. It does let you know that you are detecting dust mite allergen or that dust mites are in the environment. I wish this test were a little bit closer to 90–100% accurate. If the test comes back negative, some owners ask 'Do I really need to treat the environment?' What we have been doing is really getting away from testing the environment unless the owner is extremely interested. When we have a known area that is positive with this test, we have followed up testing after environmental treatment and have gotten negative results post-treatment in all cases that we have tested.

Anthony Chadwick   How about on the animal?

Wayne Rosenkrantz   For the animal, there is a shampoo product that has the same active ingredient, Allerase Shampoo. We have also been using the environmental spray product on the pets as well, without irritant reactions. I know it is the goal of the company to come out with some type of residual lotion or cream rinse that has the active ingredient, which seems like a logical product to use as a means of denaturing HDM allergen on the pet.

Ken Kwochka   I would like to thank ICF for their sponsorship and all the speakers and participants.

References

1 Griffies, J.D., Mendelsohn, C.L., Rosenkrantz, W.S., Muse, R., Boord, M.J., Griffin, C.E. Topical 0.1% tacrolimus for the treatment of discoid lupus erythematosus and pemphigus erythematosus in dogs. *Journal of the American Animal Hospital Association*, 2004; **40**: 29–41.
2 Codina, R., Lockey R.F., Diwadkar R., Mobley, L.L., Godfrey, S. Disodium octaborate tetrahydrate (DOT) application and vacuum cleaning, a combined strategy to control house dust mites. *Allergy*, 2003; **58**: 318–324.

Index